THE SUCCESSFUL MATCH 2017

RULES FOR SUCCESS IN THE RESIDENCY MATCH

RAJANI KATTA MD
SAMIR P. DESAI MD

FROM THE AUTHORS OF SUCCESS ON THE WARDS

PUBLISHED BY
MD2B
HOUSTON, TEXAS

www.MD2B.com

The Successful Match 2017: Rules for Success in the Residency Match is published by MD2B, PO Box 300988, Houston, TX 77230-0988.

www.MD2B.com

NOTICE: The authors and publisher disclaim any personal liability, either directly or indirectly, for advice or information presented within. The authors and publishers have used care and diligence in the preparation of this book. Every effort has been made to ensure the accuracy and completeness of information contained within this book. The reader should understand, however, that most of the book's subject matter is not rooted in scientific observation. Many of the recommendations made within this book have come from the authors' personal experiences and interactions with faculty, residents, and students over a period of many years. Since the selection process varies from one residency program to another, the recommendations are not universally applicable. No responsibility is assumed for errors, inaccuracies, omissions, or any false or misleading implication that may arise due to the text.

Printed in the United States of America

9781937978075

Dedication

As we've progressed in our careers, we are constantly reminded that no matter how hard we've worked, and continue to work, our success would not be possible without the help of so many individuals.

To our teachers and mentors, who provided so much knowledge, guidance, and, especially, inspiration

To our mentors and colleagues, who have written letters of recommendation, provided much-appreciated career guidance, and have acted as advocates at critical points in our careers

To our students, who constantly challenge us to improve and who inspire us to keep learning. And who make us very proud to be working with the next generation of empathetic, conscientious, dedicated physicians

To our patients, who remind us of the vital importance of life-long learning and inspire us to constantly seek out improvements in diagnostic techniques, treatments, and education

To our friends, who have helped us in many concrete, practical ways, and who are a continuous reminder that friends are one of the best antidotes to stress

To our families, who have helped us and supported us. Without everything that you've done, and continue to do, our success would not be possible.

Thank you.

A portion of proceeds from the sale of each of our books is donated to charities supporting education and the fight against hunger.

Do You Offer Any Other Resources To Help With Residency Matching?

We do offer other resources, in different formats. This allows us to periodically update these throughout the year.

1) Our podcast: Our podcast "Success in Medicine" covers several areas in medicine, including residency match success. We'll be sharing stories of successful residency applicants and strategies for success, as well as interviews with key decision-makers. You can access the podcast at iTunes or TheSuccessfulMatch.com.

2) Articles: We've written articles about the residency selection process. These can be accessed at TheSuccessfulMatch.com.

3) Our course: If you're seeking more interview preparation beyond the chapters in this book, we've created an online course to help guide you further on how to develop winning answers to residency interview questions. Visit TheSuccessfulMatch.com for course information.

4) Our blog: Keep up-to-date about the residency selection process by visiting our blog, available at (you guessed it) TheSuccessfulMatch.com.

ABOUT THE AUTHORS

Samir P. Desai, M.D.

Dr. Samir Desai serves on the faculty of the Baylor College of Medicine in the Department of Medicine. He has educated premedical students, medical students, residents, and international medical graduates, work for which he has received numerous teaching awards. As a member of the Clerkship Directors in Internal Medicine, he is deeply committed to medical student education. He has served on the medical school admissions and residency selection committees at the Baylor College of Medicine and Northwestern University.

He is an author and editor, having written 18 books that together have sold over 250,000 copies worldwide. The inspiration for his books often comes from his experiences as a mentor, and he has a deep desire to help students and applicants overcome the challenges of the medical school admissions, residency selection, and fellowship selection processes.

In 2009, he co-authored *The Successful Match*, a well-regarded and highly acclaimed book that has helped thousands of residency applicants match successfully. His commitment to helping medical students reach their professional goals led him to develop the website, TheSuccessfulMatch.com. The website's mission is to provide residency and fellowship applicants with a better understanding of the selection process. His book *Medical School Scholarships, Awards, and Grants* has been identified as a high-value resource by the AAMC Group on Student Affairs.

Dr. Desai is deeply committed to enhancing the quality of patient care, reducing medical error, and decreasing health care costs. This desire led him to write the book *Clinician's Guide to Laboratory Medicine*, a resource widely used in the curriculum of medical, PA, and nurse practitioner schools, and listed as one of the "Best Medical Books of All Time" by The Medical Media Review. At Baylor, he is investigating ways in which technology can be used by residents and students to enhance patient care. One initiative currently underway is "Creating and Implementing a Patient Safety Checklist App for Residents and Students on Medicine Wards," a project that was awarded an Innovations Grant by the Alliance for Academic Internal Medicine. He is also a member of the Centers for Disease Control (CDC) Mobile Application Project Team.

After completing his residency training in Internal Medicine at Northwestern University in Chicago, Dr. Desai had the opportunity of serving as chief medical resident. He received his M.D. degree from Wayne State University School of Medicine in Detroit, Michigan, graduating first in his class.

He resides in Houston with his wife (and co-author) and their two children. He keeps fit by weight-lifting and biking with his children, and continues to follow his favorite team: the Detroit Tigers.

Rajani Katta, M.D.

Dr. Rajani Katta is an award-winning educator who is deeply passionate about patient, medical student, and physician education.

She served as Professor of Dermatology at the Baylor College of Medicine for over 17 years, and founded the Baylor College of Medicine Contact Dermatitis Clinic. In 2015 she left to establish her own practice dedicated to allergic contact dermatitis.

She has authored over 60 scientific articles and chapters, and has lectured extensively both nationally and locally on dermatology and contact dermatitis to students, residents, and physicians. She served as Course Director for dermatology in the basic science years for 15 years, and previously served as Clerkship Director of dermatology.

On a national level, she has worked closely to advance the mission of the American Contact Dermatitis Society, serving on the Education Committee and serving on the Board of Directors (2013-2016).

Having advised many students over the years regarding the dermatology match process, she was determined to become an expert in this area. In 2009 she co-authored the first edition of *The Successful Match: 200 Rules to Succeed in the Residency Match*. The book quickly became the best-selling title in this field. It has been recommended as Suggested Reading in the AAMC Careers in Medicine Student Guide and identified as a high-value resource by the AAMC Group on Student Affairs.

She has co-authored a total of 5 books. One of these books, *Success on the Wards: 250 Rules for Clerkship Success*, has helped thousands of medical students make the difficult transition from the preclinical to clinical years of medical school. *Success on the Wards* is a required or recommended resource at many US medical schools.

She has a strong interest in preventive dermatology, and is currently at work on her latest book, on the link between diet and dermatology. She maintains a blog and podcast on this topic at www.KattaMD.com. Her goal is to help foster better dietary choices by emphasizing the effects of diet on the skin.

After graduating with honors from Baylor College of Medicine and completing her internship in internal medicine, she completed her dermatology residency at the Northwestern University School of Medicine.

She and her husband Dr. Samir Desai (her co-author) have two children and one frog and reside in Houston, Texas. They enjoy hiking, and love to hear about great hikes.

CONTENTS

Chapter 1

Introduction

What does it take to match successfully? What does it take to match into the specialty and program of your choice?

Over 42,000 applicants registered for the 2016 NRMP Match, making it the largest Match on record. Competition is intense, and some applicants are unsuccessful.[1]

In competitive fields such as general surgery, dermatology, plastic surgery, and orthopedic surgery, over 25% of U.S. senior allopathic applicants failed to match.

Overall, while nearly 94% of U.S. allopathic senior applicants matched, the number of unmatched seniors reached an all-time high of 1,130 applicants. The numbers are significantly worse for osteopathic and international medical graduates (IMGs). Failure to match rates are shown in the following tables.

Percentage of U.S. Allopathic Senior Applicants Who Failed to Match in Competitive Specialties (2016 NRMP and AUA Match)[2-3]	
Specialty	**% of U.S. Seniors Failing to Match**
Dermatology	28%
General Surgery	27%
Orthopedic Surgery	26%
Plastic Surgery	25%
Neurological Surgery	25%
Urology	23%
Radiation Oncology	19%
Otolaryngology	13%

Failure to Match % by Applicant Type (2016 NRMP Match)[2]	
Applicant Type	**% Failing to Match**
Osteopathic applicants	20%
U.S. citizen IMGs	46%
Non-U.S. citizen IMGs	50%

Did you know?

The failure to match rates reported by the NRMP for competitive specialties don't take into account the following:

- Applicants who give up on their preferred specialty choice because they feel that their chances of success are low.
- Applicants who apply to their preferred specialty choice but fail to receive an interview.

These applicants don't officially enter the match for their preferred specialty, and are therefore not included in these statistics. Some researchers have therefore looked at "intent to match" failure rates, and those rates are indeed significantly higher.

As an applicant, your goal is to match into your preferred specialty, and ideally your preferred program.

The evidence indicates that it has never been more difficult to reach these goals.

Over a decade ago, in response to an anticipated physician manpower shortage, allopathic and osteopathic medical schools increased student enrollment. New schools were also established. However, the number of residency positions has not increased at a corresponding rate. As more and more graduates have entered the Match, the competition for available residency positions has intensified.

Did you know?

In a 2015 survey of medical school deans, the AAMC asked "What is your level of concern about your incoming students' ability to find a residency training position of their choice upon completion of medical school?" 50% of the deans surveyed indicated having "major" or "moderate" concern. Of note, the percentage reporting this degree of concern rose from 35% in 2012 to 50% in 2015.[4]

What does it take to match successfully in such a fiercely competitive environment?

The issue is a hotly debated one, and surveys of students, reviews of student discussion forums, and discussions with academic faculty all find sharp divisions on the topic. Try entering this subject into a search engine, and you'll receive thousands of conflicting opinions.

I was speaking to a colleague, and I brought up this question and my work on this book. Her response? "A book on matching? What's there to write about? Get good grades and a great score on the USMLE. That's the book!"

Her response was sadly misinformed.

There's no doubt that medical school grades and USMLE Step 1 scores are very important, but focusing only on those two factors certainly doesn't tell the full story. If that were the case, it wouldn't explain these cases:

- A student with a Step 1 score of 260, membership in AOA, and published dermatology research, was only invited to interview at 2 dermatology programs (one of which was his home school).
- Another student, with a Step 1 score of 230 and no AOA membership, was invited to 9 dermatology interviews.
- Another student with great scores – but minimal dermatology research – was invited to interview at over 20 dermatology programs.

From a scientific approach, what are the factors that account for so much of the variability in match outcomes?

That's an interesting question, but I'm very interested in this topic for a far more personal reason. How can I help this student, sitting across my desk, match into dermatology? This is a very important, personal question for me.

After 17 years as a faculty member, and at a school that fields a high number of dermatology applicants (some years we've had as many as 12 applicants), I've advised many applicants. Dr. Samir Desai has advised a wide cross-section of applicants, from applicants with 15 interview invitations to those reapplying for the 4th time. Together, we've advised hundreds of applicants.

I certainly don't think you need an incredible USMLE score to be a great dermatologist, and yet that's being used as a screen by so many programs. I think we're missing some great applicants because of it. My goal is to help those applicants who I think will make great contributions to the care of their patients and to the specialty: conscientious, thorough, empathetic, and with a strong sense of intellectual curiosity. How can I, as an advisor, help such students? How can you, as that type of student, reach your professional goals?

The first edition of this book was published in 2009, and while the core strategies for a successful match remain the same, some important changes have occurred. The most relevant is that the competition is more intense.

With increased competition, it has become even more important to ensure that your application stands out from the other 499 applications that your dream program has received.

What does it take to achieve a successful match? It takes the right strategy. It also takes significant advanced planning and hard work, above and beyond the intense coursework of medical school.

In the following 600 plus pages, we answer the question of what it takes to match successfully. We also provide specific evidence-based advice to maximize your chances of a successful match.

Our recommendations are based on data from a full spectrum of sources. We present evidence obtained from scientific study and published in the academic medical literature. The results of these studies can provide a powerful impetus for specific actions. We present anecdotal data and advice that have been published in the literature and obtained from online sources. We also take an insider's look at the entire process of residency selection based on our experiences, the experiences of our colleagues in the world of academic medicine, and the experiences of the students and residents with whom we've worked.

We focus on the important questions that define the optimal match strategy. Who are the decision-makers? What criteria do they value? How can you ensure that your application materials highlight these criteria?

Who actually chooses the residents? We review the data on the decision-makers. What do these decision-makers care about? We review the data on the criteria that matter to them. How can you convince them that you would be the right resident for their program? We provide concrete, practical recommendations based on this data. At every step of the process, our recommendations are meant to maximize the impact of your application.

In Chapters 23 - 44, we present specialty-specific data. Given the high failure to match rates for certain specialties, is there any literature available to applicants to guide them through the residency application process? For each specialty, we present the results of those studies. For example, in urology, a survey of residency program directors (PDs) obtained data from 76 directors on the criteria that programs use to select their residents.[5] What criteria did these directors rank as most important in deciding whom to interview? Which selection factors were most important in determining an applicant's place on the program's rank order list? What were the factors that led programs to downgrade applicants? This evidence-based information is critical to developing an application strategy that maximizes your chances of a successful match.

We review each component of the application in comprehensive detail in the following chapters. Each and every component of your application can be created, modified, or influenced in order to significantly enhance your overall candidacy. We devote the next 600 plus pages of this book to showing you, in detail, exactly how to do so.

Overview of Book

The first edition of this book was written in 2009, and we've seen a sharp rise in the competitiveness of many specialties since that time. This has translated to applicants applying more widely and extensively than ever before. This means that programs are receiving a record number of applications, and it's become ever more difficult to stand out in this sea of applications.

Increasing Competition for Residency Positions	
Residency Program	**Comments**
Department of Anesthesiology Ohio State University	"Anesthesiology is not the most competitive field, but it has become a lot more competitive in recent years."[6]
Department of EM UCSF	"Emergency Medicine residency programs are becoming increasingly more competitive. This field is more popular than in the past, leading to a robust number of applicants each year. There are generally very few positions to 'scramble' into each year."[7]
Department of Surgery University of Colorado	"Over the past five years, general surgery has become quite competitive."[8]

Did you know?

In the 2016 Match, 47% of all U.S. allopathic senior applicants failed to match at the program of their choice.[2]

This has led applicants to submit a larger number of applications to programs, as shown in the following table.

Average Number of Applications Per Applicant (2011 Versus 2015)[9]		
Specialty	**Average Number of Applications Per Applicant (2011)**	**Average Number of Applications Per Applicant (2015)**
Dermatology	40	60
Emergency Medicine	27	35
Obstetrics & Gynecology	32	40
Orthopedic Surgery	47	67
Otolaryngology	38	46
Radiation Oncology	28	35
Urology	44	58

The larger number of applications means more challenges for programs. Programs are finding it difficult to reduce this large group of applicants into a smaller, more manageable number who will receive interview invitations. "These additional applications…cause congestion in the application review process," writes Dr. Steven Weissbart. "Therefore program directors may overlook preferred applicants as a result."[10]

Did you know?

"As medical schools have increased their class sizes to address the demand for physicians and the number of residency slots has largely remained the same, students are forced to navigate the application process more strategically to match into residency programs."[11]

G. Scott Waterman, M.D.
Former Associate Dean for Student Affairs
University of Vermont

Personal Statement

For many students the most dreaded aspect of the residency application is the personal statement. If the words "personal statement" raise your anxiety level, you are certainly not alone. In a study of students at a single medical school, 85% agreed or strongly agreed with the following statement:[12]

I am anxious about writing the personal statement for my residency application.

Individual specialties, residency programs, and application reviewers assign varying degrees of importance to the personal statement. In the screening phase, reviewers whittle down a large applicant pool to a select group that is ultimately extended interview invitations. At some programs, the personal statement is used minimally, if at all, during this screening phase. In others, the personal statement is considered very important:

- "Program directors read a lot of personal statements, so make yours stand out," writes Dr. Jennifer Oman, former program director of the UC Irvine Emergency Medicine Residency Program. "This is something that you want to pour your heart into and give your full attention…Take the time to do this right. It can save a borderline application from being thrown into the rejection pile."[13]

- "The personal statement helps us to get to know you, and we read it with great care," writes Dr. Dempsey Springfield, Program Director of the Harvard Combined Orthopedics Program.[14]

- "This is your only chance to 'talk' to us – make the most of it…a really good statement could be just enough to tip the balance in your favor and move you into the interview pool," writes the Wake Forest University Department of Orthopedic Surgery.[15]

- The website for the University of Washington Family Medicine Residency states that the "personal statement is the primary component that will be used to select applicants who are invited for an interview. Please write a careful and thoughtful document."[16]

Adding to the importance of the personal statement is this fact: a poorly conceived and executed personal statement may be detrimental to your application. Otherwise excellent candidates have been ranked lower, or even rejected, because of a poorly written statement. As reinforced by the University of Alabama at Birmingham Department of Obstetrics and Gynecology – "poorly written personal statements may detract from an otherwise excellent application."[17] Even when statements are free of glaring errors, far too many are viewed as neutral, and this represents a lost opportunity to impress the program.

Applicants are urged by advisors and PDs to create thoughtful and unique statements. Crafting a compelling personal statement requires reflection and creative writing. The evidence indicates that many students are uncomfortable doing just that. In the aforementioned survey, only 29% agreed or strongly agreed with the following statement:[12]

I am comfortable with creative and reflective writing.

It is very frustrating trying to put into words your vision for your medical career. Most students don't understand one basic fact about the personal statement, though. Unlike just about every other aspect of the application, you have complete control over the personal statement. You decide the content, the structure, and the form of the statement. This is a unique opportunity to impress the selection committee. In your statement you can showcase your strengths and those qualities that set you apart from other candidates. You can weave in evidence that confirms your qualities. You can use this opportunity to convince a faculty member that you would be an ideal candidate for their particular program. This is information that is not readily apparent to programs from their review of other application components.

When you create a personal statement, you need to consider your audience. When reading a personal statement, what do faculty members look for? What are they trying to determine? Consider the following:

- In a study evaluating the content of personal statements, members of the radiology residency selection committee at Wayne State University ranked eleven content areas from least to most important.[18] Most important was a candidate's explanation as to why they chose to pursue a career in radiology. Personal attributes was second in importance, while perception of radiology defined as the applicant's ability "to explicitly state what he/she feels are the most important characteristics of either radiologists or the practice of radiology" was third.

- In a survey of orthopedic surgery PDs, 43% agreed that "the most important aspect of a personal statement is to learn more about the candidate's personal interests and backgrounds," while 32% stated that "the most important aspect of a personal statement was to gain insight into an applicant's ability to write and to communicate effectively."[19]

- Among 47 themes identified in an analysis of dermatology personal statements, three were found to be emphasized more often by applicants who matched (studying cutaneous manifestations of systemic disease, contributing to the literature gap, and investigating the pathophysiology of skin diseases).[20]

- At the website for the Wayne State University pathology residency, the program writes that "your personal statement should summarize your particular background and interests and depict you as a person. You should indicate in your personal statement why you are interested in Pathology, what kind of experience you have had with Pathology, and what career path you plan to follow after training."[21]

In our chapter on the personal statement (Chapter 7), we review in more detail what programs seek in the personal statement. We review different approaches and provide a springboard to brainstorming and developing your own statement. We review in detail how to conceive and execute a personal statement that reflects your individual strengths and skills, while convincingly conveying your excellent fit with the specialty and with the individual programs in a convincing manner.

Letters of Recommendation

Letters of recommendation (LORs) are a critical component of the residency application. In the 2014 NRMP Program Director Survey, 86% of programs in 22 specialties cited LORs as a factor in selecting applicants to interview.[22] The only factor cited more frequently by PDs was the USMLE Step 1 / COMLEX Level 1 score.

Since you won't be directly writing these letters yourself, it may seem as if you have no control over their content. In reality, you wield more influence than you realize. In our chapter on letters of recommendation, we detail the steps that you can take in order to have the best possible letters written on your behalf. These steps include choosing the correct letter writers and asking in the correct manner. We also discuss the type of information to provide, and the manner in which to provide it, in order to highlight those qualities that you hope your letter writer will emphasize.

The purpose of these letters is to emphasize that you have the professional qualifications needed to excel. The letters should also demonstrate that you have the personal qualities to succeed as a resident and, later, as a practicing physician. Since these letters are written by those who know you and the quality of your work, they offer programs a personalized view. In contrast to your transcript and USMLE scores, they supply programs with qualitative, rather than quantitative, information about your cognitive and non-cognitive characteristics.

What do the faculty members reviewing applications look for in a letter of recommendation? The first item noted is the writer of the letter. In a survey of PDs in four specialties (internal medicine, pediatrics, family medicine, and surgery), it was learned that a candidate's likelihood of being considered was enhanced if there was a connection or relationship between the writer and residency program director. "In cases where there was both a connection between the faculty members and in-depth knowledge of the student (i.e., personal knowledge), the likelihood was that the student's application would be noted."[23] In a survey of 109 PDs of orthopedic surgery residency programs, 54% of directors agreed that the most important aspect of a letter was that it was written by someone they knew.[19]

In another study, the academic rank of the writer was found to be an important factor influencing the reviewer's ranking of the letter, with 48% of the reviewers rating it as important.[24] A survey of physical medicine and rehabilitation (PM&R) PDs asked respondents to rate the importance of letters of recommendation in selecting residents.[25] The study showed that the "most important letters of recommendation were from a PM&R faculty member in the respondent's department, followed by Dean's letter, and the PM&R Chairman's letter." Next in importance were letters from a PM&R faculty member in a department other than the respondents', followed by a clinical faculty member in another specialty. The University of Texas-Houston Medical School Career Counseling Catalog gives this advice: "letters of recommendation from private physicians or part-time faculty, and letters from residents are generally discounted."[26]

For international medical graduates (IMGs), this issue becomes even more important. A survey of 102 directors of internal medicine residency programs sought to determine the most important predictors of performance for IMGs.[27] When rating the importance of 22 selection criteria, the lowest rated criterion was letters of recommendation from a foreign country, with 93% of PDs feeling that such letters were useless.

What else do the faculty members reviewing applications look for in a letter of recommendation? They seek evidence of an applicant's strengths and skills. Most applicants assume that their letter writers know what to say and what information to provide in a letter to substantiate their recommendation. However, that's a dangerous assumption. In an analysis of 116 recommendation letters received by the radiology residency program at the University of Iowa Hospitals and Clinics, reviewers noted the following:[28]

- 10% were missing information about an applicant's cognitive knowledge.
- 35% had no information about an applicant's clinical judgment.
- 3% did not discuss an applicant's work habits.
- 17% did not comment on the applicant's motivation.
- 32% were lacking information about interpersonal communication skills.

In another review of recommendation letters sent to the Department of Surgery at Southern Illinois University, writers infrequently commented on psychomotor skills such as "easily performed minor procedures at the bedside," "good eye-hand coordination in the OR," "could suture well," and so on.[29]

Our chapter on letters of recommendation (Chapter 6) reviews strategies to locate letter writers who will be most helpful to your candidacy.

We review how to identify these writers and how to approach them. Most importantly, we describe the type of evidence you can provide the writer and the professional manner in which to provide it. Your letter writers want to write the best letter possible, and you can do much more than you realize to make this a reality.

Medical Student Performance Evaluation (MSPE)

Applicants must submit a letter from the Dean as part of their application. Known previously as the Dean's letter, this letter is now termed the Medical Student Performance Evaluation (MSPE). The typical MSPE contains an assessment of both a student's academic performance and professional attributes. The MSPE is particularly helpful when used as a tool to compare your performance in medical school relative to your peers.

Because this component is written by the Dean, students often don't realize the steps that they can take to influence its content:

- The "Unique Characteristics" section of the MSPE is found on the first page of this document, and is a brief statement about your background and experiences (e.g., leadership positions, involvement in research, community service activities). Schools may ask students to draft this section of the MSPE, and then utilize the draft to create the final product.

- Narrative information about your overall performance on each core clerkship and elective rotation will be placed in the "Academic Progress" section of your MSPE. Schools will often include comments taken verbatim from clerkship evaluations. As you move from clerkship to clerkship, we urge you to monitor your academic file. Keep up with your evaluations, and make note of any lukewarm or negative comments. If you feel that the comments are unfair, discuss it with the clerkship director. Addressing such issues well before the MSPE is created may allow for removal of the comments from your academic record.

These are just two ways in which you can influence the MSPE's content. The bottom line is that, at many schools, students *are* involved in the development of this letter. In Chapter 8, we review the steps that applicants can take to maximize the quality of the MSPE, from possibly choosing an MSPE writer, to providing the correct type of information, to the follow through.

Curriculum Vitae (CV)

Curriculum vitae is a Latin expression meaning the "course of one's life." Known as CV for short, this document provides an overview of a candidate's academic and professional background. While similar to a resume, a CV includes additional information such as research experience, publications, and presentations.

Programs within most specialties require applications to be submitted through the Electronic Residency Application System (ERAS). Using ERAS, applicants take information on the CV and enter it into the ERAS application form (MyERAS application). While this process limits what you can do with the look of your CV, the presentation of the information retains the same importance.

Applicants also need to generate a formal CV, as this will be used by letter writers and may be needed by faculty when interviewing.

From the standpoint of a residency selection committee member, reviewing a vast number of CVs from applicants is a difficult process. Therefore, in many cases your CV will be skimmed. Since you have a limited opportunity to impress the residency selection committee, every line, word, and number of your CV becomes important. In Chapter 9, we review how to describe and position experiences and achievements in order to maximize their impact. We review techniques such as utilization of numbers and action verbs to highlight your accomplishments. We review how to create a professional CV, how to utilize the correct structure and format, and how to maximize the impact of every word, line, and number.

Audition Elective

An "audition" elective essentially serves as an extended interview and should be regarded as such. For students applying to competitive specialties or programs, audition electives are considered a must by some programs. These rotations offer students the chance to highlight skills and qualities that aren't easily judged by the typical application materials. Students can showcase their clinical acumen, their skills in patient interaction, their abilities to work with colleagues and faculty, and their enthusiasm for the particular program and specialty. These electives also offer additional opportunities to highlight a student's qualifications for the program. Opportunities include deeper investigation of difficult cases, performing thorough literature searches, volunteering to give presentations, or seeking opportunities to publish in their chosen field.

In some specialties, particularly those that are more competitive, audition electives become very important:

- In a survey of program directors representing multiple specialties, Wagoner and Suriano found that 86% of PDs would give preference to students who had performed at a high level in an audition elective.[30]

- In a survey of plastic surgery PDs, respondents ranked away rotation performance as the most important factor in the residency selection process. 27% of positions were awarded to away rotators.[31]

- In a survey of orthopedic surgery PDs, *the most important criterion in the resident selection process* was considered to be an applicant's performance during a rotation at the director's program.[19] Of note, applicants were also asked about their impressions regarding the importance of these factors, and this factor was not cited among the top three.

- In another survey of orthopedic surgery PDs, performance on a local rotation was considered the most important attribute in obtaining a residency. This was followed by class rank and the interview.[32]

- In a survey of dermatology applicants, the audition elective was similarly important. A total of 53% of applicants matched at a program in which they had some prior experience. Of these, 29% matched at an institution affiliated with their own medical school, 18% matched with an institution where they had done an audition elective, and 6% matched with a program where they had done a research elective/fellowship.[33]

In other specialties, by contrast, the audition elective may not have much of an effect. Our chapter on the audition elective (Chapter 10) describes each advantage of the audition elective, and details how to derive the maximum benefit from each. We review what factors to consider when choosing an elective and describe how to deliver an outstanding performance.

The Competitive Edge

If you're planning on applying to a competitive program or a competitive specialty, you'll need to bring into play all of the recommendations throughout this book. In Chapter 4, we review in detail how to add an extra competitive edge to your application. For competitive programs, publications may boost the strength of your application. The possibility of being published in the medical literature is available to all students. We tell you how to locate such opportunities and walk you through the steps needed to submit an outstanding product.

We also discuss research. Many applicants who apply to competitive programs will have participated in research. *Those applicants are your competition.*

In 2014 the NRMP published data on how applicant qualifications affect match success. Included among the data were the percentage of U.S. seniors who had participated in research projects and the percentage with publications. In highly competitive fields such as dermatology, orthopedic surgery, plastic surgery, and radiation oncology, over 97% of U.S. seniors had participated in research projects. Even in the fields that are not the most competitive, including the fields of anesthesiology, pathology, and pediatrics, over 85% of U.S. seniors had participated in research projects.[34]

The Interview

Contrary to common belief, the purpose of the interview is *not* to determine if you have the qualifications needed to be a resident at the institution. By granting you an interview, the program has already made that determination. Rather, the purpose of the interview is to assess fit. Are you the right fit for the program? Is the program the right fit for you?

Although the CV, personal statement, letters of recommendation, and other aspects of the application are all of great importance, there is no disputing the fact that the interview is possibly the most critical step of the residency application process. While the other elements of the application will help you get an interview, your interview performance will strongly influence your ranking.

Surveys of program directors over the years have consistently found the interview to be a major factor used to rank applicants. In fact, the results of multiple studies indicate that the interview is the *most* valuable factor used in the ranking of applicants.

Unfortunately, many otherwise qualified applicants lose any chance of matching into the residency program of their choice because of a poor interview. In a study of internal medicine residency applicants, 1/3 of applicants were ranked less favorably following an interview.[35] In a study of emergency medicine residency programs, with data obtained from 3,800 individual interviews, a total of 14% of interviews resulted in unranked applicants.[36] The conclusion here is that the interview has the potential to destroy your chances. Preparation is critical.

Unfortunately, we find that most applicants don't give interview preparation the priority that it deserves. Applicants spend months of intense study in preparing for the USMLE exam. They then turn around and spend a few casual hours preparing for interviews. This one critical mistake can ruin your chances of matching successfully.

We devote a full six chapters to the interview process. In these chapters, we review the type of research that must be done before each interview. We review what to expect from the typical interview day and the different types of interviews you may encounter. We discuss what to say and how to say it. We review the common interview questions and delve into the intent behind the questions so that you can prepare your responses. We prepare you for what to say when you don't know the answer. These chapters will prepare you for what to do before, during, and after the interview.

Before the Interview

A significant degree of advance planning is necessary to excel during an interview. You need to understand what interviewers are looking for when they speak to applicants. What are they trying to determine? What qualities are they seeking in their future residents? How can you project these qualities? How can you guide the interview to a discussion of your achievements that emphasize these qualities?

A survey of plastic surgery PDs asked them to rank 20 items that were used in the evaluation of applicants during the interview process.[37] The survey showed that the highest ranked criteria were leadership qualities, apparent maturity, answers to questions, candidate's interest in teaching/academics and attitude toward questions. Sixth in importance were questions posed by applicants.

A study of PM&R PDs asked about the importance of different applicant characteristics assessed during the interview.[24] Ranked highest were compatibility with the program, ability to articulate thoughts, ability to work with the team, ability to listen, and commitment to hard work.

We will show you how to take this knowledge and use it when preparing your interview responses. Have you held leadership positions? Does your prior employment or volunteer experiences demonstrate a commitment to hard work? A review of your strengths and advance preparation are necessary to guide the interview in a direction that emphasizes these strengths. We also review the advance prep work that you'll need to perform for each program and each interviewer. As emphasized in the University of Chicago Pritzker School of Medicine Residency Process Guide, "If granted an interview, run a Medline search of the faculty's publications. Get some notion of who your interviewers are likely to be, and what their program emphasizes."[38] We review effective ways to research each program as well as each interviewer. Gaining this knowledge well in advance of the interview can help you create rapport and allow you to ask the specific, customized types of questions that are most likely to create a favorable impression.

Chapter 13 also tells you what to expect in an interview. You'll learn what to expect from the standard traditional one-on-one interview. You'll also be prepared for the increasingly used behavioral interview, as well as the panel interview and the conversational interview.

Interview Questions

In Chapter 15, we review common interview questions and delve into the intent behind the questions. Does the faculty member really care about your flight into town? Why do they want to know where you see yourself in 10 years? How can you best respond to the intent behind the question?

We also prepare you for specific areas of caution. Were you ready to talk about perfectionism as your greatest weakness? That response joins the other trite, overused responses that leave faculty with a negative impression. Many interviewers end their questioning with "do you have any questions for me?" "Questions asked by applicants" is actually a criterion used by some programs in evaluating applicants. This question can be used as an opportunity to emphasize your interest in the program, and your fit with the program. It's also the type of question that can sink your chances. We provide a full table of potential questions, and specifically review the ones that should never be asked of a faculty member.

Interview Day

A successful interview involves much more than anticipating interview questions and preparing the content of your answers. While most applicants focus their attention on content, nonverbal communication skills are just as important. It's estimated that 65% to 90% of every conversation is interpreted through body language.[39] Of concern for applicants, high levels of anxiety have been shown to adversely affect a variety of nonverbal communication factors, including eye contact, body language, voice level, and projected confidence.[40] Even small details can alter perceptions. In the *Lancet* article "Getting a Grip on Handshakes," it was reported that "a strong correlation was found between a firm handshake – as evidenced by strength, vigor, duration, completeness of grip, and eye contact – and a good first impression…"[41]

In Chapter 14, we talk about steps you can take to decrease anxiety, and the steps you need to take to manage the nonverbal messages during an interview. In her article, "Anxiety Patterns in Employment Interviews," Young wrote that "Anxious individuals are less likely to be hired…possibly because interviewers perceive highly anxious people to be less trustworthy, less task-oriented…than low anxiety interviewees."[42]

We also suggest what to say and what to do when you don't know the answer to a question. We review how to handle the situations that you may not be expecting, such as a silent interviewer or inappropriate or illegal questions. These occur more often than you might expect. A survey of urology residency applicants found that "being asked about marital status was recalled by 91% of male and 100% of female, if they had children by 25% of male and 62% of female, applicants, respectively."[43] These two questions are illegal. We review these types of scenarios, since advance awareness and preparation are the keys to interview performance.

After the Interview

Post-interview communication is a critical component of the interview process. However, many applicants don't recognize this fact. In one study, only 39% of applicants sent follow-up communication to every program with which they interviewed; 55% communicated only with select programs.[44] In Chapter 16, "After the Interview," we review the three cornerstones of post-interview communication and how to correctly thank a program for the opportunity to interview. We review what to say when a program contacts you. Statistics reveal that this is a common occurrence.

We also help you plan how to communicate and what to say to the top programs on your list. We elaborate further on the fact that your expressed interest in a program can, in some cases, impact their interest in you. Is there a chance that your communication with a program following the interview can influence your ranking? Absolutely. Not for every faculty member, and not for every program, but there is a chance that at some programs, expressed interest in the program may influence your ranking.

How would your interest in a program affect their interest in you? Your negative interest can provide a negative influence. Negative interest can be perceived as the lack of any communication from the applicant following the interview. Some programs don't wish to rank highly those applicants who have no interest in the program, because that lack of interest can be an indicator of a poor fit.

A positive interest can be a positive influence. An applicant who ranks a program highly is likely to feel that the program would be a good fit for her interests and abilities, which is what a program seeks. An applicant who plans to rank a program highly would be thrilled to match there, and that hopefully translates to an enthusiastic, hard-working resident. It is also a point of pride for many programs to match those applicants at the top of their own rank list. In a study examining communication between programs and applicants, the authors wrote that "some program directors appear to construct their match lists with the goal of 'matching well' i.e., not having to go far down their lists. To achieve this, knowing where applicants plan to rank them is a high priority."[45]

However, programs do differ widely in their beliefs on the value of post-interview communication. For some programs, what you say following the interview will have no effect whatsoever on the program's decision-making process. In a study looking at recruitment behavior, the authors wrote that "program directors were very skeptical of student ranking assurances."[46]

However, the authors felt that such assurances had an effect on ranking decisions at some programs. They felt that the impact of the rank order list was "limited to one third of programs." Such information is clearly important to some programs.

Surveys of applicants support this belief. When Miller and his colleagues surveyed graduating students at ten U.S. medical schools, they found that 23% were asked how they planned to rank a program, and 21.7% were told that their level of interest would have bearing on their ranking.[45]

Surveys of PDs support this belief as well. In one study, emergency medicine PDs were asked to rate the importance of 20 items in the resident selection process. An applicant's expressed interest in the program was found to be a moderately important selection factor. In this study, it ranked of higher importance than the USMLE Step 1 score, although the standard deviation was high, indicating that there were significant differences in how PDs viewed this factor.[47]

Ranking Residency Programs

Even at this late phase of the application process, applicants need to be aware of dangerous potential pitfalls. Most applicants agonize over the top three programs on their list, but don't spend equivalent time with the bottom three programs on their list. Per the words of the San Francisco Matching Program: "Pay attention to the bottom of your list! Each year some applicants tell us that they omitted a lower choice because they overestimated their chances elsewhere. They ended up unmatched because the omitted program turned out to be their only offer. The only reason not to list a program is that you would rather remain unmatched to explore other options after the match."[48]

Applicants sometimes create a rank list that is too short, or don't follow through with all the programs at which they interviewed, in the mistaken belief that they are a "lock" at a specific program. In their Statement on Professionalism, the NRMP writes that each year it is "contacted by applicants who believe that an error has occurred in the Match because they did not match to programs whose directors had promised them positions (i.e., had promised to rank them high enough to ensure a match). In every case, the NRMP has determined that the applicant did not match to the desired program because, contrary to the applicant's expectation, the program did not rank the applicant high enough on the program's rank order list for the applicant to match there."[49]

Do PDs actually promise positions to applicants? Studies have shown that students often do believe they have received informal commitments from programs. In a survey of fourth-year students at three schools, 43% felt that they had received informal commitments from at least one program.[44] In a survey of urology residency applicants, 40% felt that they had received informal commitments.[43] In Chapter 17, we review other potential pitfalls at this late, yet critical, stage of the process.

Additional Chapters

Special considerations arise for applicants in certain groups. For those at risk of not matching, it's important to have a strategy in place prior to Match week. The NRMP has a program in place called the Supplemental Offer and Acceptance Program (SOAP) for applicants who fail to match. The competition during the SOAP is very intense, and it's important to have a strategy in place far before that date. Chapter 19 reviews the SOAP in detail.

While many of the recommendations in this book are the same for allopathic and osteopathic applicants, there are some additional considerations for osteopathic applicants. This ranges from COMLEX scores to considerations for the separate AOA Match. We present this topic in significant detail in Chapter 20.

A number of different variables come into play if you are an international medical graduate (IMG). Your match strategy will require significant advanced planning, and additional factors. The strategies utilized by U.S. citizen IMGs and non-U.S. citizen IMGs will vary as well. This information is detailed in Chapters 21 and 22.

The other unique group of applicants is those going through the Couples Match. Considerations for these applicants are presented in Chapter 18.

The Successful Match

There are no shortcuts and no easy answers when it comes to a successful match. The residency application process is prolonged and difficult, and while success is never guaranteed, our evidence-based advice and insiders' perspectives provide the specific, concrete recommendations that will maximize your chances of achieving the ultimate goal: that of a successful match.

A Few Notes On How To Read This Book

"Over 600 pages? I'm never going to finish!" No, this is not that type of book. You do not have to read the entire book, and certainly not in one sitting.

- As you start to plan your match strategy, begin with the first three chapters, which include this introduction chapter, The Basics, and The Selection Process.
- If you're applying for a more competitive specialty or a more competitive program in a less competitive specialty, your advance reading should definitely include the chapters The Competitive Edge and The Right Fit. I also suggest that you read the chapter on letters of recommendation, because this is a very important pillar of your match strategy. You may also wish to read the CV chapter in advance, because you'll need to submit a CV to be considered for some research opportunities. It may also help highlight any weaknesses in your application. If you're applying for a competitive specialty, we recommend audition electives, and Chapter 10 provides important recommendations.
- The last section of the book (close to 200 pages) is included as reference material. It covers every specialty in far more specific detail. You can use this section to explore your specific specialty choice (you can ignore the others).
- There are also a lot of pages devoted to references. We referenced over 750 sources in this book. We looked at, and excluded, many, many more. While we summarized and quoted many studies, editorials, and anecdotes within the book, many of these are fascinating primary sources, and may serve as important resources for your application strategy.
- One other point. We made every effort to improve the readability of this book. Therefore, please don't rely on our writing as an example of correct grammar for professional writing. Our frequent use of contractions and dangling participles, as well as numerals at the start of a sentence, is a conscious choice to improve reading fluency.
- Some chapters were primarily authored by myself, and some were primarily authored by Dr. Desai. Pronouns, including gender pronouns, vary accordingly.
- Even though this is a very comprehensive book, we obviously can't cover every last topic here. Please check our website www.TheSuccessfulMatch.com for links to other materials and for our blog. We're also starting a podcast, and we'll be linking to it there. One of our first topics will be a more in-depth discussion of ways to locate research opportunities.

We wish you the best of luck with your residency match.

Sincerely,

Dr. Rajani Katta and Dr. Samir Desai

References

[1]Results Of 2016 NRMP Main Residency Match Largest On Record As Match Continues To Grow. Available at: http://www.nrmp.org/press-release-results-of-2016-nrmp-main-residency-match-largest-on-record-as-match-continues-to-grow/. Accessed April 23, 2016.
[2]Advance Data Tables: 2016 Main Residency Match. Available at: http://www.nrmp.org/match-data/main-residency-match-data/. Accessed April 23, 2016.
[3]2016 Urology Residency Match. Available at: https://www.auanet.org/common/pdf/education/specialty-match/Match_Statistics_2016_Updated_011916.pdf. Accessed April 23, 2016.
[4]AAMC Results of the 2015 Medical School Enrollment. Available at: http://members.aamc.org/eweb/upload/2015_Enrollment_Report.pdf. Accessed May 9, 2016.
[5]Weissbart S, Stock J, Wein A. Program directors' criteria for selection into urology residency. *Urology* 2015; 85(4): 731-736.
[6]Ohio State University Department of Anesthesiology. Available at: http://anesthesiology.osu.edu/11429.cfm. Accessed April 23, 2016.
[7]UCSF Career Information: Emergency Medicine. Available at: http://meded.ucsf.edu/ume/career-information-emergency-medicine. Accessed April 23, 2016.
[8]University of Colorado Department of Surgery. Available at: http://www.ucdenver.edu/academics/colleges/medicalschool/education/studentaffairs/studentgroups/SurgicalSociety/Pages/FAQ.aspx. Accessed April 23, 2016.
[9]Electronic Residency Application Service. Available at: https://www.aamc.org/services/eras/stats/359278/stats.html. Accessed April 23, 2016.
[10]Weissbart S, Kim S, Feinn R, Stock J. Relationship between the number of residency applications and the yearly match rate: Time to start thinking about an application limit? *J Grad Med Educ* 2015; 7(1): 81-85.
[11]University of Vermont College of Medicine. Available at: http://www.uvm.edu/medicine/. Accessed March 2, 2015.
[12]Campbell B, Havas N, Derse A, Holloway R. Creating a residency application personal statement writers workshop: Fostering narrative, teamwork, and insight at a time of stress. *Acad Med* 2016; 91(3): 371-375.
[13]American Academy of Emergency Medicine Resident Section. Available at: http://www.aaemrsa.org/pdf/rulesoftheroad_students.pdf. Accessed January 30, 2013.
[14]Harvard Medical School Department of Orthopedic Surgery. Available at: http://www.hms.harvard.edu/ortho/apps/index.html. Accessed April 30, 2012.
[15]Wake Forest University Department of Orthopedic Surgery. Available at: http://www.wakehealth.edu/School/Orthopaedic-Surgery/Tips-for-Senior-Medical-Students.htm. Accessed April 30, 2012.
[16]University of Washington Department of Family Medicine. Available at: https://depts.washington.edu/fammed/residency/fellowships/global-health/applicant-information/. Accessed April 23, 2016.

[17]University of Alabama at Birmingham Department of Obstetrics & Gynecology. Available at: http://www.obygn.uab.edu/medicalstudents/obgyn/uasom/documents/2005ResidencyGuidelines.pdf. Accessed March 2, 2009.
[18]Smith E, Weyhing B, Mody Y, Smith W. A critical analysis of personal statements submitted by radiology residency applicants. *Acad Radiol* 2005; 12: 1024-1028.
[19]Bernstein A, Jazrawi L, Elbeshbeshy B, Della Valle C, Zuckerman J. Orthopedic resident-selection criteria. *J Bone Joint Surg Am* 2002; 84-A (11): 2090-2096.
[20]Olazagasti J, Gorouhi F, Fazel N. A critical review of personal statements submitted by dermatology residency applicants. *Dermatol Res Pract* 2014; Epub 2014 Sep 14.
[21]Wayne State University Department of Pathology. Available at: http://www.med.wayne.edu/Pathology/residencytraining/FAQ.htm. Accessed April 23, 2016.
[22]Results of the 2014 NRMP Program Director Survey. Available at: http://www.nrmp.org/wp-content/uploads/2014/09/PD-Survey-Report-2014.pdf. Accessed March 3, 2015.
[23]Villanueva A, Kaye D, Abdelhak S, Morahan P. Comparing selection criteria for residency directors and physicians' employers. *Acad Med* 1995; 70(4): 261-271.
[24]Greenburg A, Doyle J, McClure D. Letters of recommendation for surgical residencies: what they say and what they mean. *J Surg Res* 1994; 1994; 56(2): 192-198.
[25]DeLisa J, Jain S, Campagnolo D. Factors used by physical medicine and rehabilitation residency training directors to select their residents. *Am J Phys Med Rehabil* 1994; 73: 152-156.
[26]University of Texas-Houston Medical School Career Counseling Catalog. Available at: https://med.uth.edu/. Accessed January 1, 2008.
[27]Gayed N. Residency directors' assessments of which selection criteria best predict the performances of foreign-born foreign medical graduates during internal medicine residencies. *Acad Med* 1991; 66 (11): 699-701.
[28]O'Halloran C, Altmaier E, Smith W, Franken E. Evaluation of resident applicants by letters of recommendation: a comparison of traditional and behavioral-based formats. *Invest Radiol* 1993; 28: 274-277.
[29]Fortune J. The content and value of letters of recommendation in the resident candidate evaluative process. *Curr Surg* 2002; 59(1): 79-83.
[30]Wagoner N, Suriano J. Program directors' responses to a survey on variables used to select residents in a time of change. *Acad Med* 1999; 74: 51-58.
[31]Drolet B, Brower J, Lifchez S, Janis J, Liu P. Away rotations and matching in integrated plastic surgery residency: Applicant and Program Director Perspectives. *Plast Reconstr Surg* 2016; 137(4): 1337-1343.
[32]Bajaj G, Carmichael K. What attributes are necessary to be selected for an orthopedic surgery residency position: perceptions of faculty and residents. *South Med J* 2004; 97(12): 1179-1185.

[33]Clarke J, Miller J, Sceppa J, Goldsmith L, Long E. Success in the dermatology resident match in 2003: perceptions and importance of home institutions and away rotations. *Arch Dermatol* 2006; 142 (7): 930-2.
[34]Charting Outcomes in the Match (2014). Available at: http://www.nrmp.org/wp-content/uploads/2014/09/Charting-Outcomes-2014-Final.pdf. Accessed March 3, 2016.
[35]Gong H, Parker N, Apgar F, Shank C. Influence of the interview on ranking in the residency selection process. *Med Educ* 1984; 18(5): 366-369.
[36]Martin-Lee L, Park H, Overton D. Does interview date affect match list position in the emergency medicine national residency matching program match? *Acad Emerg Med* 2000; 7(9): 1022-1026.
[37]LaGrasso J, Kennedy D, Hoehn J, Ashruf S, Pryzbyla A. Selection criteria for the integrated model of plastic surgery residency. *Plast Reconstr Surg* 2008; 121(3): 121e-125e.
[38]University of Chicago Residency Process Guide. Available at: http://pritzker.uchicago.edu/current/students/ResidencyProcessGuide.pdf. Accessed January 2, 2008.
[39]Cole K. *The Complete Idiot's Guide to Clear Communication*. Published by Alpha Books in 2002.
[40]Freeman T, Sawyer C, Behnke R. Behavioral inhibition and the attribution of public speaking anxiety. *Communication Education* 1997; 46: 175-187.
[41]Larkin M. Getting a grip on handshakes. *Lancet* 2000; 356: 227.
[42]Young M, Behnke R, Mann Y. Anxiety patterns in employment interviews. *Communication Reports* 2004; 17(1): 49-57.
[43]Teichman J, Anderson K, Dorough M, Stein C. Optenberg S, Thompson I. The urology residency matching program in practice. *J Urol* 2000; 163(6): 1878-1887.
[44]Anderson K, Jacobs D. General surgery program directors' perceptions of the match. *Curr Surg* 2000; 57(5): 460-465.
[45]Miller J, Schaad D, Crittenden R, Oriol N, MacLaren C. Communication between programs and applicants during residency selection: effects of the match on medical students' professional development. *Acad Med* 2003; 78(4): 403-411.
[46]Carek P, Anderson K, Blue A, Mavis B. Recruitment behavior and program directors: how ethical are their perspectives about the match process? *Fam Med* 2000; 32(4): 258-260.
[47]Crane J, Ferraro C. Selection criteria for emergency medicine residency applicants. *Acad Emerg Med* 2000; 7(1): 54-60.
[48]San Francisco Matching Program. Available at: www.sfmatch.org. Accessed May 2, 2008.
[49]National Resident Matching Program. Available at: www.nrmp.org. Accessed May 2, 2008.

Chapter 2

The Basics

The residency application process starts with some basic yet essential information. You may have chosen a specialty, but have you realistically evaluated your chances of matching into that field? How do you decide which programs you should apply to? How do you locate and actually work with a specialty-specific advisor? How do you actually start the application process? In this chapter, we consider basic information needed to start the application process.

Choice of Specialty

Your residency application starts with your selection of a specialty. Once you decide on a specialty, you must determine:

- The competitiveness of your chosen specialty
- Your competitiveness for that specialty
- The matching program that administers the match process in your chosen field
- The right advisor to help you reach your career goals

Assessing the Competitiveness of Your Chosen Specialty

To develop the optimal match strategy, you must take into account the competitiveness of your chosen specialty. Listed in the following table are the numbers of U.S. allopathic seniors who failed to match in each specialty (2014 NRMP Match). We've also included the percentage of positions in the specialty filled by U.S. allopathic seniors, as opposed to IMGs or graduates of osteopathic schools.

The other columns present the mean USMLE Step 1 scores among matched applicants and the percentage of applicants in the Alpha Omega Alpha Honor Medical Society (AOA) for each specialty.

Assessing the Competitiveness of Specialties Participating in the NRMP Match				
Specialty	**U.S. seniors who failed to match**	**Fill rate (U.S. seniors)**	**Mean USMLE Step 1 score for matched U.S. seniors**	**% AOA**
Anesthesiology	49 (4.4%)	73%	230	10.6%
Dermatology	111 (24%)	91%	247	50.8%
Emergency Medicine	106 (7.2%)	79%	230	12.0%
Family Medicine	49 (3.6%)	44%	218	8.0%
General Surgery	158 (15.4%)	80%	232	15.3%
Internal Medicine	105 (3.1%)	49%	231	16.4%
Medicine/Pediatrics	11 (3.8%)	84%	233	22.1%
Neurological Surgery	50 (21%)	90%	244	28.3%
Neurology	10 (2.6%)	55%	230	12.8%
Obstetrics/Gynecology	89 (8.6%)	80%	226	12.6%
Orthopedic Surgery	190 (22.7%)	94%	245	32.2%
Otolaryngology	91 (24.7%)	95%	248	38.9%
Pathology	5 (1.9%)	47%	231	11.0%
Pediatrics	73 (3.9%)	71%	226	12.9%
PM&R	26 (11.3%)	61%	220	5.5%
Plastic Surgery	52 (29.2%)	92%	245	39.0%
Psychiatry	26 (3.7%)	57%	220	4.9%
Radiation Oncology	20 (10.6%)	82%	241	23.6%
Radiology	12 (1.5%)	50%	241	21.8%
Vascular surgery	4 (10.8%)	84%	237	22.6%
Adapted from Charting Outcomes in the Match (2014). Available at: http://www.nrmp.org/wp-content/uploads/2014/09/Charting-Outcomes-2014-Final.pdf.				

Using this information, specialties can be divided into three groups:

- Highly competitive (> 15% of U.S. allopathic applicants fail to match)
- Moderately competitive (5 – 15% of U.S. allopathic applicants fail to match)
- Less competitive (< 5% of U.S. allopathic applicants fail to match)

Competitiveness of Specialties		
Highly Competitive	**Moderately Competitive**	**Less Competitive**
Dermatology General Surgery Neurological surgery Ophthalmology Orthopedic Surgery Otolaryngology Plastic Surgery Urology	Emergency Medicine Obstetrics/Gynecology Physical Medicine & Rehabilitation Radiation Oncology Vascular Surgery	Anesthesiology Family Medicine Internal Medicine Medicine/Pediatrics Neurology Pathology Pediatrics Psychiatry Radiology

Among the highly competitive specialties, dermatology, neurological surgery, orthopedic surgery, otolaryngology, plastic surgery, and urology had the highest failure to match rates, ranging from 21% (neurological surgery) to 29.2% (plastic surgery).[1]

> **Note...**
>
> For highly competitive specialties, you need a back-up plan. What do you plan to do if you don't match? Interviewers often ask about back-up plans to learn about the depth of your commitment to the specialty. A well thought out back-up plan that allows reapplication implies a deeper commitment to the specialty. Some students apply to two different specialties, using one as a back-up to the other. However, in a survey of general surgery PDs, 75% felt that knowledge of an applicant interviewing in multiple specialties would have a negative effect on the applicant's rank order.[2]

Assessing Your Competitiveness for Your Chosen Specialty

It's of critical importance to realistically assess your academic credentials and qualifications. Periodically, the NRMP publishes two important documents that applicants may use to assess their competitiveness for specialties participating in the NRMP Match:

- NRMP Program Director Survey[3]

  On a biennial basis, the NRMP surveys all program directors participating in the Match. Respondents are asked to rate the importance of criteria used to select applicants to interview. PDs are also asked to rate the importance of criteria used to rank applicants. In the 2014 survey, approximately 53% of PDs responded to the survey.

- Charting Outcomes in the Match[1]

  In this document, the qualifications of matched and unmatched applicants are presented by specialty.

It's also important to discuss your academic credentials and qualifications with those who are knowledgeable about the selection process. It's both necessary and important to seek the opinions of your dean, department chairman or PD in your chosen specialty, your advisor, and other key faculty. With their assistance, you can develop a more informed and objective view of your competitiveness for the specialty. Through this process, some applicants recognize the necessity of a back-up plan.

Just as some specialties are more competitive than others, some programs within a specialty are far more selective than others. Again, discussions with experienced advisors can help you learn about program selectivity. In developing a list of programs to apply to, we encourage you to apply to those programs which you consider your "dream" programs. Every year, applicants match to programs for which they thought they had little or no chance. However, your list definitely needs to include a sufficient number of programs which are sure bets.

Tip # 1

Ask key faculty members at your school for their thoughts on the number of programs to which you should apply. Based on your credentials, have you considered enough programs for which you're competitive?

Tip # 2

Strategize about concrete steps that you can take to strengthen your application. Should you take the USMLE Step 2 CK exam before applying? Can you participate in research? Should you do an elective with a distinguished professor to secure another strong letter of recommendation? Would an audition elective help?

As you review your competitiveness for the specialty and for particular programs, you must strategize on how to strengthen your candidacy. If you're reading this book early in your medical education, you have the advantage of time. However, even if you're in the midst of the application process, there are multiple ways to enhance your credentials.

Tip # 3

Make sure you apply to enough programs. If you receive a plethora of interviews, you can always cancel some.

Matching Programs

While most specialties participate in the National Resident Matching Program (NRMP), the ophthalmology and urology matches are handled by the San Francisco Matching Program and the American Urological Association, respectively. Osteopathic applicants may also choose to participate in the AOA Match administered by National Medical Services (see Chapter 20). Both allopathic and osteopathic applicants can participate in the Military Match.

National Resident Matching Program (NRMP)

In 1952 the National Resident Matching Program, commonly referred to as NRMP, was established through the efforts of its sponsoring groups, which included the American Medical Association, the Association of American Medical Colleges, and the American Board of Medical Specialties. Before its inception, medical students were pressured by residency programs to accept residency training contracts early in their medical training, sometimes as early as the second year of medical school. Many students were forced to make specialty decisions before they were ready.

With the establishment of the NRMP the process became much more ordered, and today there's general agreement that the process is much easier. What did the NRMP do to improve this process? The NRMP requires both applicants and programs to create a rank list. Applicants submit a list of programs they would be willing to attend, in order of preference. Programs also submit their own lists, ranking the candidates they've interviewed in the order in which they would extend offers to fill their residency program. Match results are produced by a computer which matches each applicant to the highest ranking program (on the applicant's rank list) which has offered him or her a position in their program. The results are announced throughout the country in mid-March on "Match Day."

Programs and applicants are expected to honor the results of the Match. To participate in the Match, applicants must agree with the policies and rules of the Match Participation Agreement. When a match occurs between a program and an applicant, both parties have a binding commitment to one another. If either party does not honor the commitment, it is considered a breach of the agreement and results in an NRMP investigation.

In the 2016 NRMP Match, there were over 42,000 registrants vying for just over 30,000 first-year positions.[4] Over 18,000 of these applicants were U.S. allopathic seniors. The remaining applicants were considered "independent applicants" and included graduates of U.S. medical schools, students at osteopathic schools, Canadian students, and IMGs.

To participate in the Match, applicants must first register for the NRMP at the organization's website. Applicants can register at the site by completing a form, agreeing to the terms and conditions of the Match, and paying the registration fee.

Other Matches

Ophthalmology and Urology do not participate in the NRMP. The ophthalmology match is administered by the San Francisco Matching Program (www.sfmatch.org) while the urology match is handled by the American Urological Association (www.aua.net). Both matches take place earlier than the NRMP match and are often referred to as "early matches." Results of these matches are announced in January.

Some Important Terms in the Match...

Categorical Residency Positions: Refers to programs in which residents complete their first year, or internship, as part of the training program. After completing internship, residents remain there to finish training.

Advanced Residency Positions: Refers to positions which begin 1-2 years after the Match, and require completion of preliminary training. Applicants must arrange for this initial period of training separately.

Preliminary Residency Positions: Internal medicine, pediatrics, OB/GYN, and general surgery residency programs may offer preliminary residency positions. These one or two-year positions fulfill the initial training requirements for certain specialties (see Advanced Residency Positions above).

Transitional Year Positions: Refers to a one-year position during which the trainee rotates through various specialties, including internal medicine, surgery, pediatrics, and emergency medicine. Of note, some specialties allow their trainees to complete a transitional year in lieu of a preliminary year. For example, prior to starting dermatology residency, trainees can complete either a transitional or preliminary year.

Note...

Applicants participating in other matches (i.e., ophthalmology or urology) will often register in the NRMP for several reasons. First, many of these residency programs require applicants to arrange for their first year of training (preliminary year) separately. Second, since both specialties are highly competitive, applicants will often apply to a second choice specialty as a back-up plan in the event that they fail to match.

Electronic Residency Application Service (ERAS)

In 1995, the Electronic Residency Application Service (ERAS) was founded by the Association of American Medical Colleges (AAMC). Through ERAS, applicants complete a single application which is transmitted electronically to designated programs. Presently, all specialties participate in the ERAS program, with the exception of ophthalmology, which participates in the San Francisco Matching Program Central Application Service (CAS).

ERAS allows for transmission of all application components, including the common application, personal statement, MSPE, letters of recommendation, and transcripts. For applicants participating in the NRMP Match, September 15 is the earliest date ERAS applications may be submitted to programs.

Note...

All specialties with the exception of ophthalmology use ERAS. Note that, while the urology match is administered by the American Urological Association, urology programs also use ERAS. Ophthalmology, however, participates in the Central Application Service (CAS). A few programs within ERAS participating specialties do not use ERAS. If so, you will need to obtain the application directly from the program.

Did you know?

You can track the status of your ERAS application by using the Applicant Document Tracking System (ADTS). You can determine when supporting documents have been uploaded, and the dates on which residency programs downloaded these documents.

Selecting an Advisor

Insider advice is invaluable. Students recognize that the help of an advisor in guiding them through the complex residency application process can be an important factor in boosting the strength of their application. In a survey of third- and fourth-year medical students at UCSF, 96% of all participants rated mentors as important or very important.[5] Unfortunately, recognizing the value of a mentoring relationship is a far cry from developing such a relationship. Although 96% of the participants rated mentors as important, only 36% actually reported having a mentor.

The value of advising is recognized in all fields. The literature in the fields of business, education, and medicine all support its value. Although they're at an advanced level in their career, even medical school faculty describe the need for advisors. Comments made by medical school faculty emphasize the value of an advising relationship:[6]

- "I had a difficult time learning the rules of the game."
- "Without a mentor…I had no idea really what to expect from academic medicine. I have been feeling my way through the tunnels because I don't know where the roadblocks are. I just kind of deal with them when I get there."

These comments mirror those we hear from applicants. It's difficult to learn the rules of the game when they're not written down. "I didn't know you could customize your personal statements for different programs." "I didn't know I should have sent an e-mail thank you immediately after the interview, especially since I was planning to send a note later."

It's particularly difficult when you learn the rules of the game too late to make a difference. "I didn't know that matched applicants to neurosurgery in the NRMP data had reported, on average, nearly 12 abstracts, publications, or presentations. I'm in my fourth year now, and it's probably too late."

As you'll see throughout this book, we often recommend seeking the opinions and advice of your advisors. Their insider advice and specific knowledge about the specialty is clearly very valuable. However, how do you, as an applicant, actually locate such an advisor?

Some medical schools recognize the importance of advising students and have responded with the development of mentoring and advising programs. These programs differ widely in structure and scope. At some schools, highly organized programs have been developed. At other schools, the mentoring process is more informal, consisting of students being given a list of faculty members willing to serve as advisors, and then encouraged to cultivate relationships. As one student in a survey of UCSF students stated, "I create the relationship, and then I follow it. I sort of take the risk."[7]

While some students are able to create such relationships, it can be difficult, and some students blame themselves for not being assertive enough to find a mentor. "I just didn't know how to go about setting myself up for a good thing to happen."[7] Other students maintain that the problem lies with the system, citing the short duration of courses and clerkships as impediments to developing relationships with faculty.

Did you know?

In a recent study of academic plastic surgeons, researchers had medical students at different institutions place e-mail requests for mentorship with faculty at the same institution. Nearly 25% of plastic surgeons never responded despite students sending 2 separate e-mail requests. The report also shed light on how quickly faculty respond to student e-mails. After the initial e-mail contact, the mean response time was 36 hours. The mean response time following the second e-mail reminder was 72 hours. Of note, 23.1% of responses occurred after the second reminder, emphasizing the importance of follow-up if no response is received after initial contact. Researchers also noted that younger faculty members, those at top 20 medical schools, and members of the American College of Surgeons were more likely to respond.[8]

How have other students met potential mentors? In one study, 28% of students met their mentors during inpatient clerkships, 19% through research activities, and 9% during outpatient clerkships.[5] If you're lucky, you'll be assigned to an inpatient or outpatient clerkship in which you learn and excel, and through that process develop a relationship with your attending. If so, you may seek a letter of recommendation from your attending, or ask for advice with your career choices and application.

Many students won't find a mentor through randomly assigned clerkships and courses. One option is to choose a particular elective or clerkship for the chance to work with a specific attending. A discussion with other students, upperclassmen, or residents in your chosen field should help identify those faculty members who are known to be excellent advisors. If you're not able to work with these individuals directly in a clinical setting, you may be able to contact them for opportunities to work on research projects or publications. In some cases, potential advisors may be willing to meet with you outside of clinical activities.

Did you know?

The importance of the mentor in the residency selection process was highlighted in a recent study of EM residents. Researchers found that residents who reported "greater mentor effectiveness were more likely to match to their first or second choice." Of note, 1/3 of respondents indicated that they didn't have a mentor during medical school. Osteopathic and IMG applicants were less likely to have mentors than their allopathic counterparts.[9]

Using the Mentor Effectiveness Scale (MES) to Choose Among Potential Mentors

While many students ask upperclassmen about potential mentors, the conversation is often short on specifics. To make more informed decisions about your choice of mentor, consider using the Mentor Effectiveness Scale created by researchers at Johns Hopkins University. Ask past student mentees to rate potential mentors on a scale of 1 (strongly disagree) to 5 (strongly agree) using the following 12 behaviors.

My mentor was accessible.
My mentor demonstrated professional integrity.
My mentor demonstrated content expertise in my area of need.
My mentor was approachable and easy to talk with about concerns.
My mentor was supportive and encouraging.
My mentor provided constructive and useful critique of my work.
My mentor motivated me to improve my work product.
My mentor was helpful in providing direction and guidance on professional issues (e.g., networking).
My mentor answered my questions satisfactorily (e.g., timely response, clear, comprehensive).
My mentor was helpful in providing advice on work/school and personal life.
My mentor suggested appropriate resources (e.g., experts, contacts, source material).
My mentor challenged me to extend my abilities (e.g., risk taking, try a new activity, draft a section of an article).

Through this tool, you'll be able to more accurately identify strengths and weaknesses of potential mentors.

Berk R, Berg J, Mortimer R, Walton-Moss B, Yeo T. Measuring the effectiveness of faculty mentoring relationships. *Acad Med* 2005; 80(1): 66-71.

It can be difficult to ask a faculty member for their help. Understandably, students often hesitate to burden faculty members who are already clearly very busy. However, while faculty members have many demands placed on their time, there are faculty at every medical school who find mentoring and advising students enjoyable and rewarding. While these individuals are sometimes recognized publicly for their work, it's more typical that they go about their work diligently but quietly. You should make every effort to identify these types of motivated, dedicated individuals.

In many departments, students applying to a particular field will be advised that they should start the process by setting up a meeting with the clerkship director, program director or chairman of the department. The intent of this meeting is to state that you're planning to apply to the field. From there, the meeting can go in several directions. You can ask for recommendations on potential advisors. You can ask for recommendations on the application process, given the strength of your credentials. You can seek opportunities to work on a case report, to work on a research project, or to arrange a research elective.

Some schools lack residency programs in certain specialties. That poses obvious difficulties for students applying to that specialty. One option would be to seek advisors elsewhere, such as during an audition elective. In addition, local or national organizations may provide assistance. The Society of Academic Emergency Medicine (SAEM) has a virtual advisor program (EAdvisor) open to medical students at all institutions. Through this program, students can query experienced individuals about a variety of issues, including the EM residency application process.

Finding the right advisor can be difficult. Even with a formal system for assigning advisors, the advisor won't necessarily be the right fit for the student. If you encounter this problem, seek guidance from other faculty members. Even classmates, upperclassmen, and residents can serve as additional advisors, although they shouldn't be your sole source of information. Few advisors have the answers to every question, and it's often to your advantage to have several opinions on certain issues. As one student told us, "My faculty advisor was very helpful when it came to writing my letter of recommendation and giving me advice on where to apply. However, two of the upperclassmen who had matched into my field were very helpful when it came to my application itself. They told me which faculty members were the ones to work with, who might have papers that I could work on, and how I should be customizing my personal statement. I wish that I'd had the guts to approach the other faculty that I had worked with for their thoughts on the subject. I also really wish I had asked one of them to help me with a mock interview."

Did you know?

Although you might expect that mentors in a single specialty would agree on the nature of advice delivered to residency applicants, research has not shown this. In one study, researchers designed and distributed a survey to all family medicine residency programs. Respondents were asked to indicate their level of agreement with various advising statements that faculty may offer to students applying to programs. Respondents were asked to use a 4-point Likert scale (strongly agree, agree, disagree, strongly disagree) with each advising statement. Of the 24 items in the survey, consensus was only achieved for 7/24 items. "Lack of shared understanding about factors being used to determine success of applicants presents a significant barrier," wrote the authors of the study. This is yet another reason to consider having multiple mentors.[10]

A Note for Shy Students Searching for Mentors

If you're shy, or you just hate having to ask for a favor, please read this.

I was testing out a talk one year, and I gave a practice lecture on the successful match to five 4th-year medical students. One student had several questions following the lecture, because her match efforts weren't going well. In the following week, I received emails from two of the other students. Both asked me to review their personal statements. Both were stellar. Neither needed my help.

The student who clearly could have used my help, though, never contacted me. I had hoped she would. I had several suggestions for her, but I try not to give unsolicited advice. I just wish she had contacted me with a simple email:

Hello Dr. Katta,

I enjoyed your lecture today, and it raised several points that concern me about my own application. Is there any way you might be able to meet with me for 15 minutes during the next two weeks to discuss my application? If you're too busy at this time, I understand, but thank you for considering it.

Regards,

It's always difficult reaching out to individuals in positions of power. It's especially difficult when you're asking for a "favor." Here are my suggestions:

1. Express appreciation when you ask. "Thank you for taking the time to consider my request."

2. Express appreciation afterwards. "Thank you so much for taking the time to meet with me today. I appreciated your advice on..."

3. Be very clear about what it is that you're asking for, and make it clear what kind of time commitment will be involved. "Would you be able to meet with me for 15 minutes to discuss..."

4. If you're asking for potential case reports or research projects, then remember that your offer of hard work may be just what your attending needs at that point in time. If so, it's not a favor: you're offering a valuable contribution.

5. Your request may be met with silence, or with a polite "not at this time." Much of this, as in so much of life, is about timing. Don't take it personally, because it's not.

6. If you're asking to participate in a research project, how many phone calls/emails/meetings will it take before you're offered an opportunity? If your department is actively involved in research, maybe just 2-3. If you're seeking opportunities outside of your home department, maybe 10-20. If you're not a current medical student, maybe 100. Yes, that's correct. A family friend, an IMG, knocked on over 100 doors before she was given the opportunity to write a case report. She parlayed that into more opportunities, and is now finishing her Cardiology fellowship.

7. Lastly, don't hesitate to ask for help if you need it. Please remember that many faculty members are very happy to advise and support medical students, because they find it to be a fulfilling, rewarding aspect of their jobs. I find it very fulfilling to mentor and support individuals whom I believe have great potential. After 17 years as a faculty member, a number of former medical students and residents are now colleagues and friends. I refer friends and family members to some of the dermatologists whom I trained. These are individuals who are caring, empathetic, diligent, and conscientious - in short, the type of physician I admire. I'm proud of these individuals, and I'm happy that I had a part in their training.

Did you know?

Have you ever wondered what forms the basis for the advice offered by mentors and advisors? In one study of pediatric clerkship directors, researchers inquired about the resources which informed advising strategies for applicants. Approximately 40% of respondents reported using subjective resources alone, including their own experiences as an applicant, input from former students, and discussions with colleagues. Less than half indicated that they used objective resources such as NRMP data.[11]

Did you know?

In a study of over 70 medical students mentored by radiation oncology faculty at a single institution, researchers assessed the impact of the mentorship program. Mentees delivered 75 presentations at national conferences, and published a total of 53 manuscripts. Mentees were also noted to have received numerous medical school and national awards for their work and involvement. The authors concluded that mentorship can have a positive effect on research productivity.[12]

Did you know?

Will your mentoring needs be met by your assigned mentor? Factors to consider include the number of mentees served by the mentor and time spent per month. In a study of 14 newly established schools since 2006, researchers found that the ratio of mentors to mentees ranged widely from 1:1 to 1:20. Time spent in hours per month varied considerably, from as few as 1-2 hours to over 10 hours.[13]

As you consider possible advisors, you should be aware of problems that can occur in the advisor-advisee relationship. Chief among these is the potential conflict of interest that can occur with a faculty member who advises a student and also serves on the residency selection committee (at a program affiliated with the student's medical school). In a survey of 740 graduating medical students from 10 U.S. medical schools, Miller found that nearly half met with their advisors during or following the interview season.[14] The results indicated that:

- 31.8% were encouraged to rank the advisor's program highly.
- 10.3% were asked which programs they planned to rank highly.
- 4% were asked how they planned to rank the advisor's program.

Students reported varying degrees of discomfort with these queries. One respondent stated that "it felt very uncomfortable to talk to him about my own strengths and weaknesses and about which programs I preferred knowing that he would later be evaluating me in comparison with many other applicants and deciding whether or not to advocate for me to be accepted." Faced with such dilemmas, some students felt pressured to make misleading statements. Miller went on to raise some important questions. "What is safe for applicants to tell their advisors? Can applicants be sure that their advisors will put their interests first in these situations?" You need to consider how you would respond to these types of queries, since you may be placed in a similar situation.

Studies of medical students, advising, and the match are sparse, but our experience has demonstrated that having an effective advisor is invaluable. Advisors can help students with career decisions, evaluate potential residency programs, review *curriculum vitae* and personal statements, write letters of recommendation, and conduct mock interviews. Since faculty members often sit on residency selection committees, many can offer insight into the selection process that is not available elsewhere. By analyzing and comparing your credentials with those of students who have matched in previous years, advisors can identify ways in which you can strengthen your application and work with you to develop an overall strategy for success. Applicants should work hard to identify the right advisors, since these relationships can be invaluable in ensuring a successful match.

Adapted with permission from our column, "The Successful Match," available at www.studentdoctor.net

Mentors as Inspiration

We've focused in this section on mentors who can provide career guidance and who can help with career advancement, but their most important role may be that of role models. Mentors can show us the type of physicians that we can choose to become.

When I was a 3rd-year medical student, I did a rotation at our county hospital. I remember presenting the case of a 12-year-old girl with atopic dermatitis. It was very routine. The resident asked me what medications she was on, and then refilled her prescriptions. As I was discussing a different case with the attending, Dr. D., the young girl walked out of the room. Dr. D. asked me what we had done for the patient. She then proceeded to teach me.

She asked me to look at the girl's posture. She made me see her downcast gaze, her slow gait, and her overall sense of defeat. I saw the angry flare of dermatitis on her face. Why were we refilling her medications, when they so clearly weren't working?

She asked me to bring the patient back to the room. We sat down with her and revised her treatment regimen. We worked on giving her hope.

I remember thinking, at that moment, that this was the kind of doctor I wanted to be.

Medical School Resources

If you are currently in medical school, you can and should take full advantage of the resources available at your institution. The scope and quality of these resources vary greatly, and you'll need to research to discover what resources are available. Many schools will offer meetings on the residency application process, with a particular emphasis on deadlines. These meetings typically review the institutional resources available to help students match successfully.

However, the support offered by medical schools varies greatly. In speaking with students and residents, we've heard of schools that cover the whole spectrum. In one school, no group meetings were offered, and no individual meetings with the Dean were arranged. Instead students were reminded of application deadlines by e-mail. "The information was handed down from the residents and upperclassmen, and you were pretty much expected to arrange your own advisors."

At another institution, every student meets with the Dean during the third year. The student's strengths and weaknesses are reviewed, especially as it relates to the student's chances of matching into his or her chosen field. An annual workshop is offered, which pairs a group of students with a recently matched applicant who offers informal advice. At another school, a series of lectures reviews deadlines and the application process itself.

Some schools provide more extensive resources. The Mercer University School of Medicine has a specific Career Counseling and Residency Planning Program. The University of Chicago Pritzker School of Medicine offers an online residency planning guide, which provides specific recommendations from each of the departments. Some schools offer formal mentorship programs. Others offer workshops or assistance with writing a CV or personal statement. Some offer interview skills workshops or mock interviews.

It reflects well on a medical school when their students match well. Therefore, the administration is interested in providing the necessary resources to help their students achieve that goal. Interest expressed by the students can spur the development of further resources. You can also be involved in the creation of additional resources. You can approach the Dean's office. Would they be able to suggest a faculty member to give a lecture on interviewing skills? Would they be able to suggest several advisors to run a mock interview workshop? What about arranging for an annual workshop that takes place after Match Day and provides a forum for matched applicants to advise students applying to the same field? Can the student government approach the Office of Student Affairs about the feasibility of offering these types of programs?

Such programs can also be offered within individual departments. We've interviewed the founders of internal medicine or dermatology interest groups at individual schools. Such interest groups are ideal platforms from which to approach the department. Would the chairman or program director be able to suggest residents who could participate in an informal workshop with the students to offer their insights into the process? Is there a faculty member who would be interested in participating?

Timeline

To match successfully with the specialty of your choice, it's critical that you remain well organized throughout the entire process. Of key importance is knowing and meeting critical deadlines. Timelines for the NRMP, San Francisco Match (ophthalmology), and Urology Match are presented on the following pages.

Note...

In recent years, the residency match has become more competitive. If you're reading this book as a preclinical student and are considering a career in a competitive specialty, consider contacting faculty for shadowing, research, and other opportunities. With so many highly qualified applicants to choose among, programs also look for involvement in extracurricular activities, community service, and research. The preclinical years are an excellent time to build these credentials. In our companion book, *Success in Medical School: Insider Advice for the Preclinical Years*, we provide you with a detailed blueprint on how to stand out in these areas as it relates to the specialty you're considering.

Application Timeline for NRMP Match	
Months	**Task**
January – April (3rd Year)	Attend school meetings regarding residency selection process Plan fourth year schedule Determine USMLE Step 2 CK/CS dates Determine if you'll do any away electives; if so, obtain information from schools' websites, and apply early Begin writing CV and personal statement (may need to include as part of away elective application and for MSPE Questionnaire) Complete MSPE Questionnaire
April – May (3rd Year)	Attend school meetings regarding residency selection process Attend specialty-specific workshops (if offered by your school) and/or meet with specialty-specific advisor to develop application strategy. Ask graduating 4th-year students about their experiences Continue writing CV and personal statement Request letters of recommendation Meet with your school's MSPE writer Complete applications for away electives
June – August	Research programs Develop preliminary list of residency programs Identify each program's application deadline (aim to submit application as early as possible to maximize chances) Meet with advisors to discuss programs on your list Continue writing CV and personal statement Review CV and personal statement with advisor Review transcript for accuracy Request LORs Meet with your school's MSPE writer Arrange for application photo Begin preparing ERAS application Register with NRMP
August – September	Request LORs (if not yet done) Review MSPE Applications may be transmitted on September 15 Track status of application using ADTS Schedule interviews (accept interview invitations quickly)
October	National release date for MSPE – October 1 Track status of application using ADTS Participate in mock interviews with faculty advisors Schedule interviews (accept interview invitations quickly)
November – February	Interview (send thank you notes following)
January – February	Complete last interviews Review rank order list with advisor Submit rank order list to NRMP
March	Match day usually in mid-March Applicants notified of their status (matched vs. unmatched) 4 days before Match Day SOAP for unmatched applicants

Application Timeline for Ophthalmology Match (San Francisco Matching Program)	
Months	**Task**
January – April (3rd Year)	Plan fourth year schedule Determine USMLE Step 2 CK/CS dates Determine if you'll do any away electives; if so, obtain information from schools' websites, and apply early Begin writing CV and personal statement (may need to include as part of away elective application and for MSPE Questionnaire) Complete MSPE Questionnaire
April – May (3rd Year)	Ask graduating fourth-year students about their experiences Continue writing CV and personal statement Request LORs Meet with your school's MSPE writer Complete applications for away electives
June – August	Registration for SF Match opens (early June) Research programs Develop preliminary list of residency programs Identify each program's application deadline (aim to submit application as early as possible to maximize chances) Meet with advisors to discuss programs on your list Continue writing CV and personal statement Review CV and personal statement with advisor Review transcript for accuracy Request LORs Meet with your school's MSPE writer
August – September	CAS Target/Deadline Date (early September) Review MSPE Schedule interviews (offers begin late September)
October	National release date for MSPE – October 1 Participate in mock interviews with faculty advisors Schedule interviews (accept interview invitations quickly) Begin interviews
November – December	Interview (send thank you notes following)
January - February	Rank list submission deadline for SF Match (early January) SF Match results announced (mid-January)

Application Timeline for Urology Match	
Months	**Task**
January – April (3rd Year)	Plan fourth year schedule Determine USMLE Step 2 CK/CS dates Determine if you'll do any away electives; if so, obtain information from schools' websites, and apply early Begin writing CV and personal statement (may need to include as part of away elective application and for MSPE Questionnaire) Complete MSPE Questionnaire
April – May (3rd Year)	Ask graduating fourth-year students about their experiences Continue writing CV and personal statement Request LORs Meet with your school's MSPE writer Complete applications for away electives
June – August	Registration for Urology Match opens at AUA website (early June) Research programs Determine if programs participate in ERAS Develop preliminary list of residency programs Identify each program's application deadline (aim to submit application as early as possible to maximize chances) Meet with advisors to discuss programs on your list Continue writing CV and personal statement Review CV and personal statement with advisor Review transcript for accuracy Request LORs Meet with your school's MSPE writer Begin ERAS application
August – September	Review MSPE Schedule interviews (offers begin late September)
October	National release date for MSPE – October 1 Participate in mock interviews with faculty advisors Schedule interviews (accept interview invitations quickly) Begin interviews
November – December	Interview (send thank you notes following)
January - February	Rank list submission deadline for Urology Match (early January) Urology Match results announced (mid-January)

Researching Programs

Once you determine your specialty choice, you can consider individual residency programs. Applicants utilize a variety of resources to research individual programs:

- Fellowship and Residency Electronic Interactive Database Access (FREIDA Online)

  FREIDA Online has been a principal source of residency program information for many years. Applicants can access this directory at www.ama-assn.org at no charge. Information contained in the directory comes directly from residency programs. Every year, programs are surveyed by the AMA and AAMC and the data is loaded onto FREIDA. Currently there are nearly 10,000 residency and fellowship programs in the database, and the system easily allows for searching by specialty or state.

  Through FREIDA, applicants can identify the PD and obtain contact information for both the director and coordinator. Generally, applicants are asked to contact the program coordinator for additional information. A link to the program's website is usually included. Applicants may also learn about a program's size, primary teaching sites, interview period, earliest and latest dates for submitting applications, work and call schedules, educational conferences and lectures, employment policies/benefits, compensation and leave, and medical benefits.

- Specialty Organizations

  Specialty organizations often have a section on their websites for medical students. In some cases, links to and information about residency programs are included.

- Printed Brochures

  Before the internet age, programs routinely printed brochures with program information. With the advent of the web, fewer programs are producing brochures. This information has now been moved to program and departmental websites. Some programs have made brochures available online.

- Residency Program Websites

  FREIDA Online often contains links to program websites. However, these links are not always functional. In a study of general surgery residency program websites, only 71% of programs listed in the database had viable links.[15] When links are nonfunctional, program websites can still be found through search engines. In a survey of applicants who were invited for interviews at the Oregon Health and Science University internal medicine residency program, 79.6% of respondents found these sites helpful in deciding where to apply, while 68.5% found the sites useful in deciding where to interview.[16]

- Accreditation Council for Graduate Medical Education (ACGME)

  At the ACGME website, applicants can determine the accreditation status of residency programs, including the date of the most recent site visit.

- Advisors/Colleagues

  Faculty and resident advisors, as well as colleagues, can be a valuable source of information about residency programs. Advisors can provide insider information not readily available elsewhere.

Using these resources, develop a list of programs that are of interest. Base your list on the factors most important to you. Consider reputation, competitiveness of the program, geographic location, type of hospital (university affiliated, community), program emphasis (academic), setting (urban, rural, suburban), future plans (desire to pursue fellowship training), and your family's needs, in addition to a host of other factors.

Review your list of programs with your advisor. Ask if your list is realistic. While you shouldn't hesitate to apply to a program that would be considered a long shot, there should be a sufficient number of programs on your list which are within reach. Your advisor can estimate your chances of matching with programs on your list, taking into account the competitiveness of the specialty, the competitiveness of the programs on your list, and your academic qualifications and non-academic credentials.

Tip # 4

To remain organized, we recommend that you start a filing system. Keep a file (physical or electronic) for each residency program with program information, application requirements, deadlines, and copies of all correspondence and communication.

The Basics: Common Sense Rules

> Why would an applicant approach an attending for a letter of recommendation, and then say "By the way, the deadline is next week." Why would a student ask to work on a case report, take from the attending the case details, photos, and preliminary literature on the topic, and then never turn in an actual case report? Why would an applicant interview at a program and not send a thank-you letter?

One would think that the actions in the box would be obvious mistakes. *We* would think that these would be obvious mistakes. And yet…we can quote from actual experience and anecdotes from colleagues, each of these mistakes made by multiple applicants. A student asking for a LOR and then not providing the attending any time to work on it. Was the applicant thoughtless, or desperate? Never turning in a final product? Was the applicant paralyzed by perfectionism? In the case of thank you letters, only 39% of applicants in one study sent a thank you letter to every program with which they interviewed. Did they believe it wasn't worth the hassle because the program wasn't going to be high on their list anyway?

We can only guess and try to keep further applicants from making the same mistakes. Some of these mistakes may seem like violations of common sense, and we fully agree. We've included rules that start with "Don't lie," words one should never have to say to future physicians. However, we quote from multiple studies that indicate that dishonesty in the residency application process occurs, and more often than you would think. In a review of 134 applications to the emergency medicine residency program at Washington University, of the 14 applicants claiming AOA membership, 5 claims were found to be inaccurate.[17] In the same study, of the 15 applicants claiming advanced degrees, 4 claims were inaccurate.

We've included these obvious rules because we see them every year, and the literature supports the fact that they occur.

Pay attention to the rules that only an insider would know well. Pay equal attention to the rules that are so obvious that they may be overlooked.

References

[1]Charting Outcomes in the Match (2014). Available at: http://www.nrmp.org/wp-content/uploads/2014/09/Charting-Outcomes-2014-Final.pdf. Accessed March 3, 2016.
[2]Anderson K, Jacobs D. General surgery program directors' perceptions of the match. *Curr Surg* 2000; 57(5): 460-465.
[5]Results of the 2014 NRMP Program Director Survey. Available at: http://www.nrmp.org/wp-content/uploads/2014/09/PD-Survey-Report-2014.pdf. Accessed March 3, 2015.
[4]Results Of 2016 NRMP Main Residency Match Largest On Record As Match Continues To Grow. Available at: http://www.nrmp.org/press-release-results-of-2016-nrmp-main-residency-match-largest-on-record-as-match-continues-to-grow/. Accessed April 23, 2016.
[5]Aagaard E, Hauer K. A cross-sectional descriptive study of mentoring relationships formed by medical students. *J Gen Intern Med* 2003; 18: 298-302.
[6]Jackson V, Palepu A, Szalacha L, Caswell C, Carr P, Inui T. "Having the right chemistry": a qualitative study of mentoring in academic medicine. *Acad Med* 2003; 78(3): 328-334.
[7]Hauer K, Teherani A, Dechet A, Aagaard E. Medical students' perceptions of mentoring: a focus-group analysis. *Med Teach* 2005; 27(8): 732-734.
[8]Silvestre J, So A, Lee B. Accessibility of academic plastic surgeons as mentors to medical students. *Ann Plast Surg* 2015; 74(1): 85-88.
[9]Dehon E, Cruse M, Dawson B, Jackson-Williams. Mentoring during medical school and Match outcome among emergency medicine residents. *West J Emerg Med* 2015; 16(6): 927-930.
[10]Crossman S, Gary J, Flores S, Bradner M, Sabo R. Residency faculty opinions about medical student advising. *Fam Med* 2015; 47(2): 134-137.
[11]Ryan M, Levine L, Colbert-Getz J, Spector N, Fromme H. Advising medical students for the Match: A national survey of pediatrics clerkship directors. *Acad Pediatr* 2015; 15(4): 374-379.
[12]Hirsch A, Agarwal A, Rand A, DeNunzio N, Patel K, Truong M, Russo G, Kachnic L. Medical student mentorship in radiation oncology at a single academic institution: A 10-year analysis. *Pract Radiat Oncol* 2015; 5(3): e163-168.
[13]Fornari A, Murray T, Menzin A, Woo V, Clifton M, Lombardi M, Shelov S. Mentoring program design and implementation in new medical schools. *Med Educ Online* 2014; 19: 24570.
[14]Miller J, Schaad D, Crittenden R, Oriol N. The departmental advisor's effect on medical students' confidence when the advisor evaluates or recruits for their own program during the match. *Teach Learn Med* 2004; 16(3): 290-295.
[15]Reilly E, Leibrandt T, Zonno A, Simpson M, Morris J. General surgery residency program websites: usefulness and usability for resident applicants. *Curr Surg* 2004; 61(2): 236-240.
[16]Embi P, Desai S, Cooney T. Use and utility of Web-based residency program information: a survey of residency applicants. *J Med Internet Res*; 5(3): e22.
[17]Roellig M, Katz E. Inaccuracies on applications for emergency medicine residency training. *Acad Emerg Med* 2004; 11(9): 992-994.

Chapter 3

Selection Process

In order to plan the optimal strategy and position your application for maximum impact, you need to first understand the selection process. Strategizing for a successful match hinges on the answers to these three questions:

- Who chooses the residents?
- What do they care about?
- How can you convince them that you would be the right resident for their program?

Who chooses the residents?

This first question really should be broken down further.

- Who selects the applicants to interview?
- Who ranks the applicants?

The two processes are markedly different, and the criteria for interview selection and candidate ranking are markedly different as well.

Who selects the applicants to interview? The committee may be composed of one individual – the program director, the chairman, a designated faculty member, or another designee. In this case, one individual has the power to choose all of the applicants that will be asked to interview. Their criteria become all-important if you have any hope of making it past the screening process.

Alternately, the committee may be composed of several individuals. If so, the committee members decide how to review applications, and this process varies. In some cases, the committee members divide up the applications randomly. In this case, again, only one individual will see your application, and their criteria become all important. In other cases, the committee reviews applications jointly, and discusses the applicants as a group.

What criteria do these decision-makers utilize?

In the process of reviewing hundreds of applications, screening criteria are used frequently. It is a daunting task to review over 400 applications in order to choose 30 candidates to interview, as is the case at some programs. In a sea of qualified applicants, it's difficult to choose a small fraction to interview.

Did you know?

"Many RPDs use ERAS software tools to set parameters that confine the number of applications downloaded by setting filters that screen for minimum USMLE scores, clerkship grades, citizenship, and geographic location. Applicants whose credentials do not meet the spectrum of criteria set for automatic download from ERAS may never have their applications seen by faculty on a selection committee."[1]

Kenneth Grundfast, M.D.
Chief
Department of Otolaryngology
Boston University School of Medicine

Personal knowledge of an applicant's skills and strengths can trump numbers alone. In highly competitive programs, applicants who are personally known to the program and its faculty have an advantage from that standpoint alone. The sole faculty member deciding whom to interview, out of hundreds of excellent applicants, will naturally give preference to a student she personally knows and respects. In fact, excellent performance on an audition elective at the program is frequently mentioned as an important resident selection criterion. Personal knowledge may also come in the form of a strong LOR from a program's own faculty member. A strong LOR from a faculty member outside the program, but well-known to the members of the selection committee, can also be very persuasive.

However, when personal knowledge of an applicant isn't available, objective criteria, of necessity, take on more importance. Particularly when screening large numbers of applications, objective data is more easily mined. As a broad generalization, objective data is typically more important when making decisions on which applicants to interview. Subjective criteria take on more importance when making decisions on how to rank applicants.

By objective data, we mean factors that are easy to determine and quantify, such as grades in the specialty rotation, USMLE scores, clerkship grades, number of honors grades, and AOA status. Although grades in rotations themselves are based on a combination of objective and subjective factors, the grade itself is easily compared. In the following pages, we discuss the factors used by programs in the residency selection process. Please also visit our specialty-specific chapters for detailed information that pertains to your specialty of choice.

USMLE Scores

The residency selection process can be divided into two phases – screening and ranking. In the screening phase, programs whittle down a large applicant pool into a smaller group. The members of this group will be offered interview invitations. The USMLE Step 1 score is frequently used in the screening process. In the 2014 NRMP Program Director Survey, the USMLE Step 1 / COMLEX Level 1 Score was cited by 94% of residency programs in 22 specialties as a factor used in selecting applicants to interview. No other factor was cited by a higher percentage of programs (When compared to 2008 NRMP data, every specialty in the 2014 survey showed a rise in the percentage of programs utilizing the score in the screening process, as shown in the table below).[2-3]

% Residency Programs Citing USMLE Step 1 / COMLEX Level 1 Score as a Factor in Selecting Applicants to Interview in 2014 Versus 2008

Specialty	2008	2014
Anesthesiology	81%	99%
Dermatology	76%	92%
Emergency Medicine	85%	97%
Family Medicine	85%	91%
General Surgery	83%	97%
Internal Medicine	81%	92%
Med/Peds	89%	94%
Neurology	87%	90%
OB/GYN	78%	97%
Orthopedic Surgery	75%	95%
Otolaryngology	87%	98%
Pathology	84%	94%
Pediatrics	81%	98%
Physical Medicine & Rehabilitation	87%	91%
Plastic Surgery	80%	94%
Psychiatry	82%	87%
Radiation Oncology	72%	95%
Radiology	82%	99%

Adapted from:

Results of the 2014 NRMP Program Director Survey. Available at: http://www.nrmp.org/wp-content/uploads/2014/09/PD-Survey-Report-2014.pdf. Accessed March 3, 2016.

Results of the 2008 NRMP Program Director Survey. Available at: http://www.nrmp.org/wp-content/uploads/2013/08/programresultsbyspecialty.pdf. Accessed March 3, 2014.

PDs are interested in your Step 1 score because it's a good measure of content knowledge, and that's of obvious importance to training programs. Programs are also interested because it offers them some insight into whether you're capable of passing the specialty board certification examination. "Low USMLE scores concern program directors that the applicant may have difficulty passing Step III (which is needed for medical licensure) and may ultimately have difficulty passing the pediatric board exam (which may reflect poorly on the residency program)" writes Dr. Su-Ting Li, Program Director of the Pediatrics Residency Program at the University of California Davis School of Medicine.[4] Research done in multiple specialties has shown that performance on the Step 1 exam is predictive of performance on board certification exams. Another reason why these scores are so highly valued by programs is that they allow for easier comparison of students from different schools. Finally, programs are receiving a higher number of applications than ever before, and this flood of applications can easily tax programs. The USMLE allows for winnowing of a large applicant pool into a smaller, more manageable group.

Many residency programs have established threshold or target scores, and applicants who exceed these scores remain in consideration for interview offers. Dr. Sandra Oldham, Program Director in the Department of Diagnostic and Interventional Imaging at the University of Texas Medical School at Houston, provides this information on the process: "The ERAS applications are first viewed by the Program Coordinator who filters out those I should read from the many I don't need to read. Ms. Roberts looks at several things in each ERAS application – the dreaded USMLE Step 1 score and grades from the medical school transcript. We set the minimum USMLE Step 1 score each year as the main filter for which applications move on to my computer and which do not."[5] The Office of Residency and Career Planning at the Case Western University School of Medicine concurs. "Board results are most important for the very competitive specialties. A number of the programs set a threshold Step 1 score level that must be achieved in order to receive an invitation for an interview, such as the national mean of about 220 or even one standard deviation above the mean. The same is true for some of the most outstanding and sought-after residency programs in less competitive specialties."[6] Data from the NRMP shown on the following page indicates the percentage of programs with threshold scores by specialty.

% Residency Programs Citing Use of USMLE Step 1 / COMLEX Level 1 Target Scores in Selecting Applicants to Interview in 2014

Specialty	Percentage
Anesthesiology	85%
Dermatology	82%
Emergency Medicine	69%
Family Medicine	42%
General Surgery	91%
Internal Medicine	71%
Med/Peds	76%
Neurological Surgery	79%
Neurology	60%
OB/GYN	75%
Orthopedic Surgery	93%
Otolaryngology	80%
Pathology	63%
Pediatrics	56%
Physical Medicine & Rehabilitation	48%
Plastic Surgery	86%
Psychiatry	30%
Radiation Oncology	73%
Radiology	86%
Vascular Surgery	81%

Adapted from:

Results of the 2014 NRMP Program Director Survey. Available at: http://www.nrmp.org/wp-content/uploads/2014/09/PD-Survey-Report-2014.pdf. Accessed March 3, 2016.

Did you know?

Dr. Ellis, the program director of the dermatology program at the University of Michigan, wrote that "last year, more than 100 of our applicants had achieved the top percentile on the United States Medical Licensing Examination."[7]

Students ask us all the time about the importance of the USMLE score, and whether they have what it takes to get into a certain field. For low-scoring applicants, these are some of the most difficult conversations to have. What we tell them is that, although the USMLE exams were developed for licensure purposes, the reality of the situation is that these scores do play an important role in the selection process at most programs. It's possible that the time will come when these scores carry less weight in the selection process. In fact, there is a growing group of educators and leaders trying to transform the process. "We do not believe that USMLE Step 1 scores should continue to be the major determining factor in the selection of graduating medical students for interview for graduate medical education programs," writes Dr. Charles Prober, Senior Associate Dean for Medical Education at Stanford School of Medicine. "Although using numbers as a filter is a convenient way to screen large numbers of applications, USMLE Step 1 scores do not come close to reflecting the totality of attributes critically relevant to a candidate's potential performance during residency training."[8]

What do we recommend for applicants with lower scores who seek careers in competitive specialties? We offer advice based on the available data so that students can make informed decisions. We remind them that some programs in every specialty are more holistic in their approach to evaluating applications. We also remind applicants that there are ways to overcome low scores, but that they should also give serious thought to what they will do if they fail to match. What is their back-up plan?

Overcoming a Low USMLE Step 1 Score: 10 Strategies

1 Although the USMLE Step 1 score is of major importance to residency programs, this score is only one component of your application. Strengthening other components is essential to overcoming this obstacle. Dr. Andrew Lee, Chairman of Ophthalmology at the Houston Methodist Hospital, offers the following advice. "Getting the program to ignore a subpar score is challenging but not impossible...Applicants with a subpar score should do everything possible to demonstrate their value in other ways...if you have a less optimal score you must demonstrate to the interviewer or the screener that you offer something else in your application that can justify looking away from the score alone."[9]

2 Perhaps the most common advice low-scoring applicants will hear is to take and do well on the USMLE Step 2 CK exam. This exam, which is generally taken in the fourth year of medical school, assesses clinical knowledge. Since residency programs do use the Step 2 CK score in the residency selection process, a high score on this exam can put to rest any concerns that programs may have about your low Step 1 score.

3 Dr. Vicki Marx, Program Director of the radiology residency program at the USC Keck School of Medicine, recommends that "the student work hard over a sustained period of time in the third year of medical school to excel on clinical rotations. Clinical rotation scores of Honors and High Pass carry significant weight in screening ERAS applications."[10]

4 Demonstration of leadership ability is another way to strengthen your application. A survey of emergency medicine PDs revealed that having a "distinctive factor," such as being a medical school officer, was one of three factors more predictive of residency performance.[11] In a survey of plastic surgery PDs, leadership qualities were the most important subjective criterion used to evaluate applicants during the interview process.[12] In a study done to determine the predictors of otolaryngology resident success using data available at the time of the interview, candidates having an exceptional trait such as leadership experience were found to be rated higher as residents.[13]

5 A mentor in your chosen field can be a powerful advocate. Dr. Roy Ziegelstein, former Program Director of Internal Medicine at the Johns Hopkins Bayview Hospital, writes that "In the modern era, sports agents have emerged as powerful figures...Modern sports figures need an agent if they are going to get the mega-contract...A medical student needs an agent too. The student has to do well in school, but that is often not enough. The student needs someone, or preferably more than one person, to trumpet his or her accomplishments."[14]

6 Letters of recommendation are an important component of the application, and you will request these letters from faculty. Preclinical students can develop relationships with faculty, and cultivating these relationships over time may lead to the development of a stronger letter later. Dr. Ziegelstein writes that the "best letter is from an individual who is very well known, who has evaluated hundreds or perhaps thousands of students over several decades, who knows you well and who believes you are one of the best students ever."[14]

7 Applicants who have a red flag in their application, such as a low USMLE score, may address the issue in their personal statement. "I recommend that a student for whom a low Step 1 score is an aberration in performance explain their academic strengths very clearly up front in their personal statement," says Dr. Marx.[10] Dr. Lee offers similar advice. "Another tactic is to tackle the problem head on in the personal statement and to highlight other alternative evidence of performance and intelligence in their record."[9] For applicants who failed the Step 1, Dr. Li states that "if failure of Step 1 was due to unusual circumstances (e.g., applicant's parent died immediately prior to Step 1), the applicant should explain the unusual circumstances in their personal statement…"[4]

8 Exceptional service to the community may help overcome the low USMLE score obstacle. Community service is valued by some programs, and your involvement provides information about your non-cognitive attributes, such as teamwork, leadership ability, maturity, seriousness of purpose, and conflict resolution skills. These are all skills vital to resident success.

9 Significant contributions to research are yet another way to strengthen the residency application. Although some surveys of PDs have suggested that research is less important in the selection process, Dr. Marianne Green, Associate Dean for Medical Education at Northwestern University, writes that "Personally I believe that depth in any area can make a student stand out."[15]

10 As a clinical student, you'll be able to arrange "audition," or away, electives at residency programs. Your performance during an audition rotation can have a profound impact on your chances. According to Dr. Lee, "The away elective offers the applicant the opportunity to shine at a prospective institution and introduces the student to the faculty at that specific institution in a real world setting that can create a relationship that leads to an interview or even a higher ranking for the match."[9]

Adapted from the companion book *Success in Medical School: Insider Advice for the Preclinical Years*.

Did you know?

The website for the radiology program at the University of California at San Francisco (UCSF) states: "We review each application as a whole, and we do not have a threshold value for USMLE scores. However, in recent years, most of our interviewees have had three-digit scores of 240 or higher on Step 1. The small number of our interviewees with Step 1 scores between 200 and 239 have had offsetting factors such as a combination of top clinical grades at a competitive medical school and extraordinary research experience and academic promise."[16]

Clerkship Grades

Clerkship grades are also a major factor in the residency selection process. In March 2009, Dr. Marianne Green, Associate Dean for Medical Education and Competency at Northwestern University, published the results of her survey submitted to over 1,200 program directors across 21 specialties. She and her colleagues sought to determine the relative importance of various residency selection criteria. Grades in required clerkships were found to the most important academic selection factor.[17] Although the study was not designed to determine the reasons why so much importance is placed on clerkship grades, Dr. Green offered us her thoughts. "Program directors and selection committees are looking for people who are going to become excellent physicians, with the primary emphasis on patient care and teamwork," said Dr. Green in an interview with us published on the *Student Doctor Network.* "A student's performance on a clinical team in the direct care of patients is perceived to be the best assessment of these skills."[15]

Since Dr. Green's study, the NRMP has released several program director surveys. In the most recent survey of nearly 1,800 program directors, published in 2014, 70% cited clerkship grades as an important factor in making interview decisions. Respondents rated it 4.0 in terms of importance on a scale of 1 (not at all important) to 5 (very important).[2]

Many medical students underestimate the importance of clerkship grades. In fact, 44% of students surveyed at the University of Colorado, University of Utah, and Vanderbilt University felt that these grades were moderately, mildly, or not important at all.[18]

Particularly important is the number of honors clerkship grades. This is especially true for highly competitive specialties, as shown in the table on the following page. Most students don't realize this; only 14.7% of students in Brandenburg's survey rated the number of honors grades as extremely important.[18]

Clerkship grades are also a major determinant of class rank. The most competitive specialties rate class rank among the most important selection criteria. Here again, a significant difference was noted between PDs and students regarding its importance. Surprisingly, 49.3% of students felt that class rank was mildly important or not important at all.[18] For more details on how to excel during rotations, please see our book *Success on the Wards*.

Importance of Clerkship Grades in the Residency Selection Process		
Specialty	**% Programs Citing Honors in Clinical Clerkships as a Factor for Making Interview Decisions**	**Mean Rating***
Anesthesiology	75%	4.0
Dermatology	76%	4.3
Emergency Medicine	82%	4.0
General Surgery	78%	4.0
OB/GYN	72%	4.2
Orthopedic Surgery	87%	4.3
Otolaryngology	85%	4.4
Plastic Surgery	76%	4.2
Radiation Oncology	72%	4.2

*Scale of 1 (not at all important) to 5 (very important)

Adapted from: Results of the 2014 NRMP Program Director Survey. Available at: http://www.nrmp.org/wp-content/uploads/2014/09/PD-Survey-Report-2014.pdf. Accessed March 3, 2016.

Importance of Clerkship Grades: Perspectives of Residency Programs	
Residency Program	**Comments**
Department of Medicine University of Washington	"Do well in your clerkship. Yes, this is obvious - and easier said than done - but it's also important. Most residency programs look closely at the third-year clerkship grade when selecting applicants."[19]
Department of Surgery University of Colorado	"Most surgery programs look very favorably on an 'Honors' grade in your MS3 surgery clerkship rotation and may factor in the grades you received in your Medicine and Ob/Gyn rotations."[20]
Department of OB/GYN UC Davis	"USMLE scores and clerkship grades (especially in ob/gyn, surgery, and internal medicine) are considered factual data and ranked high."[21]
Dr. Tobias Kohler Program Director Department of Urology Southern Illinois University	"Most institutions utilize board score and clerkship grade cut points to help narrow the field."[22]
Dr. Michael Wu Director of Medical Student Education Dept. of Ophthalmology University of Washington	"Academic performance, particularly on the core clerkships and the USMLE Step 1, may limit a student's ability to match successfully in ophthalmology."[23]
Department of Radiology Stanford University	"Successful candidates will have demonstrated outstanding performance in the core clinical clerkships."[24]

Awards

Election to the Alpha Omega Alpha Honor Medical Society (AOA) is perhaps the most well studied award as it relates to residency admission. Eligibility is limited to only allopathic medical students, and members are selected based on academic achievement, leadership, professionalism, and commitment to service. Members are elected by individual chapters, and this process may vary significantly from chapter to chapter. According to the AOA Constitution, no more than 1/6 of the graduating class can be elected into the school's chapter. In 2014, the NRMP surveyed nearly 1,800 residency programs representing 21 specialties about the importance of various residency selection criteria.[2] Overall, membership in AOA was cited by 61% as a factor in selecting applicants to interview. Membership in AOA was also an important factor in ranking. Overall, it received a mean rating of 4.0 on a scale of 1 (not at all important) to 5 (very important). Data for individual specialties is presented below.

Percentage of Residency Programs Citing AOA as a Factor in Selecting Applicants To Interview by Specialty

Specialty	% of Programs
Anesthesiology	69%
Dermatology	64%
Emergency Medicine	75%
Family Medicine	31%
General Surgery	70%
Internal Medicine	58%
Neurosurgery	81%
Obstetrics & Gynecology	62%
Orthopedic Surgery	84%
Otolaryngology	83%
Pathology	54%
Pediatrics	62%
Physical Medicine & Rehabilitation	42%
Plastic Surgery	79%
Psychiatry	51%
Radiation Oncology	60%
Radiology	77%

Adapted from 2014 NRMP Program Director Survey. Available at: http://www.nrmp.org/wp-content/uploads/2014/09/PD-Survey-Report-2014.pdf. Accessed March 3, 2016.

Although osteopathic students are not eligible for AOA induction, both allopathic and osteopathic students may be elected into the Gold Humanism Honor Society (GHHS). Started in 2002 by the Arnold P. Gold Foundation,

GHHS honors medical students for "demonstrated excellence in clinical care, leadership, compassion and dedication to service."[25] In a study conducted to determine if GHHS membership influences residency selection, the authors wrote that "membership in GHHS may set candidates apart from their peers and allow PDs to distinguish objectively the candidates who demonstrate compassionate medical care."[26] In the 2014 NRMP Program Director Survey, 27% reported using Gold Society Membership as a factor in selecting applicants to interview.[2]

AOA and GHHS are not the only awards or honors viewed favorably by residency programs. In a survey of over 1,200 PDs in 21 specialties, Dr. Marianne Green determined the relative importance of various residency selection criteria.[17] Dr. Green found that medical school awards (non-AOA) were 10th in importance among a group of 14 criteria. Although not as important as USMLE Step 1 scores, clerkship grades, and LORs, awards were ranked higher than such factors as preclinical grades, research while in medical school, and published medical school research.

Benefits of winning medical school awards and scholarships include:

- Awards can provide a significant boost to the strength of your application, and distinguish you from your peers. Awards and scholarships can easily be placed in the residency application, MSPE (Dean's Letter), LORs, and CV. We've found that interviewers often ask about awards during residency interviews.

Did you know?

In 2013, Justin Berk, a medical student at Texas Tech University School of Medicine, received the American Medical Association Foundation Leadership Award. "For Justin, it's obviously a huge accolade and something that will follow him for the rest of his medical career," said Dr. Tedd Mitchell, President of Texas Tech Health Sciences Center, in an interview with *The Daily Toreador*. "As he's applying for residency programs, it will stand out."[27]

Did you know?

Alexander Gallan, a medical student at the Boston University School of Medicine, was the recipient of the 2012 American Society of Clinical Pathology Academic Excellence Award. "The award was a common topic during my residency interviews. I believe it helped my residency application immeasurably by providing justification for all the hard work I have done."[28]

- Competitive specialties and residency programs value students who've been recognized with awards. Educators believe you have the potential to make similar contributions as a trainee.

Did you know?

When Casey DeDeugd, a medical student at the University of Central Florida, won the Medical Student Achievement Award from the Ruth Jackson Orthopedic Society, she enhanced her visibility in the field. "Your accomplishments thus far are very impressive!" wrote Dr. Gloria Gogola, Chair of the Society's Scientific Committee. "We look forward…to welcoming you to our field of orthopedic surgery."[29]

Did you know?

In 2008, Brian Caldwell, a medical student at the University of Arkansas for Medical Sciences, was the winner of the Dr. Constantin Cope Medical Student Research Award from the Society of Interventional Radiology. "Brian carried the whole project with very little help and really did a nice job," said Dr. William Culp, Professor of Radiology and Surgery. "I am so pleased that he won the national SIR award, because his participation in the conference introduced him to national leaders in interventional radiology and will help jumpstart his career."[30]

- You gain visibility in your school, and bring recognition to the institution.

Did you know?

When Ramy El-Diwany, an M.D./Ph.D. student at Johns Hopkins University, won the 2014 Excellence in Public Health Award from the U.S. Public Health Service (USPHS) Physician Professional Advisory Committee, his institution was also lauded. "This award is a testament to the education provided by the Johns Hopkins University School of Medicine and to the high caliber of its students," wrote USPHS Lt. Cmdr. Kimberly Smith. "We hope that this award will encourage other Johns Hopkins faculty and students to continue their strong work in public health."[31]

Did you know?

After Rahul Vanjani received the AMA Foundation Leadership Award, Dr. Scott Schroth, Senior Associate Dean of Academic Affairs at George Washington University, took pride in his student's accomplishment. "Rahul's commitment to the community and leadership of service efforts are unparalleled. He exemplifies the sort of creativity and dedication that we look for in medical students at GW, and we are extraordinarily proud of him as a winner of the AMA Foundation's 2011 Leadership Award."[32]

- Recipients have found that awards have made them more competitive for other awards and scholarships. Awards follow you throughout your career, and can make you more competitive for future opportunities, programs, and employment.

- You further your professional reputation and enhance your credibility in the areas that form the basis for the award.

- Winning an award or scholarship can give you the confidence to pursue other goals.

- Applying for an award requires the support of advocates who become reference letter writers. Strengthening these relationships over time allows faculty members to write strong LORs for residency.

Did you know?

In applying for awards, you often have to submit reference letters. Over time, your letter writers become even stronger advocates, with a vested interest in furthering your career. After David Leverenz won the Southwestern Medical Foundation Ho Din Award, his mentor had this to say: "Dr. Leverenz has done exceptionally well in medical school, performed research, worked, volunteered, and completed multiple mission trips," said Dr. David Balis, his faculty mentor at UT Southwestern Medical Center. "But what strikes me most about David is his caring, sincere, compassionate personality." Dr. Leverenz is now a resident at Vanderbilt University.[33]

It's clear that there are compelling reasons to pursue medical school scholarships, awards, and grants. To help maximize the chances of winning awards and scholarships, I wrote the book *Medical School Scholarships, Grants & Awards: Insider Advice on How to Win Scholarships.* Although this book includes an extensive list and description of scholarships and awards, I've also placed considerable emphasis on strategy. These recommendations are based on data from a full spectrum of sources. Whenever possible, I've included evidence obtained from scientific study and published in the academic medical literature. I also take an insider's look at the entire process based on our experiences.

For years, we've helped applicants match successfully into competitive specialties and residency programs. We've worked with medical students at all levels, and we always try to identify scholarship and award programs that will bolster their credentials. In the process of helping students win scholarships and awards, we've gained insight into the factors that lead to success. There's much that can be learned from your predecessors, and the book includes multiple profiles of past scholarship winners. Two copies of this book were mailed to every medical school in the United States, so hopefully it's available as a resource in your library or at your Office of Financial Aid.

Other criteria

Criteria such as USMLE thresholds, AOA status, or class rank are typically used by the most competitive specialties and programs to narrow their applicant pool. Even in these types of programs, though, some decision-makers will choose to look more thoroughly at an application, even during the initial screening process. They may give weight to a variety of different factors, such as the personal statement or LORs indicating leadership qualities or community involvement. As we stated earlier, personal knowledge of an applicant's skills and strengths can also be a powerful factor for those deciding whom to interview.

We emphasize that these types of objective criteria may not be in standard use by less competitive specialties or programs. The personal statement takes on more importance for family practice PDs, for example. At the website for the University of Washington Family Medicine residency program: The "personal statement is the primary component that will be used to select applicants who are invited for an interview. Please write a careful and thoughtful document."[34] Recent studies continue to emphasize the importance of the statement in the family medicine residency selection process. In the 2014 NRMP Program Director Survey, 87% cited the statement as a factor in making interview decisions. Among criteria, only the USMLE Step 1 score was cited by a higher percentage of programs.[2]

> **Did you know?**
>
> In one study, 17% of PDs in the surgical specialties used social networking sites in the screening of residency applicants. 1/3 of this group reported lowering the ranking of applicants due to inappropriate content.[35]

How can you determine if you have the minimum requirements to be selected to interview?

Chapters 23 – 44, on specialty-specific information, provides some concrete numbers to review, including average USMLE scores and the percentage of applicants below a threshold who still matched into the specialty. The NRMP data from 2014 indicated that for applicants to emergency medicine, the mean USMLE Step 1 score was 230. Of the applicants with Step 1 scores below 210, 166 of 208 matched. Of U.S. seniors who matched, 12% were members of AOA. Of 2014 applicants reporting no prior research experience, 162 of 175 matched.[36] Such concrete numbers can provide perspective on the strength of your own application.

A review of program websites may also provide very useful and specific information. Even within a competitive specialty, some programs are far more competitive than others, and criteria such as USMLE thresholds or AOA status may vary greatly. These criteria may not matter at all for less competitive specialties.

Probably the most important advice on this subject will come from your residency advisor. Advisors who participate in the residency selection process have a well-informed sense of the qualifications of other applicants and how you compare with your competition. Therefore, an advisor who's a program chairman, a residency program director, or a faculty member on the residency selection committee can provide valuable insight into your chances. Other advice may come from the Dean's office, residents in the specialty, or recently matched students or upperclassmen who've researched the issue.

However, selecting applicants to interview is a very different process from ranking those who interview. In speaking with students and reviewing the discussion forums, we don't think enough students grasp this critical point. Great USMLE scores may get you in the door, but when it comes to ranking, they often don't play as much of a role. From the UCSF Department of Radiology: "Once an applicant is selected for an interview, USMLE scores have little bearing on the final rank."[16]

Who is actually ranking the applicants?

In 2006, researchers surveyed 145 radiology PDs about the process for ranking candidates.[37] A total of 77 directors responded to the survey. In 88.1% of the programs, all members of the interviewing body vote in the ranking of candidates. Of interest, in 76.5% of programs, residents and fellows serve as interviewers. While the interviewing body is responsible for making the final ranking in 62.9% of the programs, the PD has the final word in 33.8%.

Some programs have published information about their own selection process.

- At the general surgery residency program at the Medical University of South Carolina, Brothers wrote that "...all surgical faculty are given equal input, with individual members providing insight into applicants whom they interviewed."[38]

- Dr. Cruz, former chairman of the department of dermatology at the University of Texas Southwestern Medical Center, stated "Because we are committed to a democratic process, each faculty member who participates in interviews (residents as well as the chief resident) has an equal opportunity to influence the match ranking...During a dedicated meeting, each applicant is discussed and her or his ranking is refined by consensus."[39]

- The website for the department of radiology at UCSF states that "the selection committee meets in late January...we formulate our rank order list based on consensus."[16]

- The department of anesthesiology at the University of Pittsburgh states that their selection committee meets as a group, discusses each applicant, and then ranks the applicant. The scores are then averaged to yield a final score which is used to form the program's rank list.[40]

- Creation of the rank list for the University of Washington otolaryngology residency program "involves all members of the residency selection committee. Each member will develop his or her own rank list…A meeting of the residency selection committee will be held in February to develop a consensus rank order and which candidates will not be ranked. The program director and Chair may review and revise the final list if needed."[41]

What do these decision-makers care about?

The short answer to this question is that it varies from program to program, and from individual to individual. In some programs, the decision-makers have made an effort to provide objective grading of subjective criteria. In these programs deciding criteria are identified, and a standard scoring system is used to grade the applicant on each criteria.

In other programs the process of ranking applicants can be very subjective. In the study by Otero cited above, 15 directors stated that the "fit" of the candidates and a "gut feeling" were the most important criteria for admission decisions.[37] Dr. Moore, Chair and Program Director at the University of California-Davis Department of Anesthesiology, feels that an applicant's performance during the interview "is the deal breaker/maker."[42]

Remember that every candidate invited to interview has already met the standards for acceptance. At this stage, subjective measures of personal characteristics become more important. Studies have shown that behavioral and noncognitive skills have significant value in predicting resident performance, while measures such as USMLE scores may be poorly predictive of clinical performance.[43-44] Therefore, at this stage of residency selection, indicators of noncognitive skills become very important. The Office of Residency and Career Planning at the Case Western University School of Medicine states "Remember it is performance on the clinical services reflected by your grades and, above all, by the evaluation comments that program directors consider most important in ranking their applicants. These parameters are considered to be the best predictors of how well an applicant will do as a resident…the highest board scores will not guarantee a position in a program if the comments from your attendings are negative…"[6]

As we alluded to earlier, interview performance is the one criterion that becomes magnified in importance at this stage of the process (ranking). The interview is of such important that one study found that 1/3 of internal medicine residency applicants were actually ranked less favorably following an interview.[45] In a 2002 survey of orthopedic surgery PDs, researchers found that once invited for an interview, 22% of programs place candidates on equal footing, with ranking decisions based solely on interview performance.[46] A survey of 361 family practice PDs found that the interview was the most important element of the resident selection process.[47] One study performed at the Children's Hospital of Philadelphia pediatrics residency program, a highly competitive program, offered insight into the importance of the interview at their program.[48] The authors wrote that "interview scores were the most important variable for candidate ranking on the NRMP list."

What are the qualities that programs seek in a resident and are therefore searching for in the application components and interview?

Further chapters delineate these qualities more thoroughly, but in short, the qualities that make for an outstanding clinician are the same as those that make for an outstanding resident. Programs look for evidence that a student not only possesses high levels of intelligence, but also has a very strong work ethic, is compassionate, is enthusiastic about their chosen field, and is able to handle an intense workload. Beyond that, the criteria for each program and for each individual decision-maker at that program will vary.

Furthermore, the evidence required to demonstrate these criteria will vary for each decision-maker. For example, what evidence best demonstrates a strong work ethic? Is it clinical grades, or letters of recommendation? What evidence best demonstrates high levels of intelligence? Is it USMLE scores, or overall grades in clerkships?

Your research should begin with a review of the individual program websites. These may provide insight into the program's goals and criteria for residency selection.

- The website for the radiology program at UCSF states that "One of our primary goals is to train academic radiologists, especially clinician-scientists…Most of our interviewees have had research experience…We should emphasize that because ours is a clinically rigorous program, we prefer applicants who have shined on the wards as well as in the laboratory."[16]

- Dr. Flemming, Program Director of the Penn State Hershey radiology program, states, "As for the qualities we seek most of you will have demonstrated more than adequately, your academic abilities with success in exams, good board scores…Beyond academics, there are two important qualities we expect. These are creative thinking and character. Radiology is divorcing itself from the descriptive nature of the art. It is becoming one in which it is important to analyze, develop an opinion, and express this thought process to our other clinical colleagues. It is imperative that you possess the ability to communicate and to understand your role as a communicator…Character is equally important in our resident selection process. We expect trainees to understand their professional responsibility as a physician radiologist, their pivotal role in patient care, and their commitment to fulfill these expectations. It is clear then that we not only look at the merit of your application, but the interview process is all-important."[49]

- The website for the psychiatry department at the Stony Brook University Hospital states that applicants should have "high intelligence, excellence in both written and verbal self-expression, superior ability to understand both verbal and non-verbal communications from others, exceptional curiosity about the human mind and human behavior, and psychological mindedness."[50] The website provides further information on the members of the selection committee, interview questions, and a copy of the applicant rating form used by evaluators.

- The Department of Anesthesiology at the University of Pittsburgh outlines the criteria that interviewers use to rank the applicants, which include such diverse criteria as "grades and honors," "knowledge of Pitt program," "quality of answers," "quality of questions, "enthusiasm, energy, liveliness" and "articulateness, communication skills."[40]

After sitting through years of selection committee meetings, we can state that the impact of selection factors varies markedly from faculty member to faculty member. Beliefs about which types of evidence prove certain traits also vary markedly. Meetings of the selection committee can be heated, and arguments about the importance of the different selection factors are common. What best predicts how well a candidate will perform as a resident? Our arguments during the ranking process can be as heated as any discussion forum on the topic.

The following paraphrased comments provide an insider's look at a residency selection committee meeting:

Behind the Scenes at a Residency Selection Committee Meeting

Applicant	Selection Committee Comments
# 1	"Her USMLE score is the lowest score of all the students we've interviewed this year." "Who cares? Her score is high enough that we don't have to worry about her passing the boards. I don't care about the numbers, as long as the enthusiasm and work ethic is there."
# 2	"That letter of recommendation was lukewarm, and I consider that a red flag." "But are you taking that comment out of context? The evaluations from his senior electives were outstanding."
# 3	"That interview was great, but the letter of rec from Dr. Grant wasn't exactly gushing. Amy, don't you know him? Can you e-mail him to find out more?"
# 4	"Did you see what the attending on his Internal Medicine rotation wrote about him? That's very concerning." "Maybe there were personality issues? I certainly didn't see that repeated anywhere else, so I think we need to take that into account."

# 5	"You all know that work ethic is my number one priority, and the fact that this student couldn't even write a case report after two derm electives is a bad sign." "I know that everyone else we've interviewed today has been published, but maybe you need to cut him some slack. Maybe at their institution, there just aren't many opportunities to work on case reports." "That doesn't mean that much to me, because there are opportunities everywhere if you try hard enough."
# 6	"Based on that interview, I just don't think he'd fit in well here." "I know what you mean, but I think you're jumping to conclusions. Take a look at the letter from Dr. ____. He worked with him for one month, and that's a much more meaningful impression than one interview." "After that interview, I don't think any letter is going to convince me."
# 7	"That personal statement, to me, seems to emphasize lifestyle factors." "I certainly didn't see it in that light."

In the following chapters, we delve more deeply into these questions. What do the individuals making the decisions care about? What are the qualities they seek in a resident?

More importantly, how can you demonstrate that you embody those qualities? *How can you convince them that you would be the right resident for their program?*

The remainder of this book is devoted to maximizing the impact of your application. Each component of your application can be created, modified, or influenced in order to significantly strengthen your overall candidacy. We devote the following pages to showing you, in detail, exactly how to do so.

References

[1]Kaplan A, Riedy K, Grundfast K. Increasing competitiveness for an otolaryngology residency: Where we are and concerns about the future. *Otolaryngol Head Neck Surg* 2015; 153(5): 699-701.
[2]Results of the 2014 NRMP Program Director Survey. Available at: http://www.nrmp.org/wp-content/uploads/2014/09/PD-Survey-Report-2014.pdf. Accessed March 3, 2014.
[3]Results of the 2008 NRMP Program Director Survey. Available at: http://www.nrmp.org/wp-content/uploads/2013/08/programresultsbyspecialty.pdf. Accessed March 3, 2016.

[4]The Successful Match: Getting into Pediatrics. Available at: http://studentdoctor.net/2011/05/the-successful-match-getting-into-pediatrics/. Accessed September 2, 2012.
[5]University of Texas Houston Department of Radiology. Available at: http://www.uth.tmc.edu/med/adminsitration/student/ms4.2003CCC.htm. Accessed September 21, 2012.
[6]Case Western University School of Medicine. Available at: http://casemed.case.edu/CareerPlan/USMLE%20&%20The%20Matches.htm. Accessed November 2, 2008.
[7]Kia K, Gielczyk R, Ellis C. Acaademia is the life for me, I'm sure. *Arch Dermatol* 2006; 142: 911-913.
[8]Prober C, Kolars J, First L, Melnick D. A plea to reassess the role of United States Medical Licensing Examination Step 1 scores in residency selection. *Acad Med* 2016; 91(1): 12-15.
[9]The Successful Match: Getting into Ophthalmology. Available at: http://studentdoctor.net/2009/08/the-successful-match-interview-with-dr-andrew-lee-ophthalmology/. Accessed September 20, 2012.
[10]The Successful Match: Getting into Radiology. Available at: http://studentdoctor.net/2010/10/the-successful-match-getting-into-radiology/. Accessed April 26, 2012.
[11]Hayden S, Hayden M, Gamst A. What characteristics of applicants to emergency medicine residency programs predict future success as an emergency medicine resident? *Acad Emerg Med* 2005; 12(3): 206-210.
[12]LaGrasso J, Kennedy D, Hoehn J, Ashruf S, Pryzbyla A. Selection criteria for the integrated model of plastic surgery residency. *Plast Reconstr Surg* 2008; 121(3): 121e-125e.
[13]Daly K, Levine S, Adams G. Predictors for resident success in otolaryngology. *J Am Coll Surg* 2006; 202(4): 649-654.
[14]The Successful Match: Interview with Dr. Roy Ziegelstein. Available at: http://studentdoctor.net/2009/06/the-successful-match-interview-with-dr-roy-ziegelstein/. Accessed September 5, 2012.
[15]TheSuccessfulMatch: Interview with Dr. Marianne Green. Available at: http://www.studentdoctor.net/2009/05/the-successful-match-interview-with-dr-marianne-green/. Accessed February 26, 2016.
[16]UCSF Department of Radiology. Available at: http://radiology.ucsf.edu/residents/apps. Accessed March 3, 2008.
[17]Green M, Jones P, Thomas J. Selection criteria for residency: results of a national program director survey. *Acad Med* 2009; 84(3): 362-7.
[18]Brandenburng S, Kruzick T, Lin C, Robinson A, Adams L. Residency selection criteria: what medical students perceive as important. *Med Educ Online* 2005; 10: 1-6.
[19]University of Washington Department of Medicine. Available at: http://depts.washington.edu/medclerk/drupal/pages/Internal-Medicine-Residency-Application-FAQ. Accessed September 15, 2012.
[20]University of Colorado Department of surgery. Available at: http://www.ucdenver.edu/academics/colleges/medicalschool/education/studentaffairs/studentgroups/SurgicalSociety/Pages/FAQ.aspx. Accessed April 30, 2012.

[21]University of California Davis Department of Obstetrics and Gynecology. Available at: *www.ucdmc.ucdavis.edu/gme/ppts/Residency_advice_1.pps*. Accessed February 10, 2013.
[22]Department of Urology at Southern Illinois University. Available at: http://www.urologymatch.com/node/1361. Accessed March 22, 2016.
[23]Department of Ophthalmology at University of Washington. Available at: http://ophthalmology.washington.edu/. Accessed January 2, 2012.
[24]Department of Radiology at Stanford University. Available at: http://med.stanford.edu/xray/AP/timeline.html. Accessed March 22, 2016.
[25]Arnold P. Gold Foundation. Available at: http://humanism-in-medicine.org/. Accessed June 22, 2014.
[26]Rosenthal S, Howard B, Schlussel Y, Lazarus C, Wong J, Moutier C, Savoia M, Trooskin S, Wagoner N. Does medical student membership in the gold humanism honor society influence selection for residency? *J Surg Educ* 2009; 66(6): 308-13.
[27]The Daily Toreador. Available at: http://www.dailytoreador.com/news/article_4512fb50-758f-11e2-a99f-0019bb30f31a.html. Accessed June 3, 2014.
[28]American Society of Clinical Pathology. Available at: http://www.ascp.org/Newsroom/ASCP-Academic-Excellence-Award-Crucial-to-Medical-Students-Career-Path.html. Accessed June 24, 2014.
[29]University of Central Florida College of Medicine. Available at: http://today.ucf.edu/ucf-medical-student-wins-national-orthopaedic-award/. Accessed June 2, 2014.
[30]University of Arkansas for Medical Sciences. Available at: http://www.uams.edu/update/absolutenm/templates/news2003v2.asp?articleid=7594&zoneid=15. Accessed June 2, 2014.
[31]Johns Hopkins Medicine. Available at: http://www.hopkinsmedicine.org/news/media/releases/johns_hopkins_mdphd_student_wins_us_public_health_award. Accessed June 23, 2014.
[32]George Washington University School of Medicine. Available at: http://smhs.gwu.edu/news/gw-medical-student-wins-prestigious-ama-leadership-award. Accessed June 23, 2014.
[33]UT Southwestern Medical School. Available at: http://www.utsouthwestern.edu/newsroom/center-times/year-2013/may/award-ho-din.html. Accessed June 3, 2014.
[34]University of Washington Department of Family Medicine. Available at: https://depts.washington.edu/fammed/residency/fellowships/global-health/applicant-information/. Accessed March 22, 2016.
[35]Go P, Klaassen Z, Chamberlain R. Attitudes and practices of surgery residency program directors toward the use of social networking profiles to select residency candidates: a nationwide survey analysis. *J Surg Educ* 2012; 69(3): 292–300.
[36]Charting Outcomes in the Match- 2014. Available at: http://www.nrmp.org/wp-content/uploads/2014/09/Charting-Outcomes-2014-Final.pdf. Accessed March 2, 2016.

[37]Otero H, Erturk S, Ondategui-Parra S, Ros P. Key criteria for selection of radiology residents: results of a national survey. *Acad Radiol* 2006; 13: 1155-1164.
[38]Brothers T, Wetherholt S. Importance of the faculty interview during the resident application process. *J Surg Educ* 2007; 64(6): 378-385.
[39]Cruz P. Residency selection: The Southwestern experience. *Arch Dermatol* 2001; 137(6): 808-811.
[40]Metro D, Talarciso J, Patel R, Wetmore A. The Resident Application Process and its correlation to future performance as a resident. *Anesth Analg* 2005; 100: 502-505.
[41]University of Washington Department of Otolaryngology. Available at: http://depts.washington.edu/otoweb/training/residency/policies/index.shtml. Accessed March 22, 2008.
[42]Moore P. A guide to the perplexed: residency guide. Available at www.ucdmc.ucdavis.edu. Accessed December 4, 2008.
[43]Boyse T, Patterson S, Cohan R, Korobkin M, Fitzgerald J, Oh M, Gross B, Quint D. Does medical school performance predict radiology resident performance? *Acad Radiol* 2002; 9(4): 437-445.
[44]Bell J, Kanellitsas I, Shaffer L. Selection of obstetrics and gynecology residents on the basis of medical school performance. *Am J Obstet Gynecol* 2002; 186(5): 1091-1094.
[45]Gong H, Parker N, Apgar F, Shank C. Influence of the interview on ranking in the residency selection process. *Med Educ* 1984; 18(5): 366-369.
[46]Bernstein A, Jazrawi L, Elbeshbeshy B, Della Valle C, Zuckerman J. Orthopedic resident-selection criteria. *J Bone Joint Surg Am* 2002; 84-A(11): 2090-2096.
[47]Galazka S, Kikano G, Zyzanski S. Methods of recruiting and selecting residents for U.S. family practice residencies. *Acad Med* 1994; 69(4): 304-306.
[48]Swanson W, Harris M, Master C, Gallagher P, Maruo A, Ludwig S. The impact of the interview in pediatric residency selection. *Amb Pediatr* 2005; 5 (4): 216-220.
[49]Penn State Hershey Department of Radiology. Available at: http://www.pennstatehersey.org/web/radiology/education/residency. Accessed March 2, 2008.
[50]Stony Brook Department of Psychiatry. Available at: http://www.hsc.stronybrook.edu/som/psychiatry/selection_procecess.cfm. Accessed March 22, 2012.

Chapter 4

The Competitive Edge

If you plan to apply to a competitive program or a competitive specialty, you'll need to bring into play all of the recommendations throughout this book. In this chapter, we go further and review in detail how to add an extra competitive edge to your application. To begin with, you should make every effort to be published in your field. Such opportunities are available to every student, although they can be difficult to locate. We review how to find these opportunities as well as the process of writing for the medical literature. We also review the topic of research. If you're applying to a competitive field, NRMP data indicate that the vast majority of your competition will have participated in research. We review how to locate research opportunities and how to excel.

Rule # 1 **If you're applying to competitive programs, you should make every effort to be published in your field.**

In every academic medical center, there are ample opportunities to publish. We meet many medical students who would choose to describe themselves as "self-starters." Opportunities to publish only go to those students who truly are self-starters.

Locating these opportunities is often the hardest step, because there are no hard and fast rules. Different types of opportunities to publish exist at the medical school level, even if you've never been involved in formal basic science or clinical research. A few include:

- The case report of a classic case
- The case report of an interesting case
- A case series
- A review article

The case report is typically the entry point for medical students who lack experience in research. Even if you've researched and published extensively, it can be important to have additional scientific study in your chosen field. This confirms your interests in the specialty and your ongoing commitment to scientific pursuits.

How can a case report strengthen your application?

- By seeking out the opportunity, you've demonstrated your drive and enthusiasm.
- You've confirmed your interest in the specialty.
- You've confirmed your thirst for additional knowledge.
- Just the act of seeking out the opportunity demonstrates commitment to the field.
- Seeking out opportunities to publish provides a professional way in which to speak with or meet residents, faculty, and PDs in the institution.
- On a basic level, you've added to, or at least started, the publication section of your CV.
- By writing the case report, you have become an expert in one specific area.
- Your expertise becomes a potential topic of discussion in interviews.
- Your publication may also act as a point of commonality in interviews that can build rapport. "I'm very pleased to meet you, Dr. Lo. I referenced your work on…when writing my review article on…"
- Writing provides an ideal opportunity to showcase your work ethic, your drive, and your skills.
- By writing the case report in record time and by producing outstanding results, you'll be able to highlight your skills to your attending, an individual who can influence your acceptance to the residency program.
- Faculty members with concrete knowledge of your skills may use this specific example in their rotation evaluation, and in their letters of recommendation.
- Such faculty members can also act as vocal advocates for your candidacy for their own program.

Students who produce outstanding case reports in record time are also more likely to be considered for more substantial research projects or publications. More substantial projects are difficult to locate on the medical student level, but obviously are much more valuable in strengthening your application. An attending who's been asked to write a book chapter for the new edition of a well-respected textbook will only collaborate with individuals of known merit. By showcasing your skills, you've increased your chances of being awarded such valuable opportunities.

Rule # 2 Possibilities for publishing abound.

In general, medical students can be involved in publishing two types of case reports. The first type is what we term "classic" cases. These are typical examples of certain diagnoses, and may be published in a variety of journals in sections entitled "diagnostic puzzles," "clinical pearls," "grand rounds," or others.

The other type of case report describes rare or distinctive clinical findings. "This represents the first case of pseudoporphyria due to the medication sulindac."

If an opportunity to publish has been presented to you by your attending, then they'll typically advise you on journal selection. Certain types of clinical material are appropriate for different journals. However, as we discuss the process of publishing on the medical student level, we'll start with a discussion of opportunities in different journals.

Peer-reviewed and indexed journals are preferred, as they signal a higher level of scientific scrutiny. This information will typically be found in the journal's front pages, or online under the instructions for authors. Journals indexed in PubMed are preferred. If the journal is found when searching on www.pubmed.com, it's indexed on PubMed.

Many options are available within this category of peer-reviewed and indexed journals. However, on a medical student level, an opportunity to publish in any medical journal is significant. Publication in a non-peer reviewed, non-indexed medical journal is still quite an accomplishment, and will be regarded as such.

Your residents and faculty advisors are the best source of suggestions for appropriate sections of journals to which to submit. These may include specialty-specific or non-specialty specific journals. For example, in the field of dermatology alone, we can list a dozen journals that accept classic cases that are published for the education of the reader. These types of classic cases are often seen in a typical week at an academic dermatology outpatient clinic. A case of epidermolysis bullosa acquisita, for example, may not be all that interesting to the dermatology attending, but may prove to be an interesting case for submission to the Photo Quiz section of *American Family Physician*.

We could list many examples of medical journals that students may wish to investigate further. *Journal of Medical Case Reports* is available online without a subscription, and is indexed and peer-reviewed. *Consultant* is a peer reviewed journal which has short features such as "What's Your Diagnosis?" "Photoclinic," Photo Quiz," and "Dermclinic." Other journals to explore include the *American Medical Student Research Journal* and *Student BMJ*. These are simply a few of the many journals that accept case reports of classic or interesting cases. Again, your faculty advisor is the best source for suggestions, particularly for specialty-specific journals. In the table on the next page, we've presented journals to consider for case report submission, organized by specialty. Note that this is not an exhaustive list, but rather a starting point for your own research.

Residents and faculty are very helpful in suggesting clinical material that's appropriate for publication. However, with both the case report of an interesting case and the discussion of a classic case, students can take the lead in suggesting a publication. You may see an interesting case, perform a thorough literature search in order to learn more about the disease, and recognize its potential for publication. You can then suggest the case and ask your resident and attending for their thoughts about its potential acceptance.

Journals Publishing Case Reports By Specialty	
Specialty	**Specialty Journals Publishing Case Reports**
Anesthesiology	A&A Case Reports Case Reports in Anesthesiology Anaesthesia Cases Journal of Anaesthesia and Critical Care Case Reports
Dermatology	Case Reports in Dermatology Images in Dermatology
Emergency Medicine	Case Reports in Emergency Medicine Academic Emergency Medicine
Family Medicine	American Family Physician Journal of Family Practice Journal of the American Board of Family Practice
Internal Medicine	ACP Hospitalist American Journal of Medicine American Journal of the Medical Sciences Annals of Internal Medicine Archives of Internal Medicine Case Reports in Gastroenterology Case Reports in Nephrology Case Reports in Oncology Clinical Medicine Insights: Case Reports Consultant Endocrinology, Diabetes & Metabolism Case Reports Hospital Physician Images in Clinical Medicine (NEJM) Journal of General Internal Medicine Lancet New England Journal of Medicine Southern Medical Journal
Neurology	Case Reports in Neurological Medicine Epilepsy and Behavior Case Reports Case Reports in Neurology
Neurological Surgery	Journal of Neurological Surgery Reports
Obstetrics & Gynecology	Gynecologic Oncology Case Reports
Ophthalmology	Retinal Cases & Brief Reports Case Reports in Ophthalmology
Orthopedic Surgery	Journal of Knee Surgery Reports
Pediatrics	Case Reports in Pediatrics Journal of Pediatric Surgery Case Reports European Journal of Pediatric Surgery Reports
Radiation Oncology	Practical Radiation Oncology
Radiology	Case Reports in Radiology Images in Radiology Radiology Case Reports Journal of Radiology Case Reports BJR Case Reports
Surgery	Thoracic and Cardiovascular Surgeon Reports Journal of Surgical Technique and Case Reports Journal of Surgical Case Reports Journal of Pediatric Surgery Case Reports International Journal of Surgery Case Reports European Journal of Pediatric Surgery Reports
Urology	Urology Case Reports Case Reports in Urology Pediatric Urology Case Reports Journal of Case Reports and Images in Urology

Case series are more substantial publications, but will require a faculty member asking you to collaborate using their clinical material. Reviews are articles which are also typically identified by the faculty member. Clinical and basic science research projects require a more formal and in-depth commitment. While there are some one-month clinical and basic science research electives, many research projects require much more of a commitment. In order to participate in research, you'll need to identify a faculty mentor who can support and educate you about the process. We review research later in this chapter.

Note that we've only focused on opportunities to publish. Many of these opportunities, however, can also translate into opportunities to present a poster at a national meeting, or to make a presentation at a local, regional, or national meeting. Can this case be presented at the monthly meeting of the Atlanta Pediatric Society? Can it be submitted as a clinical vignette for the national American College of Physicians meeting? Your faculty advisor can advise you of any potential opportunities.

Rule # 3 In order to publish, you need to locate an opportunity.

In some departments, students are frequently involved in publishing case reports, case series, review articles, and book chapters, even if they haven't formally participated in basic science or clinical research. In such departments, students will find it easier to locate opportunities to publish, because the path to doing so is relatively clear-cut. They can often locate opportunities just by discussing the situation with their classmates or upperclassmen.

In other departments, it may be uncommon for students to be involved on such a level. While there may not be a track record at your program of students authoring publications, ample opportunities to do can still be found. Students can easily be involved in publishing case reports, which simply describe a clinical case. There are ample cases of interest in any academic medical center. You need to be extremely motivated and ready to work independently, but you can still successfully publish in your field.

How can you identify opportunities to publish? As we mentioned, there are no hard and fast rules, and you really need to exhibit the skills of a self-starter to even be given the opportunity to start writing. Speak to other students, especially in the class ahead of you. They can relay their own experiences, and how they found their opportunities to publish. Speak to the residents, and let them know your interest in strengthening your application. They can identify clinical material that is interesting and appropriate for the medical literature. They can also, most importantly, direct you to the appropriate faculty members.

Certain faculty members are prolific writers, and have an interest in adding to the medical literature. Such faculty may be willing to work with you on case reports. They may have clinical material in their files that is awaiting an eager medical student to perform a literature search and prepare it for publication. Alternately, they may ask you to keep an eye out for interesting clinical cases during your time on the elective. Such faculty members are often asked to collaborate with colleagues in their field. They may have been asked to write a book chapter, or a review article. Such opportunities are ideal for medical student collaboration, and many faculty welcome interest by medical students.

In some institutions, it would be appropriate to send an e-mail to the faculty in your department highlighting your interest in working on a paper. Depending on your circumstances, you may seek to work on a paper during your elective or at any time during your third year. Many motivated students complete papers during their time on other rotations. Some students arrange time for a research elective, and then search for a faculty member to work with. In these cases, it is also appropriate to schedule a meeting with the chairman or program director to seek their advice.

Another ideal way to locate opportunities to publish is by participating in an away elective. Certain programs are well-known to provide ample opportunities for student participation in such projects, and your away elective can be chosen with this goal in mind. As with much of this section, there's no single best method to locate such programs. You can speak to the residents, your faculty advisor, and the PD. You can participate in online forums, or even scan journals to note which programs publish work with student authors.

Locating an opportunity to write is an accomplishment in and of itself. Congratulations. Now do everything in your power to maximize this opportunity.

Rule # 4 Finish what you've started.

The first and most important point about identifying opportunities to be published in your field is a simple one. Once you've identified an opportunity to write, you need to submit a finished product.

The reason we choose to discuss such an obvious rule is that somehow, despite its obvious nature, students just don't always finish projects. We've witnessed for ourselves many cases in which students don't complete a project. We've heard many negative comments from our colleagues about students who don't complete a project. We've sat in faculty meetings where the inability to complete a project is used as evidence of a student's poor fit for a residency program.

It's not just that you'll have lost out on an incredible opportunity to impress your attending and strengthen your application. Unfortunately, your inability to complete the project will convey a lack of commitment, a lack of dedication, and a poor work ethic.

It's rare that students in this situation actually have a poor work ethic and lack commitment. In many cases, students become paralyzed by their own perfectionism. They're not sure what they're doing, are insecure about the results they've produced and can't bear to turn in a final product that's not perfect. As a student, though, hardly anyone has experience with preparing cases for publication. You need to read extensively, plan to work hard, and move forward. We've outlined the process in more detail here.

Rule # 5 Before you write, you need to read.

A great deal of literature exists on designing and conducting medical research, but not so much when it comes to writing a straightforward case report or review of the literature. We've outlined the process in more detail below.

Learning how to write medical papers starts with reading medical papers. Read the articles in your targeted journal. If you'll be writing a case report, pay close attention to that section. Get a feel for format, sentence structure, and word usage. Move on to articles written in prestigious medical journals. Review articles written in specialty-specific journals. This type of reading provides the foundation for your medical writing.

Rule # 6 It may be one of the most important papers you've ever written, but it's not easy to write an outstanding case report.

Arrange to meet with your attending before you start. You need to obtain several key pieces of information. To which journal will you be submitting the paper? Which section in that journal? What is the anticipated timeline for submission of the paper? How would your attending prefer that you communicate with her? Would an e-mailed first draft be acceptable? If submitting a case report, what makes your case unique and compelling to the readers? Can your attending provide more information on what makes the case worthwhile for publication? These are all critical to the creation of a compelling, publishable report, and we review each of these points in further detail.

Rule # 7 Your publication must include a "hook."

What important point are you trying to convey to your readers? What makes this case unique or compelling to the readers? What is the point of publishing this case?

If you're submitting the case of a patient who presented with the classic features of Wegener's granulomatosis, you are presenting the case for the further education of your readers, so that they can recognize such cases in the future. As we discussed, many journals have sections in which they present examples of classic cases to their readers.

If your case is the first reported case of pseudoporphyria due to sulindac, then your hook is this: "We present this case of pseudoporphyria due to sulindac. While pseudoporphyria often occurs due to NSAIDs, this is the first reported case due to the medication sulindac. Therefore, this medication must be added to the possible causes."

If you're presenting a syndrome or disease that is well-described in the medical literature, then you need to search more deeply for what makes your case either unique or worth publishing. This can be difficult. It may be a fascinating syndrome, but if there's not a compelling point to make, then many journals won't see what use the information will have for their readers.

The insight and extensive clinical experience of your advisor will be critical in this situation. Was the last reported case of this syndrome 20 years ago? Then a reminder of its features may be useful. Does this case demonstrate a new association? Did the patient respond to a previously undescribed therapeutic measure? Did you note an interesting clinical finding that may serve as a clue to the diagnosis? "This case illustrates a complication of systemic amyloidosis and emphasizes its utility in reaching a timely diagnosis." Your point is that this information has educational or clinical significance for the readers.

Another option is to write a case report and review of the literature. "We present a case of Dowling-Degos disease and review and summarize the medical literature, with an emphasis on clinical and histologic presentations." What is the point of this type of publication? You describe an interesting case and summarize the medical literature to date, so that your readers will be fully educated on all aspects of this condition.

Rule # 8 For extensive projects, you need to establish a timeline.

"What timeline did you have in mind for this project?" If you'll be working on an extensive project, this question becomes very important. In your mind, a review article with over 200 references may take at least eight weeks. Your advisor may expect it in four, especially if she herself was given a deadline for submission. If you have a prior commitment, such as Step 2 in four weeks, then it's important to let your advisor know that you won't be able to meet that deadline. Be specific about your reasons, offer an alternative timeline, and ask if that would be acceptable.

We're going to emphasize an important point here. The date you're given is NOT a deadline. Some students will delay, then work feverishly for the week before, and then turn in a first draft on that date. That represents a wasted opportunity. The date you're given is actually an indication of your advisor's expectations, and is really an opportunity to exceed those expectations. Once you've heard the expected timeline, plan to cut it significantly. Turning in an outstanding finished product that exceeds expectations in terms of both quality and timeliness is an impressive accomplishment.

As a final note, a lack of timeline is not an excuse to delay. Many attendings won't have a timeline in mind. "Just do your best, and we'll work with it." Other attendings will say the same, but are in actuality judging your work ethic.

Note that we specified asking for an expected timeline in the case of extensive projects. Case reports are a different situation, because they should be completed and submitted promptly. Realistically, many case reports can be completed in one very lengthy weekend spent at the library and at your computer. This is particularly true for presentations of a classic case, which take less time to research and write. Submitting a high-quality case report at that speed will get you talked about.

Rule # 9 Model your report on others in your targeted journal.

Find the right journal for your submission. This is easier when your attending has a concrete idea of where your article should be submitted. Find out what journal you'll be submitting to. Seek out the instructions for authors. Seek out prior examples of publications for that section. Model yours using that format.

Rule # 10 You cannot write a strong case report without becoming an expert on your topic.

Perform a thorough literature search. You cannot write a strong case report without becoming an expert on the topic. You should begin by reading the textbooks. You can then move on to online sources such as emedicine (www.emedicine.com), which are regularly updated textbooks. You should then seek out review articles that summarize the literature on the subject. Lastly, you should review prior case reports on the topic.

Some students, when first writing a case report, heavily reference the major textbooks. However, such references are not ideal. For general information on the topic, it would be better to reference a review article, ideally one which is more recent, up to date, and in-depth. Including such a review article is helpful to your readers, as they can use that reference to obtain more information on the topic. However, review articles should never be used as substitution for the primary source of a piece of information. "Pseudoporphyria has been described as occurring due to ibuprofen, naproxen, and diclofenac.[1]" While it would be easier to include one reference that summarizes this information, such as a review article, it would be more appropriate, and in some cases more helpful for your readers, to include examples of publications that described each of these cases. "Pseudoporphyria has been described as occurring due to ibuprofen[1], naproxen[2] and diclofenac.[3]"

We assume that by this point in your career you've learned to navigate PubMed. You may find it helpful, however, to further maximize your knowledge of PubMed and the various search options available. Our own medical library offers multiple classes on maximizing the use of PubMed, and online tutorials are available as well.

Rule # 11 Write the case.

Once you pinpoint why your case would be compelling to readers, the work of writing the case report becomes more straightforward. For a case report, you'll typically write an introduction, a description of the case, and a discussion. The introduction will be brief, but should capture the reader's attention. Why would they care to read about your case?

In summarizing the clinical features of the case, make sure you review other cases previously published in your target journal. Your description of the clinical features of the case, including the depth of detail included, should be modeled after that type of case report.

In the discussion, just as in a typical college review paper, you will summarize and present the existing literature on this subject, with an emphasis on the important take home points learned from the case. Learning the appropriate focus and level of detail in the report is a skill that can take years to develop. "Should I focus on the clinical features of pseudoporphyria in general, and how to make the diagnosis, or should I just limit myself to a discussion on the prior reports of the NSAIDs that have triggered pseudoporphyria? Do I need to go into the pharmacological details of the different NSAIDs?

The level of detail included will depend, in large part, on the goals of your advisor and the limitations of the journal. The instructions to authors specify a range of word counts, and it's very important to adhere to these guidelines. Hopefully, the meeting with your advisor will have clarified the focus of the report. If in writing the discussion, though, you sense that you can go in two directions with your focus, you should contact your advisor for further guidance.

Rule # 12 Even your first draft should conform to the journal's exact specifications.

The first draft that you turn in to your attending must be perfect. As always, every aspect of your performance is up for scrutiny, and you need to be sending a consistent message throughout the application process. And yes, without a doubt, writing a paper is part of that process. Your message is that you bring excellence to whatever task you perform, and that your attention to detail is impeccable. Proof your paper for grammatical and spelling mistakes, especially with medical terms for which neither you nor your spell-checker are familiar. Submit a title page that adheres to the journal's specifications. Ensure that the format of your paper adheres to these specifications as well. If the journal requires an abstract for case reports, then submit an abstract of the specified length. Instructions for clinical photos, radiologic or other images, tables, and graphs should all be studied closely. Journals vary in their requirements for listing of references. Follow these requirements exactly.

Since this is a first draft, your content will be revised. Therefore, you should maintain two versions of your first draft. In the draft submitted to your advisor, the references should be formatted according to the instructions of the journal. In many cases, this means that references would be numbered and superscripted as directed, and the references section would include the numbered references in order of their inclusion in the body of the report. In the other draft version, you would note the author after the sentence, and avoid numbering your references at all. The references section would then list the authors in alphabetical order. This way, if your advisor suggests a change in the order of the content, the work required for significant renumbering of your references won't be as difficult. The second version would be for your use only.

Sulindac has been described as a cause of many different types of cutaneous reactions. (Smith, Jensen).

Rule # 13 The follow through is just as important.

Most students feel a tremendous sense of relief when they can finally turn in a paper and say they're done. However, follow through is just as important. Always offer to make any necessary revisions. Provide explicit instructions on how to reach you in the months to come. "I'll be doing an away elective in the month of February, but please feel free to contact me by e-mail, because I'd like to make whatever revisions are necessary without delay."

Sometimes the revisions suggested by your advisor can be lengthy and painful. Your ability to complete suggested revisions, and to do so promptly, will be noted. If a paper is submitted and subsequently accepted, there are almost always required revisions to be completed before the paper will be published. Be available for these revisions as well.

While your revisions should be submitted promptly, the converse won't always be true. Some attendings may take a great deal of time to respond to your first or second draft of an article. While you should have made it clear that you are available to work on any suggested changes, you cannot do much more than that to speed up the process. Some students, after working so hard on a paper, are understandably impatient for the paper to be submitted, accepted, and published in time to help their application. However, it's easy to annoy an attending when you check in too often on the status of your paper.

Research

In the last section, we focused on being published in your field. Opportunities to publish case reports are easily available to motivated, driven students, and as we outlined, simply publishing a case report can boost your application. In this section, we focus on research opportunities. These can more significantly strengthen your application, but opportunities to participate in research projects are more difficult to locate and complete.

Rule # 14 Many applicants who apply to competitive programs or a competitive specialty will have participated in research. Those applicants will be your competition.

Participation in research can significantly strengthen your application. However, it's not a requirement. A survey of PDs in multiple specialties found that in most fields, published medical school research and participation in research were two of the lowest ranked criteria in the residency selection process.[1] In most fields, many applicants without publications or research experience will still match. In radiology, for example, only 4 of the 125 U.S. allopathic applicants lacking publications failed to match (2014 NRMP Match).[2]

However, there are several important caveats. If the majority of students applying to your field have research experience, your lack of experience will make you stand out. While it may be ranked behind factors such as class rank and strength of LORs, research experience will still carry great weight with certain programs. In the fields of pathology and radiation oncology, published medical school research was among the top three academic criteria important to the residency selection process.[1]

In many fields, including the highly competitive fields and those considered not as competitive, your competition will have participated in research. In 2014, the NRMP published data on how applicant qualifications affect match success. Included among the data were the percentage of U.S. seniors who had participated in research projects and the percentage with publications. In highly competitive fields such as dermatology, orthopedic surgery, otolaryngology, plastic surgery, and radiation oncology, over 97% of U.S. seniors had participated in research projects. Even in specialties that are not the most competitive, including the fields of anesthesiology, emergency medicine, and radiology, over 85% of U.S. seniors had participated in research projects.

Percentage of U.S. Seniors in the 2014 Match Participating in Research and Reporting Publications by Specialty

Specialty	% U.S. seniors involved in research projects	% U.S. seniors with abstracts, presentations, or publications	Of note...
Anesthesiology	91%	74%	99/109 with no research experience matched.
Dermatology	97%	97%	Only 13 applicants had no research experience. Of the 297 applicants with > 5 publications, 58 did not match.
Emergency Medicine	87%	69%	Nearly all applicants with > 5 pubs matched (94%). Applicants with no publications matched at a similar rate (91%).
General Surgery	93%	79%	91% with > 5 publications matched. 77% with no publications matched. 67% (47/70) with no research experience matched.
Neurosurgery	99%	95%	67% of matched applicants reported > 5 publications. Only two applicants reported having no research experience.
OB/GYN	90%	76%	92% with > 5 publications matched. 89% (210/236) with no publications matched. 86% (83/97) with no research experience matched.

Orthopedic Surgery	99%	88%	63% (60/96) with no publications matched. 84% (293/350) with > 5 publications matched.
Otolaryngology	99%	94%	63% of matched applicants reported 4 or more publications.
Pathology	93%	81%	Only 1/101 with > 5 publications did not match. Only 1/48 with no publications did not match. 94% (16/17) with no research projects matched.
Pediatrics	87%	69%	94% of applicants reporting no research experience matched.
PM&R	90%	72%	87% (20/23) reporting no research experience matched. 83% (53/64) reporting no publications matched.
Plastic Surgery	99%	94%	Only 1 applicant reported no research experience. 77% of applicants reporting > 5 publications matched. Mean number of pubs among matched versus unmatched applicants varied considerably (12.5 versus 6.4).
Psychiatry	86%	73%	91% (82/90) of applicants with no research experience matched. 168 applicants with no publications matched.
Radiation Oncology	98%	98%	Only 3 applicants with no publications matched.
Radiology	94%	83%	98% (46/47) applicants with no research experience matched.

Data Adapted from Charting Outcomes in the Match- 2014. Available at: http://www.nrmp.org/wp-content/uploads/2014/09/Charting-Outcomes-2014-Final.pdf

Rule # 15 Participate in a research project for the right reasons.

We've emphasized that your competition will have participated in research projects. We've emphasized that such projects can significantly enhance the strength of your application. However, you should never participate in a research project for those reasons alone. If buffing up your CV is your only motivation, this will be transparently obvious to your colleagues and preceptor. Your project can then become detrimental to your chances of matching successfully.

Your main motivation for participation in a research project should be that it can help you become a better doctor. Upon completion of a research project, students often report an increased ability to formulate a hypothesis, conduct a literature search, critically appraise the literature, collect data, analyze results, and prepare a manuscript. Some students find the experience so intellectually satisfying that it leads them into a career with a heavy emphasis in research.

Others find that the experience provides them with the foundation to practice evidence-based medicine. Since research is the foundation of evidence-based medicine, exposure to research and scientific methods will strengthen your critical thinking skills. You'll be in a better position to critically analyze and interpret scientific advances, and then translate those findings into improved patient care.

Rule # 16 Participation in a research project provides a number of distinct benefits.

Some students who participate in a research project will focus on the advantages to their CV. A research project can be listed under research experience. Publications or presentation may also result, further enhancing a student's CV. However, there are a number of other distinct advantages:

- Participation in a research project provides invaluable experience, as we've already discussed. Many accomplished investigators credit research experience in medical school as the impetus for their present careers. Even physicians who ultimately decide not to make research a focus of their career still speak highly of their experience. These clinicians report an enhanced ability to search the literature, answer clinical questions, and analyze and interpret scientific data.

- Students who perform research through a research elective in their third or fourth year of medical school will receive credit for the course. Your research preceptor will assign a final grade, which will appear on your medical school transcript. The formal evaluation with written comments and the transcript itself can all strengthen your application.

- Working closely with your research preceptor presents a unique opportunity to highlight your abilities. Your preceptor can become familiar with the quality of your work, your communication skills, and you skills in research. Such close interaction can lead to a strong LOR.

- Your research preceptor may become a career advisor or mentor. In a survey of third- and fourth-year medical students at one medical school, UCSF, 96% of all participants rated mentors as important or very important.[3] Mentors provide invaluable guidance and advice, and their recommendations alone can significantly strengthen your application.

- Your research preceptor's connections at other program may open doors for you, as in opportunities to participate in audition electives or other research projects. In some cases, research preceptors who have advocated on behalf of their students have been able to increase the chances of a successful match in a particular specialty or program.

Rule # 17 Research involves a number of different processes. You may be involved in any or all of these.

What do we mean when we use the term "research?" Taber's *Cyclopedic Medical Dictionary* defines research as "scientific and diligent study, investigation, or experimentation in order to establish facts and analyze their significance."[4]

In a more general sense, research involves answering a question. The scientific process involved in answering that question can be quite complex, and consists of a number of different processes.

Steps Involved In The Process Of Research

Review of literature
Hypothesis generation
Study design
Requesting approval from the institutional review board
Data collection
Data tabulation
Data analysis
Manuscript preparation and revision
Manuscript submission/resubmission

Years ago I saw a child with cutaneous mucormycosis at the site of an intravenous catheter. I had never seen a case before in a child. Despite a thorough literature search, I was left with a number of questions. How often did such cases occur in children? What were the risk factors involved? What was the ideal therapy, and what was the usual outcome? I designed a simple (relatively speaking) study to try to answer some of these questions, which consisted of a retrospective chart review. I obtained Institutional Review Board (IRB) approval to do a chart review at Texas Children's Hospital. Obtaining IRB approval can be an in-depth, complicated process in and of itself, as the IRB ensures that the study is safe and effective for human participation. IRB approval is necessary even for a chart review.

Once I obtained IRB approval, I had to locate and contact the point person who could perform a computerized search of the pathology records. We limited our search to ten years' worth of data, and searched for biopsies of skin that carried a diagnosis of "fungal" or "mold." We read each of these biopsy reports, and only included those that demonstrated hyphae extending into the dermis. We then contacted the medical records department, and asked for the complete chart on each of these cases. A review of these charts excluded some of these patients from our series. For the remainder of the cases, we created a data collection form.

What information were we seeking on the cases? Our data collection form included demographic information (gender, age) in addition to the clinical factors that we wished to study, including clinical appearance, underlying medical conditions and medications, other predisposing factors, treatment, and outcome.

Once the medical records were reviewed, we collected all of this clinical information. We created tables that summarized the information. We analyzed the data, and in doing so came to several conclusions about cutaneous mold infections in children, the risk factors involved, and the outcomes. We prepared the manuscript, submitted the manuscript, made the requested revisions, and our study was ultimately published.[5]

As a medical student, you may find yourself in any of these aspects of research. While this is an example of clinical research, you may have the opportunity to participate in either clinical or basic science research. While you may be able to work on a project from inception to publication, as described above, that is unusual on the medical student level.

The typical entry point to medical student research is the identification of a faculty member who is willing to involve you in a study of their design. The type of involvement may vary quite a bit. You may be involved in the literature search and IRB approval process. Your involvement may be a relatively simple, one-time involvement in data collection. For example, during your one-month research elective, you may participate in reviewing medical charts and collecting information from those charts. You may even be involved in analyzing the results, drawing conclusions, and preparing a manuscript. Whatever aspects of the research process you ultimately participate in, you should make every effort to understand all aspects of the research process and all aspects of your particular project.

Rule # 18 **If you're able to participate in a research project, it's not enough to understand the background literature on your particular subject. You must be able to describe the question that you are attempting to answer, the specific methodology used, the results, the weaknesses of the study, and the ultimate relevance of the research.**

Students are often asked about their research at interviews. Some are unable to describe the relevance of their research, let alone the specific methodology used. While the reasons for this are many, chief among these reasons is not having a solid understanding of the project. According to Dr. Michelle Biros, editor-in-chief of *Academic Emergency Medicine*, there are certain questions every student should be able to answer when embarking on a project.[6]

Important Questions To Answer About Your Research Project

Why was this research topic chosen?
What is the background that makes this question important?
What is the specific study hypothesis?
What is the study design?
Why was it designed this way?
What are the methods that will be used to answer the question?
Why was this method developed for this research question?
How is the data to be collected and managed?
If the data is collected and managed properly, will the study hypothesis really be answered?
What are the unanswered questions?

From Biros M, Adams J. Medical students and research: getting started in emergency medicine research (www.saem.org).

If you'll be participating in any type of basic science or clinical research, you should be reading more extensively on scientific methods. Even a simple chart review or questionnaire study entails a great deal of work, from study design, to IRB approval, to data analysis. Although many decisions will be made by your advisor, you should be able to understand the basis for those decisions and offer your own input. You can start by reading introductory texts on the subject. Further study would include formal courses and more advanced textbooks. This is in addition to asking questions of your advisor.

As we mentioned previously, participating in a research project should not be limited to the one aspect of the project in which you are directly involved. While you may participate only in the chart review, you should read and ask questions in order to develop a full understanding of the research question, the study design, the results, and the relevance of those results. You should understand and be able to intelligently discuss your research.

Rule # 19 Locating a research project can be a significant project in and of itself.

Locating opportunities to participate in a research project can be difficult. The advice in this section is very similar to that for locating opportunities to publish. You can't just look up job postings on medstudentresearch.com. You will need to be motivated and persistent in order to locate these types of opportunities. While projects may be difficult to locate, in many schools there are ample opportunities to participate in research on the medical student level.

Start by seeking information and advice from your peers. Your classmates may already be involved in research. Upperclassmen at your school may have participated in projects, and can provide additional information. The residents in your program may also be involved in, or aware of, different research projects.

Your institution will often have resources available. Many schools keep an updated database in which faculty members are listed, along with their projects. Most schools have a research office, and the members there may be able to offer additional information and insight.

You may also schedule an appointment with the clerkship director, program director, or chairman of your own program. Ask them for advice about potential research opportunities. Be prepared to provide your CV, and be prepared to respond to questions about your anticipated time frame for research and prior experience. In some institutions, it may also be considered appropriate to e-mail all of the faculty members in the department to let them know of your interest in participating in a research project. In this case, you would attach your CV.

As we discussed in the section on case reports, the best opportunities may not be available for the asking. However, once you've demonstrated your skills and abilities during a rotation or with a case report, faculty members may be more willing to work with you. If you've worked with any faculty members during a clerkship or on an outside project such as a case report, you should approach them for additional guidance. You can ask if they have any ideas of research projects that you could work on, or if they know of any potential opportunities within the department.

Rule # 20 If you plan to participate in research in a meaningful way, you'll need advance planning.

Starting and finishing a research project takes considerable time. Students who are new to research often believe that two or three months are sufficient. In reality, while a several month block of time is helpful, research projects usually require a much greater commitment of time.

Students who are sure of their specialty choice when entering medical schools have the advantage of being able to start a project early in their education. However, while many students have an idea of the specialty they wish to pursue, surveys have shown that this specialty choice often changes. In AAMC surveys of students graduating in 1991 and 1994, 80% chose to pursue a career in a different specialty from what they had declared at the time of medical school matriculation.[7]

Most advisors will suggest that you dedicate a block of time to devote to research, rather than trying to find time for a project during busy rotations. While you may schedule a research elective during your fourth year, it would be to your advantage to do so earlier. While the research itself may be completed at an earlier date, preparing for presentation and publication can add significantly to the length of the project, and much of the follow up work will be done past the completion of your elective. If your school allows flexible scheduling, you may consider breaking up your core clerkships with a research elective in your third year.

Rule # 21 Maintain realistic expectations about your chances for publication.

Many students who participate in research have the expectation that their work will lead to publication. However, research is a difficult and complex process, and you need to maintain realistic expectations. If you're planning to participate in a research project and are purely focused on completing that project so that you can add a publication to your CV, you are likely to be disappointed. Students may sign up for a one-month, or even a two-month, research elective, and hope to complete a project in that time. However, that depends greatly on the nature of the question you hope to answer.

Even one year of full-time research may not be sufficient. The Clinical Research Training Program at the National Institutes of Health (NIH) and the Doris Duke Clinical Research Fellowship are prestigious programs that immerse students into one year of full-time experience in clinical research. In one study, only 23% of fellows in either program had publications in print by 6 months post-fellowship.[8] This date was chosen to indicate publications that could be included in residency applications, as fellows usually participated between their third and fourth year of medical school. While a variety of factors may account for this, in an anonymous survey of the Doris Duke Clinical Research fellows, 18% felt that their research question was not well suited to the time available.[9]

The conclusion is that not all research experience will result in a publication to add to your CV. However, research experience can be an invaluable addition to your application. It demonstrates your dedication to the field, may result in stronger LORs, and provides a topic of discussion in interviews. Most importantly, the value of research experience extends far beyond what it can do for your application.

Rule # 22 Hard work and follow through are critical.

Once you commit to working on a research project, your preceptor will expect a significant commitment. While some projects may be a part-time commitment, others require long days and work on weekends. As a student free of other responsibilities, you need to be willing and able to work the long hours that are required.

Follow-up is critical as well. A month or two of research is rarely a sufficient period of time to complete a project, although this depends on the nature of the project. Once the research itself is completed, significant work is still required to bring the study to publication. Therefore, it will be important to remain involved in the project, even after your research block has ended. If you have participated in a research elective, make it quite clear to your preceptor that you would like to be involved in further stages of the project. Provide explicit directions on how you can be reached.

Rule # 23 **Finish what you start.**

Finish what you start. The same rule that we listed for publications applies to research projects. If you hear of an opportunity to participate in a research project, make sure you fully understand what is required. Before committing to a project, make sure you clearly understand the time frame and degree of work involved. If you can't get the project done in the eight-week period of time before you start your surgery rotation, you can't commit to the project. Let your potential advisor know your schedule.

Estimating the time frame on a project can be difficult in some cases. If the project in question is a chart review that involves extracting clinical information, then it will be easier to estimate the investment of time. Other projects may require a year of intermittent work to complete. You may have to wait until specific goals and objectives are defined, the methodology to perform the research is established, funding is secured, and approval from the institutional review board is granted. Some projects, especially laboratory-based projects, require the acquisition and development of specialized skills. Acquiring these skills may take a considerable investment of time.

Rule # 24 **Be prepared for your initial meeting with a potential research preceptor.**

During an initial meeting about a potential research project, the following issues will be discussed:

- Previous research experience

  You may be asked about your background and previous research experience, particularly if you'll be involved in bench research or in a clinical research project from inception that would involve IRB approval. Have you done research before? If so, are you grounded in the basic research concepts?

- Your timetable

  Issues related to scheduling should be discussed before the project begins. Inform your advisor when you would be able to start, the time you have to devote to the project, and when your research block will end. Discuss any potential interruptions, such as vacation, exams, or clerkships. Your timetable will help your advisor determine the most suitable project for you.

- Questions

  Be ready to ask questions and take notes. What aspects of the project will you be involved with? What will be your duties and responsibilities? How often and in what fashion would your advisor like to be kept apprised of your progress? What is their anticipated timetable for the completion of your portion of the project?

Rule # 25 **You should make it explicitly clear that you are willing and hoping to participate fully in all aspects of the project.**

When embarking on a research project, you'll discuss with your advisor the aspects of the project in which you will participate. For example, it's relatively easy to involve an inexperienced student in data collection for a chart review. However, you should always attempt to participate more fully in a project. At the very least, you should work on data tabulation, after asking how your advisor would like the data to be presented. You should also let your advisor know that you are willing and hoping to participate fully in all aspects of the project. Ideally, you would play a role in all aspects of the project, including data collection, analysis of the results, and development of the manuscript. This won't be possible with all research projects, particularly those that are more complex or large in scope, but your willingness to be involved in further aspects of the project should be clearly conveyed.

Some students participate in a research project in a very limited fashion. They may perform the chart review, collect the data, and then hand it to their advisor. However, if you're hoping for additional participation in a research project, such as inclusion as an author or participation as a presenter, then you need to be fully involved in the project. If you did the grunt work, but didn't analyze or interpret data, present results, or write the paper, you can't expect to receive the honor of first authorship.

References

[1]Green M, Jones P, Thomas J. Selection criteria for residency: results of a national program director survey. *Acad Med* 2009; 84(3): 362-7.
[2]Charting Outcomes in the Match (2014). Available at: http://www.nrmp.org/wp-content/uploads/2014/09/Charting-Outcomes-2014-Final.pdf. Accessed March 3, 2014.
[3]Aagaard E, Hauer K. A cross-sectional descriptive study of mentoring relationships formed by medical students. *J Gen Intern Med* 2003; 18: 298-302.
[4]Taber's *Cyclopedic Medical Dictionary.* Available at: http://www.tabers.com/tabersonline/. Accessed March 3, 2016.
[5]Katta R, Bogle M, Levy M. Primary cutaneous opportunistic mold infections in a pediatric population. *J Am Acad Dermatol* 2005; 53(2): 213-219.
[6]Biros M, Adams J. Medical students and research: getting started in emergency medicine research. Available at: http://www.saem.org. Accessed January 2, 2008.
[7]Kassebaum D, Szenas P. Medical students' career indecision and specialty rejection: roads not taken. *Acad Med* 1995; 70(10): 937-943.
[8]Cohen B, Friedman E, Zier K. Publications by students doing a year of full-time research: what are the realistic expectations? *Am J Med* 2008; 121: 545-548.
[9]Gallin E, Le Blancq S. Clinical Research Fellowship Program Leaders. Launching a new fellowship for medical students: the first years of the Doris Duke Clinical Research Fellowship Program. *J Investig Med* 2005; 53: 73-81.

Chapter 5

The Right Fit

In this chapter we focus on the final question of the application process:

How can you convince the decision-makers that you would be the right resident for their program?

In order to convince those making the decisions, you need to strategize, and you need to start early. Strategic planning begins and ends with outstanding patient care. If you want to match at the residency program of your choice, then the first step is to learn how to be an outstanding clinician. Your ultimate message for any residency program is that you will be an outstanding physician, and that you would make an outstanding resident. Our advice is to start by being the absolutely best clinician. You came to medical school to be a doctor. Learn how to be the best.

Excellence in patient care translates to better clinical evaluations and stronger letters of recommendation. These translate to a stronger transcript, a more positive MSPE, a higher class rank, and AOA candidacy. Evidence of outstanding patient care in an audition elective may even translate to a match at that program.

How do you excel at patient care? The process starts with the recognition that the skills needed to excel in clinical rotations are very different from those required for the basic science years. Our companion book, *Success on the Wards: 250 Rules for Clerkship Success*, lays out in full detail how to perform at an outstanding level in the clinics and on the wards. Chapter 10 of this book, "The Audition Elective," provides further information on how to excel during your clinical experiences.

We outline the strategizing that continues throughout the application process. Your ultimate goal is to convince those making the decisions that you would be the right resident for their program. In order to do so, you need to confirm that you would be the right fit for their program.

"Fit" is one of those concepts that students don't realize is such an important criterion. In a survey of radiology PDs, 15 directors stated that the "fit" of the candidates in the program along with a "gut feeling" were the most important criteria for deciding admission.[1] In another survey, PDs wrote that they sought to find applicants who were "people like us."[2]

Importance of "Fit" to Residency Programs

You will see the word "fit" time and time again on program websites, highlighting its importance in the selection process. Representative comments are shown below.

"Our application process is designed to…determine your specific interests and 'fit' in our program."[3]

- University of Buffalo Department of Anesthesiology

"We are recruiting the applicants at the same time we are interviewing them to try to discern which applicants are the best fit for our residency program."[4]

- University of Michigan Department of Dermatology

"We interview candidates whose academic and personal strengths indicate they would be a good fit for our program."[5]

- Morristown Medical Center Department of Medicine

"The personal interview is very important in assessing all components important to a good 'fit' for both the applicant and the program."[6]

- Wayne State University Department of Neurosurgery

The goals of the interview are to "assess the 'fit' of the applicant…weed out applicants who are a poor fit."[7]

- Duke University Department of Anesthesiology

"We are looking for an applicant that will fit well within our department and training program."[8]

- LSU Department of Obstetrics & Gynecology

"Candidates are assessed based on perceived intellectual ability and personality fit to the Department of Orthopedics."[9]

- West Virginia University Department of Orthopedics

"The program seeks candidates who are committed to their education and training, and have personality traits that fit with existing staff and residents."[10]

- University of California Davis Department of Urology

Other residency programs use the term "compatibility with the program." In a survey of PM&R PDs, DeLisa found that compatibility with the program was one of the three most important candidate traits, along with the ability to articulate thoughts and work with others.[11] In yet another study, PDs in 14 different specialties were asked to rank the importance of 6 personal and professional characteristics.[12] Compatibility with the program was highest. This was followed by commitment to hard work, fund of knowledge, empathy and compassion, and communication skills.

What are PDs looking for when they search for applicants with the right fit for their program? "Fit" can refer to qualities of the applicant that faculty members feel are essential to success in their program. In one study done by faculty in the department of radiology at the Baylor College of Medicine, the five qualities "deemed most appropriate for training radiologists" at Baylor were interpersonal skills, recognition of limits, curiosity, conscientiousness, and confidence level.[13]

"Fit" can also refer to qualities of the applicant that would help the program reach its goals. Some programs are committed to training future clinician-educators. Students with a stated interest and experience in areas of teaching and education, such as through their work or volunteer experience, would more convincingly demonstrate their fit with the program.

When strategizing for your application, you should plan to utilize techniques that will confirm your fit with a program. This begins with thorough research to determine the traits valued by the specialty. This is followed by thorough research of individual programs to determine valued traits and departmental goals. Although you already performed a thorough self-evaluation in the process of preparing your application, you need to repeat this step. What strengths do you exhibit that are highly valued by your specialty and targeted programs? At this point, you can formulate a compelling message as to why you would be the right resident for the program. Of course, your message doesn't mean anything without evidence to back it up. You must locate and present the evidence that confirms your fit with the program in the most compelling fashion possible.

Rule # 26 Research the specialty: What traits are valued by the specialty?

What traits are necessary to excel in your chosen field? What traits are valued by the members of the specialty? The chart on the following page shows some essential attributes in selected specialties.

By speaking with specialists in the field and researching specialty-specific websites, you can generate a similar list for your chosen specialty. Analyze your list. Which qualities do you share, and how have you demonstrated these qualities?

Essential Skills and Personal Qualities for the Future Resident in Selected Specialties	
Anesthesiology	Good manual dexterity Skillful at procedures Meticulous Ability to remain calm under stressful situations Ability to make quick decisions Warm and caring
Emergency Medicine	Good manual dexterity Ability to work with and manage a team Compassionate Ability to establish rapport quickly with variety of people Ability to multitask Strength to make tough decisions Ability to make quick decisions Prioritizes well Ability to remain calm during stressful situations Recognizes one's own limits and is not afraid to seek help
Family Medicine	Character traits that make a good family physician were identified by the Association of Family Medicine Residency Directors:[14] Compassion Enthusiasm to learn Excellent interpersonal skills Good work ethic Honesty
Neurology	Intellectual curiosity Diligent attitude Patience Comfort with ambiguity Openness to new diagnostic tests and treatments Intense interest in patient's story Fascination with nervous system
Neurological Surgery	In a survey of neurological surgeons, respondents were asked to rate the importance of 22 skills and attributes needed for successful completion of residency training. The top five characteristics identified were honesty, motivation, willingness to learn, ability to problem solve, and ability to handle stress. Although critical thinking, manual dexterity, and communication skills were also important, neurosurgeons believed that these skills could be more easily taught in contrast to the top characteristics.[15]
OB/GYN	Excellent interpersonal skills Communicate effectively with patients Ability to quickly adapt to different environments Enthusiasm Energy
Ophthalmology	Compassion Meticulous attention to detail Excellent manual dexterity

Orthopedic Surgery	In one article, qualities which the authors felt were anecdotally associated with better performing residents included trustworthiness, hard-working, efficient, detail-oriented, and personable.[16]
Otolaryngology	Ability to work well as part of a multidisciplinary team Good manual dexterity Superb technical skills Ability to quickly make sound clinical decisions Effectively listening to patients' problems and concerns
Radiology	Ability to interact effectively with a wide variety of clinicians and patients Good written and spoken communication skills Willingness to seek help when necessary Meticulous Thorough Good problem-solving and decision-making skills

Rule # 27 Research the individual programs.

By virtue of training many residents over the years, directors of residency programs have identified qualities they believe are essential to a resident's performance at their institution. Your application should emphasize the fact that you embody the traits that the residency program seeks in a resident.

In the table below is a partial list of personal qualities that are valued by residency programs (also included in Chapter 13: Before the Interview). In each section of this book, we've reviewed these traits, and how to successfully emphasize them. These traits form the foundation of how well you would fit with a residency program.

Personal Qualities Valued by Residency Programs		
Ability to work with a team Ability to solve problems Ability to manage stress Enthusiasm Energy Flexibility Effective time management Efficient problem-solving Confidence without arrogance Recognition of limits Responsibility	Willingness to admit error Perseverance Initiative Intelligence Maturity Motivation Communication skills Conscientiousness Listening skills Professional competence	Positive attitude Reliability Honesty Dedication Compassion Curiosity Determination Work ethic High values Poise

All programs value these personal qualities, and your application in its entirety should project them. Some programs will further delineate qualities they find most valuable in a resident. For example, the Department of

Orthopedic Surgery at Duke University states that "residents are selected for interview on the basis of preparedness, ability, aptitude, academic credentials, communication skills, and personal qualities such as motivation and integrity...Important intangibles which are fundamental to the selection process include leadership, work ethic, communication skills, and enthusiasm."[17]

For many programs, valued qualities won't be that clearly defined. You'll need to determine any distinguishing characteristics that are not clearly stated. For example, a program centered in a multi-ethnic community serves a diverse population. Obviously, this program would value individuals with experience or an interest in serving a diverse population. Excellent communication skills and the ability to handle added obstacles in this type of population are critical. Characteristics of a program's patient population may be described on the program's website or in informational brochures. You may be able to determine the traits most valued by the program based on its features and the areas where the program's resources are concentrated.

Unique Features of Selected Residency Programs
Cooper University Hospital Internal Medicine Residency: Among the unique features of this program is its "Resident as Teacher Curriculum." This curriculum "covers a range of topics including team leadership, bedside teaching, leading effective rounds, and giving and receiving feedback. Resident-led work rounds are frequently observed by senior medical educators, after which residents are provided with brief and focused feedback designed to foster leadership and management skills that would otherwise not be addressed in any formal curriculum."[18]
East Carolina General Surgery Residency: "One year of the residency is devoted to research. The research year sharpens technical skills, provides rigorous training in research methodology, ensures an academically competitive curriculum vitae, fosters national research networking opportunities, and provides time for reflection and creativity. In cooperation with the ECU School of Business we have implemented a program to allow the optional use of the surgery research year to obtain the MBA degree."[19]
Christ Hospital / UC Family Medicine: "Our program is known nationally for its longitudinal training in Global Health...Our curriculum reflects this commitment, featuring integrated global health rotations, monthly global health conferences, diverse scholarship opportunities, and strong community medicine experiences...Residents enjoy fully funded trips during their first two years and $2000 towards a third-year experience. Our dedicated faculty members have broad experience as long-and short-term medical providers in Honduras, Cambodia, Cameroon and Armenia."[20]

Another component of fit is dependent on the goals of the department. For example, if the program is committed to producing future clinician-educators, would you be the ideal candidate to help them reach their goal? If the program is committed to an understanding of the mind-body dynamic in treating medical illness, would your strengths and achievements suggest that you could help the program attain this goal? Other goals may include the training of future leaders in the specialty, enhancement of physician-patient communication, enhancement of care for rural populations, or enhancing the practice of evidence-based medicine, among a host of other goals. These goals may be reflected in the program's mission statement, may be described in their informational materials, or may be voiced by their faculty.

Rule # 28 **Evaluate your experiences in order to emphasize your unique, individual qualities.**

In a sea of extremely well-qualified applicants, how do you distinguish yourself? You can't rely on your class rank and great USMLE scores, because for competitive programs, those alone won't set you apart and won't make application reviewers sit up and take notice. You need to emphasize your individual strengths. Ideally, you'll emphasize to selection committee members that you embody all the traits that they are seeking in a resident.

One of the first steps in the application process is an analysis of your career to date. What have you accomplished? What have your attendings written about you in your formal evaluations? What comments have residents or attendings made about your performance on rotations? (For example, "highly inquisitive" "very compassionate" "excellent teacher to junior students" "dedicated" "meticulous") What have you been recognized for by your attendings? By your peers? What have you studied? Where have you worked? What did you bring to your work? What did you accomplish at work? Where have you volunteered? What did you learn about yourself from your volunteer experience? What extracurricular activities have you been involved in? What leadership positions have you held? What activities do you participate in outside of medicine?

At the end of this analysis, you need to answer this question: What types of qualities do these activities highlight? Rules 1 and 2 delineate some of the qualities valued by specialties and programs. Use these lists as a springboard for performing your self-evaluation.

Corollary to this Rule

The corollary to this rule is just as important. You can ask yourself, "What am I known for?" However, you also need to ask yourself, "What do I wish to be known for?"

What do you envision as the qualities of the ideal physician? What would you like others to say about you as an individual and as a physician? The processes of self-evaluation and striving for improvement should always remain a priority.

Rule # 29 **Formulate your message. Make sure that each component of your application reinforces this message.**

"We have so many good applicants this year. Tell me why we should accept you."

The entire residency application process boils down to this one question. And yet, when we've asked this question in interviews, we've received so many truly unconvincing answers:

- "I think you'll find that I'm a real team player."
- "I realize that everyone today has great scores, or they wouldn't have been invited to interview. I think you should accept me because I have a very strong work ethic, and I've always brought 100% to whatever I do."
- "I'm sure it must be very difficult for you to decide, because everyone going into derm is so strong. I'm a very hard worker, and I would do whatever is needed to be done."
- "I'm very enthusiastic, and I would get along very well with the other residents."
- "I'm a very fun person to be with, and I would bring that to the program."
- "Well, you're right, you have excellent applicants. I'm sure everyone has great credentials. You'll find that I'm a real people person, and I work well with my colleagues no matter where I am."
- "I'm a very hard worker, and you'll find that I would come to work every day on time, ready to get the work done."
- "I'm a real team player."

Are some of these sounding good to you? Decent answers, the kind you yourself might give? Sorry, but no. These answers could be given by just about any applicant, and they tell us nothing about you as an individual. They provide no evidence. They don't tell us *why* you would be an ideal fit for our program. They don't tell us specifically what you as an individual could bring to our program.

In some dermatology programs, there are well over 100 applicants for each residency position. We're not thinking about what we can do for each individual applicant. Our focus is on the program. How well will this applicant match the goals of our program? How well will they fit with our program? What can this applicant bring to the specialty? Certain baseline qualities are assumed. To have gotten this far in your career, you are assumed to be hard-working, enthusiastic about your work and calling, and able to get along well with others. To stand out from other applicants, you must have an individual, convincing message.

As you start the application process, one of your primary goals is to formulate your message. Give a concise answer as to why the program should accept you. *Every aspect of your application must reinforce this message.*

Many books and articles have been written about creating a compelling message, and there are many different ways of approaching the same basic objective. Marketers write entire books on the subject. What makes your product so special? Can you convince a customer to buy your product? For entrepreneurs they call it the "elevator pitch." You meet a venture capitalist in the elevator. Can you convince her to invest in your company? Workplace experts call the same process "self-branding." What are you known for? How can you bring value to a company?

When formulating your message for a residency selection committee, you need to convince them that you would be the right resident for their program. What type of physician will you be? Compassionate, hard-working, focused, driven? Will your goals mesh with those of the program? What unique strengths and qualities do you possess that can help the residency program achieve its goals?

Your message may not gel until you've done the initial work of the application process. Brainstorming for your CV and your personal statement are critical components, especially as this process will highlight your own strengths and accomplishments. The substance of the message will be based on the work you've already done. If you're in your fourth year, you may not recognize the evidence that exists in your past experiences and evaluations. If you're still in your third year, even better: you have time to provide tangible evidence to support your message about your fit for the program.

Case 1

Joyce is a student from a middle tier medical school with an average transcript and an average USMLE score. She's applying to several competitive internal medicine programs. When asked why the program should choose her, she could say that she's a hard worker, and would get along well with the other residents, and that would be entirely true. Instead, her response:

"You'll find that I give 100% to my patients, and I try very hard to involve the patient and their family in their own care. Several of my attendings have half-jokingly commented on my 'second job' in the patient education resource center at our teaching hospital, but several of the letters I've gotten back from former patients have made it worth it. I know that Lutheran General emphasizes an understanding of the family and community dynamic in the care of each individual patient, and that's one of the reasons that I would love to be here."

Her message: She is passionate about the care of her patients and works very hard to see that they're taken care of. She is very interested in patient education as part of that process.

Each piece of her application reinforces this message:

- Several of her attendings have included supporting comments in the written section of her formal clerkship evaluations. "Joyce works very hard to see that her patients are well taken care of, in all respects. I saw one of my patients in the clinic, and he related to me how much Joyce had helped him with the materials that she provided from the American Cancer Society."

- Joyce asked for LORs from two of the attendings who had commented on this quality in her end of clerkship meeting.
- The MSPE, in the narrative section summarizing attending evaluations, included two such comments verbatim.
- In her CV, she highlighted her past experiences of volunteering for the American Cancer Society on an ongoing basis for two years and her involvement in multiple health fairs.
- She did an elective with a well-regarded preventive medicine attending and specifically asked for opportunities to participate in a case report or other publication. Dr. Seveta asked her to author a patient information brochure that was to be published in a nursing journal, and it was accepted for publication.
- Her personal statement discussed a memorable patient who was only partially compliant with diabetes care recommendations.
- She came prepared to reinforce this message during her interviews. What's your greatest strength? Tell us about a memorable patient. What are you looking for in a program? Where do you see yourself ten years from now? Each of her answers was supported by evidence.

Case 2

Rita was a very soft-spoken student with average grades and average scores. During the interview, when asked about her publications, she simply replied that one was a review article on reactions to chemotherapy, and one was a case report about an interesting patient she had seen in clinic.

When asked where she saw herself in ten years, she simply replied that she wanted to go back to her hometown rural community, which lacked dermatologists. She stated that she would have liked to be more involved in academics and teaching, but there were not academic programs in the area. The overall impression she created was that of a nice, average applicant.

I quizzed her more extensively in an informal meeting, and here her message came across much stronger. She was very nice and soft-spoken, but was also passionate about patient care and the field of dermatology. Her strong work ethic was already evidenced by her LORs and her publications, but she needed to send that message more clearly during the interview. She was ready to emphasize that her goal was to practice in a rural, underserved area, and to become a source of expertise for the primary care physicians in the area.

Interviewer: Tell me about one of your publications.

One of the most interesting publications I worked on was the review article on cutaneous reactions to chemotherapy. Dr. Sentry needed to submit the final publication in four weeks, and I was concerned because it was the first dermatology article I had worked on. But once I got started, the information was fascinating, and even though it was a challenge, we submitted it on time. The finished publication had over 100 references, and I'm very proud that it was such a thorough review.

Interviewer: Tell me about an interesting patient you had.

Stella was a one-year old girl with a large hemangioma on her face. She was seen by her pediatrician in a rural area that didn't have any dermatologists, and the pediatrician was used to dealing with dermatology cases on his own. The parents were told that hemangiomas eventually resolve on their own, and no treatment was needed. However, the hemangioma was obstructing her vision, a key criterion for aggressive therapy. Stella was now blind. I was so saddened to think that this was an entirely preventable case of blindness, and it really emphasized to me how much access to a specialist would have helped that baby and that pediatrician, and how there are still underserved areas in this country.

Interviewer: Where do you see yourself in ten years?

I've always wanted to go back to my rural community to practice. I really see myself serving as a source of information to the primary care physicians and nurse practitioners in the area. I've spent a lot of time working and volunteering in tutoring and educational programs, as you can see from my CV, and I'd like to create some formal programs of education in the area.

Rule # 30 Your message doesn't mean much without the evidence to back it up.

If you're applying to a competitive specialty, you'll hear statements like the following:

- "Don't even bother to apply unless you're AOA."
- "They screen out applications based on minimum USMLE scores."
- "You need to have an outstanding transcript, or they won't even look at your application."

There is some truth to these statements.

Programs that receive an overwhelming number of applications are forced to seek out tangible evidence of a student's qualifications. Membership in AOA, USMLE scores, and the MSPE summary statement: all of these provide easily quantified data.

However, students sometimes focus exclusively, and erroneously, on such academic criteria. The assumption is that once you've reached a certain academic level, getting into the residency program of your choice is guaranteed. However, personal traits are given greater weight than applicants usually realize.

Programs want residents who can learn the material and pass the boards. However, it takes a lot more than that to be an outstanding resident. Programs seek residents who: are hard-working, excited about patient care, compassionate, involved in patient education, interested in improving their communities, exhibit manual dexterity, are able to handle the pressures of residency, will contribute to the specialty in some meaningful fashion, and on and on. All of these criteria are important to programs, and none can be easily quantified. How do you prove you're hard-working? How do you prove you're passionate about the field of anesthesiology? How can a program know how well you get along with others?

Your job is to provide the evidence that backs up each of these claims. A program isn't going to just take your word for it. Anybody can say that they're hard-working, and pretty much everyone does. You're going to have to provide tangible evidence. Many of the most important criteria are those for which tangible evidence is not easy to come by. That's why students who can convincingly capture the presence of these qualities and support them with evidence are so notable.

Your past experiences contain many such examples of evidence. It can be difficult to initially recognize them as such. Your work as an anatomy teaching assistant, for example, was far more than just employment experience. Analyze your work experience. What did your experience reveal about your strengths and about you as an individual? How can you successfully highlight this evidence? Do the same with all of your honors, work experience, volunteer experience, research experience, publications, presentations, and outside activities.

Following are examples of how applicants presented information in ERAS and the message conveyed by this information. By changing the emphasis, adding crucial details, or expanding upon the information, the applicant can substantiate their message. The information can then serve as evidence to back up their message. In the following examples, the use of evidence sends a message with greater impact.

Information in ERAS: Work experience September 1999-December 1999 Served as an anatomy teaching assistant.
Message: This student has teaching experience.
Evidence: September 1999-December 19999 Anatomy teaching assistant; position awarded to two students per year by invitation of anatomy faculty. Instructed first-year medical students in anatomy lab, created 10 dissection lesson plans, and led an additional 10 discussion sessions.
Message: This student has successfully emphasized that he values teaching, and was recognized for his abilities to teach. The preparation of ten lesson plans is a significant commitment of time, energy, and effort, and his transcript confirms that he was able to maintain excellent grades during this time period.

Information in the personal statement: I'm a very hard worker, and one of my strengths is attention to detail. I bring these qualities to everything that I do, especially in issues of patient care.
Message: This student believes she is a hard worker.
Evidence: *With all my might, I tightened the knob one last time. Bending over the gas tank, I placed my nose just millimeters away from the connection site and took in a deep breath. No smell of gas could be detected. With drops of water on my palms, I rubbed a bar of soap for a couple of minutes. I coated the soap suds over the connection site and waited for signs of bubbling but saw none. Gingerly, I turned on the stove and lit a match. What a sigh of relief! No explosion.* I am always systematic and detailed in my work. Whether the job is a routine replacement of the portable gas tank for the stove, gathering data for my research projects, or taking care of my patients at the hospital, my performance has always been thorough.
Message: This student is systematic and detailed, and has demonstrated these traits in multiple ways.

Information in the interview: What is your greatest strength? I'm a very hard worker and I bring 100% to everything that I do.
Message: This student believes she is a hard worker.
Evidence: What is your greatest strength? I think my perseverance. When I first conceived of the idea of the pre-natal and post-natal classes in the city school district, the faculty were on board immediately, but we hit a lot of logistical issues with the school administration. I had to work through a number of issues, but I'm very proud of the fact that our first classes started this year.
Message: This student is innovative, persistent, and willing to work hard to reach a goal.

Information in ERAS: The Erin Kelley Award 2006
Message: This student won an award.
Evidence: The Erin Kelley Award 2006 – awarded to one student per year who embodies compassion in patient care; voted on by peers.
Message: This student is known for her compassion, to the point that she was the single individual recognized by her peers for her compassion in patient care.

Information in ERAS: Work experience 2003-2004 Physician Director, Karachi Ob/Gyn Associates, Karachi, Pakistan. Supervised a team of healthcare professionals.
Message: This physician has clinical experience as an Ob/Gyn.
Evidence: Work experience 2003-2004 Physician Director, Karachi Ob/Gyn Associates, Karachi, Pakistan Supervised team of 20 healthcare professionals in clinic responsible for the care of 3000 obstetrics and gynecology patients.
Message: The concrete numbers and action verbs used in this CV provide evidence of the responsibility she was entrusted with as a physician director, and documents her significant clinical experience and the type of heavy workload to which she is accustomed.

Information in ERAS: Hobbies and interest: Varsity college volleyball player
Message: This student played college volleyball.
Evidence: In the personal statement, this student fleshed out the lessons she learned from her time in collegiate athletics. She wrote about her work ethic, ability to handle a challenging schedule, her lessons in prioritizing, and lessons on teamwork.
Message: The traits she developed and displayed through her time in varsity college volleyball are the same traits that a program seeks in its residents, and are the traits that have contributed to her reputation as an excellent clinician, as per her MSPE and clinical evaluations.

Information in ERAS: Participant in the Susan A. Albert junior-senior mentor program 9/2014-5/2015.
Message: This applicant served as a mentor.
Evidence: Invited by the faculty panel to serve in the Susan A. Albert junior-senior high mentor program. Mentored two adolescent middle-schoolers with learning disabilities. Met weekly with mentee, discussed any personal or academic school issues, and tutored in the subjects of English and science.
Message: The applicant was invited to serve, and thus this is recognition of his abilities. He gained tutoring experience. Serving as a mentor to a child for a one-year time period, and meeting weekly, is a significant effort and demonstrates commitment.

The concept of presenting evidence in your application is easy to understand. It sounds great. And we make it sound so easy. However, we do recognize the difficulties involved. How can you identify and present evidence when you're not even sure what you're really known for? What if it seems as though you're not that outstanding?

Each section of this book walks you through this process. Your experiences in patient care provide the best opportunities to demonstrate those qualities that would make you an outstanding resident. Each rotation provides multiple opportunities to demonstrate your work ethic, your compassion, your commitment to patient education, your ability to work well with a team, and many other traits. After you've demonstrated your skills in patient care, add in other experiences that can serve to illustrate your best traits. Make presentations during your rotations. Look for opportunities to be published in your field. Reflect on your past work experiences. Seek out opportunities for clinical or basic science research, depending on your interests. Continue your volunteer commitments. Don't neglect your outside pursuits.

We discuss how to strengthen your application in this type of concrete fashion in much greater detail throughout this book. Our companion book, *Success on the Wards: 250 Rules for Clerkship Success*, reviews how to excel in clinical rotations. In this book, Chapter 10, "The Audition Elective," goes into further detail on how to excel during an audition elective. Opportunities to give talks may arise during clerkships or audition electives and should be fully utilized. Our companion book also provides explicit directions on how to give an outstanding talk. In this book, Chapter 4, "The Competitive Edge," provides further guidance on how to locate opportunities to participate in publications and research, and how to make the most of these opportunities. If you're applying to a competitive residency program, these sections are a must. Strengthening your application is much easier if you have sufficient lead time. If you're reading this book in your third year, you can make significant strides in improving your candidacy. However, even as a fourth-year student, you can actively create and present further evidence. These same opportunities exist for residents applying to a different field, or for practicing physicians seeking additional training.

Rule # 31 Present it all in a powerful package.

In each section of this book, we discuss how to create a perfect package. By perfect, we mean *perfect*. This is a painstaking process, and you need to follow the guidelines exactly. Your CV and personal statement must be in the proper format, the correct length, and completely free of any grammatical or spelling errors. When members of a residency selection committee are reviewing hundreds of applications, even a single such error can be grounds for exclusion. If this applicant made a mistake on such an important document, how are they going to handle the tenth admission of the night?

The perfect package also means that your application is noticed. You may have great grades and great scores, and your application may be free of errors, but that won't always be enough to make members of the residency selection committee notice your application. You need to include the type of information that convinces committee members that you would be the right resident for their program, and you need to highlight that information in such a way that they notice it.

We've discussed how to formulate your message and how to collect the evidence that backs it up. In Rule # 30, we've given examples of how the same experience, presented in a different manner, can send a completely different message. The remainder of this book goes over, in comprehensive detail, how to prepare each component of your application so that your candidacy is presented in a powerful package.

References

[1]Otero H, Erturk S. Ondategui-Parra S, Ros P. Key criteria for selection of radiology residents: results of a national survey. *Acad Radiol* 2006, 13: 1155-1164.

[2]Villanueva A, Kaye D, Abdelhak S, Morahan P. Comparing selection criteria for residency directors and physicians' employers. *Acad Med* 1995; 70(4): 261-271.

[3]University of Buffalo Department of Anesthesiology. Available at: http://www.smbs.buffalo.edu/anest/residency_application_process.php. Accessed January 22, 2016.

[4]University of Michigan Department of Dermatology. Available at: https://wiki.umms.med.umich.edu/display/DERM/Resident+Selection+Process. Accessed February 2, 2016.

[5]Morristown Medical Center Department of Medicine. Available at: http://www.atlantichealth.org/morristown/for+professionals/residents+&+fellows/residency+programs/internal+medicine/application+process/. Accessed February 2, 2016.

[6]Wayne State University Department of Neurosurgery. Available at: http://neurosurgery.med.wayne.edu/resident_selection.php. Accessed February 2, 2016.

[7]Duke University Department of Anesthesiology. http://anesthesiology.duke.edu/wp-content/uploads/2013/08/AIG-how-to-interview.pdf. Accessed February 2, 2016.

[8]LSU Department of Obstetrics & Gynecology. Available at: https://www.medschool.lsuhsc.edu/ob_gyn/residency.aspx. Accessed February 2, 2016.

[9]West Virginia University Department of Orthopedic Surgery. Available at: http://medicine.hsc.wvu.edu/ortho/residency/application/. Accessed February 2, 2016.

[10]University of California Davis Department of Urology. Available at: http://ucdmc.ucdavis.edu/urology/education/residency_program/index.html. Accessed February 2, 2016.

[11]DeLisa J, Jain S, Campagnolo D. Factors used by physical medicine and rehabilitation residency training directors to select their residents. *Am J Phys Med Rehabil* 1994; 73: 152-156.

[12]Wagoner N, Suriano J, Stoner J. Factors used by program directors to select residents. *J Med Educ* 1986; 61(1): 10-21.
[13]Lamke N, Watson A, Fisher R. Radiology resident selection: objective restructured interview to assess five essential attributes. *SQU Journal for Scientific Research: Medical Sciences* 2003; 5(1-2): 27-30.
[14]Robinson M, Callaway P, Palmer E, Kozakowski S, Jones S, Carr S, Carek P, Cobb S, Gravel J, Balachandra S. Core character traits for family medicine. *Ann Fam Med* 2008; 6(3): 278.
[15]Myles S, McAleer S. Selection of neurosurgical trainees. *Can J Neurol Sci* 2003; 30(1): 26-30.
[16]Nemani V, Park C, Nawabi D. What makes a "great resident": the resident perspective. *Curr Rev Musculoskelet Med* 2014; 7: 164-167.
[17]Duke University Department of Orthoapedic Surgery. Available at: https://ortho.duke.edu/education-and-training/residency/orthopaedic-surgery-residency/apply. Accessed February 2, 2016.
[18]Cooper University Hospital Internal Medicine Residency. Available at: http://www.cooperhealth.edu/residencies/internal-medicine/clinical-experience. Accessed February 2, 2016.
[19]East Carolina General Surgery Residency. Available at: http://www.ecu.edu/cs-dhs/surgery/residency/. Accessed February 2, 2016.
[20]University of Cincinnati Department of Family and Community Medicine. Available at: http://www.familymedicine.uc.edu/education/residency/christ.aspx. Accessed March 2, 2016.

Chapter 6

Letters of Recommendation

Letters of recommendation are a critical component of the residency application. The purpose of these letters is to demonstrate to programs that you have both the professional and personal qualities to succeed as a resident and, later, as a practicing physician. Since these letters are written by those who know you and the quality of your work, they offer programs a personalized view. In contrast to your transcript and USMLE scores, they supply programs with qualitative, rather than quantitative information, about your cognitive and non-cognitive characteristics. A number of studies have shown that behavior, attitude, and other non-cognitive skills are important predictors of resident success. As such, programs place great importance on these letters in evaluating your application.

Since you will not be directly writing these letters, it may seem as if you have no control over their content. In reality, you wield more influence than you realize.

Rule # 32 Letters of recommendation are extremely important in some specialties.

In a 2006 study of medical students at the University of Colorado, University of Utah, and Vanderbilt University, participants were asked to rate the importance of sixteen residency selection criteria.[1] While 65% of survey participants rated the letters of recommendation extremely important, 35% felt that letters were either moderately, mildly, or not important at all. This underlines the misconceptions that students hold about the selection process. Although awareness of letters' importance in the residency selection process has increased over the past ten years, our experience has shown that many students continue to underestimate the value placed on letters by programs.

In a NRMP survey of nearly 1,800 program directors across 21 specialties, 86% cited letters as a factor used to make interview decisions (versus 75% in 2008). Letters of recommendation received a mean rating of 4.2 on a scale of 1 (not at all important) to 5 (very important).[2] A number of studies have looked at the importance of recommendation letters in the residency selection process. These studies have demonstrated that letters are an important factor in selecting candidates for interview and in the development of the program's rank list.

Importance of Letters of Recommendation in Residency Selection	
Study	**Findings**
In personal research performed by Greenburg, surgical residency program directors were surveyed. Directors were asked to rank the various factors they consider important when ranking candidates.[3]	Recommendation letters from surgical faculty were the second most important factor following only the interview. Letters from nonsurgical faculty were fifth most important.
Questionnaire sent to all PM&R program directors in the U.S. asking about the relative importance of various application factors. Directors were asked to rate factors on a scale of 1 to 5 with 1 being unimportant and 5 being critical.[4]	Letters of recommendation were the second most important candidate criteria (3.7 + 0.9) that program directors use as they complete their Match list, second only to the interview.
Questionnaire sent to emergency medicine program directors asking them to rank 20 application items on a scale of 1 to 5, with 5 being most important.[5]	Letters of recommendation were fourth most important (mean score of 4.11) following emergency medicine rotation grades, interview, and clinical grades.
Review of every letter of recommendation for the emergency medicine residency program at the Christ Hospital during the 1998-1999 application cycle.[6]	Offered insight into the match list ranking process at one residency program. Letters of recommendation accounted for 16% of an applicant's score.
Survey sent to all radiology residency program directors asking them about the criteria that departments use for selecting their residents.[7]	Letters of recommendation were the fourth most important criterion in selecting candidates for interview, behind USMLE scores, Dean's letter, and class rank.
Survey of dermatology residency program directors. Participants were asked to rate 25 criteria on a scale of 1 (not at all important) to 10 (extremely important).[8]	Criteria were subdivided into four groups based on the rating. Only two criteria were considered very important – interview and letters of recommendation.
Survey of neurosurgical residency program directors[9]	Most important factors identified in the selection process were the interview, USMLE Step 1 scores, and letters of recommendation.
Survey of ophthalmology residency program directors[10]	Four factors were deemed most important in the selection process – interview, clinical course grades, letters of recommendation, and board scores.

Rule # 35 **Your letter writers can make your career, so choose the correct ones.**

Your goal is to secure a glowing letter of recommendation. You'll never know exactly what a potential letter writer would say about you, so this poses a challenge. First, seek out attending physicians who gave you an honors evaluation. Because most students will be able to review their clerkship evaluations at the end of the rotation, this is straightforward. However, it's only the start. You must take into consideration a number of other issues. If you can answer the following questions with a "yes," then consider the individual to be a potential letter writer:

- Did I do well in the letter writer's rotation?
- Does the writer think highly of me?
- Did I work closely with the writer?
- Can the writer include specific experiences from our work together that reflect my strengths?
- Does the writer care about me and my future?
- Can he or she write a letter that will best reflect my background and strengths?
- Does the writer have good communication skills?
- Is the writer known to reliably meet deadlines?

We agree fully with the advice of Dr. Greenburg of Brown University. In his article on recommendation letters, he writes that "students need to select someone whom they feel knows them and their performance well and who is concerned and committed enough to the student's career to write a well thought out, detailed, and positive appraisal of them. We have seen that some letters, written on behalf of excellent applicants, did not do them justice because their authors were brief, vague, and/or noncommittal."[3]

Did you know?

In a survey of writers who wrote letters for applicants applying to a baccalaureate-M.D. program, participants were asked about how they would handle a request for a letter from an applicant with whom they had little contact.[13] Sixteen percent stated that they would write a letter, but that it would be generic, containing little detail. It's likely that many medical school faculty would do the same, an important point to note as you decide whom to ask for a letter.

Rule # 36 **Request letters from medical school faculty**

Avoid asking residents, interns, family, friends, or basic science professors. Solicit letters from faculty members of U.S. medical schools who are familiar with your clinical skills. You may also choose to request a letter of recommendation from a faculty member you assisted in performing research, if he knows you well, and especially if you plan on making research a big part of what you do in the future. Faculty members in the department of emergency medicine at the University of California San Diego and University of California Irvine wrote that "research mentors can provide effective letters of recommendation, assuming they also know the clinical skills of the applicant."[14] Your other letters of recommendation, however, must come from clinical faculty.

Tip # 9

Before you request a letter from a resident or a private physician, consider the words of Dr. Mark Farnie, director of the internal medicine/pediatrics residency program at the University of Texas Medical School at Houston, who wrote that "letters of recommendation from private physicians or part-time faculty, and letters from residents are generally discounted."[15]

Did you know?

Directors of 102 internal medicine residency programs were surveyed to determine the most important predictors of performance for international medical graduates Directors were asked to rate the importance of 22 selection criteria. Rated lowest were letters of recommendation from a foreign country. "Only 7% of the program directors disagreed with the statement that such letters are useless." In another words, 93% of the program directors agreed that such letters were useless. The results of this study confirm that international medical graduates are better served by submitting letters of recommendation from U.S. faculty.[16]

Rule # 37 **Choose a writer who knows how to write a letter of recommendation**

Writing effective letters of recommendation is both an art and a science. Unfortunately, few faculty members have received training in this area. Your letter writer should be aware of the norms of letter writing by persons of professional standing. Also of importance is the person's writing ability. A professor may have very positive things to say about you, but if he can't express himself well, he won't be able to effectively convey his favorable views.

How can you possibly learn about a professor's writing ability? Examine your clerkship evaluation. Pay close attention to how well the attending has worded your evaluation. A favorable evaluation that has been eloquently worded suggests a comparable letter. If at all possible, ask upperclassmen about their experience.

Rule # 38 Choose a writer who actually cares about your career.

When choosing among possible writers, select faculty members who care about you and your future. Such faculty members will spend the time and energy necessary to write an effective, well thought out, and carefully written letter. They will be committed to you and your goals, and will want to provide you with whatever assistance is needed in order to help you succeed. Ideally, they will also be available to handle any phone inquiries from the residency program.

At every medical school, there are many professors who have a sincere interest in mentoring, advising, and helping their students reach their professional goals. As you progress through clerkships, have your radar up for these faculty members. Some will be easy to spot, such as the professor who is so impressed with your performance that he volunteers to write you a letter of recommendation. With others, question if the professor has shown interest in your work, goals, and plans.

Tip # 10

If you haven't had the opportunity to work with someone whom you feel cares about you and your goals, ask upperclassmen and fellow students about faculty members who take an active interest in the careers of their students. Once you've identified these individuals, arrange to work with them.

Rule # 39 The professional status of a letter writer is important, but isn't everything.

How important is the letter writer's professional status? Clearly it's an important consideration. A glowing letter written by a distinguished full professor carries more weight than one written by an associate professor. Likewise, a letter written by an associate professor is preferred over one written by an assistant professor. Clinical instructors and chief residents would be options of last resort. Many feel that an applicant should never request a letter from a resident.

Did you know?

In a survey of program directors in four specialties (internal medicine, pediatrics, family medicine, surgery), it was learned that a candidate's likelihood of being considered was enhanced if there was a connection or relationship between the writer and residency program director. "In cases where there was both a connection between the faculty members and in-depth knowledge of the student (i.e., personal knowledge), the likelihood was that the student's application would be noted."[17] In another survey, 54% of orthopedic surgery program directors felt that the most important aspect of a letter was that it was written by someone they knew.[18]

Did you know?

In one study, academic rank of the writer was found to be an important factor influencing the reviewer's ranking of the letter. Forty-eight percent of the reviewers rated it as important.[3]

Why does professional status matter? Acclaimed professors are likely to have developed relationships with faculty at other institutions. In fact, they often interact at conferences, collaborate on projects, and publish papers based on shared work. When program directors and members of the resident selection committee receive a strong letter of recommendation from a colleague whom they know and trust, it can make a tremendous difference. Obviously, the letter carries more weight than a similar letter from a junior faculty member whom they don't know. The following table taken from a survey of PM&R program directors supports this belief. This study showed that the "most important letters of recommendation were from a PM&R faculty member in the respondent's department, followed by the Dean's letter, and the PM&R chairman's letter."[4]

Results of Mean Ratings of the Importance of Letters of Recommendation in Selecting Residents

	Mean Score
Clinical PM&R faculty member in respondent's department	4.0
Dean's letter	3.7
Chairperson of a PM&R department	3.7
PM&R faculty member in a PM&R department other than the respondents	3.6
Clinical faculty member in another specialty	3.0
Basic scientist's letter	2.6

DeLisa J, Jain S, Campagnolo D. Factors used by physical medicine and rehabilitation residency training directors to select their residents. *Am J Phys Med Rehabil* 1994; 73: 152-6.

Many people in the academic community also feel that it is easier to impress junior rather than senior faculty members. Although this isn't necessarily true, those reviewing your application may be operating under that assumption. It that's the case, a letter from a junior faculty member won't be given the same weight as one from a full professor.

Having said this, you may be tempted to request letters from renowned figures. Unless that individual knows you well, resist the temptation. A stellar letter written by a junior faculty member with whom you've had significant interaction is much better than a lukewarm letter written by a senior faculty member of high stature. Applicants often lose sight of this fact, thinking that a letter written by Professor Bigwig, irrespective of its content, will do wonders for their application. In reality, a lukewarm letter will weaken your application.

Requesting a letter of recommendation from a professor who knows you well may prevent a letter of "minimal assurance." Messner and Shimahura defined this as a letter "missing one or more of the following attributes: 1) specific distinguishing information about an applicant 2) information about an applicant's academic record 3) an evaluation or comparison of the applicant's traits or accomplishments."[19] In their study of letters written on behalf of 204 applicants to the Stanford University otolaryngology residency program, 13.2% and 10.8% of female and male applicants, respectively, had a letter of "minimal assurance."

Tip # 11

While name recognition and status is important, it does you no good to submit a neutral or lukewarm letter from a well-known or distinguished faculty member. It is far better to submit a strong letter from a less known junior faculty member.

Did you know?

In the document titled "How to request a letter of recommendation," found on the website of the David Geffen School of Medicine at UCLA, advisors at that school state that "the ideal letter of recommendation is from an individual who:

Is a national recognized figure in your specialty of choice and is well known to other program directors in your field;

Has personally worked with you clinically;

Thinks you are a star; and

Came from the institution to which you are applying."[20]

Did you know?

In an article written by faculty in the departments of emergency medicine at the University of California San Diego and University of California Irvine, the authors wrote that "an exceptional letter from a respected faculty member may sway residency program directors to offer an applicant with non-competitive scores and evaluations an interview due to the importance programs place on clinical abilities. Therefore, it is valuable for a student to orchestrate time to work with a well-known EM faculty member, such as program director or assistant program director, clerkship director, research director, or Chief/Chair.[14]

Rule # 40 **Discuss your list of possible letter writers with your residency advisor or dean of student affairs**

Because they have counseled many students over the years, residency advisors and deans are often knowledgeable about professors who write great letters of recommendation. They may also steer you away from professors who are not good letter writers, including those who have missed deadlines in the past. Always discuss your list of possible letter writers with your advisor.

Tip # 12

Show your advisor or dean your list of potential letter writers. Ask them which of the professors on your list have been known to write timely, thoughtful, and positive letters.

Rule # 41 **The number of letters requested from faculty in the same specialty varies. Be familiar with the general recommendations for your specialty but realize that some programs will not follow these rules.**

Among the most common questions we receive from applicants at TheSuccessfulMatch.com is "How many letters do I need to get from faculty within my chosen specialty?" The answer to this question varies widely from specialty to specialty. As a general rule, the less competitive specialties ask for 1 or 2 letters from physicians in the field. Check with each program's website to ensure compliance with their policy.

Number of Letters Recommended From Faculty Within the Specialty	
Specialty	**Number of Letters**
Anesthesiology	1
Dermatology	At least 2
Emergency Medicine	2
Family Medicine	1
General Surgery	All
Internal Medicine	2
Neurology	1-2
Neurosurgery	2-3
Obstetrics & Gynecology	2
Ophthalmology	1
Orthopaedic Surgery	All
Otolaryngology	At least 2
Pathology	1-2
Pediatrics	At least 2
PM&R	1-2
Plastic Surgery	All
Psychiatry	1-2
Radiation Oncology	At least 2
Radiology	1
Urology	All

Rule # 42 **The chair's letter may be critical to your application. Plan accordingly, especially if you've never even met the chair.**

Some specialties either mandate or recommend that one of your letters come from the department chairman. If you've worked closely with the chairman during a clinical or research rotation and performed at a high level, this won't be a problem. Approach the chairman the same way you would any other faculty member.

However, many students haven't had the opportunity to interact with, let alone work with, the chairman. Don't worry if you've never met the chairman. Departments understand that many students interested in their specialty won't have had this opportunity. They typically have a policy in place for the writing of the chair's letter. To determine the policy at your school, call the department office.

Depending on the program, the chairman or his designee will write the letter. In order to do so, the chairman will typically ask for a CV, review your clerkship evaluation forms, and meet with you to learn more about you and your goals. Treat any meeting with the chairman as you would a formal interview. Bring with you any supporting materials that might be useful in the development of your letter, such as copies of journal articles or summaries of presentations.

Specialties Requiring Chairman's Letter	
Specialty	**Chairman's Letter Required?**
Anesthesiology	No
Dermatology	No
Emergency Medicine	No
Family Medicine	No
General Surgery	Recommended
Internal Medicine	Yes
Neurology	No
Neurosurgery	No
Obstetrics & Gynecology	Yes
Ophthalmology	No
Orthopedic Surgery	Yes
Otolaryngology	Yes
Pathology	No
Pediatrics	No
PM&R	No
Plastic Surgery	Yes
Psychiatry	No
Radiation Oncology	No
Radiology	No
Urology	Yes

Why would programs place such importance on the chairman's letter, given that most students don't even work with the chairman? In the article "Factors used by program directors to select residents," Wagoner and Suriano offered some possible reasons. They "speculated that the chairman is perceived as feeling less compelled to act as an advocate for the student and can, therefore, present a more factual portrayal of the student's performance in courses of that specialty. Further, because department chairmen are often in personal contact with each other by telephone and at professional meetings, the authors believe that it is important to the program directors to maintain their credibility with each other by giving credible evaluations."[21]

Did you know?

If you're applying for a specialty that doesn't require a Chairman's Letter, understand that there may be a few programs that are exceptions to the rule.

Rule # 43 **When asking for a letter, provide your writer with an out.**

There is a right way and a wrong way to request a letter of recommendation. Many students have approached us for a letter with "could you write a letter of recommendation for me?" *Anyone* can write you a letter, but the key question is whether they know you well enough to write a *strong* letter of recommendation. The correct way to phrase the question is this: "Dr. Desai, do you feel you know me and my work well enough to write me a strong letter of recommendation?"

By phrasing the request in this manner, your letter writer can politely opt out if he doesn't feel comfortable writing you a letter. Don't despair. A negative or even lukewarm letter written and sent can sink your application. Count yourself lucky to avoid that fate.

Even if a writer says that he will support your application with a letter, gauge their level of commitment. If they seem hesitant or ambivalent, then the recommendation letter may not be as positive as it could be. In this case, simply thank them for their time and let them know that you will ask another professor.

Tip # 13

Don't just ask for a letter of recommendation. Ask for a strong letter. Otherwise, you might have a faculty member simply agree to your request, not because he is a fervent supporter of your application, but because he feels it is another one of his many job responsibilities. This could lead to a poor letter.

Tip # 14

Writing an effective letter of recommendation takes time and effort. Not all letter writers are able to make that type of commitment. You, of course, would like to know that up front. How can you find out? Politely and delicately tell the letter writer that you realize he is busy, you understand how much effort and time it takes to write a letter, and you will understand if he can't make that commitment to you right now. This provides an easy way to opt out.

Rule # 44 **Ask for a letter of recommendation in the correct fashion.**

Never ask an individual for a letter of recommendation by:

- Asking in the hallway
- Passing a note under the door
- Leaving a note in the mailbox

- Asking him or her on the phone
- Leaving a voice mail message
- Sending an e-mail
- Approaching at a busy time, such as in between patients
- Making your request at the last minute

Doing any of the above is unprofessional and may make a difference in the strength of your recommendation letter. The best way to ask for a letter is by making an appointment.

Dr. Murthy, I would like to meet with you for fifteen minutes to get some advice on my career plans. Would you be able to meet with me, and if so, when would be a good time?

Remember that you are asking for a favor, one that takes time and effort. Don't take the request lightly. Be sensitive, polite, cordial, and formal.

Asking for a letter of recommendation in person also allows you another advantage – you can gauge the professor's level of interest in writing the letter. If you have any doubts at all about the letter writer, you must meet face to face. If there is any hesitancy, indifference, reluctance, or aversion on the letter writer's part, it will be more apparent to you in person than by phone or e-mail. Should this occur, simply thank the letter writer for his time and move on to the next potential writer on your lsit.

Tip # 15

Always ask for a letter of recommendation in person. Why? Not only is it more polite but it offers several other advantages. A face to face meeting reminds the faculty member of who you are and how you excelled. And last, but certainly not least, it allows you to gauge the person's response to your request.

Rule # 45 Empty praise means nothing. Your job is to provide the evidence that backs up the adjectives.

Unfortunately, many letters, while complimentary, are simply full of adjectives. They lack examples, stories, and anecdotes that support the adjectives used. Letters that include evidence to support the writer's opinions are much more effective and powerful than letters that simply praise. Details often convince the reader that the praise is actually true.

Typical recommendation: Lisa's intellectual curiosity was refreshing. In fact, few of my medical students have been as inquisitive. During rounds, this quality enriched the entire team's educational experience.

Powerful recommendation: Lisa's intellectual curiosity was refreshing. In fact, few of my medical students have been as inquisitive. During rounds, this quality enriched the entire team's educational experience. For example, she performed a literature search on a relatively newly described microorganism, *Leclercia adecarboxylata*, after our team took care of a pyelonephritis patient whose urine grew out this organism. Her search revealed that there were 21 published articles on this organism. She not only brought us each one of these abstracts, but she even had one article, which was published in French, translated into English.

To maximize the chances that your letter writers will provide evidence to support their opinions, choose writers who know you well enough that they can include specific anecdotes. Examples of evidence:

- She performed a literature search on a newly described microorganism.
- She was a great source of comfort to a family with newly diagnosed breast cancer. She provided patient information booklets from the hospital library, and when the patient expressed interest in attending a support group, investigated the options. The family wrote a heartfelt note of thanks at the end of the patient's stay.
- He was very enthusiastic about the learning process, and early in the rotation expressed his interest in writing a case report. When I identified a potential case, he had a first draft ready within 72 hours, with a full discussion, references, and very few revisions needed.
- I had asked for a volunteer to make a short presentation on diagnostic techniques for pulmonary embolism. He was the first to volunteer, and a few days later gave an outstanding presentation on the topic. He even provided handouts and an excellent reference article.
- As a sub-intern, she had a heavy case load and many duties. However, she clearly made quite an effort to help guide and educate the third-year students on the team.

Rule # 46 **You cannot tell your letter writer what to say. However, there are professional ways in which you can emphasize your strengths and the evidence that backs those up.**

Most applicants assume that their letter writers know what to say. That's a dangerous assumption to make. In an analysis of 116 recommendation letters received by radiology residency program at the University of Iowa Hospitals and Clinics, reviewers noted the following points:

- 10% of letters were missing information about an applicant's cognitive knowledge
- 35% of letters had no information about an applicant's clinical judgment
- 3% of letters did not discuss an applicant's work habits
- 17% of letters did not comment on the applicant's motivation
- 32% of letters were lacking information about interpersonal communication skills.[22]

In another review of recommendation letters sent during the 1999 application season to the Department of Surgery at Southern Illinois University, writers infrequently commented on psychomotor skills such as "easily performed minor procedures at the bedside," "good eye-hand coordination in the OR," "could suture well," and so on.[23]

If you simply assume that a letter writer knows precisely what to say about you, you may be doing yourself a disservice. To increase the chances that your letter writer will submit a letter commenting on those qualities valued by programs in your chosen specialty, you must first determine these qualities. In the following table, we have included qualities valued by program directors in four specialties.[17]

Skills and Personal Qualities Frequently Identified by Residency Program Directors in Defining an Applicant's "Fit"	
Family Medicine	Good communicator, interpersonal skills, team player, lifelong learning skills, empathic, interested in community practice, non-judgmental, active in the program, experience with underserved populations
Internal Medicine	Good communicator, interpersonal skills, team player, hands-on patient care, potential positive impact upon program, reliable and stable, warm and humane, demonstrated commitment to specific area (music, sports), well-organized, ability to get along with others, resourceful
Pediatrics	Good communicator, interpersonal skills, team player, well-organized, well-rounded, mature, independent, sense of professionalism, flexible (ability to change), enthusiastic, ability to cope with stress and change, positive attitude (views glass "half full")
Surgery	Good communicator, compulsive, neat, high energy, honest and straightforward, confident, hardworking, demonstrated commitment to specific area (music, sports)
Villanueva A, Kaye D, Abdelhak S, Morahan P. Comparing selection criteria for residency directors and physicians' employers. *Acad Med* 1995; 70(4): 261-71.	

If you are applying to a surgical residency, it would be great if your letter commented on your ability to perform procedures, suture in the OR, and maintain a high level of energy. However, directly asking the writer to comment on your abilities in these areas is presumptuous, and will be viewed negatively.

A more professional approach is to list patient encounters from your rotation. Include those encounters that highlight your strengths in these areas, and emphasize how these patient encounters impacted your training.

Sample Patient List

Dear Dr. Tung,

During our month together, I cared for a number of patients. Below are a few of these patients, along with my role in their care and the impact these patients had on my training:

1) Mr. J – 72-year old male with dementia with was hospitalized with small bowel obstruction due to adhesions from previous surgery. Managing the bowel obstruction was challenging because Mr. J sometimes became agitated, particularly at night. On three occasions, he pulled out his nasogastric tube. I had the opportunity to reinsert the tube each time and became quite comfortable inserting these tubes. I also learned how to better evaluate delirium in a patient with dementia.

2) Ms. H – 52-year old female with alcoholic cirrhosis who developed spontaneous bacterial peritonitis following incision and drainage of a skin abscess. To confirm the diagnosis, I was given the opportunity to perform the paracentesis under the supervision of Dr. Jones. Analysis of the ascitic fluid revealed findings consistent with monomicrobial bacterial ascites, prompting us to repeat the procedure 48 hours later. After performing the second tap, we were able to diagnose him with spontaneous bacterial peritonitis when his neutrophil count returned > 250.

3) Mr. F – 64-year old male with history of intravenous drug abuse who was admitted with appendicitis. Shortly after admission, his IV fell out. The nurses on the floor had difficulty inserting a new IV. Understandably, Mr. F was quite upset with these failed attempts and was reluctant to have anyone try again. After much discussion, he agreed to let me try. Having had considerable experience placing IVs as part of a hospital IV team before starting medical school, I was able to successfully insert the IV and build great rapport with the patient. I was thereafter known on our team as the "IV man."

I learned so much during my rotation, from these patients, from others, and from your teaching. Thank you very much for your teaching and for your letter of recommendation, and please let me know if you need any further information.

Sincerely,

Jorge Rubio

An attending reading the above might be inclined to comment on your ability to perform procedures. If he had forgotten about your involvement in Mr. J's care, your list will help to jog his memory. You should never assume that the writer remembers as much as you do.

This approach may facilitate the development of a letter highlighting certain skills or qualities. Include these examples in the letter of recommendation packet you give to your writers.

> **Tip # 16**
>
> In a survey of program directors in 14 specialties, directors were asked to rank the importance of six personal and professional characteristics.[24] Compatibility with the program was highest. This was followed by commitment to hard work, fund of knowledge, empathy and compassion, and communication skills. Provide your letter writers with patient examples that highlight your strengths in these areas.

> **Did you know?**
>
> In a study done to assess how faculty, specifically clerkship directors, rate letters of recommendation, researchers found that the most important factors were depth of understanding of the trainee (98% essential or important), numerical comparison to other students (94%), grade distribution (92%), and summary statement (91%).[25]

Rule # 47 Faint praise is just as bad as no praise

If your letter writer shares the letter with you, examine it carefully. It's a given that the writer will praise you. However, you need to be vigilant for faint praise. This is defined as praise that appears positive at first glance, but may not be viewed as such by a residency program. In an article discussing letters of recommendation for pediatric residency applicants, Dr. Morgenstern of the Mayo Clinic wrote that "some words, seemingly positive, are often considered ref flags. Calling a student's performance very good, so solid, may be viewed by program directors as a warning to avoid ranking the student very highly."[26] Below are other examples.

Faint Praise – What Does It Really Mean?	
Statement	**Translation**
"Shilpa's write-ups were solid."	Shilpa's write-ups were solid but not exceptional in any way.
"Roberto's knowledge base was above average."	Roberto's knowledge base was above average but not very far above average.
"Glen's oral case presentations clearly improved throughout the course of the rotation."	Glen's oral case presentations were subpar to begin with and required considerable work.
"As far as I'm aware…"	I don't want to wholeheartedly back this applicant because I don't know him that well.

Using the word "improved" can also be considered a red flag. While every student would be expected to show improvement during the course of a rotation, apparently the inclusion of the word "improved" suggests that the writer did not feel that the applicant was very strong in that area.

Notice how these comments on the surface seem to say good things about an applicant. However, the use of the above adjectives, rather than stronger ones, may lead the reader to wonder why the writer wasn't more enthusiastic about his choice of words.

As an applicant, you may wonder why your letter writer would "damn you with faint praise." While faint praise may be intentional, more often than not its use is entirely unintentional. Some writers are simply unaware that an unofficial hierarchy of superlatives exists. These well-intentioned writers may wish to give their highest recommendation to an applicant, but may unknowingly use an adjective considered by program directors to be a second or third-tier superlative.

Dr. Fortune of Southern Illinois University, in his article analyzing the content of recommendation letters, described this unofficial hierarchy of superlatives.[23] He commented on the fact that letter writers will often sum up an applicant using a particular adjective as in "Randy will make an exceptional house officer." He categorized these adjectives as shown:

Single Adjective Summary	
Outstanding	Outstanding, superior, exceptional, best, phenomenal
Excellent	Excellent, superb, great, terrific, wonderful
Good	Good, strong, solid, fine, valuable, splendid
OK	Asset, successful, delightful, distinguished, capable, effective, qualified, well rounded
Fortune J. The content and value of letters of recommendation in the resident candidate evaluative process. *Curr Surg* 2002; 59(1): 79-83.	

Fortune also writes about how writers generally provide, usually in the last paragraph, an indication of their comfort level of recommendation for the candidate. Examples include "enthusiastically recommend," "give my outstanding recommendation," and "without reservation I recommend." These qualifiers are categorized below.

Level of Recommendation	
Highest	Highest, most enthusiastically, wholeheartedly, strongest, outstanding, stellar, superior
Strongly	Strongly, highly, enthusiastically, heartily, very highly, excellent
Without reservation	Without reservation, no hesitation, unqualified
Recommend	Recommend, no hesitation, unqualified, comfortable, support, endorse, pleased.
Fortune J. The content and value of letters of recommendation in the resident candidate evaluative process. *Curr Surg* 2002; 59(1): 79-83.	

The risk of faint praise emphasizes two points. To avoid being the recipient of faint praise, always ask the letter writer if he feels comfortable writing you a strong letter of recommendation. While an enthusiastic "yes" does not offer any guarantees, it significantly reduces the risk. Secondly, if you view a letter that includes faint praise, seek out additional letter writers.

Did you know?

In a study evaluating the content of recommendation letters, the comment, "I hope we can attract ______ to our own residency," was viewed very favorably. On the other hand, the commonly used phrase, "If I can provide any additional information, please call…" was generally viewed as a negative comment. It was believed that its inclusion meant that the letter writer had additional things to say but did not feel comfortable discussing them in the letter.[3]

Did you know?

In a review of letters written on behalf of applicants to the Stanford University otolaryngology residency program, the authors wrote about how disclosure of a personal relationship between the letter writer and applicant could affect the way in which the letter is viewed. "Disclosed personal relationships…can also raise doubt in a reader's mind, constituting a doubt raiser (e.g., 'I coached him in little league,' 'I have known his parents for many years'). While the letter writer is appropriately stating his/her credentials to evaluate the candidate, revelations such as these lead to questions in the reader's mind whether the recommendation is impartial or based on a personal relationship."[19]

Rule # 48 Short letters of recommendation may harm you

In a review of 966 letters of recommendation sent during the 1999 application process to the Department of Surgery at Southern Illinois University, the average length of the recommendation letter was 13.7 sentences, with a range of 4 to 36 sentences.[23] Is there any correlation between the length of a letter and its value to program directors?

In a study designed to determine the aspects of letters that programs find useful screening and selection, the letters which received the best scores were generally twice as long (363 versus 150 words) as those letters rated lowest.[3] This makes sense, as letters that contain stories and anecdotes to support a writer's praise will be longer than letters that simply praise.

Tip # 17

If your letter writer shares the letter with you, pay attention to its length. If it's too short, you may not wish to submit it.

Rule # 49 **Waive your right to review the letter.**

In 1974, with the passage of the Family Educational Rights and Privacy Act (FERPA), students were given some important rights regarding their educational records. These rights, which also apply to letters of recommendation, include the following:

- Students have the right to inspect their educational records.
- Students have the right to challenge any information in the educational records that they feel is inaccurate or incorrect.
- Students have the right to keep the educational records private or confidential.

With the granting of these rights, no institution can force you to waive these rights. It is fairly standard, however, for students to be given a form in which they are asked to indicate whether they waive or retain the right to review the recommendation letter. Before making the decision, review the following table, which discusses the advantages and disadvantages of waiving your right to see the letter.

Letters of Recommendation: To Waive Or Not To Waive?	
Advantages of retaining your rights	**Advantages of waiving your rights**
By knowing the content of the letter, you will know exactly what the residency program knows about you.	You will have no need to explain why you retained your rights, if asked in an interview.
You will have less stress and anxiety because you know the contents of the letter.	The letter writer may not write you a letter if you have retained your right to view the letter
You will also be able to identify mistakes before the letter is sent. You can then give the writer an opportunity to correct these errors.	The selection committee may feel that the letter is more candid because waived your rights.
You can use the comments in the letter to maintain your strengths and work on your weaknesses.	The selection committee may feel that you have nothing to hide and that you are not concerned about what the faculty member might say.
You can make sure that an unfavorable letter is not sent.	The letter writer may be less inhibited in praising you if you have waived your right.

Most advisors, including ourselves, recommend that applicants waive their right to review the letter. In a study cited previously, a review of letters written on behalf of 204 applicants to the Stanford University otolaryngology residency program in 2006 found that only one applicant "was recorded as 'not waiving' her right to see the letters."[19] Many residency programs consider confidential letters to have greater credibility. Because of this, they may be given greater weight in the application process. When rights are not waived, programs may assume that you only sent letters that painted you in a very positive light.

If you are reluctant to waive your rights, consider the reasons for your reluctance. If you have heeded the advice in this chapter, you can be very confident that the letter writers you have chosen will write you a strong letter of recommendation, in which case you should feel comfortable waiving your right to review the letter. If there is any concern that the writer may submit a letter that is not flattering or frankly negative, then you should be asking that individual for a letter of recommendation.

Tip # 18

Waiving your right to see the letter of recommendation does not prohibit you from reading your letter if the writer chooses to share it with you. However, if you've waived your right to see the letter, then don't ask to see the letter. That would be poor etiquette, and you risk annoying the letter writer. If the writer offers to show it to you, however, then by all means accept.

Tip # 19

If you have applied for a grant, award, or scholarship during medical school, you may have been asked to submit letters of recommendation as part of the application process. Think back to that time. Were you asked to sign a waiver? If not, you should have full access to the letters of recommendation. You may even have been asked to submit the letters along with the rest of the application, in which case you may have the letters in your possession. Review the letters to gauge their strength. Since writers will often use a previous letter as a template for future letters, you will know which letter writers will be most supportive of your residency application.

Did you know?

In a study done to assess how often applicants waived their rights to view recommendation letters, researchers examined 264 applications submitted to a single emergency medicine residency program by U.S. medical students. Rights were not waived in only 6% of the submitted standardized letter of recommendations.[27]

Rule # 50 Do not hesitate to ask for a letter of recommendation.

Students are often hesitant to approach professors to ask for letters. Some students feel they are imposing. However, faculty members realize that this is just one of their many professional responsibilities. Professors expect to be asked to write letters for goo students. Other students are hesitant because they fear refusal. If the letter writer refuses, what's the worst that could happen? You just move on to the next person on your list of potential letter writers.

Did you know?

Letter writers can do more than write a letter. If a writer ever asks you "Is there any other way I can be of assistance?" always respond with a "yes." Can they conduct a mock interview with you? Do they know anyone on the faculty of your top-choice programs? Would they be willing to give them a call on your behalf?

Rule # 51 **In this section, perhaps more than any other, you cannot procrastinate.**

In this section, perhaps more than any other, you cannot procrastinate. You do not have the ability to make up for lost time, as your letters are not under your direct control. Students often procrastinate when deciding whom to ask and how to ask for a letter of recommendation. Procrastination makes things much more difficult. Professors who may have been willing to write a letter may not be able to do so when asked on short notice. Provide the writer with adequate time, preferably one or two months, to write the letter. Professors have other tasks and responsibilities, so contact them as early as possible.

Tip # 20

Don't procrastinate when it comes to asking for letters of recommendation. Faculty members expect to be asked to write these letters. However, giving short notice is not only poor form; it also increases your risk of a suboptimal letter.

Rule # 52 **Don't even bother asking for a letter unless the writer has sufficient time to do an outstanding job.**

As a general rule, you should give the letter writer at least one to two months to write and send the letter. If possible, give the letter writer more time. Nothing is more irritating than being asked to write a letter of recommendation under pressure. Remember that letter writers do have other responsibilities. You don't want them to do shoddy work, which you risk if you don't provide enough advance notice.

Rule # 53 **Always provide all of the relevant information.**

Even if a professor tells you that he will write a strong letter of recommendation, the letter may turn out to be mediocre. Many professors are just not proficient at writing effective letters. They may lack a firm understanding of what residency programs are seeking, or may not know how to advocate strongly for their students. For example, a well-intentioned letter writer may produce a letter full of generalities. Although the overall tone and content will be supportive, a letter that is short on specifics that back up the praise will do little to differentiate you from other candidates.

Tip # 21

Larkin wrote that "some writers invest significant time and effort into writing an accurate narrative with examples and evidence to support their conclusions. Others write quickly and superficially, in generic, nonverifiable terms that seem to lack substance."[28]

Therefore, you need to make it as easy as possible for the writer to produce a strong letter of recommendation. You can do so by providing the writer with a packet, containing the following:

- Cover letter thanking them for writing your letter, along with a summary of the packet's contents (see following example)
- Letter Request Form if you are applying through the Electronic Residency Application Service (ERAS). These are forms that can be generated as early as May through MyERAS.
- Your reasons for applying to the specialty
- Anecdotes, stories, and examples from your rotation together (see Rule # 46)
- Curriculum vitae (CV)
- Personal statement
- Transcript
- Clerkship evaluation form completed by the letter writer
- Write-up or other assignment given a high grade or evaluation by the same professor
- Ways to reach you in the event more information is required or a question arises
- Deadline

If you are applying through the Electronic Residency Application Service (ERAS), note that the process of uploading letters for applicants has changed. For years, letter writers submitted their letters to the applicant's medical school administration which, in turn, uploaded letters into the ERAS system. With

ERAS 2016, the process of uploading letters has changed. ERAS 2016 requires letter writers (or their designees) to directly upload letters into the system. The process can begin as early as May when applicants are permitted to generate Letter Request Forms through MyERAS.

If you are applying through the Central Application Service (San Francisco Match), you will have to obtain your letter directly from the writer in a sealed envelope to include as part of your application. If you will need the letter writer to mail the letter directly, then you should provide stamped envelopes with neatly typed addresses of the residency programs.

Sample Cover Letter

Dear Dr. Egbert,

Thank you for writing me a letter of recommendation for orthopedic surgery residency. I know how busy you are, and I sincerely appreciate your support of my application. I am including additional information to help you as you write the letter. Included are the following:

- This cover letter
- CV
- Personal statement
- Two write-ups that you reviewed during the clerkship
- Handout from the talk I gave on pulmonary embolism
- Several cases from our month together that impacted my training

I am hoping to have my entire application completed by September 15. If you have any questions or require any other materials from me, please let me know. I can be reached by phone (555-1212) or e-mail (lisa.ray@gmail.com).

Thank you,

Lisa Ray

This packet provides the writer with all the facts needed to write an effective letters. The information in the packet will help the writer include specifics and examples that convince the reader that the praise is true. We agree with the words of Dr. Lotfipour, a faculty member in the Department of Emergency Medicine at the University of California Irvine, who wrote that "the easier the letter-writing process is, the more positive the letter is likely to be."[14]

Tip # 22

If you are applying to two or more specialties, make sure that your letter writer is recommending you for the right specialty.

Rule # 54 **You may be asked to write your own letter of recommendation. Take great care if you've presented with this option.**

Don't be surprised if you encounter a professor who asks you to draft your own letter of recommendation. While some students are disappointed or even insulted by this type of response, others view it as an incredible opportunity. If you are presented with the opportunity to write your own letter, you may choose to accept the offer. Do so with great caution, and only after deliberation, for the following reasons:

- By asking you to write the letter, the professor has already made it clear to you that he is not that enthusiastic about you and your application. What will this individual say if a selection committee member calls to ask more questions?
- You probably haven't been asked to write a letter of recommendation before. Having the ability to write a strong letter of recommendation is not an innate ability – it is one that is learned through practice. Letters of recommendation written by seasoned professors have a certain tone and perspective. Your inexperience may result in the development of a weak letter.
- A letter that you write may end up being similar to your personal statement and may not add much to your application. In contrast, letter writers who use their own words will offer multiple perspectives on your performance, achievement, and strengths.
- Some application reviewers view this act as unethical.

Tip # 23

If your letter writer asks you to draft your own letter of recommendation, consider the negatives. Program directors, having seen thousands of letters, may be able to spot a letter written by an applicant. This may lead the director to call the letter writer. If it is learned that you wrote the letter and the professor merely signed it, your risk having your application taken out of consideration. In a survey of family practice directors inquiring about candidate deception, it was learned that 15% of deceptive acts were related to the letter of recommendation.[26] While the article did not describe these acts of deception in any detail, writing your own letter may be viewed as such.

Rule # 55 Say "Thank you."

When you're caught up in the stress and anxiety of completing applications, then interviewing, then making critical decisions about your future, it's easy to forget about the people who got you this far. You must convey your appreciation for all of their work, because they deserve to know. You must also provide them with follow up on your career plans, because faculty are always interested in their students' successes. And while you may think that once medical school is done, it's over, you may need the assistance of your mentors and letter writers in the future.

After the recommendation letters have been sent, send each of your letter writers a personal thank-you note. In your note, express your appreciation for their support. You should also provide your letter writes with follow up. Let them know how the application process is going, and ultimately, where you match.

Tip # 24

As you progress through residency, stay in touch with your letter writers. This doesn't involve tremendous effort or time on your part. A short e-mail or postcard with a comment or two about your progress will suffice. Your letter writer has shown a desire to help you, and the time may come when his assistance will be needed again.

References

[1]Brandenburg S, Kruzick T, Lin C, Robinson A, Adams L. Residency selection criteria: what medical students perceive as important. *Med Educ Online* 2005; 10: 1-6.
[2]Results of the 2014 NRMP Program Director Survey. Available at: http://www.nrmp.org/wp-content/uploads/2014/09/PD-Survey-Report-2014.pdf. Accessed March 3, 2016.
[3]Greenburg A, Doyle J, McClure D. Letters of recommendation for surgical residencies: what they say and what they mean. *J Surg Res* 1994; 1994; 56(2): 192-198.
[4]DeLisa J, Jain S, Campagnolo D. Factors used by physical medicine and rehabilitation residency training directors to select their residents. *Am J Phys Med Rehabil* 1994; 73:152-156.
[5]Crane J, Ferraro C. Selection criteria for emergency medicine residency applicants. *Acad Emerg Med* 2000; 7(1): 54-60.
[6]Harwood R, Girzadas D, Carlson A, Delis S, Stevison K, Tsonis G, Keng G. Characteristics of the emergency medicine standardized letter of recommendation. *Acad Emerg Med* 2000; 7(4): 409-410.
[7]Otero H, Erturk S, Ondategui-Parra S, Ros P. Key criteria for selection of radiology residents: results of a national survey. *Acad Radiol* 2006; 13: 1155-1164.
[8]Gorouhi F, Alikhan A, Rezaei A, Fazel N. Dermatology residency selection criteria with an emphasis on program characteristics: a national program director survey. *Dermatol Res Pract* 2014; 692760.
[9]Khalili A, Chalouhi N, Tjoumakaris S, Gonzalez L, Starke R, Rosenwasser R, Jabbour P. Program selection criteria for neurological surgery applicants in the United States: a national survey for neurological surgery program directors. *World Neurosurg* 2014; 81(3-4): 473-7
[10]Nallasamy S, Uhler T, Nallasamy N, Tapino P, Volpe N. Ophthalmology resident selection: current trends in selection criteria and improving the process. *Ophthalmology* 2010; 117(5): 1041-7.
[11]UMMS Resident Applicant Reference Guide. Available at: http://medstudents.medicine.umich.edu/sites/default/files/downloads/Residency_Applicant_Reference_Guide.pdf. Accessed January 4, 2016.
[12]Queens Hospital Center Department of Medicine. Available at: https://icahn.mssm.edu/education/residencies-and-fellowships/consortium-of-graduate-medical-education/directory/queens-hospital-center/internal-medicine-residency/frequently-asked-questions. Accessed January 4, 2016.
[13]Mavis B, Shafer C, Magallanes B. The intentions of letter writers for applicants to a baccalaureate-M.D. program: self-report and content analyses of letters of reference. *Med Educ Online* [serial online] 2006; 11:6. Available at: http://www.med-ed-online.org.
[14]Lotfipour S, Luu R, Hayden S, Vaca F, Hoonpongsimanont W, Langdorf M. Becoming an emergency medicine resident: a practical guide for medical students. *J Emerg Med* 2008; Jun 10 (epub).

[15]Farnie M. Career counseling: internal medicine. Available at: http://www.uth.tmc.edu/med/administration/student/ms4/2003CCC.htm. Accessed November 3, 2008.
[16]Gayed N. Residency directors' assessments of which selection criteria best predict the performances of foreign-born foreign medical graduates during internal medicine residencies. *Acad Med* 1991; 66(11): 699-701.
[17]Villanueva A, Kaye D, Abdelhak S, Morahan P. Comparing selection criteria for residency directors and physicians' employers. *Acad Med* 1995; 70(4): 261-71.
[18]Bernstein A, Jazrawi L, Elbeshbeshy B, Della Valle C, Zuckerman J. Orthopedic resident-selection criteria. *J Bone Joint Surg Am* 2002; 84-A(11): 2090-2096.
[19]Messner A, Shimahara E. Letters of recommendation to an otolaryngology/head and neck surgery residency program: their function and the role of gender. *Laryngoscope* 2008; 118: 1-10 (epub).
[20]David Geffen School of Medicine at UCLA. Available at: http://www.medstudent.ucla.edu/offices/sao/academic-career/how_lor.cfm. Accessed January 4, 2016.
[21]Wagoner N, Suriano J, Stoner J. Factors used by program directors to select residents. *J Med Educ* 1986; 61(1): 10-21.
[22]O'Halloran C, Altmaier E, Smith W, Franken E. Evaluation of resident applicants by letters of recommendation: a comparison of traditional and behavioral-based formats. *Invest Radiol* 1993; 28: 274-277.
[23]Fortune J. The content and value of letters of recommendation in the resident candidate evaluative process. *Curr Surg* 2002; 59(1): 79-83.
[24]Wagoner N, Suriano J. Program directors' responses to a survey on variables used to select residents in a time of change. *Acad Med* 1999; 74: 51-58.
[25]DeZee K, Thomas M, Mintz M, Durning S. Letters of recommendation: rating, writing, and reading by clerkship directors of internal medicine. *Teach Learn Med* 2009; 21(2): 153-8.
[26]Morganstern B, Zalneraitis E, Slavin S. Improving the letter of recommendation for pediatric residency applicants: an idea whose time has come? *J Pediatr* 2003: 2: 143-144.
[27]Diab J, Riley S, Overton D. The Family Education Rights and Privacy Act's impact on residency applicant behavior and recommendations: a pilot study. *J Emerg Med* 2011; 40(1): 72-5.
[28]Larkin G, Marco C. Ethics seminars: beyond authorship requirements – ethical considerations in writing letters of recommendation. *Acad Emerg Med* 2001; 8(1): 70-73.
[26]Grover M, Dharamshi F, Goveia C. Deception by applicants to family practice residencies. *Fam Med* 2001; 33: 441-446.

Chapter 7

Personal Statement

One of the most dreaded aspects of the residency application, for many students, is the personal statement (PS). In a survey of medical students at a single school, 85% agreed or strongly agreed with the statement "I am anxious about writing the personal statement for my residency application."[1] It can be very frustrating trying to put into words your vision for your medical career.

Most students don't understand one basic fact about the personal statement, though. Unlike just about every other aspect of the application, you have complete control over the personal statement. You decide the content, the structure, and the form of the statement. This is a unique opportunity to impress the selection committee. In your statement you can showcase the strengths and qualities that set you apart from other candidates. You can weave in evidence that confirms your qualities. You can use this opportunity to convince a faculty member that you would be an ideal candidate for their particular program. This is information that is not readily apparent to programs from their review of other application components.

With sufficient time and effort, you can create a personal statement that effectively sells yourself to the residency program. While a well-written statement can strengthen your application, a poorly written one can eliminate you from further consideration, even if you are at the top of your class.

Rule # 56 Recognize the importance of the personal statement to some specialties

Individual specialties, residency programs, and application reviewers assign varying degrees of importance to the PS. In the screening phase, reviewers whittle down a large applicant pool to a select group that is ultimately extended interview invitations. Applicants often believe that the personal statement is used minimally, if at all, during this screening phase. While this is true at some programs, you can't assume that's the case with all programs:

- At the website for the University of Washington Family Medicine Residency, the "personal statement is the primary component that will be used to select applicants who are invited for an interview. Please write a careful and thoughtful document."[2] In fact, a study of family practice residency program directors showed that the personal statement ranked second only to the Dean's letter for making decisions about whom to interview.[3] With regard to the ranking of applicants, it was third in importance, following only the interview and the Dean's letter.

- At the Wake Forest University Department of Radiology, members of the selection committee use the personal statement along with the rest of the application to place candidates into one of five groups – interview (high priority), interview (normal priority), interview (low priority), hold for additional information, and do not interview (reject).[4]
- "Personal statement is read by each of our orthopedic faculty members, and is considered by our faculty to be a very important part of the application process," writes the Department of Orthopedic Surgery at the University of Texas-Houston Medical School. "It is often used as a point of departure for interviewing the student."[5]
- "Assuming the consummate applicant has impeccable curriculum vitae, letters, and grades, the personal statement takes on immense importance," writes Dr. Warren Heymann, Head of the Division of Dermatology at Cooper Medical School."[6]

In further support of the importance of the PS in screening applicants for interview are the results of the 2014 NRMP Program Directors Survey. The percentage of programs citing the statement as a factor used to make interview decisions is shown in the following table.[7]

Importance Of The Personal Statement In Selecting Applicants For Interview

Specialty	% Programs Citing Statement As A Factor
Anesthesiology	78%
Dermatology	85%
Emergency Medicine	67%
Family Medicine	87%
General Surgery	72%
Internal Medicine	66%
Medicine/Pediatrics	71%
Neurological Surgery	78%
Neurology	71%
Obstetrics & Gynecology	81%
Orthopedic Surgery	82%
Otolaryngology	74%
Pathology	83%
Pediatrics	70%
Physical Medicine & Rehabilitation	79%
Plastic Surgery	85%
Psychiatry	92%
Radiation Oncology	84%
Radiology	74%
Vascular Surgery	80%

Adapted from Results of the 2014 NRMP Program Director Survey. Available at: http://www.nrmp.org/wp-content/uploads/2014/09/PD-Survey-Report-2014.pdf.

Tip # 25

Some specialties, programs, and application reviewers attach great importance to the PS, while others may only glance at it. Because you'll have no way of knowing how your PS will be read or weighted, it's important to create a compelling statement.

Did you know?

Offering advice to the dermatology residency applicant, Dr. Heymann wrote that "assuming the consummate applicant has impeccable curriculum vitae, letters, and grades, the personal statement takes on immense importance. Who is this person? Is it someone I want to meet face-to-face? Tell me about yourself candidly. What do you want to contribute to the discipline in the course of your professional lifetime? In short, make me want to meet you."[6]

Rule # 57 **Programs don't always want a generic statement. Read the instructions carefully.**

While many programs give applicants complete control over the statement's content, some programs do ask the applicant to address specific questions. At the website for the San Francisco General Hospital internal medicine residency (primary care track), applicants are asked to write "a personal statement specifically addressing why you want to work in a public hospital setting and care for a vulnerable and medically underserved population."[8] The dermatology residency program at the University of Utah informs applicants that the "personal statement should summarize how your qualifications and goals mesh with those of our Department."[9] At the website for the University of Oklahoma orthopedic surgery residency program, the following advice is given to applicants:

"It is desirable for the statement transmitted to our program to include information on:

1) Any involvement you have had with the State of Oklahoma or the surrounding region, the purpose being for you to consider and then translate to us why you believe you would be satisfied living and training in Oklahoma for five years.
2) Your class standing if your school ranks students.
3) An accounting for any breaks greater than three months in your education since high school."[10]

Tip # 26

Before you write, carefully review any personal statement directions the program may have. While most programs leave the content of the statement completely up to you, others may make specific requests. Failure to follow the instructions may lead the program to assume you will have the same difficulty as a resident, thus removing your application from further consideration.

Tip # 27

In their article "Crafting a Great Personal Statement," Drs. McGarry and Tammaro, program directors of the internal medicine residency at Brown Medical School wrote that "a great personal statement will make the program director eager to meet you and potentially work with you... A poorly written PS can cast doubt on your education and focus for a demanding profession like medicine...The PS that falls between these two extremes may be neutral in its overall effect, but represents a missed opportunity to add luster to your candidacy...While no personal statement can substitute for an excellent academic record throughout medical school, it may help you and your application stand out from the pack and win you an invitation to interview or gain a few points on a program's rank list."[11]

Rule # 58 **Know your audience. Convince them that you embody the qualities that they are seeking in a future resident.**

Before drafting your PS, consider your audience. Your audience is the residency program director, your interviewers, and other members of the selection committee. An effective personal statement must focus on what the audience is seeking. In this case, the reviewers seek to learn more about you as an individual to help them determine if you have the qualities they are seeking in a future resident. What are they seeking in a future resident? How can you convince them that you embody these qualities?

There are several ways to make a convincing argument. Consider addressing the following questions in your personal statement.

- **Why did I choose this specialty?**

  Programs seek deeply committed residents. Therefore, they are interested in learning about the factors that led you to pursue the specialty. What is it about the specialty that appeals to you? Is it the nature of the work? Is it the intellectual challenge? Were you motivated by a personal, family, or clinical experience, or a combination thereof? Give specific reasons why you are interested in the specialty. In answering this question, show them that you are deeply committed to the field. There should be no ambiguity. If you are unable to communicate a clear understanding of, and commitment to, the specialty, your application may be removed from further consideration.

We emphasize that you should be writing about the factors that led you to pursue the specialty, with the emphasis on you. As Dr. Oldham, the program director of the radiology program at the University of Texas Medical School at Houston, writes: "...please do not regale me with how much you like Radiology. I like it too and don't need convincing about how great a specialty it is – you would be preaching to the choir."[5] At the end of this chapter, we list reasons which lead applicants to pursue careers in different specialties. This information will help you develop content to answer the question "Why did I choose this specialty?"

Did you know?

In a study evaluating the content of personal statements, members of the radiology residency selection committee at Wayne State University ranked 11 content areas from least to most important. Most important was a candidate's explanation as to why he or she chose to pursue a career in radiology. Personal attributes was second in importance. Third in importance was perception of radiology, defined as the applicant's ability "to explicitly state what he/she feels are the most important characteristic of either radiologists or the practice of radiology."[12]

Tip # 28

Applicants often write about the reasons that led them to become physicians. However, residency programs aren't interested in why you chose to become a doctor. Instead, focus on why you have chosen a career in that specialty.

- **What am I looking for in a residency program?**

  Programs seek out residents who will be a good "fit" for the program. Be specific about what you seek in a residency program. "Given my goals of providing health services to underserved communities, I'm seeking a residency program that..."

  Don't forget the corollary, which can be easy to do when you're applying to large numbers of programs. Don't confirm the fact that you would be a poor fit for the program. "I am very interested in continuing my basic science research on matrix metalloproteinases, and I hope to eventually make significant contributions in the field." You've also just made it clear that you're a poor fit for this clinically oriented program that has no time set aside for research endeavors.

- **What are my professional goals in the field I have chosen?**

  Some residency programs have institutional goals. They may aim to train doctors who will serve in primary care, who will serve underserved populations, who will serve as clinician-educators, who will advance research, or who will achieve any other number of goals. Programs understand that these goals evolve with time, so you don't need to have absolute certainty. However, including your future goals in the statement gives the program some idea of your motivation and knowledge of the specialty.

- **What are my strengths?**

Every specialty values certain qualities in their residents. Studies have outlined some of these qualities, and many specialty websites publish information about the qualities necessary to succeed in the field.

Examples of Skills and Personal Qualities Frequently Identified by Residency Program Directors in Defining an Applicant's "Fit"	
Family Medicine	Good communicator, interpersonal skills, team player, lifelong learning skills, empathic, interested in community practice, non-judgmental, active in the program, experience with underserved populations
Internal Medicine	Good communicator, interpersonal skills, team player, hands-on patient care, potential positive impact upon program, reliable and stable, warm and humane, demonstrated commitment to specific area (music, sports), well-organized, ability to get along with others, resourceful
Pediatrics	Good communicator, interpersonal skills, team player, well-organized, well-rounded, mature, independent, sense of professionalism, flexible (ability to change), enthusiastic, ability to cope with stress and change, positive attitude (views glass "half full")
Surgery	Good communicator, compulsive, neat, high energy, honest and straightforward, confident, hardworking, demonstrated commitment to specific area (music, sports)
Villanueva A, Kaye D, Abdelhak S, Morahan P. Comparing selection criteria for residency directors and physicians' employers. *Acad Med* 1995; 70(4): 261-71.	

Study these lists. Determine which you can claim as your own strengths, and weave these into your personal statement. As always, naked statements don't mean much. Always include evidence in the form of personal anecdotes, clinical experiences, or other forms to back up your claims.

Program Directors Speak...

"Please also include a personal statement with your application. Tell us why you have chosen radiation oncology as your specialty. The selection committee is most interested in what special qualities and experiences you have and what you hope to do with your radiation oncology training. The personal statement helps us to know you, and we read it with great care."[13]

Harvard University Radiation Oncology Residency Program

- **What accomplishments should I highlight?**

  Programs seek certain traits and qualities in their residents. Every program wants hard-working, enthusiastic, focused residents. They want individuals with proven skills of communication, perseverance towards a goal, and the ability to work with all types of people to achieve a common goal. The PS can be used to highlight different types of accomplishments that underscore your stellar qualities. You can highlight your commitment and dedication by discussing your long-term volunteer commitments. Areas such as occupational history and outside interests may be woven in. What did you accomplish in the two summers that you worked as an EMT? What type of qualities can you highlight from your one year working as an engineer?

- **What contributions can I make to the specialty?**

  In a very competitive field like dermatology, it is a given that applicants will all have extremely strong academic records. Since programs can pick and choose among so many academically stellar candidates, they have the luxury of looking for more. Programs seek out applicants who can actually contribute to the discipline as a whole. This becomes even more of an issue in the fields of dermatology and ophthalmology, which have seen a rise in applications as lifestyle issues become more important to medical school graduates. Look at it from the program's standpoint. If you're interviewing so many outstanding applicants, why choose the ones who are going to graduate with the intention of working the least amount of hours for the most amount of money?

  Since programs seek out applicants who will contribute to the discipline as a whole, emphasize your own strengths, skills, and experiences and how these will aid you in contributing to the specialty. Do you have a background in research? What do you plan to do with that background? Have you done a fellowship and accumulated significant experience in clinical trials? What do you plan to do with those skills? Do you have significant volunteer experience in tutoring? Have you created educational materials or programs? Have you worked with cancer prevention programs or do you have an interest in preventive medicine strategies? Have you spent time working with underserved populations?

Do you have additional skills, such as computer database management or graphic design experience that can be used to benefit the specialty in some way? Think long and hard about how you as an individual plan to contribute to your field when you finish residency training, and write about your individual skills and strengths that will help you accomplish those goals.

- **Why would I be a great fit for this particular residency program?**

  Most applicants write one statement that they then have ERAS forward to all programs. However, some students write several different statements. Students with research experience may choose to emphasize a different skill set for different programs. They may send a research-oriented statement to programs which place great emphasis on research, but send a statement that emphasizes their outstanding skills as a clinician to other programs.

  Some applicants will actually write a different statement for each program, tailoring their statement to each individual program. In doing so, they can successfully answer the question "Why am I interested in your program?" This approach demonstrates to PDs that you are genuinely interested in their program and are knowledgeable about the program's strengths.

- **What are my outside interests?**

  Again, your outside interests can be used to highlight desirable qualities, as in the marathon runner who is a focused, determined individual used to setting goals and working hard to achieve them. Your unique interests can also leave a memorable impression. Are you working on hiking all the state parks in Texas? Restore classic cars in your spare time? Do you specialize in cooking Thai cuisine? Tell a memorable story, and use it as a hook by which people will remember you.

Program Directors Speak...

"We look for how you present yourself in your personal statement, your involvement in academic and civic organizations, your volunteerism, and anything that sets you apart from the rest of your peers," writes the Adena Health System. "I look for young proven leaders willing to serve, and young professionals proven to work well in group settings."[14]

Did you know?

In a survey of over 700 ophthalmology residents, 32% had hobbies or interests that they felt would make them successful in ophthalmology. These generally involved the use of fine motor skills or hand-eye coordination, and included such hobbies as jewelry, crafting, woodwork, carving, calligraphy, music, sewing, sculpture, and sports. Approximately 5% reported an interest in photography.[15]

Program Directors Speak...

"One of the things I hate most when reading a personal statement is when the student spends the whole time telling me why they like EM. I hate this because they all sound the same and they really don't tell me much. I recommend to students that they write their personal statement from the perspective of a job applicant (sometimes the students forget that this is what they are). Sit down and think about your strengths and how they will fit into EM and then start writing. Your personal statement should tell me about your experiences and accomplishments and how they will make you a successful EM physician. For instance, leadership positions taught you how to work with a variety of people and successfully accomplish your goals. This is extremely important in EM because you will be leading a team in the department and these skills are invaluable. When it comes to the common application form my advice is pretty similar. Don't just list what you're accomplishments are, tell me a little about your role and involvement."[16]

Dr. Jamie Collings (Former Program Director of Northwestern University Emergency Medicine Residency)

"I think the main point is that this can't be a recitation of what's already in other parts of the application. I'll get to the positive side, but one of the main things that bothers me with personal statements is reading about that first I did this, and then I did that, and I wrote this paper, and I did this research, and I published it in this journal, and I did this volunteer work. It's all in the CV already and the whole statement becomes 'I, I, I.'

But while the personal statement is just that – personal – if it's all going to be about delineating accomplishments that are covered in other places, then that simply isn't helpful. What is helpful is to draw a picture of yourself that can't be obtained from anywhere else in the application. It should be personal - this is who you are, this is what makes you excited, these are your special interests. Sometimes it may be outside of medicine, sometimes it may be a volunteer experience that is expanded upon, or it could be a personal connection that stimulated the applicant to want to do something more, such as a specific part of Dermatology down the line. You might express your future goal, as that is something that wouldn't be revealed in other parts of the application.

It certainly has to be sincere. If everyone just says at the end of their statement 'I want to be an academic dermatologist' and there's nothing else in the application that tells a reason for this, it's not believable...Overall, your statement has got to be personal, sincere, and bring out information not available in other places."[17]

Dr. William James (Program Director of University of Pennsylvania Dermatology Residency)

"More than anything else, I look at the personal statement to answer the questions: 'Why is this student interested in ob/gyn, and does this interest seem to ring true?' Certainly if the personal statement tastefully and artfully presents some unique aspects of the student without being awkward or bizarre, then all the better. As a program director, I am looking for a solid responsible resident who will be committed in a demanding specialty to the end. I am not looking for a literary or creative genius. Grammar, spelling, and diction, however, are important. Sometimes spell check can create strange words, so a careful read is mandatory."[18]

Dr. Eugene Toy (Program Director of OB/GYN Residency at the Houston Methodist Hospital)

Rule # 59 Never exaggerate.

Students sometimes overstate their role in a research project. When asked about their work during the interview, some are unable to discuss the project in any depth, thus harming their credibility. Resist the temptation to exaggerate.

Under no circumstances should you lie in your personal statement. Unfortunately, some students will, and the following box demonstrates how surprisingly often this occurs. Although some lies may escape detection, most don't. An application reviewer may note a discrepancy between the PS and other components of the application, such as the letter of recommendation. In other cases, the lie is discovered when an interviewer probes the applicant further.

Did you know?

In a study of family practice PDs over a 5-year period, directors were asked about candidate deception. 339 cases of deception, accounting for 56% of all deception acts, involved the personal statement. Of the recognized incidents of deception, 89% were discovered before the Match, either during the interview or when programs made efforts to verify application information.[19]

Rule # 60 Don't ever plagiarize.

Don't "borrow" any part of a PS for a starting point or for a framework, even if the rest of the statement is all yours. If you're not sure whether what you've done is sufficiently different from another's personal statement, then consider that a warning – a reader may also have concerns. In recent years, many examples of statements have been posted on different websites. While reading the statements of others can be useful, never copy part of another statement. Be careful about writing services which may recycle words, phrases, or text. ERAS has noted that personal statement plagiarism is an increasingly common issue. Sites that have been plagiarized include www.medfools.com, www.usmleweb.com, www.medstudentcafe.com, and www.aipg.info.[20]

Did you know?

Drs. Lehrmann and Walaszek, psychiatry faculty at the Zablocki VA Medical Center and the University of Wisconsin School of Medicine in Milwaukee, wrote about finding a "personal statement development website for U.S. and international medical students which displayed example personal statements." They were shocked to see that they "actually recognized some of them. We had received several nearly identical personal statements that had been plagiarized."[21]

Researchers at the Brigham & Women's Hospital analyzed essays written by applicants to their institution's anesthesiology, emergency medicine, general surgery, internal medicine, and obstetrics & gynecology residency programs between 2005 and 2007. By using specialized software, researchers were able to determine if essays had similarities to website content, print resources, and previously submitted statements. Approximately 5% of essays included text which had more than 10% overlap with other content.[22]

Did you know?

In a letter to the editor following publication of Dr. Segal's work, Dr. Moxie Stratton-Loeffler offered some reasons why applicants may plagiarize, including "competition, lack of confidence in writing and communication skills, lack of skill, exhaustion and lack of inspiration from fatigue during medical school, stymied creative expression due to long hours and overwork, and a widely held belief that no one actually reads the personal statements. There is also doubt among students that a program will decide anything on the basis of the essay."[23]

Did you know?

In a more recent study, researchers screened personal statements submitted by 467 applicants to a single anesthesiology residency program using Viper Plagiarism Scanner software.[24] Unoriginal content was defined as 8 or more consecutive words. The analysis revealed that 4% of statements submitted by U.S. medical school graduates contained plagiarized material. A higher percentage of essays (13.6%) submitted by IMGs contained plagiarism. In response, the authors indicated that their institution will begin screening essays of applicants applying to all of their residency programs. Any applicant found to have plagiarized content will be rejected.

Applicants who have been found to plagiarize may suffer serious consequences. ERAS has a program (Integrity Promotion Investigations Program) in place to handle complaints of unethical behavior on the part of applicants.[25] After a complaint is received, an investigation is launched to learn more about the alleged fraudulent activity. Applicants deemed to be in violation are added to a violator database and the final report generated from the investigation is sent to each residency program applied to, along with the applicant's medical school. Furthermore, ERAS states that the report will also be sent to programs applied to in future application cycles.

Rule # 61 **Finish your personal statement early in the application cycle.**

Some of your letter writers will request a copy of your PS, so plan your schedule accordingly. Your deadline will be the date that you provide information packets to your letter writers, and not the date for submission of applications.

It may not take that long to actually crank out a one-page statement. However, we recommend that you start the process a minimum of two months out. Brainstorming and outlining should be done in multiple sessions, especially since you need to provide multiple opportunities for inspiration to hit. You'll also need to give your reviewers sufficient time to complete their work, and to provide yourself enough time to process their comments and to make multiple revisions.

Tip # 29

Don't wait until the last minute to start your PS. Start early so that you give yourself enough time to develop a high quality statement. Many letter writers will ask you for your PS before writing your letter of recommendation.

Did you know?

Some institutions and programs require students to submit personal statements as part of their application for away electives. Since these applications are due well before the residency application, you may need to have a PS written in your third year.

Rule # 62 Start the process by brainstorming.

Writing the PS is a daunting task, period. Most applicants have no idea where or how to start. Without a plan, you may be stuck waiting for random inspiration. A specific strategy can make this entire process easier by breaking a large task into smaller, more manageable components.

Your first step is to brainstorm. One goal is to pinpoint a unique or distinctive item about yourself that will pique the selection committee's interest. Take a piece of paper or sit in front of your computer, and plan to start writing down everything that you can think of, without any editing. It may even be better to record your answers to these questions on a tape recorder, since transcribing the text may provide further inspiration. Now ask yourself the following questions:

- When did I become interested in this specialty?
- What experiences, events, or factors led me to develop this interest?
- How did my interest in this specialty evolve? What specific turning points can I identify?
- What have I learned about the field and myself while exploring it?
- Was there a particular patient that I cannot forget? What was it about him or her that made such an impact?
- What are my professional goals and aspirations?

- What qualities do I possess that will enhance my chances for success in this specialty?
- What makes me stand out from the rest of the candidates?
- What are my strengths and skills?
- What is unique or distinctive about me or my life story (undergraduate, medical school, personal events, work experience, volunteer experience, teaching experience, research, hobbies, languages, travel, sports, etc.)?
- Why should the selection committee be interested in me?
- Was there a challenge or hardship that I had to overcome? How did this experience shape me?
- Are there any gaps or deficiencies in my record that need to be explained?

If you find it difficult to answer any of these questions, look over your CV. Discuss your accomplishments and experiences with a friend, family member, or advisor. Those close to you may be able to identify accomplishments which have escaped your attention. Consider polling those close to you while writing your statement. The following questions may be used as springboards for discussion:

- What is it about me that the residency selection committee absolutely needs to know?
- What is it about me or my background that you find distinctive?
- Are there any events or experiences in my background that would be of interest to a selection committee?
- Which of my qualities or skills should I showcase in my statement? How do you think these qualities or skills have helped me in the past? How might they help me be successful in residency and in my chosen field?

Tip # 30

Are you having difficulty coming up with a unique characteristic, experience, or subject to write about in your personal statement? Many students are anxious to complete their statement, and consider sitting around and "reflecting" to be a waste of time. Many therefore skip this critical step.

Tip # 31

Don't neglect any attribute that makes you extraordinary or unusual. If you are an accomplished musician, leader of a student organization, or top-level athlete, you should discuss this in your statement. Focus on the traits and lessons learned and how these relate in particular to your chosen specialty. Programs are interested in knowing how you differ from others.

Did you know?

In a study designed to determine predictors of otolaryngology resident success, Daly found that candidates having an exceptional trait, such as leadership qualities, were not only ranked higher but were also found to be more successful during their residency training than those without exceptional traits.[26]

Rule # 63 Plan on multiple drafts.

After you've completed your outline, you're ready to take on your first draft. This is only a draft, and should be approached as such. Creation of a high quality personal statement takes considerable time, and you can't expect a polished product after one draft. Qualified applicants often approach the first draft with the same perfectionist attitude that got them this far. In this case, though, just focus on getting something reasonable down on paper.

Tip # 32

The first draft is always the hardest. Do not approach this first draft with a perfectionist attitude. Instead, aim to get something reasonable down on paper, and plan on many revisions.

There are a million ways to start drafting your PS. Some applicants begin with the introduction, while others prefer to write the ending first, and others just attack the body of the statement. Start wherever you feel comfortable.

After you've written your first draft, set it aside for a few days. Then look at it again and ask yourself the following questions:

- Have I answered the questions that PDs ask?
- Does it flow logically?
- Is it too long? Is it too short?
- Do I need to add more details?
- Do I need to remove some details?

Now revise. With subsequent drafts, ask these questions once again. You'll also start to deal with other issues such as sentence structure and transitions between paragraphs. Expect multiple drafts before you end with a product you like.

Tip # 33

Although you can type your PS directly into ERAS, it's more useful to complete your statement using your word processing software. This allows you to take advantage of editing features such as the spell checker. Once you have a polished product, save the statement as a text file, which you can then cut and paste into ERAS. Don't submit the statement to programs until you have printed a copy for your review. Only after you've carefully proofread your printed copy should you copy it into ERAS.

Tip # 34

You can solicit feedback from others at any point in the writing process; there's no need to wait until you have a polished product. Having others look over your first draft can be invaluable. One caveat: try to submit a polished product when seeking feedback from a faculty member.

Rule # 64 Submit a personal statement of the correct length.

Do whatever it takes to create a PS that is the "right" length. First, comply with all rules regarding the length of the statement. Second, don't go on and on. Your audience includes faculty members and PDs. These are busy individuals who have neither the time nor the patience to read through lengthy tomes.

Tip # 35

When you print your PS from the ERAS system, does it fit onto one page? If not, your statement is too long. Keep in mind that most PDs will spend just 2-3 minutes on average reading your statement.

Tip # 36

Application reviewers appreciate sentences that are concise and direct. Avoid using extraneous or unnecessary words. Choose your words carefully, using the right word rather than the longest word possible.

Don't submit a PS that is too short, either. A short statement suggests that you did not expend much time, energy, and effort in its creation. The natural assumption is that this would extend to your performance as a physician.

Rule # 65 Learn the art of effective self-promotion.

Some applicants downplay their successes in the statement. They hesitate to make strong statements about their strengths and skills for fear that it might be perceived as self-serving. While humility is an admirable quality, it shouldn't be the aim of your PS. You must be able to write about your accomplishments, skills, and strengths in a way that emphasizes that you are a desirable candidate. If you received numerous compliments during your surgery rotation about your manual dexterity, then you should find a way to include this in your PS for surgery residency. Applicants often don't realize that while exaggeration and overstatements can be damaging, so can understatements. The latter prevents the selection committee from getting a better sense of who you are, what you have done, and what you have to offer.

Program Directors Speak...

"Do not be modest. If you believe you have done exceptional things or have an interesting background, tell us!"[27]

UC Davis Pediatrics Residency Program

Did you know?

In a study evaluating the content of personal statements, Smith and colleagues wrote that "although some candidates might hesitate to explicitly define their personal attributes for fear of seeming conceited, the fact that the members of the committee rated this category highly demonstrates that this is not the case. The committee members instead implied that they felt this type of self-promotion was an important part of the personal statement..."[12]

Rule # 66 Leave out your entire life story.

In the one page that you have for your PS, you cannot, and should not, try to write your life story. Some applicants write about all the experiences and events that they consider significant. It is far better to describe a few events or accomplishments in some detail, and emphasize what these experiences meant to you, and how they reflect upon your individual strengths. A laundry list of experiences, events, and honors has no significance.

Program Directors Speak...

"A personal statement explaining your interest in psychiatry is very important. Please do not simply reiterate your accomplishments; let us know something about yourself that is not on the application."[28]

New York University Psychiatry Residency Program

Rule # 67 **Use your personal statement to highlight your outstanding communication skills.**

Programs also use the PS to learn about your writing ability. Communication skills are of obvious importance in every specialty. A poorly written statement will raise concerns about your ability to care for patients, record the results of your patient evaluations, convey important and sometimes complicated information to other health care professionals, and educate patients about their illness.

> **Did you know?**
>
> At the website for the psychiatry residency at the State University of New York in Stony Brook, the program states that "writing skills are an essential component of medical record keeping, particularly in psychiatry...The selection committee will evaluate the preparation of the application and in particular the personal statement for evidence of writing skills...Applicants with poorly written essays, e.g., multiple spelling and grammatical errors will not be invited for an interview."[29]

A poorly written personal statement is not hard to spot. Indicators include the following:

- Lack of flow (e.g., jumping from one tangent to another)
- Lack of structure. Remember that each paragraph should develop one idea or central point, and each sentence should build on the one before it.
- Spelling errors
- Grammatical errors
- The use of clichés, tired analogies, and metaphors. These bore readers and make you appear lazy or lacking imagination. Instead, use original words to convey your intended meaning.
- The use of "I" to begin every sentence.
- The use of long or run-on sentences
- The use of abbreviations. Don't assume that everyone recognizes your abbreviations.
- Not backing up descriptive comments about yourself. One classic example is writing that "I'm a very hard worker" without providing specific examples.

> **Did you know?**
>
> In a survey of orthopedic PDs, 32% stated that "the most important aspect of a personal statement was to gain insight into an applicant's ability to write and to communicate effectively."[30]

Tip # 37

Residency programs are looking for applicants who can communicate effectively. Speaking and writing English well is crucial to evaluating and managing patients, communicating with colleagues, and reading large volumes of detailed information. Your personal statement will be examined carefully for any deficiencies of written expression.

Rule # 68 Do not permit even a single spelling or grammatical mistake.

Spelling and grammatical mistakes are glaring errors that can seriously damage your candidacy. Always seek out several reviewers to read your PS before submission.

One PD we know reads every statement with a red pen in hand. He then proceeds to circle all grammatical, spelling, and punctuation errors. At the end of the statement, if he has more than a few circles, he questions the applicant's ability to pay attention to detail. Thc obvious conclusion is that the applicant may approach the care of patients in the same manner.

Tip # 38

In reviewing your statement, PDs will look at the quality of your writing, not just its content. While the proper grammar and spelling will not impress them, errors will severely weaken your application. PDs value precision and attention to detail.

To catch spelling errors, use the spell check function of your computer. However, don't rely solely on spell check. Proofread your work carefully, looking for both typographical and grammatical errors. It can be useful to put aside your statement for a few days. Reading it out loud or backwards one word at a time are other useful techniques.

Did you know?

In a study evaluating the content of personal statements, members of the radiology residency selection committee at Wayne State University ranked 5 elements of form from least to most important. Most important was a candidate's basic language skills. This was defined as the applicant's ability to "express his/her ideas in a way that is grammatically correct and free from major spelling and punctuation errors."[12]

Did you know?

Dr. Warren Heymann, head of the dermatology division at Cooper University Health Care, wrote "I may eliminate an applicant because of too many typographical errors on the application (if the applicant does not care enough to proofread his own application, will he care enough to review the chart thoroughly?)"[6]

Why Anesthesiology?

- Love of anatomy, physiology, and pharmacology, and opportunity to apply knowledge with every patient
- Importance of field to good surgical outcomes
- Immediate results of efforts and interventions
- Ability to customize plan/care during procedure to patient's situation
- Focus attention and skills fully on one patient
- Adapting to ever changing needs of the patient during surgery
- Thrill associated with quickly assessing problems and making rapid decisions in potentially life-threatening situations
- Intense patient encounters requiring ability to gain trust and confidence quickly
- Collaboration with other specialists and professionals
- Privilege to anesthetize patients, support them during surgery, and bring them back through difficult operations
- Constantly evolving specialty
- Enjoyment of airway control and resuscitation
- Satisfaction gained through reducing or relieving pain
- Hands-on nature of work requiring technical expertise

Why Dermatology?

- Intellectual challenge associated with caring for patients with challenging skin diseases
- Ability to make diagnoses without need for complex testing
- Breadth of specialty
- Diversity of patient problems
- Early detection of skin cancer, and rewards associated with cure
- Restoring self-esteem by improving outward appearance
- Results of efforts and interventions often readily visible
- Combination of medicine and surgery
- Dealing with specific problems that can often be fixed
- Development of deeper relationships with patients of all ages
- Variety of treatment options (topical therapy, systemic therapy, phototherapy, laser, cryotherapy, surgery)
- Satisfaction gained by relieving misery

Why Emergency Medicine?

- Desire to practice in high-pressure situations requiring quick life and death decisions
- Intellectual challenge of evaluating undifferentiated patients
- Enjoyment of acute care medicine and resuscitation
- Satisfaction associated with being able to handle any emergent condition
- Collaborative nature of the work and daily interactions with all specialists
- Responsibility to lead large group of professionals taking care of patients at critical times
- Variety of problems encountered (medical, surgical, trauma, psychological)
- Requiring knowledge in every single field
- First point of contact for many patients
- Diversity of patients (age, culture, ethnicity, income level)
- Lifelong learning to keep up with advances in the field
- Opportunities to perform variety of procedures

In a survey of nearly 400 EM applicants, researchers sought to determine the factors that motivated applicants to pursue a career in EM.

Factors cited included diversity in clinical pathology and emphasis on acute care. "Emergency physicians (EPs) care for patients of all ages and backgrounds and deal with life-threatening, acute and chronic problems relating to all organ systems," wrote the authors. "The scope of practice in EM is also diverse, depending on the practice setting (e.g., rural, tertiary) and the availability of specialty back-up, follow-up care and hospital equipment."

"EM encompasses procedural, interventional and diagnostic clinical medicine in dealing with the onset of new illness, the initial manifestation of injury and the acute manifestation of chronic illness."[31]

Why Family Medicine?

- Deeply meaningful and long-lasting relationships with patients
- Joy associated with bettering health over a period of time
- Opportunity to treat several generations within a family, and be a part of precious moments in their lives
- Wide range of medical problems
- Emphasis on health maintenance and preventive medicine for all ages
- Continuity of care
- Variety of problems encountered
- Caring for patients of all ages from birth to end of life
- Intellectual challenge that comes with caring for patients with chronic disease or those having multiple medical problems
- First point of contact for many patients
- Caring for the "whole person" with focus not only on physical complaints but social, emotional, and mental issues as well
- Ability to handle any undifferentiated problem
- Varied practice settings (clinic, operating room, ICU, ED)

Why General Surgery?

- Interacting and caring for patients at the most vulnerable times in their lives
- Immediate positive impact, and the chance to return patient to normal life relatively quickly
- Ability to deal with any surgical emergency
- Caring for patients with serious conditions, and the gratification that comes with observing successful recovery
- Challenge of acquiring new technical skills and incorporating new technologies
- Working with full surgical team to deliver care in collaborative process
- Caring for adult patients in both the inpatient and outpatient settings
- Diverse nature of problems
- Evaluating and managing challenging problems in critically ill and injured patients
- Providing care for patients of all ages presenting with variety of acute and chronic conditions
- Making rapid decisions regarding interventions for acutely ill patients
- Varied practice settings (clinic, operating room, ICU, ED)

Why Internal Medicine?

- Enjoyment of diagnostic process, akin to solving puzzles or working like a detective
- Emphasis on pathophysiology
- Variety of problems and symptoms encountered
- Caring for patients with acute and chronic illnesses
- Caring for adult patients in both the inpatient and outpatient settings
- Coordinating overall care of patient
- Different practice settings (clinic, hospital, ICU, nursing home, hospice)
- Long-term relationships with patients which allow involvement at important times in their lives
- Involvement in complex cases affecting multiple organ systems
- Lifelong learning
- Intellectual challenge that comes with providing comprehensive care
- Interaction with colleagues from variety of specialties
- Ability to evaluate and manage just about everything
- Emphasis on disease prevention

Why Neurology?

- Diagnostic challenges associated with assessing neurological problems
- Fascination with anatomy of brain
- Complexity of neurological system and examination
- Localizing the disease or lesion with the emphasis on the history and exam
- Thrill of making diagnoses without overreliance on technology
- Intellectual challenge involved with each case, akin to solving puzzle or unraveling mystery
- Unusual symptoms and signs which are challenging to assess
- Wide ranging specialty with varied presentations and illnesses
- Interaction with colleagues from variety of specialties
- Drawn to challenge of furthering the understanding of the brain and the diseases affecting it
- Excitement about being part of a specialty that is making strides in treatment

Why Obstetrics & Gynecology?

- Opportunities to be involved in cherished times in patients' lives
- Privilege to discuss concerns women are hesitant to share with others
- Guide women in their most intimate areas of health
- Emphasis on humanism and compassion
- Long-term and unique relationships with patients
- Special bond that develops between physician and patient/family
- Variety of patients and problems
- Care delivered in different settings (office, operating room, labor & delivery, international)
- Promotion of overall health and well-being to women
- Challenges encountered in providing care at various stages of women's life
- Caring for women of all ages
- Opportunities to educate women to make healthy choices
- Mixture of medicine and hands-on surgery
- Mix of surgeries from simple to complex and extensive
- Challenge of learning new approaches
- Opportunities to perform variety of procedures (e.g., colposcopy, LEEP, IUD insertion, endometrial biopsy, polyp removal)
- Ability to cure or improve many problems with variety of treatments

In a study of obstetrics and gynecology residents, participants were asked to rate the most appealing aspects of the specialty. Participants were also asked to rate factors on a five point scale in terms of importance (with 5 being most important). Among the factors cited were surgical opportunities (4.7), variety of clinical experience in day-to-day practice (office/surgery/labor unit) (4.6), fast-paced/high-acuity experiences (4.3), obstetric opportunities (4.2), opportunity to be a women's health advocate (4.1), and variety of patient problems (4.0).[32]

Why Ophthalmology?

- Preserving or improving vision
- Opportunity to profoundly change, sometimes very quickly, peoples' lives
- Long-term relationships with patients
- Working with hands
- Fascination with complexity of the visual system
- Love of the ophthalmological exam
- Eye examination reveals so much about the rest of the body
- Nature of surgery (detailed, delicate, challenging)
- Technologically advanced specialty which constantly adopts new innovations
- Ability to treat patients medically and surgically
- Care for patients of all ages

In a survey of over 100 U.S. third- and fourth-year medical students, researchers sought to determine the motivations to pursue a career in ophthalmology. The authors wrote that "the leading response was the importance that vision plays in one's life and specifically the ability to help people see better compared with other aspects of health." Other factors cited were performing surgery, technology, junior-year medical school ophthalmology rotation, and personal history of ocular disease.[33]

In a survey of over 700 ophthalmology residents, residents were asked to provide reasons for entering the field. Residents also ranked factors based on their effect on choosing ophthalmology as a career (1 = large effect, 5 = no effect). Among the highest rated factors were surgery (1.49), patient contact (1.83), junior/senior electives (2.24), and previous contact with ophthalmologists (2.54).

Approximately 10% of residents had a family member or relative in the specialty. Nearly 60% were patients of ophthalmologists before becoming residents. The authors wrote that some residents had "visual problems in childhood that resulted in close contact with an ophthalmologist while growing up, and that greatly influences their interest in ophthalmology."[15]

Why Orthopedic Surgery?

- Satisfaction gained from helping patients recover from injuries, and return to the activities that give them pleasure in their lives
- Surgeries and procedures performed allow for immediate positive feedback and impact
- Opportunities to improve quality of life and restore function in patients with chronic disease (e.g., arthritis requiring hip replacement)
- Love of mechanics and materials
- Enjoyment of musculoskeletal system
- Working with hands
- Technical nature of procedures
- Rapidly changing specialty involving use of advanced technology
- Combination of conservative therapy and surgical intervention if conservative options fail

In the *British Medical Journal*, Dr. Alexander Young offered reasons to pursue a career in the field. Among these reasons were the rewarding and satisfying nature of the field, ability to rapidly improve quality of life, combination of theoretical knowledge and practical skills, combination of clinical acumen and technology, appreciation and application of anatomy, immediate critique of results, and wide interaction with multidisciplinary team.[34]

Why Otolaryngology?

- Fascination with complex anatomy and physiology of head and neck
- Enjoyment of problems involving ear, nose, and throat
- Patient diversity
- Development of close physician-patient relationships as many conditions require follow-up over a period of time
- Good combination of outpatient and surgical work
- Hands-on nature of the specialty with use of variety of tools (e.g., microscopes, endoscopes, lasers)
- Large range of presenting complaints
- Diversity in type and complexity of procedures ranging from endoscopic sinus surgery to major head and neck reconstruction
- Desire to perform procedures on small areas requiring precision
- Care spans all ages
- Constantly changing field with technological advances
- Opportunities to perform procedures which have tremendous impact on lives
- Procedures in the specialty can lead to significant improvements in quality of life with respect to speech, swallowing, breathing, hearing, smell, and taste

Why Pathology?

- Each case is a new intellectual challenge, and there are surprises every day
- Requires broad knowledge base of disease processes affecting every organ
- Necessitates lifelong learning
- Desire to fully understand disease processes and know why problems occur
- Interest in visual imagery
- Enjoy problem solving nature of the field
- Exciting to arrive at diagnoses by integrating findings from gross and microscopic examination with clinical and radiologic findings
- Pivotal role in decision-making with pathological diagnoses affecting treatment and prognosis
- Cerebral field which is logical and evidence-based in nature
- Encompasses variety of areas (molecular diagnostics, clinical chemistry, etc.)
- Gratifying to assist physicians of all specialties deliver high quality care
- Collaborative nature of the field in which there are daily interactions with colleagues and opportunities to explain diagnosis
- Reliance of other specialties on the discipline of pathology for evaluation and management of patients
- Involvement in the most exciting and challenging cases
- Knowledge that one's work plays a major role in helping doctors reach correct diagnoses and impact patient care
- Opportunities to bridge basic science research with clinical medicine in ongoing efforts to develop methods and tools to improve diagnosis, treatment, and patient outcomes

Why Radiation Oncology?

- Opportunity to care for patients at the most vulnerable times in their lives, and appreciate the human spirit during the course of therapy
- Gratifying to cure patients of serious disease
- Potential for immediate benefit from therapy
- When cure is not possible, still very rewarding to help improve quality of life, alleviate pain or other symptoms, and provide comfort at a difficult time
- Rewarding to develop close relationships with patients through what are often daily encounters for weeks to months
- Combines practice in medicine with cutting edge technology
- Fascination with applied physics, technology, and delivery of radiation
- Involvement in innovative specialty which is rapidly advancing and offering patients better treatments with reduced toxicity
- Working within multidisciplinary and collaborative team of specialists in medical oncology, surgical oncology, radiation therapy, physics, and nursing to deliver best possible care
- Process of designing and planning course of treatment and tailoring the plan to the patient using advanced technology

Why Radiology?

- Requires immense depth of knowledge, and there's always something to learn
- Cerebral and analytical with focus on problem solving
- Process of combining clinical presentation with findings on imaging tests to arrive at a list of possible diagnoses
- Diagnosis and management of patients often hinges on imaging
- Breadth of specialty with cases and pathology from all areas of medicine
- Cutting edge of science and technology
- Excitement of specialty in which imaging modalities are constantly evolving and changing
- Opportunity to care for patients of all ages and genders
- Opportunity to interact with physicians from different specialties on a routine basis, and be part of a unified team to exchange ideas and find answers to difficult patient questions
- Involvement in most interesting and complex patients
- Rewarding nature of work which guides patient management in different disciplines
- Offers imaging techniques to monitor disease progression
- Satisfaction that comes with identifying disease early before tremendous harm has occurred
- Availability of minimally invasive procedures which impacts patient care and, in some cases, may be the best or only diagnostic or treatment option

Why Urology?

- Challenging specialty which combines operative experience with office practice. In a survey of approximately 250 urology applicants inquiring about the reasons to enter the specialty, 28% cited the mix of medicine and surgery / clinic and procedures. One applicant wrote that he was drawn to the specialty because of "the wide range of office, surgical, and procedural techniques used in this field."[35]

- Opportunity to care for patients of all ages and genders

- Breadth of urology in the operating room (open surgery, laparoscopic procedures, microsurgery, endoscopic procedures)

- Everything from simple to very complex surgeries

- Forefront of technological advances

- Options for treatment with nonsurgical approaches (biofeedback, radiation, cryotherapy)

- Diverse clinical problems

- Ongoing patient interaction over period of years which leads to deeper relationships with patients

- Requires patients to discuss very personal issues, and mandates bedside manner that fosters trust in the physician-patient relationship

- Gratification that comes when impact is made on a patient suffering with a chronic problem

- Constantly changing specialty which challenges its practitioners to improve with it

- Illnesses that are often curable

- Outcomes that are often very positive

- Availability of tests to help diagnose variety of problems affecting bladder, prostate, and kidneys

Sample Personal Statements

Radiology Residency Personal Statement

The coldness of the water startled me when it soaked through my clothing. I tightened my grip on our guide's head and repositioned myself more securely on his shoulders. As we waded across the river and Brazilian border, only the rippling of the water broke the silence. I could not see my parents nor my siblings in the dark. Images of lights shining down on us and voices telling us to stop haunted me. I was 8 years old.

My family first moved from Taiwan to Paraguay in 1976 in order to gain entrance into Brazil and join our relatives in Sao Miguel. Our aim was to circumvent the political sanctions which forbade our emigration. However, disillusioned with the political situation, we moved back to Paraguay after living in Brazil for one year. In search of better social and educational opportunities, we applied for permission to reside in the United States. During the five long years of waiting, my father worked 15-hour days at our restaurant while my mother walked door to door selling clothes and faux-jewelry. Since I was the oldest of three children, I was in charge of caring for my siblings while our parents were absent from home. At the age of 9, I cooked our meals and washed the dishes while my 8 year-old sister washed our clothes by hand and cleaned the house. We both acted as babysitters for our 6 year-old brother. I learned the meaning of responsibility, hard work, and self-reliance at an early age. These lessons helped me attain my dream of becoming a physician and will definitely be essential in my pursuit of a career in Diagnostic Radiology.

With all my might, I tightened the knob one last time. Bending over the gas tank, I placed my nose just millimeters away from the connection site and took in a deep breath. No smell of gas could be detected. With drops of water on my palms, I rubbed a bar of soap for a couple of minutes. I coated the soap suds over the connection site and waited for signs of bubbling but saw none. Gingerly, I turned on the stove and lit a match. What a sigh of relief! No explosion. I was 9 years old.

I am always systematic and detailed in my work. Whether the job is a routine replacement of the portable gas tank for the stove, preparing dinner for 20 guests, gathering data for my research projects, or taking care of my patients at the hospital, my performance has always been thorough. One cannot be an outstanding Radiologist without being detailed. No matter how much knowledge and experience a Radiologist has, she will undoubtedly miss the correct diagnosis if the subtle changes on the radiographic study are left undetected.

I sharpened my pencil and took another look at the model's face staring at me from the page of the magazine. Slowly, the expression in her eyes and the shape of her nose appeared on the white sheet of paper on which I had been drawing. I applied subtle shading around the cheekbones and nose in order to capture the lighting on her face. My art teacher entered my first attempt at a human portrait into the school-wide Art Contest. Surprise! I won Honorable Mention. I was 18 years old.

The ability to derive three-dimensional structures from two-dimensional pictures comes naturally to me. My grasp of the three dimensions combined with my eye for detail brought me recognition not only in the area of Fine Arts but also in other areas of my life. The wonderful taste and look of my Chinese cuisine are well-known to friends and family. They have also complimented me on my skill to bring to life a hairstyle off the pages of a magazine. I first discovered that I was such a "visual" person when I started attending school. I learned to read and write Chinese characters without difficulty because I was able to assemble and visualize very stroke in my mind. As a result, reading and writing Chinese now is no obstacle even though I received only two years of formal schooling in Taiwan. Diagnostic Radiology is a "visual" field, and the ability to extrapolate three dimensional structures from two-dimensional radiographs is indispensable.

The five year-old girl who had acute lymphocytic leukemia looked straight at me with her big brown eyes. "I am not going to cry," she said as she brought her knees onto her chest, in preparation for her usual prophylactic lumbar puncture. "I won't cry because I am a good girl...I am a good girl." She screamed as the needle entered her back but kept her body still. "I was a good girl, right? I didn't cry." She looked searchingly at me, dry-eyed. Tears welled up in my eyes, and I had to look away. I was 24 years old.

I have always been proud of the special relationship I share with my patients. Often I curse the painful procedures my patients have to experience, especially when I see innocent children suffering from their terrible illnesses. Thankfully, several advancements in radiologic imaging have curtailed the need for invasive diagnostic procedures. For example, disease staging for a number of malignancies can now be easily and painlessly obtained through computed tomography instead of exploratory laparotomies. Through my Pediatric Hematology-Oncology elective at Caring Children's Hospital, I learned the important role Diagnostic Radiology plays in the diagnosis, management, and treatment of numerous oncologic diseases. I also had the chance to appreciate the value of different imaging modalities utilized in the diagnosis of malignancies while researching for my project in both Body Imaging and Pediatric Radiology and would like to pursue further studies in these areas at the completion of my residency.

I feel I possess the qualities your program desires in a residency candidate, and I look forward to my visit to your institution.

Dermatology Residency Personal Statement

While I continued to pull through the heavy water, I heard the coxswain call out, "This is it!" My feelings of complete exhaustion and loss of breath would have to wait. Months of getting up at five in the morning for drills on the Strong River would come down to one final moment. Rowing in college had meant working hard surrounded by teammates who shared enthusiasm and drive. Although my present goal is to train in dermatology, tenets in rowing continue to serve me today: hard work and perseverance never go out of style.

As my fondness for rowing demonstrates, I love a good challenge. The opportunity for challenge and new discovery attracted me to chemical engineering and medical research as an undergraduate. While working in a lab at Harvard, I became interested in applying technology to the field of medicine. I was given many hands-on tasks including learning tissue grafting. Surgery on animals allowed us to study tumor angiogenesis and directly visualize vessel growth and regression. My talents in engineering proved to be of great use when I developed an algorithm to quantify blood flow. I had found research I truly enjoyed and this interest motivated me.

In medical school, I enjoyed the visual inspection of physical diagnosis; clearly describing what I saw came naturally. I enjoyed the focus of small, hands-on procedures. Dermatology captured my interest and by early in my fourth year, I decided I needed more time to explore the field. Following medical school, I took a two-year position at Medical University where my engineering background allowed me to contribute to the creation of a survey tool for an outcomes research study where I gained critical skills in conducting clinical trials. I became expert in FDA and IRB regulatory issues and spent a great deal of time seeing dermatology patients. Gleaning clues from subtle distinguishing features required a true love of the diagnostic process; studying disease and following treatment outcomes continued to be satisfying. Together, these experiences confirmed my enthusiasm for dermatology was worth pursuing.

The field of dermatology appeals to me for many reasons. The relationship between doctor and patient is collaborative and often ongoing. Blistering and other diseases offer a spectrum of severities and clinical challenges. Our growing understanding of the skin's immune system makes this an especially exciting time to be in dermatology. Developing new therapies is tremendously rewarding – and the end results thrilling to see.

Since completing my medical internship in June, I have worked as a Clinical Fellow with the Department of Dermatology. I continue to add to my research skills guiding a Phase III melanoma vaccine trial. I have become expert in vaccine development, manufacturing, and testing. My experience has allowed me to collaborate with world-renowned dermatologists and researchers. Skills I develop here will surely serve me well throughout my career.

My goal is to utilize my unique background in engineering to one day design and test new dermatologic therapies of my own. I would consider myself lucky to return to My University for residency and my elective only strengthened this feeling. I believe My University can offer the ideal training environment for the type of career I have chosen. The diversity of clinical settings and spectrum of disease is appealing, and training with research leaders such as Skin Doctor would offer a great perspective on evolving therapies, as well as continued mentorship. I will continue to use hard work and determination to reach my goals in dermatology and like in rowing, look forward to new challenges and discoveries ahead.

From www.medfools.com (with permission)

Pathology Personal Statement

The woman lying in Bed 14 was totally disfigured. More than half of her body was covered by deep ulcers, foul-smelling pus and thick crusts. She had lost her hair and eyelids and her cheeks were penetrated deeply. Seven years ago I was a dermatology resident at a teaching hospital in Beijing. I had the opportunity to see a wide range of cases from across the nation where I met Mrs. Yao. From her husband I learned that her ordeal started with a coin-like macule on the forearm, which was first misdiagnosed as psoriasis at a local clinic. Believing the misdiagnosis, she treated herself with herbal medicine for several years until a full eruption of skin lesions occurred. She was later diagnosed as having mycosis fungoides, a cutaneous T-cell lymphoma, and sadly passed away on our ward despite an enormous effort to save her. The tragedy was reinforced by the fact that Mrs. Yao cold have had a good chance of survival if treated early. During my residency I could not help but wonder: "How can we give every patient the correct diagnosis?" personal experience has made me fascinated with Pathology as a science and as a career and although I started my medical career in dermatology, I have realized that my calling lies in pathology.

The person who correctly diagnosed Mrs. Yao is my mentor, Dr. Xavier, a brilliant dermatologist and dermatopathologist whom I deeply admire. My training in dermatopathology with Dr. Xavier turned out to be the most exciting time in my residency. Pathology is our most powerful weapon to reach the correct diagnosis. Dr. Xavier liked to say "Pathology is the third eye of the dermatologist." Indeed, in a specialty where cases tend to be diagnosed by a mere glance at the skin, Pathology has a dramatic impact on clinical decision making. I enjoyed sitting before a microscope, browsing through our collection of slides and making discoveries. Every slide, every cell tells a story. At that time I was convinced that Pathology would always be my passion.

I also chose Pathology because of enormous research opportunities. During my first residency, I studied p53 gene mutations in skin cancers and wrote a well-received thesis while under the pressure of a tight residency curriculum. With great enthusiasm I performed most experiments at night in my spare time. This early adventure in science inspired me with great interest in scientific exploration. During the following years my adventure has gone further and deeper. It has moved from thermal cyclers to tissue culture rooms, to microarray chips, and even to supercomputers. No matter what front I work on, my goal of applying science to furthering human health has never changed. Being a pathologist would give me an enormous opportunity to bridge basic science and clinical medicine while applying the latest scientific advancements to solving the mysteries of human disease.

No specialty attracts me more than Pathology. Making diagnoses is a complex task that requires gathering and integrating information, a great intellectual challenge that I always enjoy facing. As a pathologist, I will have the unique opportunity to work with physicians of every specialty, to deal with diseases of every organ system, and to combine clinical with morphological, biochemical, and even molecular findings. It will be intellectually rewarding and will be a continuous source of learning. Above all of these, Pathology will fuel the passion of all of us who have chosen Medicine as a career, because lives can be saved by correct diagnoses.

In the future I see myself pursuing a career in academic medicine. I will dedicate myself to providing the best diagnostic service to patients while exploring young physicians and scientists. After residency I hope to pursue further training in a subspecialty. I believe a residency in pathology is a place where I can being to fulfill my professional goals.

From www.medfools.com (with permission)

PM&R Residency Personal Statement

In the banquet room of an Italian restaurant in Northern Alaska, my high school track coach addressed his team and their families at the end of the season. Most senior athletes were complimented on either a winning season or a season of hard work. I had accomplished neither. In addressing me in front of the crowd he said: “Despite what the record books show, I know Karen is the best triple jumper to ever compete for this school.” I was so proud to hear those words after a season which began with me favored to win the league title and break the school record, and ended without me having the chance. My senior season turned into months of physical therapy, sitting on the bench and hoping for a chance to get back to the form I once had. Although my injury kept me from breaking that record, the lessons I learned during that time have proven to guide me in my choice of careers.

Since then I have been drawn to a career where I am involved in helping achieve optimum function and recover from similar experiences where dreams seem lost and rehabilitation can be difficult. I had my first hands-on experience with the field of rehabilitation during college when I volunteered at the first rehabilitation hospital to open in my hometown. I worked in the Transitional

Care Unit leading activities including wheelchair aerobics, art therapy and pet therapy. The physicians and therapists I met there played a role in encouraging me to apply to medical school.

During my first two years of medical school I was able to work with three different Physiatrists who introduced me to a field where I witnessed the long-term relationships that developed between doctor and patient, as well as the opportunity to be the leader of a rehabilitation team. Both of these aspects of the specialty are important to me and coincide with my strengths, which include strong interpersonal skills and development of relationships as well as a love of organizing and motivating people. The ease with which I work with all types of people has always been one of the areas where I have been complimented most by others.

In my third year during my family medicine and internal medicine rotations I found my interest in the specialty confirmed by my enjoyment of my Workman's Compensation and orthopedic surgical recovery patients. I now look forward to broadening my exposure to the field of Physical Medicine and Rehabilitation during the two elective rotations I have in October and November.

In residency, I hope to attend a program that will provide a solid foundation in the pathophysiology as well as the clinical practice of rehabilitation medicine. I value structured training with diversity of exposure to patients and facilities. I would like to learn in an environment that encourages a close relationship with the patients as well as the other residents and faculty.

As far as my goals after residency, I would like to continue my education with fellowship training in either musculoskeletal or sports medicine. I aspire to a career in clinical medicine with opportunities to do clinical research and possibly supervise medical students and residents. I love the academic community environment and especially the constant learning that accompanies the field of medicine.

From www.medfools.com (with permission)

Emergency Medicine Personal Statement

The wind whipped through the airplane cabin as the door opened at 13,800 feet. As I sat waiting for my turn to jump, I felt more anxious and uncertain that I'd ever been in my life. "Ready?" the jump master yelled. I didn't have time to respond. My rotation in Emergency Medicine, as a fourth-year medical student, had been going well. I never imagined it would lead me to this. I had accepted an invitation to go skydiving with a couple of the residents. Suddenly, I was flipping through the sky. Only moments before, my instructor and I had discussed why I wish to become an Emergency Medicine Physician. I told him about my experiences in the field and how intense, exhilarating, and rewarding

I found Emergency Medicine. His response was, “Well, buddy, you are about to have one of the most exhilarating and intense experiences of your life!” He was right. For fifty seconds of free fall towards the Earth, I felt pure ecstasy. After pulling the rip cord, we smoothly glided down under the parachute. Everything became serene. Sailing down from the sky, the anxiety and uncertainty had disappeared. I found myself completely at peace and gratified with my decision to jump. I feel that same sense of peace about my dive into pursuing Emergency Medicine.

Emergency Medicine appeals to me as a humanistic, challenging field, offering the opportunity to provide immediate help to people in the most vital aspect of their lives: their health. The emotional rewards of helping those during their greatest times of need are intangible. Twelve years ago, I encountered this first hand as knee surgery introduced me to medicine. It was an eye-opening experience to me; then, a 14-year-old kid who, before surgery, dreamed of playing professional football. As a result of the positive impression the entire experience had on me, the medical profession emerged as my newfound desire. My employment prior to and during medical school, working as a E.M.T. and a Scribe in the Emergency Department of Saint Elsewhere Regional Medical Center in Wyoming, introduced me to the field of Emergency Medicine. It was there, as well as my experiences with the Army National Guard, serving as a flight medic, that my interest blossomed. Being tin the ED as a medical student has fortified my desire to enter the field.

Emergency Medicine offers me the opportunity to be at the forefront of medicine and to participate actively in making decisions right from the onset of patient care. I’ve learned that the ability to immediately establish rapport and make the patient feel better is not only a part of the Emergency Medicine Physician’s responsibilities, but is also one of the most satisfying aspects of the specialty. The fast pace, community involvement, and the required broad knowledge base attract me to Emergency Medicine. The Emergency Medical System comes together to help all people, including those who have nowhere else to turn. I want to be an active part of that system.

I look forward to a career in Emergency Medicine involving clinical practice, education, and research. During my own medical education, spending time in a research lab studying the response to thermal injury in a rat model, I have become increasingly aware of the importance of research. I will seek out opportunities to participate in Emergency Medicine research that will promote advancement in the field. I also feel that teaching adds a gratifying and stimulating aspect to practice that can be incorporated into almost any situation. Having the opportunity to train residents and students is something I will weigh considerably when selecting a location to practice. I hope to be in an area that allows me to serve a diverse patient population, as well as providing an environment that supports my outside interests of mountain biking, golf, basketball, scuba diving, and skiing. Skydiving doesn’t make the list just yet. These hobbies and my sense of humor allow me to keep a balance in my own life and increase my enthusiasm for practicing medicine. I'm ready to jump into residency training with this enthusiasm.

Emergency Medicine will endow me with a solid education and preparation for a profession in which I am able to deal with the entire spectrum of acute illness and injury in all age groups. I wish to enter a residency program that will provide a broad-based clinical education with a diverse patient population that emphasizes education, encourages mentoring, facilitates opportunities for research, and is intimately involved in Emergency Medical Services. I will bring to my residency program a hard working, mature individual who has a clear vision of a career in Emergency Medicine. My experiences and training have reinforced my dedication to this dynamic and exhilarating field of medicine.

From www.medfools.com (with permission)

References

[1]Campbell B, Hayas N, Derse A, Holloway R. Creating a residency application personal statement writers workshop: Fostering narrative, teamwork, and insight at a time of stress. *Acad Med* 2016; 91(3): 371-375.

[2]University of Washington Department of Family Medicine. Available at: https://depts.washington.edu/fammed/residency/fellowships/global-health/applicant-information/. Accessed January 5, 2016.

[3]Taylor C, Weinstein L, Mayhew H. The process of resident selection: a view from the residency director's desk. *Obstet Gynecol* 1995; 85(2): 299-303.

[4]Chew F, Ochoa E, Relyea-Chew A. Spreadsheet application for radiology resident match rank list. *Acad Radiol* 2005; 12: 379-384.

[5]University of Texas-Houston Medical School Department of Othopedic Surgery. Available at: www.uth.tmc.edu/med/administration/student/ms4/2003CCC.htm. Accessed on December 22, 2008.

[6]Heymann W. Advice to the dermatology residency applicant. *Arch Dermatol* 2000; 136(1): 123-4.

[7]Results of the 2014 NRMP Program Director Survey. Available at: http://www.nrmp.org/wp-content/uploads/2014/09/PD-Survey-Report-2014.pdf. Accessed March 3, 2016.

[8]UCSF Department of Medicine. Available at: http://dgim.ucsf.edu/education/sfgh/apply.html. Accessed January 4, 2016.

[9]University of Utah Department of Dermatology. Available at: http://uuhsc.utah.edu/derm/residency/residency/htm. Accessed November 4, 2015.

[10]University of Oklahoma Department of Orthopedic Surgery. Available at: https://www.oumedicine.com/department-of-orthopedic-surgery-and-rehabilitation/residency-programs/orthopedic-surgery-residency/how-to-apply. Accessed November 2, 2008.

[11]McGarry K, Tammaro D, Cyr M. Crafting a great personal statement. ACP Impact September 2006. Available at: https://www.acponline.org/medical_students/impact/archives/2006/09/perspect/ Accessed January 5, 2016.

[12]Smith E, Weyhing B, Mody Y, Smith W. A critical analysis of personal statements submitted by radiology residency applicants. *Acad Radiol* 2005; 12: 1024-1028.

[13]Harvard University Department of Radiation Oncology. Available at: http://www.harvardradiationoncologyprogram.org/application/. Accessed February 2, 2016.

[14]Adena Health System. Available at: http://www.adena.org/inside/paccar/page.dT/residency-program. Accessed February 2, 2016.

[15]Pankratz M, Helveston E. Ophthalmology. The resident's perspective. *Arch Ophthalmol* 1992; 110(1): 37-43.

[16]Getting into Emergency Medicine. Available at: http://studentdoctor.net/2010/08/the-successful-match-getting-into-emergency-medicine/. Accessed January 30, 2013.
[17]The Successful Match: Getting into Dermatology. Available at: http://studentdoctor.net/2009/10/the-successful-match-getting-into-dermatology/. Accessed April 30, 2012.
[18]The Successful Match: Getting into Obstetrics and Gynecology. Available at: http://studentdoctor.net/2010/05/the-successful-match-getting-into-obstetrics-and-gynecology/. Accessed February 10, 2013.
[19]Grover M, Charamshi F, Goveia C. Deception by applicants to family practice residencies. *Fam Med* 2001; 33: 441-446.
[20]Association of American Medical Colleges. Available at: https://www.aamc.org/services/eras/programs/policies/134636/investigation.html. Accessed January 4, 2016.
[21]Lehrmann J, Walaszek A. Assessing the quality of residency applicants in psychiatry. *Acad Psychiatry* 2008; 32(3): 180-182.
[22]Segal S, Gelfand B, Hurwitz S, Berkowitz L, Ashley S, Nadel E, Katz J. Plagiarism in residency application essays. *Ann Intern Med* 2010; 153(2): 112-120.
[23]Stratton-Loeffler M. Plagiarism in residency application essays. *Ann Intern Med* 2010; 153(11): 766.
[24]Parks L, Sizemore D, Johnstone R. Plagiarism in personal statements of anesthesiology residency applicants. A A Case Reports 2015; Oct 8 epub.
[25]ERAS Integrity Promotion – Investigation Program. Available at: https://www.aamc.org/services/eras/programs/policies/134636/investigation.html. Accessed March 16, 2016.
[26]Daly K, Levine S, Adams G. Predictors for resident success in otolaryngology. *J Am Coll Surg* 2006; 202(4): 649-654.
[27]University of California Davis Department of Pediatrics. Available at: https://www.ucdmc.ucdavis.edu/pediatrics/education/application.html. Accessed February 2, 2016.
[28]New York Medical College Department of Psychiatry. Available at: https://www.nymc.edu/departments/academic-departments/school-of-medicine/psychiatry-and-behavioral-sciences/residency-program/application-requirements/. Accessed February 2, 2016.
[29]State University of New York StonyBrook. Available at: http://www.hsc.stonybrook.edu/som/psychiatry/selection_process.cfm. Accessed June 2, 2008.
[30]Bernstein A, Jazrawi L, Elbeshbeshy B, Della Valle C, Zuckerman J. Orthopedic resident-selection criteria. *J Bone Joint Surg Am* 2002; 84-A(11): 2090-2096.
[31]Kazzi A, Langdorf M, Ghadishah D, Handly N. Motivations for a career in emergency medicine: a profile of the 1996 US applicant pool. *CJEM* 2001; 3(2): 99-104.
[32]Blanchard M, Autry A, Brown H, Musich J, Kaufman L, Wells D, Stager R, Swanson J, Lund K, Wiper D, Bailit J. A multicenter study to determine motivating factors for residents pursuing obstetrics and gynecology. *Am J Obstet Gynecol* 2005; 193(5): 1835-41.

[33]Nissman S, Kudrick N, Piccone M. Motivations and perceptions of US medical students pursuing a career in ophthalmology. *Ann Ophthalmol* 2002; 34(3): 223-9.
[34]BMJ Careers. Available at http://careers.bmj.com/careers/advice/view-article.html?id=20001442. Accessed April 30, 2012.
[35]Kerfoot B, Nabha K, Masser B, McCullough D. What makes a medical student avoid or enter a career in urology? Results of an international survey. *J Urol* 2005; 174(5): 1953-7.

Chapter 8

Medical Student Performance Evaluation (MSPE or Dean's Letter)

Applicants must submit a letter from the Dean as part of their application. Known previously as the Dean's letter, this letter is now formally termed the Medical Student Performance Evaluation (MSPE). The typical MSPE contains an assessment of both a student's academic performance and professional attributes. Residency programs find the MSPE an especially helpful tool to learn about your performance in medical school relative to your peers.

Rule # 69 Recognize the importance of the MSPE in the selection process.

In the 2014 NRMP Program Directors Survey, 84% of residency programs cited the MSPE as a factor used to select applicants to interview. Programs rated the MSPE 4.0 in importance on a scale from 1 (not at all important) to 5 (very important).[1]

Importance Of MSPE In The Residency Selection Process	
Specialty	**% of Residency Programs Citing MSPE as a Factor in Inviting Students to Interview**
Anesthesiology	87%
Dermatology	83%
Emergency Medicine	91%
Family Medicine	80%
General Surgery	79%
Internal Medicine	90%
Neurology	85%
Neurosurgery	81%
Obstetrics & Gynecology	76%
Orthopedic Surgery	79%
Otolaryngology	74%
Pathology	83%
Pediatrics	87%
Physical Medicine & Rehabilitation	88%
Plastic Surgery	62%
Psychiatry	94%
Radiation Oncology	86%
Radiology	91%
Adapted from Results of the 2014 NRMP Program Director Survey. Available at: http://www.nrmp.org/wp-content/uploads/2014/09/PD-Survey-Report-2014.pdf.	

The MSPE is also important in applicant ranking. 68% of programs cited the MSPE as a factor in ranking applicants.[1] Why do programs place so much value on this factor? There is research that indicates that the MSPE may predict future performance. In a study done to learn about characteristics of an applicant that might predict future success in an emergency medicine residency, researchers found that the MSPE correlated fairly well with overall success in residency.[2] In particular, the letter's categorical rating (outstanding, excellent, superior, very good, or good) was found to be a strong predictor of performance during residency training.

Your ultimate goal with the MSPE is to provide assistance to the Dean's office in order to develop the best letter that can be written on your behalf. Fortunately, at most schools, students are involved in the preparation of this letter.

Rule # 70 Understanding the content of the MSPE is the first step in improving it.

Although the MSPE has been a standard part of the residency application for many years, there is considerable debate about its usefulness. Some schools produce letters containing highly useful, detailed and honest information about a student's medical school performance. Others are lacking in key information that programs need to compare applicants.

Critics of the MSPE assert that these letters almost always contain positive information. They contend that significant information is often withheld or suppressed, including information about course or clerkship failure, leaves of absence, or lapses in professionalism. Supporters of the MSPE recognize these shortcomings, but maintain that the letter has value, especially in offering programs information about class rank and a comparison of students to their peers. Furthermore, they cite that schools often include an overall recommendation, usually at the end of the letter.

Because of variability in content and lack of standardization among letters from different schools, the AAMC convened several committees to make recommendations about the letter. These committees recommended that schools should not view the MSPE as a letter of recommendation predictive of future performance, but rather a letter of evaluation. As such, the letter should describe in a sequential manner a student's performance. In describing performance, the AAMC committee urged schools to include comparative performance information. In other words, how did the student perform relative to his peers?

The AAMC also recommended that the MSPE include 6 sections.

Sections Of The MSPE	
MSPE Section	**Description**
Identifying Information	Your legal name Name and location of medical school
Unique Characteristics	Brief statement about your unique characteristics (e.g., leadership positions, research abilities, community service activities). May also include information about any significant challenges or hardships you encountered during medical school.
Academic History	Month and year of initial matriculation Expected graduation date Explanations of any extensions, leaves of absence, gaps, or breaks in your medical school education Information about courses or clerkships that you were required to repeat or remediate Information about any disciplinary action you received from the medical school
Academic Progress	Your academic performance and professional attributes during basic science and clinical years of medical school Narrative information regarding your overall performance on each core clerkship and elective rotation
Summary	A summative assessment of your performance in medical school relative to your peers.
Appendices	Graphic representation of your performance relative to your peers in each preclinical course and core clerkship Graphic representation of your overall performance relative to your peers.

Did you know?

In a survey of anesthesiology PDs, researchers sought to determine which sections of the MSPE were valued most by programs in predicting successful residents. The sections found to be predictive of success included academic history summary, academic progress, and academic ranking.[3]

Rule # 71 **The Dean doesn't always write the MSPE letter. If you can, choose your writer.**

Since the writing of the MSPE is an enormous task for the Dean's office, schools have a number of administrators involved in the development of these letters. Some schools permit students to choose the author of their MSPE from this group.

Choose your writer carefully. Since the two of you will work together to develop your letter, choose a writer with whom you have good rapport. Slots with a popular writer may fill up quickly, so place your request as early as possible.

Rule # 72 **Do extensive prep work before you meet with the Dean.**

Following receipt of your student information sheet, some schools have their students meet with the Dean to discuss the letter. During this meeting, the Dean may ask you about the following:

- Your background
- Your medical school career and performance
- Your career plans, including preferred specialty and back-up plan if necessary
- Programs to which you are applying
- Any events in your medical school career that require explanation (e.g., poor grade, leave of absence)

You may also be able to discuss your competitiveness for your chosen field and overall residency application strategy.

Tip # 39

A meeting with the Dean should be regarded as a valuable opportunity. Take advantage of this opportunity to discuss your chances of matching into a particular specialty or program. Having counseled many students in the past, the dean is in a unique position to help you. He or she may be able to offer valuable insight based on the school's experience with previous students of similar backgrounds and qualifications.

Rule # 73 **You have considerable control over the Unique Characteristics section. Use it wisely.**

Students may assume that the MSPE is written by the dean using information that the school has already obtained. However, students play a much larger role in influencing the content of the MSPE than they realize. This is especially true for the Unique Characteristics section.

To develop this section, schools often ask students to complete a student information sheet, providing an opportunity for the student to highlight certain aspects of their education and activities. Deans may choose to emphasize certain aspects of a student's career if those aspects have been emphasized by a student. Prior work experience as a paramedic, a weekly commitment to volunteering in the children's education center of a homeless shelter, or an ongoing clinical research project are all activities that could be highlighted. Such items may also be emphasized when meeting with the dean in person. On the information sheet, students are asked the following:

- Undergraduate institution (major, degree, dates attended, extracurricular activities)
- Graduate education (major, degree, dates attended)
- Notable or distinguished activities prior to medical school
- Extracurricular activities during medical school
- Publications/presentations
- Employment history before and during medical school
- Leaves of absence during medical school, including reasons
- Field/specialty of interest
- Additional information you would like included

Some schools will also ask for a CV and personal statement to help prepare the MSPE. This provides yet another compelling reason to begin working on these elements of your residency application early in the process.

Just as in your CV, it's not enough to list certain accomplishments. You must highlight accomplishments that may be regarded by program directors as exceptional, such as leadership positions, athletic or artistic accomplishments, or significant volunteer work. As shown in the following box, these may be regarded as predictors of residency success.

Did you know?

In a study done to determine the factors that predict success during an emergency medicine residency, having a "distinctive factor" such as being a top-level athlete, musician, or class officer was a significant factor that predicted future success. The authors wrote that "it could be that an applicant who is capable of high-level performance in medical school and simultaneously capable of high-level achievement in sports, music, etc., is well organized and can prioritize and multitask well."[2]

MSPE Preparation: Important Tips for the Unique Characteristics Section

- Creation of the Unique Characteristics Section of the MSPE will be a collaborative effort between you and your Dean (or his designee). However, the process will differ from one school to another.
- Some schools ask students to complete a biographical information sheet or questionnaire. The MSPE writer will then use this information to write the Unique Characteristics Section.
- Other schools have their students write the Unique Characteristics section of the MSPE.
- If you'll be writing your own Unique Characteristics Section, adhere to all word limits, and write in the third person. Your Dean may edit your description for grammar, style, and content, but you'll have the opportunity to review these edits.
- Focus primarily on content from medical school, but do include particularly notable activities, service, research, scholarships, and awards from your undergraduate years.
- In terms of content, there may be some redundancy between the Unique Characteristics section and the personal statement. This is acceptable and appropriate.

Rule # 74 **Program directors will carefully read over the Academic History section. Understand that red flags may appear in this section, and you must work with your Dean to either remove concerning items or lessen their impact.**

Is there any information in your file that would be considered a red flag to residency programs? Have you experienced academic problems? Have you taken a leave of absence? Have you failed a preclinical course or clerkship? Have you received any disciplinary action for a lapse in professionalism?

These are issues that obviously concern residency programs. Programs worry that an applicant with a red flag may become a problem resident. In one study, researchers examined all residents at a single program with reported problematic behavior over a 20-year period.[4] Residency application materials were then examined closely for any areas of concern. Of all the application components, only the MSPE was found to be predictive of future problems. In particular, negative comments, even those that were mildly negative, were found to be predictive of future problems. Therefore, programs are likely to search for these in the MSPE.

Issues of concern need to be addressed with the dean. The following table outlines issues that would be considered a red flag to program directors.

Program Directors' Rankings Of Their Concerns About Selected Academic and Non-Academic Issues*	
Issue	**Mean**
Received disciplinary action in medical school	4.90
Treated for alcoholism	4.90
Received failure in a required clerkship	4.63
Took extended time to graduate for academic reasons	4.55
Has learning disability	4.47
Failed USMLE Step 1 prior to passing	4.47
Passed USMLE with minimal score	4.18
Graduated in the lower third of class	3.91
Received a failure in a preclinical course	3.73
Had mediocre preclinical grades but strong clinical evaluations	3.27
Had family responsibilities	3.00
Did not participate in extracurricular activities in medical school	2.91

*Responses from 794 residency program directors. Rating scale: 1 (no concern) to 5 (very concerned)

Wagoner N, Suriano J. Program directors' responses to a survey on variables used to select residents in a time of change. *Acad Med* 1999; 74(1): 51-8.

In a more recent study, clerkship directors were asked to rate the perceived effects of application "red flags" on the chances of matching.[5] Respondents were asked to rate each factor on a scale of 1 (no effect) to 5 (very significant effect).

Mean Scores for Perceived Effect of Application "Red Flags" on Matching in Pediatrics Residency Programs	
Factor	**Mean**
Multiple failures of USMLE/COMLEX examinations	4.98
Failed multiple core clerkships	4.95
Professionalism concerns	4.93
Failed pediatrics clerkship	4.90
Failed USMLE Step 2 CS	4.70
Failed USMLE Step 2 CK/COMLEX	4.51
Failed multiple M1 and/or M2 courses	4.67
Failed USMLE Step 1/ XOMLEX	4.38
Failed core clerkships (other than pediatrics)	4.26
Failed pediatrics clerkship NBME Subject examination only	3.78
Failed M1 or M2 course	3.68
Leave of absence	2.97

Ryan M, Levine L, Colbert-Getz J, Spector N, Fromme H. Advising medical students for the Match: A national survey of pediatrics clerkship directors. *Acad Pediatr* 2015; 15(4): 374-379.

If your medical school experience includes any of these red flags, realize that it may be included in your MSPE. Keep in mind, however, that deans have some latitude in how they present this information. In fact, several studies have shown that discrepancies between the MSPE and the official medical school transcript are common.

Did you know?

In a 1997 study looking at concordance between 532 Dean's letters and corresponding transcripts, Edmond found the following:

- Among students who failed a pre-clinical course, there was no mention of this in 27% of letters.
- Among students who failed a clinical rotation, there was no mention of this in 33% of letters.
- Among students who took a leave of absence, there was no mention of this in 40% of letters.

It was found that negative information was withheld one third of the time.[6]

There are several reasons as to why a dean would withhold negative information. One reason is that some deans argue that an otherwise strong applicant's chances of matching into the specialty or program of his choice may be damaged by including negative information, especially if the issue was not characteristic of the student's overall performance. In this case, a dean may suppress negative comments from a single evaluator if all other evaluators were glowingly positive.

Did you know?

In a survey of nearly 1,800 PDs representing 22 specialties, 65% cited evidence of professionalism and ethics as a factor in inviting students to interview. Directors rated this factor 4.5 in importance on a scale of 1 (not important) to 5 (very important).[1]

Tip # 40

If your background or record does contain a red flag, then do everything possible to make sure that your record from the remaining time you have left in medical school is impeccable. You can make a more convincing argument to the dean and in interviews if your failure is seen as an isolated incident that does not accurately reflect your abilities.

Tip # 41

Schools allow students to appeal or contest entries made in the MSPE, and you may consider exercising your right to do so. If an adverse event or red flag can't be removed, work with your MSPE writer to craft the language used to describe the problem. Doing so may help lighten its impact.

> **Tip # 42**
>
> Have you received recognition for your professionalism? If so, ask your Dean if this can be included in your MSPE. Some schools, like Temple University, identify exemplary professionalism in the MSPE.

Rule # 75 **Periodically preview your file in order to correct inaccuracies or identify red flags.**

A periodic review of your file is critical. Every few months, starting in your third year, arrange to look through your file. Several weeks before your MSPE meeting with the Dean, look over your file again. Before the dean begins to draft your letter, it is your responsibility to ensure that everything in your file is accurate, including the official transcript.

Frequent review allows you to identify inaccuracies early, and take steps towards correction before any deadlines pass. "You are strongly encouraged to monitor your academic file," writes the Stony Brook University School of Medicine. "If you have an evaluation that you believe to be grossly unfair, you may appeal it to the clerkship supervisor. Do not wait until late in the MSPE process to seek such remediation."[7]

Frequent review of your file is particularly important during the third year of medical school. You will be receiving evaluations from clinical faculty, and these comments and ratings will have great bearing on the content of your MSPE, as we'll discuss shortly. Per the University of Maryland School of Medicine: "We suggest that you read your clerkship evaluations as they come in and contact directors as soon as possible to discuss issues with evaluation content. School policy states that evaluation revisions will not be considered beyond 3 months of your receipt of the evaluation."[8]

> **Tip # 43**
>
> Search your file for any potential red flags. These types of issues are likely to be included in your letter. It's important that you note these well before you apply. You'll need to formulate a plan on how to address these issues in your application materials.

Rule # 76 **Read the narratives section very carefully. Critical review of these comments will help you identify any potential areas of concern for program directors.**

If your school follows the AAMC-recommended format, narrative information regarding your overall performance in each core clerkship and elective rotation will be included in the "Academic Progress" section of the MSPE. What is the source of this narrative information?

On clerkship evaluation forms, there's usually a section in which evaluators are asked to comment on a student's clinical performance. Comments about professionalism, knowledge, communication skills with other health care professionals, clinical reasoning, and clinical judgment are most common.[9] Often, the comments of the evaluator are taken and placed word for word in this section of the MSPE.

While comments are generally positive, evaluators may also include negative comments. Some schools have a policy to place all comments, in their entirety, within the MSPE, regardless of whether they are positive or negative. Other schools may edit out negative information, particularly if the comment reflects the thoughts of only a single evaluator.

As you review your MSPE, read the narratives section very carefully. Circle anything that might be viewed as a negative, even if it's mildly negative. Following is one example of a narrative that may be found in the MSPE:

Third-year clinical clerkships

Comments regarding Mr. Ortiz's clinical performance are given below in chronological order:

Pediatrics: High pass; "Roberto was a very earnest student. His history taking skills were at a level that was expected for his training. He progressed nicely in the quality of his oral case presentations. He brought in articles to share with the team.

Family Medicine: High pass; "Roberto has a good knowledge base. He tends to be quiet so it can sometimes be hard to realize this. He could be more involved in discussions. He worked well with team members and was always prompt at scheduled rounds.

Surgery: Pass; "Roberto was hard-working, motivated, and dedicated. Compared to other students on the service, Roberto was fairly quiet, often not being heard from for long stretches of time during rounds. He needs to work on participation during rounds. He will be a great student and physician once he develops more confidence."

In this example, a program director might be concerned about Roberto's level of participation in rounds and conferences, especially since similar comments were written by evaluators in two different clerkships. Does Roberto simply have a "quiet" personality, or does his lack of participation suggest indifference, inadequate knowledge, or lack of motivation?

Critical review of these comments will help you identify potential areas of concern for program directors. In some cases, negative information (i.e., failed clerkships) may have to be addressed in other areas of your application, such as the personal statement. Otherwise, the application may be rejected.

In other cases, the comments may be relatively minor. With minor issues, you may not want to bring any attention to them, because they may not have any effect on the strength of your application. However, you should still be ready to address these issues in case they come up during an interview.

Applicants often have a hard time deciding whether an issue raised in the MSPE requires addressing elsewhere in the application. Such issues should be discussed with your advisors.

Tip # 44

Schools make every effort to delay finalization of the MSPE until after August so that evaluations from July and August can be included in the document. It's up to you to follow up with faculty supervisors to make sure evaluations are submitted in a timely fashion.

Rule # 77 **The Summary Section of the MSPE may include a key descriptor. Make sure that the term used by your school is consistent with your class rank or standing.**

The Summary Section of the MSPE will often include a key word. This key word is of great interest to PDs. This word is known as a descriptor, and the word that is chosen provides PDs with an idea of your overall performance relative to your peers. Often schools will use a hierarchy of descriptors such as outstanding, excellent, very good, or good. Some schools will make the meaning of the word quite clear to residency programs. For example, at the University of Washington School of Medicine, "outstanding" is the highest superlative that a student can receive, and is given to only 8-15% of the class. Following this is excellent (30-36%), very good (35%), and good (8-15%).[10] This information is provided to schools in appendices which accompany the MSPE. However, not all schools are as transparent as the University of Washington. In a study of 141 medical school MSPEs, 24% of schools did not define their descriptors.[11]

As an applicant, it's important to make note of the key word that your school has used to describe you in the summary paragraph. Is the descriptor correct?

Did you know?

In one study, researchers examined the MSPEs received by three residency programs for the inclusion of the term "good" in the summary paragraph. For the institutions using this term, researchers then examined appendices to determine the percentile rankings of those students who were deemed "good." Of the 122 institutions, 28% utilized "good" as a descriptor. All of these institutions used the term to refer to students in the bottom 50% of the class. The authors concluded that the term consistently indicates below-average performance.[12]

Did you know?

The term "excellent" in the Summary Section of the MSPE can mean different things to different schools. At one top-twenty medical school (based on *US News* rankings), the term was used to describe students ranked between the 5th and 43rd percentiles (bottom half of the class). At another top-twenty school, the entire lower 75% of the class was described as excellent. Although the term "outstanding" was commonly the highest superlative, there were 12 schools that used the term as their second best.[13]

Rule # 78 Don't just assume that your final letter will be fine.

At some schools, students are able to read several drafts of the letter. More commonly, schools make only the final draft available to their students. Take advantage of any opportunity to review your letter, because it may be your only chance to make suggestions or corrections.

Tip # 45

If you will be at an away rotation when your letter is completed, make arrangements to receive this letter. Review it, make any suggestions or corrections, and return it by the date specified.

Schools will generally ask you to sign off on the final version. After signing off, you won't be able to make any further changes, and the letter will be sent to residency programs.

Did you know?

The AAMC recommends that students be allowed to correct factual errors in the MSPE but not be permitted to revise any evaluative statements. Despite this recommendation, schools often take student suggestions seriously. As far as negative comments are concerned, Deans may decide whether to exclude the comments based on the consistency of the problem and its severity.

Did you know?

In a 1992 survey, approximately 40% of deans reported that they did not always include ethical problems in their letters, 60% did not always include substance abuse, 70% did not always include emotional instability, and 75% did not always include physical illness.[14] As MSPEs have become more standardized, it's possible that these numbers have changed.

Did you know?

The MSPE will be released on October 1. Medical schools will not release the MSPE earlier, not even for applicants participating in early matches.

Rule # 79 **Do not wait until the MSPE is sent before completing the rest of your application.**

The uniform release date for the MSPE is October 1. Some applicants are under the assumption that programs won't invite applicants to interview until the application is complete. While some programs wait until they've received the MSPE, many programs extend interview invitations well before the uniform release date. For this reason, complete your application as early as possible.

Did you know?

Up until several years ago, the uniform release date for the MSPE was November 1. In a survey of 73 interviewees to the emergency medicine residency program at the Oregon Health Sciences University, applicants were asked if they received any interviews from programs before November 1 and, if so, from whom.[15] 77% of respondents reported receiving interview invitations prior to November 1. At least 44% of emergency medicine programs were found to send early interview invitations. Even though the uniform release date has changed to October 1, we continue to see programs send interview invitations in September. Therefore, applicants should submit their applications as early as possible, preferably on September 15, the earliest date for submission.

References

[1]2014 NRMP Program Directors Survey. Available at: http://www.nrmp.org/wp-content/uploads/2014/09/PD-Survey-Report-2014.pdf. Accessed November 14, 2016.

[2]Hayden S, Hayden M, Gamst A. What characteristics of applicants to emergency medicine residency programs predict future success as an emergency medicine resident? *Acad Emerg Med* 2005; 12(3): 206-210.

[3]Swide C, Lasater K, Dillman D. Perceived predictive value of the Medical Student Performance Evaluation (MSPE) in anesthesiology resident selection. *J Clinc Anesth* 2009; 21(1): 38-43.

[4]Brenner A, Mathai S, Jain S, Mohl P. Can we predict "problem residents"? *Acad Med* 2010; 85(7): 1147-51.

[5]Ryan M, Levine L, Colbert-Getz J, Spector N, Fromme H. Advising medical students for the Match: A national survey of pediatrics clerkship directors. *Acad Pediatr* 2015; 15(4): 374-379.

[6]Edmond M, Roberson M, Hasan N. The dishonest dean's letter: an analysis of 532 dean's letters from 99 U.S. medical schools. *Acad Med* 1999; 74(9): 1033-1035.

[7]Stony Brook University School of Medicine. Available at: http://medicine.stonybrookmedicine.edu/ugme/residency_match/mspe. Accessed January 2, 2016.

[8]University of Maryland School of Medicine. Available at: http://medschool.umaryland.edu/osa/handbook/mspe.asp. Accessed January 2, 2016.

[9]Pulito A, Donnelly M, Plymale M, Mentzer R. What do faculty observe of medical students' clinical performance? *Teach Learn Med* 2006; 18(2): 99-104.

[10]University of Washington School of Medicine. Available at: http://www.uwmedicine.org/education/md-program/current-students/student-affairs/career-advising/year-4-get-residency/deans-letter. Accessed January 2, 2016.

[11]Naidich J, Grimaldi G, Lombardi P, Davis L, Naidich J. A program director's guide to the Medical Student Performance Evaluation (formerly dean's letter) with a database. *J Am Coll Radiol* 2014; 11(6): 611-615.

[12]Kiefer C, Colletti J, Bellolio M, Hess E, Woolridge D, Thomas K, Sadosty A. The "good" dean's letter. *Acad Med* 2010; 85(11): 1705-8.

[13]Naidich J, Lee J, Hansen E, Smith L. The meaning of excellence. Acad Radiol 2007; 14(9): 1121-1126.

[14]Hunt D, MacLaren C, Soctt C, Chu J, Leiden L. Characteristics of dean's letters in 1981 and 1992. *Acad Med* 1993; 68(12): 905-911.

[15]Delorio N, Yarris L, Kalbfleisch N. Early invitations for residency interviews: the exception or the norm. *J Emerg Med* 2007; 33(1): 77-79.

Chapter 9

Curriculum Vitae

Curriculum vitae is a Latin expression, meaning the "course of one's life." Known as CV for short, this document provides an overview of a candidate's academic and professional background. The CV is an important component of the residency application.

Rule # 80 Your CV must create maximum impact.

Creating a good CV requires time, effort, and a thorough examination of your training and achievements. The overall appearance of your CV needs to be impeccable. The proofreading must be perfect. Each individual line should be positioned for maximum impact. Every pertinent aspect of your achievements must be included.

Students don't always recognize the importance of creating an outstanding CV. Many residency programs now require applicants to submit applications through ERAS, the Electronic Residency Application Service of the Association of American Medical Colleges. Students aren't permitted to attach their CV to the ERAS application. However, you are allowed to enter information from your CV directly into the ERAS CV format. PDs can then print out this information in a CV format.

Even though you won't be able to attach your CV to your ERAS application, you'll still need to create a professional-looking paper version of your CV for the following reasons:

- Some residency programs don't participate in ERAS. These programs will request a paper CV.
- The CV will help you fill out your Medical Student Performance Evaluation (MSPE) Data Form. Medical schools use this form to help them create your MSPE, an important component of your residency application.
- The CV will help you complete different sections of the residency application.
- The CV can be of considerable help as you begin to draft your personal statement.

- Mentors and faculty in your specialty of interest will review your CV to provide you with informed advice about how to strengthen your credentials.

- Your letter writers will rely on your CV to help them write strong LORs.

- When students apply for an elective rotation at another institution, they may be required to submit a CV. Such "away" or "audition electives are often helpful for students applying to competitive residencies. Obtaining such an elective can be a competitive process in and of itself.

- Reviewing your CV prior to the interview will remind you of your strengths and accomplishments, helping to boost confidence.

- Interviewers may request a copy of your CV at the start of an interview in order to help structure the interview. This provides an ideal opportunity to emphasize your strengths and highlight the skills you would bring as a resident.

Your CV will continue to be an important document even after you enter a residency program. It's not a static document, but rather one that needs to be updated regularly as you progress through your career.

Tip # 46

PDs are able to view and print your applicant information in an ERAS CV format. You can, and should, do the same prior to submitting your application.

Tip # 47

For programs that don't participate in ERAS, you may have to submit a paper CV. While you may be an intelligent, enthusiastic, and charming applicant, you won't have the opportunity to showcase these qualities during an interview if a poorly written, or even average, CV eliminates you from further consideration. If done well, your CV has the potential to position you above other applicants, even those who may be more qualified.

Rule # 81 **Utilize only the correct CV format and structure.**

All CVs begin with your name and contact information. Since these items will be at the top of your CV, they can contribute to a positive first impression, and so should be visually appealing. Many applicants use the same font size for the name and contact information. However, your name should be a bit bigger and even bolder than the rest of the contact information. Don't add the words "curriculum vitae" to the top of the page, as many students tend to do. The reader recognizes a CV. Why waste valuable space stating the obvious?

> **Tip # 48**
>
> Double-check your contact information to ensure that a PD could reach you quickly and easily if necessary. Since most programs will communicate with you entirely by e-mail, double check your e-mail address.

> **Tip # 49**
>
> Is your e-mail address professional? The inappropriate and immature examples we've encountered include redsoxforever@hotmail.com and ralphlaurenmd@aol.com. You've worked hard to create a specific image throughout the entire application. Need we say more? If you don't have a professional e-mail address, now is the time to create one. Your address should simply be your first and last name (e.g., meljackson@hotmail.com, jayapatel@yahoo.com).

> **Tip # 50**
>
> While most communication between an applicant and program occurs via e-mail, sometimes applicants are contacted by phone. Make sure that your answering machine or voice mail message is professional. "Hey dude, you know what to do at the tone" might suffice for your buddy, but replace this with something more professional during the application season: "Hello, this is Rodrigo Martin. Thank you for calling, but I'm not available to take your call right now. Please leave your name, telephone number, and message, and I'll return your call as soon as possible."

> **Tip # 51**
>
> A PD may contact you by phone. While most applicants now provide cell phone numbers, some forward their calls, especially if they're traveling overseas. If so, educate those answering the phone. Ask them to note the name of the person calling, the return phone number, the name of the residency program, and a good time to call back. Afterwards, have them contact you as soon as possible so you can return the call.

Following your name and contact information should be an "education" section. From here, you'll have considerable latitude in the order in which you present the remaining categories. It's preferable, however, to lead with your strengths. If you've earned honor after honor in medical school, have the "honors/awards" section follow "education" rather than placing it second to last. Weigh the impact of each section before deciding where to place it. Below are the standard sections of the CV. Not all categories are used for every CV.

Standard Sections of the CV	
Name Contact information Education Postgraduate training Employment experience Honors/awards Professional society memberships Teaching experience	Research experience Publications Presentations Committees/service Licensure and certification Extracurricular activities Volunteer activities Personal interests

Residency Programs Speak…

"The categories listed…are often included in CVs or resumes. However, no CV contains all of them, and some CVs will contain other categories that are not listed here. The basic rule is that your own unique educational and work experiences should be presented to the best effect. The first step in actually developing your CV is to write down all the relevant information - later you can organize it into categories. After you have written down all the relevant information develop a hierarchy placing the most important and relevant categories and information first. All other information can be listed in descending order of importance and relevance."[1]

Dianna A. Johnson, M.D.
Professor of Ophthalmology
University of Tennessee Health Science Center

Rule # 82 Always place items in chronological order.

Incorrect ordering is among the most common CV mistakes. In all sections of the CV, information should be presented in reverse chronological order. This means that items such as jobs and awards are listed with the most recent item first.

Rule # 83 Every section and line of your CV must impress.

If you have a section with just one item, plan on eliminating it, unless it's an impressive accomplishment. A category with a single item looks decidedly unimpressive. It also wastes valuable lines of CV space. A single item can always be woven into another category. For example, a single honor earned during medical school can be listed in the "education" section.

Rule # 84 — Each line of your CV must serve as evidence of your skills and accomplishments.

Each line of your CV must pack the maximum impact. Study your CV line by line. In many cases, a description or explanation of an item will maximize its impact.

Honors and Awards

2014 George Lambert Scholarship

Do you know what this scholarship is? The residency selection committee has no idea, either. For all we know, it's a $250 scholarship given to 35 students per class who are from a particular geographic district in the state. This version makes a far greater impression:

Honors and Awards

2014 George Lambert Scholarship
Awarded to the student with the highest academic performance during the freshman year of medical school (1/200)

> **Did you know?**
>
> As you read through your CV, ask whether the reader would understand the significance of what you have written. If not, it may be assumed to have little value.

> **Did you know…**
>
> Avoid unfamiliar acronyms or abbreviations. An abbreviation that's readily apparent to you may have no meaning to a PD. If an organization isn't readily recognizable, a brief explanation of the group and its purpose should be included.

Rule # 85 — The structure of your CV should be used to highlight all accomplishments.

While medical students review CVs with an obsessive attention to detail, the typical member of the selection committee is forced to more quickly review a CV. Part of refining your CV, then, should be the two-minute glance over. Have you captured the reviewer's attention and conveyed your accomplishments?

Professional Membership

2012 (Summer) American Medical Association, Medical Student Section (President)

Reading this, you could easily miss the fact that the applicant was president of the organization. Faculty members don't have the time to ferret out all the small print on every CV. You must structure your CV to highlight all accomplishments.

Professional Membership

2012 (Summer) President, American Medical Association, Medical Student Section

Rule # 86 Use the personal interests section to catch a reviewer's attention, but with caution.

Programs are interested in an applicant's hobbies and interests. "What is this person like? Is he or she well rounded? Interesting? What would it be like to work with this person?" Provide this information in the personal interests section of your CV, which is usually the last section.

Don't take this section lightly. Faculty often start the interview with a discussion of your interests as a way to break the ice. You may also find that you share an interest with your interviewer. This can quickly build rapport.

Certain interests are viewed positively and may enhance your candidacy. The ability to speak Spanish fluently would be a noted positive at a residency program whose institution serves a large Hispanic population. Interests may also be viewed negatively. While there are certainly student and physician members of the organization People for the Ethical Treatment of Animals (PETA), some physicians don't agree with the organization's stance against medical testing in animals.

Rule # 87 The language style you use makes a difference. Use only action verbs.

Use words that capture the reviewer's attention. The use of action verbs acts to strengthen your CV. Placed at the beginning of sentences, these verbs make more powerful statements.

In writing about your work, extracurricular, volunteer, and research experiences, use action verbs to emphasize your accomplishments. Many applicants simply describe their duties and responsibilities. It's far more powerful to stress what you accomplished.

Research Experience

2014-2015 Research Assistant, Department of Pharmacology, National Institute of Mental Health, Bethesda, MD

- Assisted professor in research related to receptors in the hippocampus
- Helped collect data

Note the impact of the changes in the revised version:

Research Experience

2014-2015 Research Assistant, Department of Pharmacology, National Institute of Mental Health, Bethesda, MD

- Isolated and characterized several receptors in hippocampus
- Elucidated function of receptors
- Sequenced amino acid composition of receptors

Utilize the following extensive list of action verbs in order to highlight your accomplishments:

A	Abridged, accelerated, accomplished, accounted for, achieved, adapted, adjusted, administered, advanced, advised, allocated, analyzed, answered, approved, arranged, assembled, assimilated, assisted, attained, augmented
B	Balanced, broadened, built
C	Calculated, calibrated, cared for, categorized, catalogued, chaired, charted, clarified, classified, coached, collaborated, collected, compared, compiled, completed, composed, conceived, condensed, conducted, consolidated, constructed, consulted, contributed, coordinated, counseled, created, critiqued
D	Debated, defined, delegated, delineated, delivered, demonstrated, derived, designed, detected, determined, developed, devised, diagnosed, directed, discovered, displayed, distributed, documented, drafted
E	Edited, earned, educated, elicited, enabled, encouraged, enhanced, ensured, established, estimated, evaluated, examined, exceeded, exhibited, expanded, expedited, explained, explored
F	Facilitated, followed, formulated, found, founded, furthered
G	Gathered, generated, guided
H	Handled, headed, helped
I	Identified, illustrated, implemented, improved, increased, initiated, innovated, inspected, installed, instituted, instructed, interacted, interpreted, interviewed, invented, investigated
J	Judged, justified
L	Launched, lectured, led, logged
M	Made, maintained, managed, mastered, measured, met, modified, monitored, motivated
O	Observed, obtained, offered, operated, organized, oversaw
P	Participated, performed, pinpointed, pioneered, planned, prepared, presented, presided, prioritized, processed, produced, programmed, proposed, proved, provided
Q	Quantified
R	Raised, realized, received, recommended, recorded, redesigned, reported, researched, revamped, received, revised
S	Scheduled, screened, searched, secured, selected, served, set up, simplified, solved spearheaded, started, streamlined, strengthened, studied, submitted, succeeded, summarized, supervised, supplied, supported, surpassed, surveyed, synthesized

T	Tabulated, tallied, taught, tested, traced, tracked, trained, translated, transmitted, tutored
U	Uncovered, undertook, updated, upgraded, used
V	Validated, verified, volunteered
W	Widened, won, worked, wrote

As you review this list, note:

- Some action verbs are more powerful than others. Use the most powerful verb you can without exaggerating your accomplishments.
- Do not downplay, diminish, or deflate your contributions by using verbs such as "assisted" or "helped."
- Avoid the much too commonly used phrases "Responsibilities for…" or "Duties included…"
- Avoid repeating the same verb if possible.
- For those activities or experiences with which you're currently involved, use the present tense. Use the past tense for completed work or past experiences.

Tip # 52

You need not, and should not, write your CV in complete sentences. Instead, use short phrases that make your points as quickly as possible. The words "I" or "me" do not belong in a CV. Articles such as "the" "a" and "an" are typically omitted as well.

Rule # 88 Use numbers to provide concrete evidence.

Provide tangible evidence whenever possible to support your claims. This means including numbers and facts to emphasize your accomplishments. Numbers can often drive home key points in ways that words can't.

Work Experience

2014-2015 Physician Director, Karachi Ob/Gyn Associates, Karachi, Pakistan

- Supervised team of healthcare professionals

In this more powerful version, note how the applicant was able to describe her experience quantitatively and specifically:

Work Experience

2014-2015 Physician Director, Karachi Ob/Gyn Associates, Karachi, Pakistan

- Supervised team of 20 healthcare professionals in clinic responsible for care of 3000 obestetrics and gynecology patients

Rule # 89 **Utilize multiple reviewers.**

It doesn't matter how many times you review and revise your own CV. You should have several individuals review your CV prior to submission. We recommend having your CV reviewed by two faculty members, if at all possible. Ideally, one would include the PD of your chosen specialty at your program. The director is likely to be an authority in this area, having seen hundreds of CVs over the years. Don't submit your CV for review to faculty, though, until you feel that it's perfect.

You should ask someone with excellent writing and editing skills to review your CV. This type of careful review may lead to the discovery of spelling or grammatical errors, mistakes that can be very damaging to your candidacy.

Finally, consider the benefits of having a family member or close friend critique your CV. Those who know you well on a personal level may point out accomplishments that you'd forgotten.

After collecting reviewer comments, consider them carefully. Compare reviewer comments with another. While you don't need to agree with all comments, if several of your reviewers make the same recommendations, take these comments seriously. If there's disagreement, solicit more opinions to help you make a more informed decision.

Tip # 53

Applicants from other countries should recognize that CV and resume styles differ from one country to another in terms of style and tone. What may be considered appropriate in your home country may be too casual or too stiff in the United States. Herein lies the importance of having the CV reviewed by someone with experience in the United States.

Tip # 54

While there's a benefit to having your CV reviewed by someone close to you, such as your mother, roommate, or significant other, understand that loved ones are usually not the best reviewers. Always have your CV reviewed by qualified individuals such as a faculty member, the PD at your institution, or advisor.

To maximize the value of others' opinions, use the following CV review form to check your own work prior to their review.

CV Review Form		
	Yes	**No**
Does the overall appearance make an excellent first impression		
Is the length of the CV appropriate?		
Is the CV easily read?		
Is the CV well organized?		
Is the font type easy to read?		
Is the font type and size consistent?		
Is the font size appropriate?		
Is the spacing consistent throughout the CV?		
Is the name and contact information presented in an appealing manner with the name being most prominent?		
Is the contact information correct and complete?		
Are the section headings lined up and consistent (i.e., font size/style, bold)?		
Is the formatting within each section consistent (spacing, font size, bullets, etc.)?		
Are the margins on each side equal?		
Are underlining, italics, and bolding used appropriately?		
Are there any grammatical errors?		
Are there any spelling errors?		
Is there any use of *I*, *my*, *me*, *a*, *an*, or *the?*		
Are the most important sections listed first?		
Is information presented in reverse chronological order?		
Are action verbs used consistently?		
Are the dates correct?		
Are there any time gaps in the work or school history?		
Is there anything in the CV that is irrelevant?		
Is the CV printed on professional, high-quality paper?		

Rule # 90 **Avoid even a single spelling, typographical, or grammatical error.**

Spelling, typographical, and grammatical errors are among the worst mistakes you can make on the CV. Even one misspelled word can make you look careless. Residency programs are searching for individuals who are motivated and compulsive. If your CV shows that you lack attention to detail, PDs fear that this will spill over into your work as a resident. Otherwise well-qualified applicants have been removed from consideration because of these errors.

Ensure your CV is free of errors:

- If you created your CV using word processing, use the spell checker. However, the spell checker won't help if you misuse a word (e.g., substituting "there" for "their"). IMGs should avoid British spellings.
- Take the time needed to proofread your CV. Read it aloud, and sound out each word, syllable by syllable. Errors not apparent during a silent read may be picked up by this method.
- Read the CV backwards one word at a time, a technique used by many professional proofreaders. This allows you to focus on each individual word.
- Set the CV aside for a day before looking at it again. This allows you to look at your work with fresh eyes.

Rule # 91 Use the correct length.

As a general rule, the CV should not exceed 1 or 2 pages. PDs don't have the patience or time to review a long CV. Occasionally the CV may be longer, particularly if an applicant has published a number of articles. If you can't place all of your information on 1 or 2 pages, ask yourself if you've been too verbose. Don't use a smaller font size or shrink the margins in order to fit more text onto a page. We've seen students attempt this technique, and it doesn't work well. Instead, use fewer words and omit information that doesn't support your application. A CV reviewer can help you edit out repetitive or unnecessary information.

Tip # 55

Placing too much information in a CV is among the most common mistakes applicants make. For most applicants, the CV should not exceed 1-2 pages.

Tip # 56

If your CV extends to a second page by a line or two, adjust the margins to fit the CV onto one page. If your CV extends to a second page but takes up only half of the second page, spread the content over the two pages to eliminate excess white space.

Tip # 57

Mark each page of your CV clearly. Place "Page 1 of 2" at the bottom of the first page. Place your name followed by the page number at the top of the second page (e.g., Reza Hourhani – Page 2).

Rule # 92 **First impressions matter, even for a piece of paper.**

The overall appearance of your CV is important as well. Programs need to whittle down a large group of applications, and therefore every piece of the application becomes magnified in importance. Before reviewing your CV, the reader will form an impression of you based on its overall appearance. These recommendations should be used to create a CV with a professional appearance.

Margins

Allow for generous margins at the top, bottom, and sides of your CV. A margin of at least 1 inch is often recommended. Shrinking the margins to anything less than an inch will make the CV difficult to read.

Font

Use a font that's easy to read. Times New Roman or Arial are appropriate choices. After selecting a particular font, stick with it. The use of multiple fonts can appear unprofessional.

Font size is also an important consideration. Avoid a font size less than 10-point or one greater than 12-point. It's acceptable to use two font sizes, a larger one for headings and a smaller one for the content under each heading. The use of more than two font sizes is discouraged.

Spacing

Be consistent with spacing. Maintain enough white (open) space, especially between sections. If you use one line space between the end of one section and the beginning of another, maintain this with all sections. If your CV exceeds one page in length, avoid splitting a section when going from page 1 to 2.

Design elements

It's acceptable to use the bold function to highlight your name and section headings (e.g., education). You can also consider bolding certain awards and leadership positions as a way to highlight these achievements. However, excessive use of the bolding technique can overwhelm the reader. If you bold an element such as "education," then you should bold similar elements as well (e.g., honors/awards). Keep headings consistent in style and size.

Limit the use of italics to the names of journals and foreign phrases such as *magna cum laude*. Underlining should also be used sparingly.

The excessive use of underlining tends to focus the eyes on the underlined portion of the CV only. Occasional use of caps may be acceptable, but some consider it to be rude, akin to shouting.

Paper quality

Print your CV on one side only of high quality 8.5" X 11" bond paper (e.g., 24 to 28 lb). Do not use unusual or multicolored paper that may appear unprofessional. Select a white, off-white, natural, or cream colored paper.

Characteristics of an Outstanding CV	**Characteristics of a Poor CV**
Visually appealing, professional look	Weathered look (e.g., bent corners, stains)
Brief and concise	Long sentences/paragraphs
Easy to read	Lack of organization
Uniform margins with none < 1 inch	Too little white space ("crowded look")
No misspelled words or typos	Typos or misspelled words
Use of action verbs	Handwritten corrections
Moderate use of bolding/underling/italics	Poor paper or printing quality

Did you know?

"Don't make them too dense, overly wordy, and disorganized and thus discouraging to read. Aim for terse, organized prose that conveys the important information succinctly. Don't crowd the page with text."[1]

Maureen Poh-Fitzpatrick, M.D., Associate Program Director of Dermatology
University of Tennessee Health Science Center

Rule # 93 **Some information has no place in a CV. Learn what to leave out.**

We've seen many CVs that include unnecessary information. The following information has no place in the CV:

- Age
- Gender
- Height/weight
- Race/ethnicity
- Social security number
- Marital status

- Name of spouse/significant other
- Children
- Religion
- Description of health

Did you know?

"It is recommended that any significant time away from the practice of medicine on the CV be explained on the CV itself and/or in the personal statement. Failure to do so can result in the applicant appearing to not be candid or attempting to hide information."[2]

Jay Harolds, M.D.
Division of Radiology
Michigan State University College of Human Medicine

Did you know?

"Because 10 % to 12% of physicians have some type of chemical dependency, any hiatus immediately suggests…that you were in a drug or alcohol rehabilitation center during that time…If you have more than a few months unaccounted…explain the gap. For example, 'took a year off to care for my dying father in Cleveland' or 'spent 6 months trekking through Southeast Asia with my fiancé.'"[3]

David Grimes, M.D.
Clinical Professor
Department of Obstetrics and Gynecology
University of North Carolina

Rule # 94 Start your CV now.

Your CV plays a key role in the residency application process. It also serves a key role in creating other components of the residency application. It is used to prepare the general application, MSPE, personal statement, and letters of recommendation. When should you start working on your CV? Some advisors will tell you to begin several months before the end of your third year of medical school. We don't recommend that you wait that long for two main reasons.

Starting early provides the time needed to create a powerful CV. Because the medical student CV tends to be a one or two-page document, many applicants mistakenly assume that they can create a CV in a matter of minutes or, at the very most, a few hours. However, if you wish to create a CV that makes a strong impact, both in content and appearance, you need sufficient time. Your reviewers also need sufficient time.

Starting early also highlights areas in your CV that can be maximized. Students who have no items to place under the heading of presentations or publications can remedy this situation with enough lead time.

There are a few other reasons to have your CV prepared now, wherever you are in the application cycle. As we discuss later, when you approach a faculty member for a letter of recommendation, you'll provide a packet of information to assist them. Your CV is a standard component of that packet. The CV you provide must be in its final, perfected form, even at this stage. You need to make an impact with these individuals, who are advocating for your candidacy and have the power to sway PDs.

If you're planning to do an audition elective, recognize that institutions may require an application, including a CV. You may also seek to approach faculty members for career opportunities, as we discuss in Chapter 4: The Competitive Edge. "Dr. Vo, I'll be applying for anesthesiology residency, and I have a one-month research elective in July. The residents suggested that I speak with you. Do you have a clinical research project that I could work on during this elective month?" Some faculty members will request a copy of your CV before entrusting you with such an opportunity. Even the simple e-mailed query about working on a review article may require further information on a faculty member's part.

Rule # 95 Don't exaggerate.

We don't include this rule lightly. However, candidates seeking residency positions in competitive specialties or programs have been known to exaggerate their research experience or even misrepresent themselves in an attempt to gain a competitive advantage. The literature is replete with studies that prove that lying on a CV is much more commonplace than students would suspect. It is also caught more often than students would imagine. In a study of applications to the radiation oncology residency program at the Roswell Park Cancer Institute, 49 applicants claimed authorship of a publication. Of those claiming authorship, 22% listed inaccurate citation information.[4] In a review of applications to the orthopedic surgery residency program at Wright State University, 20.6% of the 131 articles listed as published were in fact misrepresented.[5]

"I would never lie. This is just a slight exaggeration." "I think this should be fine – my name is mentioned in the article. If anyone ever asks me about it, I'll just explain that I didn't understand I wasn't an author." "I did work on the project, and I deserved to be listed as an author, but they couldn't include everyone due to the rules of the journal."

Most students don't set out to lie on their CV. If they do exaggerate or lie, they don't expect to be caught. While there's no universal agreement regarding the actions that should be taken if an applicant is caught in an act of misrepresentation, the possible consequences are many. At the very least, you won't be matching into that particular program. Other potential consequences include notification of the NRMP as well as the applicant's medical school and letter writers.

In some cases, applicants have claimed authorship of a publication based on participation in the research project. You cannot call yourself an author unless your name appears with the rest of the author group. Similarly, having your name cited in the acknowledgements section of an article is not synonymous with authorship.

Did you know?

You might assume that only desperate applicants would exaggerate or lie. However, Yang found that among radiation oncology residency applicants, CV misrepresentation was more common among applicants with higher USMLE scores (> 235).[4]

Other examples of misrepresentations discussed in the literature include:

- Claiming authorship of an article that does not exist in the medical literature
- Claiming authorship of an existent article when, in fact, the applicant was not listed as an author
- Moving one's name further up in the author list (i.e., listing your name as second author when, in fact, you were the sixth author)
- Listing a publication in a more prestigious journal rather than the actual journal
- Claiming membership in the AOA honor medical society when, in fact, the applicant was not a member
- Claiming receipt of an advanced degree when, in fact, the applicant did not earn the degree.

To guard against difficulties, we recommend that you bring copies of published, accepted, or submitted publications with you to the interview. Obtain your mentor's permission before bringing copies of publications that have been submitted. If you've listed an article as "in press," obtain a copy of the journal's letter of acceptance from your research mentor and bring it with you to the interview.

Did you know?

Residency programs do verify publications. In one instance, Dr. Schwartz, Chief of Dermatology at the New Jersey Medical School, came across an applicant who claimed coauthorship of a paper when in fact he had only received an acknowledgement. When Dr. Schwartz informed him that he had requested the paper through interlibrary loan for verification, the applicant withdrew his application.[6]

Rule # 96 **Take adequate time to reflect on your experiences and accomplishments.**

Most students dread the process of writing their CV; many feel they have nothing to make them stand out from other applicants. However, every applicant has individual, unique qualifications. On the other hand, the process of identifying your unique characteristics, experiences, and accomplishments is not an easy one. It's critical that you take adequate time to reflect on your experiences and accomplishments. Start with brainstorming. Begin the process by writing down absolutely everything; this is not the time to edit your thoughts. Start by taking each section of the CV, and make a list of everything that you've done that relates to that category. The standard sections of the CV are outlined in Rule # 79.

In the pages that follow, we describe each section in detail. As you complete each section, write down everything that you can possibly think of. After several initial brainstorming sessions, you should seek out other sources to help you come up with more ideas. Look at other books, websites, other examples of CVs, and speak to friends, family members, and colleagues. All of these sources may provide you with ideas. Later, you can edit this information.

Through this process, you may find that you don't have anything to list in a particular category. Don't be alarmed - you're in good company. If you don't have anything under a section, then omit the section. However, if you're reading this book well in advance of application season, you do have time to improve your situation. Discuss with your residents, your attendings, and your faculty advisor your wish to strengthen your CV. Seek out opportunities, responsibilities, or experiences that would enhance your application. The chapters on audition electives and the competitive edge outline further ways to enhance your CV.

Tip # 58

Students often have difficulty determining whether certain activities or involvement should be placed in the CV. Recognizing this, medical schools have encouraged their students to ask themselves some important questions:

- What is the item's relevance?
- Will inclusion of the item help me secure a residency interview?
- Would the information be helpful to residency programs in their decision-making process?

Although this is a worthwhile exercise, our experience advising students has shown that students are not always the best judge of type of content that programs would find useful or relevant. Our recommendation is to begin with a CV that has more rather than less, and then seek the input of your faculty advisor for paring down of content. This approach will ensure that important information is not omitted from the CV.

Rule # 97 Don't obsess over your first draft.

Once you've reviewed and written down your experiences and accomplishments, you can use this information to create the first draft of your CV. The ultimate goal is to present the information in such a way that it captures the interest and attention of the reader. However, your first draft doesn't need to be perfect.

Instead of agonizing over small details related to phrasing or formatting, take the information you've generated, transfer it to your word processing software, and arrange it in an organized manner. Once you've completed your first draft, you can then start agonizing over revisions. In the pages that follow, we present some important points about each section of the CV.

Contact Information

The CV begins with your contact information. It should include your name, address, telephone number, and e-mail address.

Did you know?

Double-check your contact information to ensure that a PD could reach you quickly and easily if necessary. Since most programs will communicate with you entirely by e-mail, double-check your e-mail address.

Did you know?

Is your e-mail address professional? You've worked hard to create a specific image throughout the entire application. You certainly don't want an unprofessional e-mail address to undo your efforts.

Did you know?

While most communication between an applicant and program occurs via e-mail, sometimes applicants are contacted by phone. Make sure that your voice mail message is professional.

Education

Detail your education in reverse chronological order (i.e., with your most recent or current place of learning first). Include the following:

- Name of institution
- Location of institution
- Area of study or concentration (major/minor)
- Dates of enrollment and completion (month/year)
- Degree(s)

For applicants in medical school, list the anticipated degree and expected graduation date. Include information about any graduate and undergraduate education. High school education is generally omitted.

If you received an honor, you can list it here (e.g., Dean's list, *magna cum laude*). If you have multiple awards, you can list them together in an "honors/awards" section. If you've completed a thesis or dissertation for a particular degree, you may wish to include it in this section.

Avoid these mistakes...

- If you hold an MBBS or medical degree other than MD, do not write MD.
- Abbreviations for degrees are the norm. Exceptions to this rule would be unusual degrees or abbreviations not widely known. If this pertains to you, provide the full degree name.
- Institutions do change their names. If your institution has changed its name, record the current name.
- Do not use abbreviations for institution names. Use the full name along with the location (city, state, country).
- The order in which you present the information is up to you but be consistent (i.e., date first, institution first, degree first).

Postgraduate Training

List all postgraduate training positions, including internship, residency, and fellowship, in reverse chronological order. Include dates and institution.

Work Experience

List jobs held during medical school, along with the dates of employment. For most applicants who have pursued a traditional path (college to medical school to residency), this is generally not an extensive section. Some applicants will have no work experience.

However, this can be an important section for medical graduates who are switching specialties, are returning to residency after practicing in another specialty, or for IMGs. In these cases, it's vital that this section is complete, and you must avoid any time gaps.

If you've had extensive work experience prior to starting medical school, you should include these jobs as well. Military service can also be placed in this section. Include your branch of service, number of years served, highest rank achieved, and any awards earned.

For each work experience, list the employer, location (city/state), job title, duties/responsibilities, and dates of employment. Give a brief description of your responsibilities using action verbs. In particular, focus on skills you gained that would enhance your value to a residency program (transferable skills). For example, tutoring may have helped you develop skills in directing, guiding, or supervising.

Tip # 59

A common mistake is to omit work experience, leaving a gap in your timeline which would be noticed by programs. Account for all time gaps.

Teaching Experience

For each teaching experience, include your position, subject taught, audience, location, frequency of teaching, and date. Don't forget about tutoring, advising, and mentoring.

Licensure/Certification

Include any licenses of health-related certificates you hold (PA, RN, EMT, ACLS). For IMGs, it's important to list ECFMG status. If you've done very well on your USMLE exam(s), list the score as well. If your performance was not stellar, you can simply state "passed." Include the date of licensure or certification. If licensure application is pending, use the phrase "application pending."

Honors and Awards

In this section, the focus should be on awards received during medical school. Awards and scholarships earned during the undergraduate years can also be included here, particularly if they're of great significance. You need not limit this section to academic awards. It's appropriate to include organizational, community, institutional, and departmental awards. If the honor is one that you feel a PD might value, then you should include it.

For awards that are not self-explanatory, include a single-sentence description to ensure that the reader understands the award's significance. Also include the date that you received the award and the bestowing organization.

What about high school awards? As a general rule, these should be omitted. An exception to this rule would be an extraordinary honor or accomplishment, such as valedictorian, National Merit Scholarship Finalist, or Eagle Scout.

Tip # 60

If you have a long list of awards and honors, consider the relevance of each award to residency programs. Important awards may be overlooked if the list is particularly long. Some applicants with numerous awards have separated items under undergraduate, graduate, and medical school.

Professional Memberships/Affiliations

List all professional organizations of which you are, or were, a member, along with the dates of your membership. It's especially important to include membership in an association that is relevant to your chosen specialty. If you are planning to pursue a career in obstetrics and gynecology and are a member of the American College of Obstetricians and Gynecologists (ACOG), you should include this in your CV. Some applicants elect not to list relevant memberships, citing their infrequent attendance at events or meetings. Even if you attended nothing more than an occasional meeting, don't let this stop you from listing membership in that organization on your CV. The fact that you're a member demonstrates a commitment to the specialty.

If you haven't yet become a member of the professional organization of your chosen specialty, do so as soon as possible. Lack of membership may indicate a lack of enthusiasm for the field. Professional memberships offer students concrete advantages, including subscription to the organization's journal, the opportunity to attend meetings at a substantial discount, and a means to network with physicians across the country. This will keep you abreast of the major issues in the field.

Leadership or committee positions within an organization are significant. Include appropriate dates for each position listed.

When listing the organization's name, do not use the abbreviation. If any organization to which you belong is considered controversial, such as PETA, you may want to consider leaving it out.

Research Experience

You should list all research experience, even if it didn't lead to a publication or presentation. Be specific in describing your duties and responsibilities. If your project was funded, list the amount and source of funding. You should always list your title/role, research mentor, and principal investigator of the project.

Publications

List all abstracts and articles that you've published. The most recent publication is listed first, followed by all others in reverse chronological order. If you've been particularly productive, the section can be subdivided into peer review journal articles, non-peer review journal articles, abstracts, and books/chapters.

Applicants often forget to include articles published in newsletters, newspapers, magazines, or the Internet. Contributions to a book, not just authorship of a book, may be listed as well. List publications in the standard format used by medical journals. Most commonly, citations are listed using the American Psychological Association or American Medical Association format.

Presentations

Although "presentations" can be combined with "publications" in one category, you may wish to create two categories. If you've only given one presentation, however, then use the joint category.

With presentations, it's particularly important to document the title, name of organization, location, and date. Include presentations given to academic societies and professional associations at the regional, national, and international level. Poster presentations should be listed here as well.

What about presentations you've given at your medical school? Presentations you were required to give should be omitted. However, occasionally a student may be asked to give a presentation because of exceptional performance. For example, if you were selected to be the sole presenter during psychiatry grand rounds, then you should include this experience.

Extracurricular activities

Residency programs take interest in an applicant's extracurricular activities. They respect the fact that students active in organizations have demonstrated an ability to balance a difficult course load with outside activities.

List activities you were involved in during medical school. Avoid listing activities prior to medical school unless they're of significance. If the type of activity isn't obvious, include a description.

Personal Interests

Few applicants give enough thought to this section. Often, two or three hobbies or interests are placed here without any consideration of how best to present the information. However, if done properly, this section can provide readers with insight into your personality and interests.

Programs are interested in an applicant's hobbies and interests. "What is this person like? Is he or she well rounded? Interesting? What would it be like to work with this person?" Provide this information in the personal interests section of your CV, which is usually the last section.

Interviews commonly begin with discussion of an applicant's personal interests as a way to break the ice. Applicants have been surprised to learn that they share the same interests as the interviewer.

Certain interests are viewed positively and may enhance your candidacy. The ability to speak Spanish fluently would be a noted positive at a residency program whose institution serves a large Hispanic population. Interests may also be viewed negatively.

While this section should not be any longer than a line or two, make every word count.

Sample CV # 1

SONIA AMIN
465 Stuyvesant Circle
Youngstown, OH 44555
(643) 844-7300
soniaamin@gmail.com

EDUCATION

Northeastern Ohio Medical University (NEOMED) 2013 – Present
Rootstown, OH
M.D., Anticipated in 5/17

University of Akron 2009-2013
Akron, OH
B.S., Biology

HONORS & AWARDS

Irwin Jacobsen Scholarship, NEOMED 2016
Awarded to top ranked student during third year

Liza Emerson Award, NEOMED 2014
Summer Research Grant 2013

EXTRACURRICULAR ACTIVITIES

NEOMED Medical Student Admissions Committee 2014 – Present
Student Chair

Dermatology Interest Group, Founder 2014 – Present

International Students Association, President 2013 – Present

RESEARCH EXPERIENCE

Case Western University School of Medicine — 2015 – Present
Department of Dermatology
Research Assistant (Supervisor: Grace Lin, M.D.)
Helped gather data on incidence of heart disease in psoriasis patients

National Institutes of Health — 2014 (Jun – Aug)
Research Assistant (Supervisor: Francisco Giovanni, M.D.)
Assisted in characterization of G2 receptor function

PROFESSIONAL MEMBERSHIPS

American Medical Women's Association — 2013 – Present

American Medical Association — 2013 – Present

Student National Medical Association — 2013 – Present

PERSONAL INTERESTS

Avid tennis player
Violin player in medical school orchestra
Traveling

COMMENTS SAMPLE CV # 1
(the good and the areas that need improvement)

Contact information: Notice how Sonia's contact information (name, address, phone number, e-mail address) is presented. In particular, her name is bolded in a larger font. The e-mail address is professional and the contact information is separated from the rest of the CV by a single, clear line.

Education: With few exceptions, CVs of residency applicants should begin with the education section. Note that Sonia has provided an abbreviation for her medical school. Throughout the rest of her CV, Sonia uses this abbreviation when referring to her school.

Honors and Awards: Following the education section, Sonia has included her honors and awards. Although she has done research and participated in several organizations, the nature of her awards is impressive. For this reason, this section should clearly follow education. Remember that readers will read your CV from top to bottom. Don't bury important information at the end of your CV.

While Sonia has properly described the Irwin Jacobsen Award, she should have done the same with the other two awards – the Lisa Emerson Award and Summer Research Grant. We have no way of knowing the significance of these awards. Was the grant given to her by the school as one of twenty grants offered to students in her class, or was it a more prestigious grant offered to five students across the country by the National Institutes of Health?

Extracurricular activities: Following the honors and awards section, Sonia continues with her extracurricular activities. She's placed this section next because it's stronger than those that follow. Of note, she has been a member of several organizations. If we hadn't been looking closely, however, we might have missed the fact that she was student chair of the admissions committee and founder of the dermatology interest group. She should have used these titles at the start of each line. She also could have bolded the words "founder" and "president" to highlight her leadership position rather than the organization name, as Robert does in sample CV # 2.

As an officer of several organizations, Sonia may have accomplished quite a bit. However, she chose not to describe her accomplishments. Her CV would have been strengthened had she done so. For example, as founder of the dermatology interest group, she could have listed her accomplishment in organizing a group of students to assist in a free skin cancer screening offered by the department.

Research experience: In the research experience section, Sonia chooses weak verbs such as "helped" or "assisted" to describe her role. We don't have any idea of her contributions to the research project. Contrast this with Robert's CV (CV # 2).

Note: Sonia's CV is spread over two pages. At the top right corner of the second page, she should have included her name and the page number, as Ashutosh did in CV # 3.

Sample CV # 2

ROBERT HERNANDEZ

1243 Huntington Drive
Chicago, Illinois 60611

rhernandez@hotmail.com

Home: (734) 222-4164
Cell: (632) 489-3500

EDUCATION

University of Oklahoma College of Medicine — 2012 – Present
Oklahoma City, OK
M.D., Anticipated 5/17
Class rank: top 10% (through junior year)

University of Central Oklahoma, Edmund, OK — 2008 – 2012
B.S., Biochemistry

RESEARCH EXPERIENCE

University of Oklahoma College of Medicine — 2014 - 2015
Department of Medicine
Clinical Research Assistant

- Developed studies investigating safety and efficacy of new antibiotic in treatment of *Pseudomonas aeruginosa*
- Strategized with leading infectious disease experts on development of study protocols
- Recruited patients through collaboration with other centers participating in multi-center study
- Collected, analyzed, and interpreted safety and efficacy data in preparation for publication and presentation
- Prepared progress reports on all aspects of study projects and presented results at monthly research meetings

PUBLICATIONS

Hernandez R, Miner Z, Costanzo T, Rainer J. The antimicrobial action of compound X5432. *J Pharm Infect Dis* 2015; 43(4): 54-59.

Costanzo T, Roberts R, Varicao C, Hernandez R, Rainer J. Susceptibility of *P. aeruginosa* to compound X5432. *J Antimic Thera* 2015; 22(3): 456-462.

PROFESSIONAL MEMBERSHIPS

Vice-President, AMSA — 2015 – Present
Member, IMIG — 2013 – Present
Member, AMSA — 2013 – Present

EXTRACURRICULAR ACTIVITIES

Intramural volleyball, soccer, and basketball — 2012 – Present

COMMENTS SAMPLE CV # 2
(the good and the areas that need improvement)

Education: With few exceptions, CVs of residency applicants should begin with the education section. Robert has chosen to include his class rank here rather than in a separate honors and awards section. This is the preferred approach for applicants who have a single honor. For applicants with multiple honors and awards, a separate section is advisable. It's not necessary to include your class rank or GPA. If it's exceptional, though, it's worth mentioning.

Also important to note is that Robert will be finishing medical school in five years. Readers will want to know why. Unfortunately, Robert doesn't make that clear. Later, in the research experience section, we see that he has done one year of research. However, we still don't know if he took one year off to do this research or if he took time off for another reason. If time was taken for a one-year research experience, it should be clearly noted in the education section.

Research experience: Robert follows the education section with research experience. Since Robert's research experience is a strong point of his application, it's appropriate to follow with this section. Note the active verbs he uses to describe his responsibilities as a clinical research assistant. Many applicants use words such as "helped" or "assisted." In many cases, this minimizes their contributions, diminishing the impact of the CV.

Professional membership: In the professional membership section, note how Robert has led with his title rather than the organization name. In leading with his title of Vice-President of AMSA, Robert succeeds in highlighting his leadership role.

In addition to membership in AMSA, Robert is an IMIG member. Readers may not be familiar with IMIG, which is an abbreviation for the Internal Medicine Interest Group. It would have been better to avoid the abbreviation in this case.

Sample CV # 3

Ashutosh Verma, MBBS

342 Webster Ave
Detroit, MI 48231
313-834-6266
averma@gmail.com

EDUCATION

2016 (Sep) Externship (Dermatology)
St. Joseph Hospital, Waco, Texas

- Interviewed and examined patients independently
- Formulated differential diagnosis and treatment plan
- Presented patients to faculty preceptor
- Wrote SOAP notes and prescriptions
- Delivered presentation on cutaneous leishmaniasis
- Published case report, "Pseudoporphyria due to Sulindac"

2014 – 2016 Master of Public Health (MPH)
University of Missouri, Columbia, Missouri

2009 – 2014 MBBS
Bombay Medical College, Mumbai, India

LICENSURE AND CERTIFICATION

2016 (July) ECFMG Certification
2016 (April) USMLE Step 2 CS – passed
2016 (March) USMLE Step 2 CK – passed (score 242)
2015 (January) USMLE Step 1 – passed (score 250)

PUBLICATIONS

Verma A, Silva I. Pseudoporphyria due to sulindac. *J Adv Derm* 2016: 31 (8): 41-43.

Page 2 – Ashutosh Verma

WORK EXPERIENCE

2013 – 2014 House Intern
Bombay General Hospital, Mumbai, India

- Rotated through departments of internal medicine, surgery, pediatrics, obstetrics and gynecology, and emergency medicine
- Conducted teaching programs for students

PROFESSIONAL MEMBERSHIPS

2014 – Present American Association of Physicians from India – Young Physicians Section

2014 – Present Michigan Association of Physicians from India – Young Physicians Section

2014 – Present American Association of Family Medicine – International Medical Graduate Section

EXTRACURRICULAR ACTIVITIES

Finished runner-up in medical school table tennis competition

COMMENTS SAMPLE CV # 3
(the good and the areas that need improvement)

Education: Note that Ashutosh is an international medical graduate. Since residency programs highly value U.S. clinical experience, Ashutosh has included his externship in the education section of this CV (although this is acceptable for the personal CV, U.S. clinical experience should not be listed under Education in the ERAS application).

Note also that Ashutosh has used the term "externship" as the title of his rotation experience rather than "observership." The former refers to an experience in which there is hands-on patient care, while the latter is strictly observational. Make sure you use the proper term. If you're unsure, ask the institution through which you rotated.

He uses bullets as a professional way to organize his responsibilities at St. Joseph Hospital.

While he has used active verbs such as "interviewed," "formulated," and "published" to describe his responsibilities, he could have taken it one step further by also including numbers. In other words, how many patients did he interview and examine per half day? How many SOAP notes did he write?

In the education section, he elected to lead with his rotation or degree rather than the institution name. An alternative approach would have been to lead with the institution name. If the institution is highly regarded, consider starting with the name rather than the degree or rotation. If you choose this option, you must begin each educational experience in the same manner.

Licensure and Certification: Ashutosh chose to follow the education section with his licensure and certification section. ECFMG status is of major interest to programs. Therefore, if you are ECFMG certified, it should be clearly stated in your CV.

If your USMLE scores are exceptional, as is the case here, include the scores in your CV. Otherwise, simply indicate that you have passed.

Work experience: Under work experience, he describes his responsibilities as an intern. Again, the inclusion of numbers would have strengthened this section.

Note: This CV is spread over two pages. At the top right corner of the second page, he has included his name and the page number. Contrast this with Sonia's CV (CV # 1).

Tip # 61

Before sending your CV to a letter writer, advisor, mentor, or PD, e-mail it to yourself to make sure there are no problems with formatting. CVs saved as certain file types may not appear the same when opened on other computers. We recommend that you convert your CV file to PDF and then submit it as a PDF file (after review). Formatting and layout will be preserved in the PDF file.

Tip # 62

Most administrators choose not to open attachments from individuals they do not know. You will need to establish contact first prior to sending attachments.

References

[1]Career Development: Information for Medical Residents. Available at: http://www.uthsc.edu/WIMS/docs/cv_pack_residents.pdf. Accessed May 23, 2013.

[2]Harolds J. Tips for a physician in getting the right job, part II: the curriculum vitae, cover letter, and personal statement. *Clin Nucl Med* 2013: 38(9): 721-723.

[3]Grimes D. Sabotaging your curriculum vitae. *Obstet Gynecol* 2010:115(5): 1071-1074.

[4]Yang G, Schoenwetter M, Wagner T, Donohue K, Kuettel M. Misrepresentation of publications among radiation oncology residency applicants. *J Am Coll Radiol* 2006; 3(4): 259-264.

[5]Konstantakos E, Laughlin R, Markert R, Crosby L. Follow-up on misrepresentation of research activity by orthopedic residency applicants: has

[6]Schwartz R. Medical student publications: a faculty mentor's perspective. *J Am Acad Dermatol* 1997; 37(4): 667-668.

Chapter 10

The Audition Elective

An "audition" elective essentially serves as an extended interview, and should be regarded as such. Audition electives are valued by programs as they provide a way to more reliably assess an applicant's cognitive and noncognitive skills and traits. For students applying to competitive specialties or programs, audition electives are considered a must by some advisors. These rotations give students the chance to highlight skills and qualities that aren't easily judged by the typical application materials. Students can showcase their clinical acumen, their skills in patient interactions, their abilities to work with colleagues and faculty, and their enthusiasm for the particular program and specialty. These electives also offer additional opportunities to highlight a student's qualifications for the program. Opportunities include deeper investigation of difficult cases, performing thorough literature searches, volunteering to give presentations, or seeking opportunities to publish in their chosen field.

Audition electives have increased in popularity as students increasingly try to gain a competitive advantage wherever possible. In response to this trend, some educators have criticized students and their medical schools for allowing applicants to do multiple audition electives. Some schools have adopted policies limiting the number of electives that students can complete in any given specialty. However, students continue to receive messages encouraging audition electives, and often these messages come directly from residency programs. Some make it clear that in order to be seriously considered, an applicant should rotate through the department. These conflicting messages are confusing. Should I do an audition elective? How many should I do? When is the best time to do one? How can I excel during the elective? Will it guarantee me an interview? We address these questions in this chapter.

Rule # 98 **In some specialties, audition electives are considered a must.**

In a survey of PDs representing multiple specialties, Wagoner found that 86% would give preference to students who had performed at a high level in an audition elective.[1] This is not surprising, since an audition elective is essentially an extended interview, during which a program can more reliably assess an applicant's cognitive and noncognitive skills and traits.

Some specialties attach great importance to the audition elective. In a survey of orthopedic surgery PDs, *the most important criterion in the resident selection process* was considered to be an applicant's performance during a rotation at the director's program.[2] The authors of the study further stated that "60% of programs reported that 50% or more of their matching residents over the previous three years had performed medical student orthopedic surgery rotations at the program prior to matching for residency." Of note, applicants were also asked about their impressions regarding the importance of these selection factors, and the audition elective was not cited among their top three. In another survey of orthopedic surgery PDs, performance on a local rotation was considered *the most important attribute* in obtaining a residency. This was followed by class rank and the interview.[3] Drs. Peabody and Manning, faculty members in the Department of Orthopedics at the University of Chicago, strongly recommend audition electives. "It's almost mandatory to do an away elective and shine."[4]

In a survey of dermatology applicants, the audition elective was similarly important. A total of 53% of applicants matched at a program in which they had some prior experience. Of these, 29% matched at an institution affiliated with their own medical school, 18% matched with an institution where they had done an audition elective, and 6% matched with a program where they had done a research elective or fellowship.[5]

In other specialties, by contrast, the audition elective may not have much of an effect. As a general rule, audition elective are less important in family medicine, internal medicine, pediatrics, neurology, and pathology. However, even within these less competitive specialties, an audition elective may be important to certain programs. This may be dependent upon other factors including the competitiveness of the program, the strength of your candidacy, and the program's familiarity with your medical school.

Rule # 99 Recognize the full advantages of an audition elective, and plan to maximize each one.

Audition electives provide many potential advantages in increasing the competitiveness of your application. However, applicants who've rotated with us and with our colleagues don't always realize the full roster of potential benefits. Before starting your elective, plan carefully so that you can take advantage of each of these potential benefits.

- An additional elective in your field can provide an unmatched clinical experience. It can allow you to work with and learn from some of the best faculty in the country. It can provide exposure to other facets of the specialty not available at your own institution.
- The audition elective serves as an extended interview. This is your chance to impress upon the program what an outstanding student you are, and what an outstanding resident you would be.
- The audition elective provides an ideal opportunity to impress upon the program how well you would fit in with their residency program. An outstanding student is not always a great fit for every program. You can

use the opportunities presented by an audition elective to emphasize those factors that make you perfect for the program, and make the program perfect for you. If you have extensive experience in basic science research and your future plans include translational research, then discuss your desire to obtain complete and thorough clinical training in order to aid you in your future translational research. If you've spent all of your formative years and education in the city of Miami, make sure the program understands that you definitely want to experience a new part of the country. If you have an interest in pediatric gastroenterology, then discuss the specialized opportunities available at this referral center.

- The audition elective provides the chance for the chairman and faculty to recognize you as an individual. With over 400 applications received for a total of three residency positions at one dermatology program, it becomes very difficult for even outstanding applicants to stand out. Just rotating through a program is not sufficient, though. You need to meet key decision-makers in the program, other faculty members, the residents, and the support staff. We discuss how to do so below.
- You've already set your application apart because of this personal experience with the program. With some applicants applying to 50 or more programs, it can be difficult for a program to gauge if a student is actually interested in the program, or if it was just one of many that a student targeted in order to increase their chances of matching. You have demonstrated a concrete interest in this particular program.
- You should plan to obtain a strong LOR from the experience. Particularly if you've chosen your elective well, you may have the support of a prominent, respected, well-known individual. Letters from such attendings can carry great weight nationally. In addition, a strong LOR from an attending within the program can be a stronger influence than a strong letter from an unknown letter writer. The section on LORs provides more guidance.
- An audition elective provides an unparalleled opportunity to directly impress your attending. Your outstanding work will hopefully impress an attending to the degree that they become your advocate in residency selection proceedings. Attendings will often argue for a certain applicant's candidacy, and often quite passionately, and that advocacy can be enough to tip the scales in your favor. Your work during the elective also provides exposure to other members of the department. Residents, nurses, and secretaries can also act as vocal advocates.
- An elective provides additional opportunities to work on a project. Seeking out case reports or review articles at the start of the elective signifies your enthusiasm and commitment to the field. Completing a project, and completing it well, signifies your skills and drive. Such work helps you stand out. It also provides additional material for your CV. It also gives your letter writer concrete information to discuss in the letter. "Soledad was a very enthusiastic student" doesn't carry all that much

weight. This statement, on the other hand, makes a reviewer take notice: "Soledad began the rotation by seeking out opportunities for articles. When we saw a case of actinic lichen planus together, she did an extensive literature search, presented her findings to me the next day, and asked if she could write up the case. I had a well-written case report on my desk three days later."

- It allows you to meet residents in your field. Residents are a great resource. Let them know on day one if you're interested in matching into this field, and if you're interested in this particular program. They can give you excellent advice on how to approach an attending, and which attendings would be best to approach, for letters or publications. They can introduce you to other faculty in the program. They can help you seek out interesting clinical cases that could serve as material for publication. They can, and often do, serve as vocal advocates for certain applicants with whom they would like to work in the future. They can sometimes be the most knowledgeable resources about programs around the country, having recently completed the application process. Let the residents know on day 30 how you feel about the program and your experience there, particularly if it's become a top choice.

Caution…

Regardless of specialty, the practice of medicine requires a broad range of skills. In addition to being intellectually capable, physicians must have the noncognitive skills necessary to effectively interact with and relate to a wide variety of patients and healthcare professionals. Just because an individual can score at high levels on a standardized test, it does not mean that they have the skills of perception and communication required to excel in areas requiring interactions, which basically encompasses almost all of medical practice.

This is a difficult area in which to counsel students, and these are skills that are difficult to teach. Many students don't even realize that they excel in these areas, because they've acquired these skills intuitively. Other students don't even realize their lack of these skills. They may only start to realize it when they are evaluated in these areas, such as during clinical rotations. It may become more apparent when they receive feedback from patients on their bedside manner, from attendings on their communication skills, and from colleagues on their teamwork.

There's a fine line between many of the qualities that are important to residency selection, and many of the qualities that are perceived as negatives, as indicated in the following list:

Assertive / Aggressive

Enthusiastic / Playing the game

Confident / Arrogant

Friendly / A suck-up

Humble / Lacking in self-confidence

Quiet / Insecure

Polite and respectful of others' turns to speak / Disinterested or lacking the knowledge required to speak

The first to volunteer to give a talk / A gunner

Meeting with decision-makers during the rotation / Too political

Obviously, we could go on and on. These negative labels may come from anyone – your colleagues, the residents, or the attendings.

How do you make sure that you're projecting the fact that you are enthusiastic about the specialty and the program without projecting an appearance of just trying to play the game? These are difficult skills to perfect, and entire books have been written about this subject in the business literature and in the career advancement genre. Some of this is beyond your control, as with some attendings who think every other elective student is trying too hard to be political. Much of it is under your control, though, even though these skills are difficult to master. The process begins with self-evaluation and close attention to feedback throughout your career.

Rule # 100 **An audition elective does not equate to an away elective. Your most important audition elective may in fact be the one at your own institution.**

Away electives are important, and can be critical to your future career. Most students recognize this fact. However, a local elective can be just as critical to your career. In terms of matching into your field, some programs will give preference to a "known commodity." In the survey of dermatology applicants described previously, 29% of applicants matched at an institution affiliated with their own medical school.[5]

As opposed to the snapshot of an applicant obtained from a 15-minute interview, faculty feel more confident in their impressions after one month of working with a student and after hearing other attendings' personal evaluations. Another important point is that faculty from your own institution, including your chairman, may be called or e-mailed by other programs for a candid opinion. The bottom line: recognize that the most important audition elective you take may be the first one you take.

Rule # 101 **An outstanding audition elective can overcome shortcomings in your application.**

We have witnessed the power of the audition elective. Residency selection committees often use screening criteria when reviewing applications. For example, a USMLE score below 200 may automatically exclude you from consideration, regardless of your transcript, Dean's letter, or letters of recommendation. However, students with such low scores can still match into competitive specialties, a fact we can attest to and a fact that is reflected in NRMP data. The audition elective is an ideal opportunity to impress upon the residency program that a low USMLE score will not prevent you from performing high-quality work and won't impact your ability to pass the specialty's board.

If you have average grades and an average USMLE score, your application won't stand out from the exceedingly strong applications under consideration at competitive programs. However, personal knowledge of your skills, qualities, and work ethic can provide a huge boost to your application.

Did you know?

Dr. Martha Terris, Program Director at the Medical College of Georgia, states that "participating in a urology rotation at an institution other than the student's home institution may be beneficial if it is a program at which the student is particularly interested in completing residency training. A visiting student rotation can give students the chance to impress the urology faculty at another institution if their clinical skills outweigh their academic record or who attend a medical school of lesser reputation."[6]

Did you know?

Some programs require applicants to do a rotation at their institution in order to be seriously considered. If you wish to match at one of these programs, you have no choice but to do an audition elective, even if you're a stellar applicant.

Did you know?

The American College of Surgeons states that "the more they like you, the better your chance of being selected. When two candidates with similar credentials are being compared, the nod will likely go to the one who performed well on-site during a senior elective. However, we certainly do not recommend more than a total of two audition electives."[7]

Rule # 102 Choose the correct audition elective.

Audition electives provide many concrete benefits, as we've outlined. If you're going to actually receive any of these benefits, however, you need to choose your elective very carefully. Consider these factors:

- During an audition elective, you may be able to work with one of the top subspecialists in the country. You may be able to work with one of the top interventional cardiologists in the country, or at one of the top clinical centers for juvenile rheumatoid arthritis. If you're interested in a particular area of medicine, this may be an unsurpassed experience.
- Some electives afford the opportunity to work with well-respected faculty members who are known to be good advisors to students, and who have excellent potential as letter writers.

Consider the negatives of certain programs as well:

- An obvious advantage to doing an audition elective is that you have the chance to make such a strong impression on a program that they will accept you as a resident. Don't waste this chance by doing an audition elective at a program where you have no chance of matching. Medical schools generally limit the number of away electives that students can do, so make sure your away electives are at institutions where you have a realistic chance of matching. If it's the top program in the country, they may be unlikely to accept a student with average grades and scores. If the program seeks out applicants with a strong basic science research background, then don't waste your time.
- Some electives are so popular that you may make no impression among a sea of other highly qualified applicants. With 5 applicants rotating during any given month, you may lose out on one of the main benefits of doing an audition elective: that of making a memorable impression.
- So many students rotate through some electives that the program becomes unable to interview such a high number of applicants. In some programs, therefore, the elective becomes an "interview" and the student won't be invited back for a formal interview. This may be a negative if you had no opportunity to meet with the other faculty, and if the faculty member with whom you did work does not serve as a vocal advocate for your application.

Choose a program where you may benefit from all of the advantages of the audition elective. Look for programs where you have a chance of making a memorable impression, where you have a chance of publishing, where you can work with outstanding faculty, and hopefully come away with a strong LOR. Choose programs where you would like to match, from a clinical and geographic standpoint. Choose a program where you actually have a chance of matching.

Choosing such a program is difficult, and there is no easy answer on how to find the perfect elective. Some of the best have become so popular that it becomes a negative – in a sea of so many students, it's difficult to make a memorable impression. Start by seeking out advice from fellow students. Some schools ask their students to complete evaluations of their away elective experiences and store them in a file to aid future students. Check with your medical school to see if such a file exists. Seek out advice from residents in the specialty. Since they've gone through the process more recently, they are valuable resources. Also discuss the issue with your faculty advisor within the specialty. If you have a particular interest within the specialty, your advisor may be able to arrange for you to work with an attending who does not offer a formal elective.

Tip # 63

Before deciding whether to do an audition elective or where to do it, it's important that you speak with your advisor. Your specialty-specific advisor will have tremendous insight based upon his or her experience with previous students.

Most medical schools provide information about the electives available to visiting students at their website. An additional source of information is the Association of American Medical Colleges (AAMC). The AAMC publishes a list of extramural electives available at AAMC-member U.S. medical schools online at https://services.aamc.org/eec/students/. This list, which is updated every January, contains a variety of information, including contact persons, application and other fees, and the earliest date at which application materials will be accepted.

Did you know?

At a workshop conducted by the Clerkship Directors of Internal Medicine, the advice given to students included the importance of doing your research before applying for audition electives. "Ask around, don't just get one where you are doomed to fail."[8]

Tip # 64

One of the disadvantages of audition electives is the costs incurred, including costs associated with travel, housing, food, and parking. Check with your school to determine if it offers any financial assistance. Some schools may have funds available to help students with these expenses. If you'll be doing an away research elective, there may be outside funding sources you can turn to.

Rule # 103 Don't underestimate the risks of an audition elective.

Here's an unfortunate truth: applicants may sometimes end up looking worse in person than on paper. A review of discussion forums found that students are sometimes given the advice to avoid audition electives, especially if their application is particularly strong to begin with. Performing at a high level can be easier said than done when you're new to an institution. Unfamiliarity with your new environment may delay or even prevent you from performing at a high level.

Some factors may be beyond your control. You may be assigned to an attending known to be a hard grader, aka "a hawk," and the high quality of your work may not be recognized. Sometimes personality factors or misunderstandings may play a role. Unfortunately, we've seen these issues at play, and we're aware of cases in which an audition elective may have worked against a student. The bottom line is that you must recognize the risks associated with the audition elective, and act accordingly to minimize those risks.

Tip # 65

If you have a very strong application, to the point that you are likely to match into a program based on the strength of your application alone, then an audition elective at that program may not be the best use of your elective time. Discuss your list of potential away electives with your advisor before deciding where to apply.

Rule # 104 Take advantage of all the key opportunities during the elective.

An audition elective should never just be about showing up for work on time and doing a great job. This is where every skill you've learned about doing well in clerkships should come into play. You should be at every meeting and conference ten minutes early. You should have a handbook or textbook (paper or digital) with you in the clinic, and you should refer to it often.

The types of patients you see in some specialty clinics or referral hospitals offer a wealth of clinical information that you may not see elsewhere, and you should take full advantage of these clinical opportunities. Search the literature after work hours and share your findings if appropriate. Actively seek out opportunities to highlight your skills and enthusiasm.

If the attending asks for a volunteer to give a talk on a subject or to research a clinical question, be the first to volunteer. If the attending is just pondering a difficult question out loud, offer to investigate further. If all elective students are expected to give a talk at the end of the rotation, then great; this is an excellent opportunity to make an impression. Talks are controlled situations in which you can research your issue, offer an excellent handout, and impress your attending and residents with your self-confidence, poise, and mastery of the material. All of this is absolutely basic third year rotation information, and yet so many elective students don't show mastery of these basics. Please see our companion book, *Success on the Wards: 250 Rules for Clerkship Success*. The book outlines how to excel in clinical rotations and how to give an outstanding presentation.

In a highly competitive field such as dermatology, elective students who can perform at this level still don't stand out. It is expected by most attendings that a student applying to our program will also be seeking out additional material. Students should speak with the residents and the attending at the start of the rotation, and make clear their wish to work on a case report, review article, presentation, or any other opportunities that might be available. For further information on locating opportunities to publish in your field or participate in a research project, see Chapter 4: The Competitive Edge.

Rule # 105 Make it a point to meet the key faculty members.

You have the best chance of matching into the program if you directly impress key faculty in the department. Key faculty members include the chairman, program director, and other members of the selection committee. In some programs, as you schedule your elective, you may be able to ask if you can be assigned to one of these individuals. In some programs, particularly smaller programs, the selection committee may consist of every faculty member. In this case, every faculty member becomes key faculty, with equal ability to affect your chances.

Even if you can't work directly with key faculty, there are still many opportunities for interaction. Learn how to introduce yourself appropriately. If you're in clinic working with one faculty member, you should introduce yourself to any other faculty members that you encounter. If you're putting away your bag in the staff room and Dr. Shell arrives at the same time, then take that opportunity. "Good morning, Dr. Shell. I wanted to introduce myself. My name is Grace Donald. I'm a visiting student from Wayne State working with Dr. Pelsky this month."

If you've attended an interesting lecture and learned useful information, then feel free to impart that information as well. Such an introduction must be done carefully, so keep it short and not too over the top. "Thank you for that lecture, Dr. Wells. I'm a visiting student from Wayne State, and we just saw a patient last week with a herald bleed, so your lecture was very helpful."

Attend all departmental conferences and journal clubs. The non-required conferences are excellent opportunities to distinguish yourself, since students taking a required rotation won't attend. If you're interested in the program, then schedule appointments with the chairman and program director to introduce yourself and express your interest in their program. These meetings should be used to ask if there are any projects that you would be able to work on during your elective.

Tip # 66

Don't ignore other faculty. You never know who may have input into the residency selection process. Also note that residents often have significant input. Take every opportunity to meet and interact with as many faculty and residents as you can.

Rule # 106 To obtain an away elective, you first have to apply.

The steps involved in the application process for an away elective are summarized here.

- The Visiting Student Application Service (VSAS) is administered by the AAMC, and allows applicants to complete a single application. With its development in 2006, VSAS streamlined the process of applying for these electives. Although allopathic and osteopathic students may utilize VSAS, the system is not available to Canadian and international medical students. Note that not all institutions participate in VSAS. For non-participating institutions, contact the appropriate person or office at the away institution for an application. In many cases, a visiting student application can be downloaded from the institution's website.
- Complete the student portion of the application and gather any supporting documents. While there are differences from one application to another, commonly requested items are the medical school transcript, immunization record, certificate of student standing, application/processing fees, documentation of health/malpractice insurance, HIPAA certificate, criminal background check, board scores, and photo ID. Make arrangements to obtain these documents through the appropriate office at your school. You may also be asked to complete your school's away rotation approval form.
- Your school may require some time to process their portion of your application. Take this into consideration to avoid any delay in the submission of your application.
- The most common reasons for failure to secure away elective positions are due to delays in application submission and receipt of all required documents.
- Be careful in your follow-up inquiries. Many students will send emails within a week of application submission. We recommend that you wait one month before making inquiries with the rotation coordinator. If you communicate too soon, the program may not have had enough time to process the paperwork. Too frequent contact too soon can be a turnoff.
- Remember to also be professional in all interactions. With the intense competition that exists for these spots, it's very easy for an applicant to be removed from consideration due to unprofessional behavior. Aim to be liked.
- Note that your application must be complete. If there's even a single item that's not available, your application may be put on hold.

Did you know?

Prior to VSAS, programs received significantly fewer applications for away electives. According to Dr. Scott Sherman, Program Director of the EM Residency at Cook County Hospital, his program received 157 applications for two spots available in August. Before VSAS, the program may have had 15 or 20 applications.[9]

Tip # 67

To enhance your chances at your most coveted institutions, ask your mentor to call or email the department about your interest in performing the away elective. With this approach, you're more likely to stand out in a sea of qualified applicants. The key with this approach is to have your mentor communicate with the program before spots are filled.

Tip # 68

If you need to cancel an away elective, do it the right way. Do not contact a program one or two weeks before your start date with notification of cancellation. In such situations, students leave programs with unfilled spots. Although you can cancel the elective by VSAS, we recommend that you also contact the program directly. You can email or phone the clerkship coordinator and thank them for taking the time to review your application. By expressing appreciation and reiterating your interest in the program in a professional manner, you will remain in consideration for an interview at the institution after you apply. Despite what you may hear, most programs don't penalize you if you must cancel your elective, as long as it's handled in a timely and professional manner.

Rule # 107 Apply early for the chance to do an audition elective.

Some of the best electives are the most competitive. Spots in less competitive electives may still be difficult to secure during the popular months of July and August. Check the institution's website and www.aamc.org to learn about the earliest date at which applications are accepted. Generally, visiting student applications are not acted upon until the schedules of the institution's own students are finalized. This typically takes place sometime in the spring. To maximize your chances of securing preferred away electives, apply in the spring of your third year. It's important that you determine the earliest date on which the program will accept the application. There's intense competition for spots, and your ability to submit applications on the earliest date possible will maximize your chances.

Tip # 69

Apply *early*. Some away elective slots fill quickly. Remember that July and August are the most popular months.

Rule # 108 Complete your local elective before taking an away elective.

Always complete your own school's rotation before you do any audition electives. The experiences that you gain will help your performance. Per the words of the Saint Louis University School of Medicine: "Conventional wisdom says that if you are going to audition externships, you would first want to do the senior year floor service or other appropriate senior year clerkship in that same discipline…to raise your skill levels up to those expected of someone who has already completed that clerkship."[10]

Tip # 70

As you prepare for an audition elective, analyze the elective that you completed at your own school. What specifically did you do well? What could you have done better? Read your faculty and resident evaluations. An analysis of your previous clerkship experience can be invaluable.

Rule # 109 Time your audition elective so that you can obtain a letter of recommendation.

A major advantage of the audition elective is the chance to secure a strong LOR. For your letter to be available at all programs before interviews are offered, you must schedule the rotation as early as possible. Keep in mind that letter writers may need considerable time to write and send a strong letter.

Tip # 71

The ideal time to do an away elective is as early as possible. If it's possible to do a rotation in your third year, after completing the rotation at your home school, then do so. Most applicants will do audition electives in July through September of their senior year due to the requirements of their medical school.

Rule # 110 Be careful with audition electives during interview season.

While you can do an audition elective during interview season, you should never schedule interviews during the rotation. Demonstrating your sense of responsibility and commitment to hard work is difficult to do when you're away interviewing at another program.

Rule # 111 **An audition elective is a great chance to impress a program. It's also a great chance to evaluate a program.**

Audition electives offer multiple benefits beyond increasing your chances of matching with a program in your chosen specialty.

- Greater exposure to the residency program allows you to make a more informed decision about your rank list.

  An audition elective provides you the opportunity to see the ins and outs of a program. How do the faculty relate to the residents? How do the residents get along with one another? What is the quality of the educational conferences? There is no better way to assess your fit for a particular program than by doing an audition elective. Among students who had done an audition elective in pediatrics, approximately 45% found the elective experience helpful in delineating the program's strengths and weaknesses, and 25% noted negatives that steered them away from the program.[11]

- The elective provides the chance to learn about the geographic area in which you will be training and quite possibly practicing for many years. Residency graduates often remain in the area to practice. An audition elective will allow you to explore the area to determine if you would enjoy living there.

- The elective may provide exposure to a specialty not available at your own medical school.

  Medical schools are not created equal. Some offer rotations in all specialties, while others don't. If you attend a school that doesn't offer a rotation in your chosen specialty, you'll have to arrange an away elective. You obviously need the experience to confirm that you've chosen the right specialty.

Rule # 112 **The audition elective does not guarantee an interview.**

You may hear that an audition elective will guarantee an interview. At many programs, all students who perform audition electives will receive an invitation to interview. However, this isn't the case at all programs. Some programs make it quite clear on their websites that they do not interview all applicants who complete an audition elective. For example, at the website for the diagnostic radiology program at the Oregon Health Sciences University, it is clearly stated: "We do not automatically interview all applicants who do an audition elective here."[12]

Findings from an Analysis of Visiting Medical Student Elective and Clerkship Programs

In a survey of 76 medical schools, researchers were able to develop a better understanding of visiting medical student elective programs:[13]

- Reasons why schools have these programs include recruitment for residency programs (90%), fulfillment of educational mission of the institution (78%), and enhancement of reputation (38%).
- In terms of eligibility requirements, 10% reported allowing third-year medical students to perform away electives, and 97% reported allowing fourth-year students to do so. 85% reported that osteopathic students were welcome to do electives. Additional eligibility requirements included documentation of immunizations (92%), previous clinical experience (85%), successful completion of the USMLE Step 1 (51%), letter of recommendation (37%), and medical school transcript (36%).
- Nearly 60% reported that international visiting medical students were allowed to do electives. For 90% of these institutions, fluency in English was required for eligibility, and some requested successful completion of TOEFL.
- 86% reported that the length of an elective was 4-5 weeks.
- At nearly half of the schools, the maximum amount of time students could rotate was 6-8 weeks.
- 78% indicated that visiting students were evaluated in the same manner as the institution's own students.
- It was not uncommon for institutions to screen prospective visiting medical students in an effort to select those who might be competitive for the GME programs.

Tip # 72

Osteopathic and international students should target away electives at institutions and programs with a track record of selecting such students as residents.

References

[1]Wagoner N, Suriano J, Stoner J. Factors used by program directors to select residents. *J Med Educ* 1986; 61(1): 10-21.
[2]Bernstein A, Jazrawi L, Elbeshbeshy B, Della Valle C, Zuckerman J. Orthopedic resident-selection criteria. *J Bone Joint Surg Am* 2002; 84-A(11): 2090-2096.
[3]Bajaj G, Carmichael K. What attributes are necessary to be selected for an orthopedic surgery residency position: perceptions of faculty and residents. *South Med J* 2004; 97(12): 1179-1185.
[4]Peabody T, Manning D. Pritzker residency process guide: orthopedic surgery. Available at: http://pritzker.uchicago.edu/current/students/ResidencyProcessGuide.pdf. Accessed November 2, 2008.
[5]Clarke J, Miller J, Sceppa J, Goldsmith L, Long E. Success in the dermatology resident match in 2003: perceptions and importance of home institutions and away rotations. *Arch Dermatol* 2006; 142(7): 930-2.
[6]Urology Match. Available at: http://www.urologymatch.com/faculty-survey-results?page=4. Accessed December 14, 2015.
[7]American College of Surgeons. Available at: http://www.facs.org/residencysearch/position/position.html. Accessed January 2, 2008.
[8]CDIM workshop "Giving advice to medical students applying for an IM residency position (October 15, 2004)." Available at: gsm/utmck/edu/IM/FAQstudent_advice.htm. Accessed January 2, 2008.
[9]EM Match Advice: VSAS 101 – Securing an Away EM Rotation. Available at: http://www.aliem.com/2015/em-match-advice-vsas-101/. Accessed March 22, 2016.
[10]St. Louis University School of Medicine. Available at: oca.slu.edu. Accessed on January 2, 2008.
[11]Englander R, Carraccio C, Zalneraitis E, Sarkin R, Morgenstern B. Guiding medical stduetns through the match: perspectives from recent graduates. *Pediatrics* 2003; 112(3): 502-505.
[12]Department of Radiology at Oregon Health Sciences University. Available at: http://www.ohsu.edu/radiology/med/index.html. Accessed January 2, 2008.
[13]Mueller P, McConahey L, Orvidas L, Lee M, Bowen J, Beckan T, Kasten M. Visting medical student elective and clerkship programs: a survey of US and Puerto Rico allopathic medical schools. *BMC Medical Education* 2010; 10: 41.

Chapter 11

Preinterview Dinner or Social Event

Surveys have shown that interactions with residents are very important to applicants. While interactions do take place during the interview day, most programs provide significant exposure to residents at social events, either before or after the interview. In a survey of fourth-year students at a single school, 96% of programs visited by applicants held a social event, usually the night before the formal interview.[1] These get-togethers are a rich source of information about the residents, faculty, and program. Even more importantly, they provide another opportunity to highlight your sparkling personality and scintillating wit.

Rule # 113 **The residency dinner or social event is important. Make every effort to attend.**

The pre-interview residency dinner or social event is an opportunity for you to meet the residents. Through these interactions, you'll be able to gauge their level of happiness. In a survey of nearly 100 matched plastic surgery residents, resident happiness was the highest rated factor influencing program ranking.[2] In a survey of orthopedic surgery applicants, similar findings were noted. The authors wrote that "applicants first and foremost wish to be happy where they match and gauge this from their observations and interactions with current residents at programs."[3] Keep in mind that the structure of the interview day may prevent you from interacting in a meaningful way with residents, which makes the dinner or social event even more important.

Did you know?

We agree with the words of Dr. Patrick Duff, Associate Dean for Student Affairs at the University of Florida College of Medicine. "If the program at which you are interviewing has a social event the night before, or the night of, your interview, you should make every effort to attend. This is your key opportunity to meet the residents on an informal basis (and vice-versa) and to learn a great deal about the day-to-day reality of working in the department... Failure to attend the event may be perceived as lack of serious interest on your part."[4]

Tip # 73

Because the websites of many great programs lack the detailed information which applicants seek, these social events are opportunities to learn more about the program. This information can be used the following day when your interviewer asks, "Why are you interested in our program?"

Rule # 114 **The social event is definitely a part of the interview. Don't drop your guard.**

Residents will form impressions of you during these events. Don't underestimate the importance of the residents in the selection process. In a recent survey of over 1,800 program directors representing 22 specialties, "interactions with house staff during interview and visit" was considered to be quite important in the ranking of applicants. It received a mean importance rating of 4.7 out of 5.0 (scale from 1 [not at all important] to 5 [very important]).[5] 88% of programs cited these interactions as a factor in ranking applicants. "We offer a dinner with the current residents the evening before all interview dates," writes the Department of Medicine at Eastern Virginia Medical School. "This is an opportunity for you and our residents to get to know each other in an informal setting. We consider this an important part of the interview process and will seek feedback on applicants from our current residents."[6]

Did you know?

The Surgical Society at the University of Colorado School of Medicine reminds applicants of the influence that residents may have in the selection process. "Take advantage of the opportunities you have to interact and communicate with the residents at those programs that intrigue you. Contact them by email after you visit and keep in touch. Many program directors ask for resident feedback about each applicant. This can be very helpful to you if you have made a good impression on those residents."[7]

Tip # 74

While these events tend to be more relaxed than the actual interview, never forget that you <u>are</u> being judged. Even if faculty members are absent, any representative of the program, including residents and support staff, may be asked for their impressions of you. Remain alert and don't let your guard down. Be cordial, friendly, and polite. Engage in conversation freely with residents and faculty. Just take care in what you reveal.

Did you know?

Dr. Andrew Lee, Chairman of the Department of Ophthalmology at the Houston Methodist Hospital, wrote that "we include a resident in our residency selection process and have found anecdotally that resident input can provide valuable information that might not be revealed in an asymmetric hierarchial faculty-applicant interview. In addition, informal feedback obtained from the residents during the social activities associated with the interview process can reach the selection committee through the resident liaison."[8]

Rule # 115 **If you're unable to attend, not all programs will be understanding.**

Social events are considered optional at most programs. "Our residents may invite you to join them for dinner the night before or following the interview day," writes the Department of Obstetrics and Gynecology at Oregon Health Sciences University. "While this may be helpful in your assessment of our residents and program, it is not part of our selection process and does not have any effect whatsoever on our applicant rankings. If you are able to attend, you'll be able to learn about our residents and program in a relaxed and informal setting. If logistics make it difficult for you to attend the dinner, you will not be at any disadvantage in the application process."[9]

Although optional at most programs, some programs feel strongly that applicants should attend social events. The Department of Orthopedic Surgery at Cleveland Clinic invites applicants to an informal social event that is well attended by residents. "This event is typically from 6pm - 10pm and is not required but highly encouraged."[10]

Tip # 75

Even if considered optional, it's to your advantage to attend these dinners. These get-togethers provide an ideal opportunity to discuss the program with the residents and gauge their level of happiness. The information you discover may help you perform better during the interview, and ask more informed questions. Keep in mind that these "optional dinners" may not be considered optional by certain faculty. Some applicants who've worked with us in the past have reported being asked, "Did you attend our dinner last night?" If you weren't able to attend the dinner, offer a good reason for your absence. Also make sure the interviewer knows that you'll be contacting residents to learn more about the program.

You will also encounter programs that require your attendance at these events. "An interview day really begins the evening before, as the applicants and spouses/significant others are invited to join a number of residents and their significant others for dinner at a local restaurant," writes the Department of Anesthesiology at Duke University. "We consider this dinner a crucial part of the interview experience. So if you're considering one of the above dates, make sure you can arrive the evening before."[11] "There is a casual dinner the evening before the interview," writes the Department of Orthopedic Surgery at the Baylor College of Medicine. "The dinner is a very important factor in the interview process."[12]

Did you know?

"The dinner and social hours that residency programs hold before interview day are a great way to learn more about the program and get a feel for the residents and faculty who may be interviewing you the next day. Even though this will be a more informal event, remember that your interactions during these pre-interview activities will be included in the program's discussion of you after you're gone...Also, some programs won't rank students who do not attend the social events as they see it as a sign that the student is not really interested."[14]

University of Washington Department of Family Medicine

Rule # 116 Be prepared for the unexpected.

In a survey of fourth-year students at one medical school, researchers were able to determine features of the social event that were disliked by applicants.[1] These included:

- Event at a resident's home
- Presence of only a single resident, and the awkwardness that results if you don't form a connection with the resident or if the resident doesn't talk much
- High applicant to resident ratio leading to competition among applicants
- Limited access to residents because of room/table structure
- Events lasting too long
- Disorganized events
- Residents arriving late
- Drunk residents keeping applicants out late
- Presence of faculty and concerns that their presence would inhibit residents from being completely open about their experiences
- Presence of residents' spouses or significant others

Tip # 76

Note the number of residents that come to these events. A large turnout may be a sign that residents are happy in the program, and enjoy interacting with one another even after a long day's work. Their presence may also indicate that they take their responsibility for resident recruitment seriously.

> **Did you know?**
>
> At these social events, you'll find that alcohol is frequently served. In the aforementioned survey, alcohol was available at 64% of the events. 92% percent of applicants did not report feeling any pressure to drink.[1]

Rule # 117 **Don't be afraid to ask about attire for the event. When in doubt, it's better to be overdressed.**

How should you dress for these events? Your decision should be guided by the invitation. Most programs indicate that these social events are casual. If that's the case, business casual attire is appropriate. If the program hasn't indicated appropriate dress for the event, you should ask.

Business Casual Attire for Social Events Hosted by Residency Programs	
	Recommended Attire
Men	Neatly pressed khaki or dark pants Neatly pressed long-sleeved buttoned shirt with conservative solid-colored or striped pattern. Tie usually not necessary Dark socks of appropriate length (mid-calf) Leather belt Leather shoes (no sandals or athletic shoes)
Women	Pants or skirts favoring solid colors (skirt length to at least knees while standing) Tailored shirt, blouse, or sweater (avoid tight or flowing) Leather or fabric shoes with color appropriate to dress (flat or low heels)

> **Did you know?**
>
> Not all social events are casual. In one survey of applicants, 14% reported attending formal dinners. In some cases, the events took place at a resident's or faculty member's home.[1]

Rule # 118 Your mother was right. Manners matter.

At conferences and meetings, we've heard multiple anecdotal stories of faux pas made by candidates at social events. Below we provide some recommendations. Some of these may seem obvious, but all have been reported at events.

- Your conversations with others at these events need not, and should not, be focused exclusively on the program. Ask the residents about themselves, and their interests.
- Your focus should be on the residents and fellow applicants. It's annoying when applicants frequently check their cell phone, take phone calls, or send texts during an events. Turn your cell phone off, and give your full attention to those in front of you.
- Have you ever received any feedback about how you look when you eat? Few people have, and therefore most have no idea of how they come across while eating. Are you the applicant who chews with his mouth open? Do you chew too loudly? Solicit feedback if needed.
- Please be polite to the wait staff. Use the words "Please" and "Thank you".
- Stay away from alcohol. If your host insists you have a drink, just take a sip here and there. Stories abound of inappropriate applicant behavior.
- Avoid messy foods like spaghetti. Avoid difficult-to-eat foods such as sandwiches, shellfish, or pizza. Stay away from foods that can easily get caught in your teeth or cause bad breath.
- Order something simple and light. Don't order the most expensive item on the menu.
- Don't be overly indecisive when you're ordering.
- Take small bites so you can quickly finish chewing if you're asked a question.
- Only reach for items that are in front of you. For items that you can't easily reach, ask someone to pass them to you.
- Don't start eating until everyone's meal has been served.
- Never complain about the food or send it back.
- The purpose of the meal is to get to know the program and for them to get to know you. Eating isn't the main goal.

Since some events are formal affairs, it's important to be aware of the norms of etiquette at such events. For more information, we refer you to the excellent post "Table manners for physicians" published on KevinMD in 2014.

References

[1]Schlitzkus L, Schenarts P, Schenarts K. It was the night before the interview: perceptions of resident applicants about the preinterview reception. *J Surg Educ* 2013; 70(6): 750-7.
[2]Atashroo D, Luan A, Vyas K, Zielins E, Maan Z, Duscher D, Walmsley G, Lynch M, Davenport D, Wan D, Longaker M, Vasconez H. What makes a plastic surgery residency program attractive? An applicant's perspective. *Plast Reconstr Surg* 2015; 136(1): 189-196.
[3]Huntington W, Haines N, Patt J. What factors influence applicants' rankings of orthopedic surgery residency programs in the National Resident Matching Program? *Clin Orthop Relat Res* 2014; 472 (9): 2859-66.
[4]University of Florida College of Medicine. Available at: http://osa.med.ufl.edu/first-year-orientation/faq/student-advice/. Accessed February 2, 2016.
[5]Results of the 2014 NRMP Program Director Survey. Available at: http://www.nrmp.org/wp-content/uploads/2014/09/PD-Survey-Report-2014.pdf. Accessed March 3, 2016.
[6]Department of Medicine at Eastern Virginia Medical School. Available at: https://www.evms.edu/education/centers_institutes_departments/internal_medicine/residencies/internal_medicine/application_process/. Accessed February 2, 2016.
[7]Surgical Society at the University of Colorado School of Medicine. Available at: http://www.ucdenver.edu/academics/colleges/medicalschool/education/studentaffairs/studentgroups/SurgicalSociety/Pages/FAQ.aspx. Accessed February 2, 2016.
[8]Lee A, Gonik K, Oetting T, Beaver H, Boldt H, Olson R, Greenlees E, Abramoff M, Johnson A, Carter K. Re-engineering the resident applicant selection process in ophthalmology: a literature review and recommendations for improvement. *Surv Ophthalmol* 2008; 53(2): 164-176.
[9]Department of Obstetrics and Gynecology at Oregon Health Sciences University. Available at: http://www.ohsu.edu/xd/education/schools/school-of-medicine/departments/clinical-departments/ob-gyn/educational-programs/obgyn-residency/application-information.cfm. Accessed February 2, 2016.
[10]Department of Orthopedic Surgery at Cleveland Clinic. Available at: http://my.clevelandclinic.org/services/orthopaedics-rheumatology/for-medical-professionals/orthopaedics/residencies. Accessed February 2, 2016.
[11]Duke University Department of Anesthesiology. Available at: http://anesthesiology.duke.edu/?page_id=818098. Accessed February 2, 2016.
[12]Department of Orthopedic Surgery at the Baylor College of Medicine. Available at: https://www.bcm.edu/departments/orthopedic-surgery/education/orthopedic-surgery-residency/admissions. Accessed February 2, 2016.
[13]University of Washington Department of Family Medicine. Available at: https://depts.washington.edu/fammed/education/advising/apply/interview-interview-day/. Accessed February 2, 2016.

Chapter 12

Scheduling Interviews

The process of scheduling interviews may seem straightforward. You receive an interview invite. You contact the program to schedule. In reality, the process is much more complicated. Year after year, students make mistakes in scheduling. Some are minor, some are major, but all have the potential to change the impression you make.

Rule # 119 Respond to the invitation as quickly as possible.

Reply promptly to interview invitations. Slots are filled quickly. We recommend that you respond to an invitation within hours of its receipt. Some candidates who've waited until the next day have found themselves on the waitlist.

Scheduling Interviews: What Do Residency Programs Recommend?	
Residency Program	**Recommendation**
Department of Surgery University of Missouri	"Please be sure to respond to an interview invitation as soon as possible to reserve a position as interview days fill up quickly."[1]
Department of Surgery Brown University	"We hold four interview dates throughout November, December, and January and these will be filled on a 'first come, first served' basis as e-mail responses to the invitations are received."[2]
Department of Medicine Louisville University	"Invitations to interview are sent from the program coordinator to applicants via email. A timely response in the affirmative reserves an interview slot for you. No response or a late response can mean losing an interview spot. A common courtesy is to reply in the negative if you have decided not to apply or interview with our program."[3]

Tip # 77

Respond to interview offers quickly, even if you're not sure of your level of interest in the program. Remember that you can always cancel the interview later.

Template For Accepting An Interview Invitation

Dear _____:

Thank you for inviting me to interview at [residency program]. I consider it an honor to be selected for an interview, and I look forward to visiting your program.

After looking over the list of possible interview dates, any of the following dates, if available, would be suitable for me:

November 14
November 18
November 23

Thank you once again.

Sincerely,

Rebecca Conley

After you've agreed on a date, you'll usually receive another e-mail from the program with further instructions, including when to arrive, where to stay, directions, and the day's events. Note the following:

- Place and time of the interview
- Directions
- Where to park
- Where to stay
- Whether you're required to bring any additional documents with you
- Whom you'll be meeting, including the names, titles, and pronunciation of all interviewers. Pay special attention to the positions of those whom you will be meeting.
- Interview itinerary (schedule of events)
- Type of interview (one-on-one versus panel, blinded versus open, number)

Tip # 78

Applicants often schedule their flight home or to another interview destination without taking into account the actual time that the interview day will end. Leaving early can inconvenience administrative staff, other applicants, and faculty, all of whom may have to rearrange their schedule. If you're going to interview at a program, then do so properly.

Rule # 120 **Be professional in all interactions with the program coordinator and other support staff.**

Prior to your interview, you'll have to contact the program's administrative staff. You may have a question or you may need to schedule your interview. Convey your utmost respect to the administrative staff, and convey your appreciation of their help. Don't be too demanding as you try to agree on a day and time for the interview visit.

Scheduling and coordinating interviews is a Herculean task for programs, and this responsibility falls largely upon the shoulders of the residency coordinator. The residency coordinator is responsible for:

- Scheduling interviews
- Identifying and scheduling faculty to conduct interviews
- Arranging tours
- Identifying resident hosts
- Preparing information packets for interviewees
- Responding to candidates seeking additional information about the program

"We interview about 170 to 200 people, so you get all those emails back, trying to get everybody scheduled in, so it's hundreds of emails and phone calls and stuff," says Amy Matenaer, anesthesiology medical education residency program coordinator at the Medical College of Wisconsin (MCW).[4]

Although the residency coordinator won't formally interview you, he or she will be forming judgments about you during every interaction, whether it occurs by phone or e-mail. These opinions may be freely shared with the program director.

Many applicants underestimate the power of the residency coordinator. At many programs, the coordinator is heavily involved in resident recruitment. "Many coordinators have some responsibility for initial screening," writes Dianna Otterstad, Education Coordinator in the Department of Radiology at the University of Texas Southwestern Medical Center.[5]

Tip # 79

When does your interview start? It starts with the first phone call you make to the residency program. When speaking with members of the administrative staff, remember to be courteous and appreciative of their help. Displaying good manners won't increase your chances of securing a position in the program. Poor manners, however, can sink your chances. Reports of a poor attitude will definitely be conveyed to the program director.

Tip # 80

Polite follow-up (and not too frequent!) with the program coordinator may help you obtain an interview or cluster interviews in the same geographic region on a single trip. "If you don't get interviews from schools that you are interested in, it doesn't hurt to contact the program coordinator/director and reiterate your interest in the program," writes the Department of Anesthesiology at the Ohio State University College of Medicine. "Many interviewees seem to have gotten interviews after calling/e-mailing (don't do this too early in the interview season)."[6]

Tip # 81

During the application process, programs become deluged with applicant e-mails and phone calls. There are typically some applicants every season who call or e-mail repeatedly to check on the status of their application. These applicants quickly become annoyances.

Rule # 121 **Consider your first interviews practice sessions. Save your most valued programs for later.**

If at all possible, avoid scheduling your first interviews with programs you highly covet. Your first interviews should be with programs that are lower on your list. The pressure won't be as intense, and you can ease into the process somewhat. You're likely to make mistakes early on, so get them out of the way here. With each successful interview, you'll gain confidence.

Tip # 82

If you have many interviews, consider placing interviews at your top choices somewhere in the middle. Don't save them for the end, because many applicants are tired of interviews by the end of the season.

Rule # 122 **In our opinion, interviewing early or late in the season does not have a significant impact on your ranking.**

Applicants often wonder if it's better to interview early or late in the season. There's never been a clear answer, and opinions vary. Those who favor interviewing late maintain the following:

- You may be better remembered and, therefore, more highly regarded.
- You'll have had lots of practice.

- Your application will be compared to the true applicant pool, since the rest of the pool has already interviewed. If your application is of higher quality when compared to the rest of the applicant pool, this could be of great benefit.
- Interviewers have a tendency to downgrade applicants who interview early because they haven't yet developed a good feel for the applicant pool.

Proponents of early interviewing maintain the following:

- You'll have more energy and enthusiasm, as will your interviewers. Neither one of you is likely to be tired of the interview process.
- Interviewing early is better because interviewers tend to choose as they go along. Some interviewers may have already made their decisions by the time the later season arrives.

For years, there was no data on this issue. In 2000, however, Martin-Lee published the results of a study involving 44 emergency medicine residency programs.[7] In this study, the date of an interview (early, middle, or late in the interview season) had no bearing on the ranking of candidates. In another study from the Department of Anesthesiology at New York University, the authors determined the interview dates for each of the applicants who matched at the program during a three-year period.[8] They found no significant association between the interview date and likelihood of matching. Since there's no evidence to suggest that interview timing has an effect on how a program ranks applicants, our recommendation is not to worry about it.

> **Tip # 83**
>
> When scheduling interviews, don't make any special requests such as asking for an interview on days the program does not interview. While the program may grant your request, it will require busy faculty to rearrange their schedules.

Rule # 123 Arrange for maximum flexibility during interview season.

Residency interviews are generally conducted from October through early February. The heaviest months are typically December and January. Some programs, particularly those that participate in an early match, may begin earlier.

While the policy on absences differs from school to school and from clerkship to clerkship, schools generally ask their fourth-year students to schedule interviews not during clerkship time. Students are asked to use vacation time, breaks, or off months. Students often take a month or two off during the interview season, especially if they're planning to interview around the country.

Despite your best efforts to schedule interviews that won't conflict with clinical work, you'll find that some programs offer little or no choice in scheduling. If so, you must contact the clerkship director for permission. Do so as early as possible. Be professional and courteous in your interactions with the clerkship director. Offer to make up any time, and be ready to provide documentation of the invitation. Once the clerkship director has granted an approved absence, inform all team members, including the attending physician, resident, and interns.

Tip # 84

Some rotations prohibit students from taking any absences at all. Plan to schedule flexible rotations that will allow you to be absent for interviews. Even with flexible rotations, though, time off is generally limited to a few days.

Tip # 85

Follow the absence policy at your school and clerkship. Failure to follow these guidelines may result in unfavorable clerkship evaluations.

Rule # 124 It's possible to reschedule an interview, but it very much depends on your approach.

Can you reschedule an interview? Most programs will try to work with you if you must. This does add work for the program coordinator, so be polite, and avoid making multiple requests at the same program. "We are happy to reschedule your interview date if need be," writes the Department of Internal Medicine at Georgetown University. "Please let our Coordinator know as soon as possible so as to have enough time to refill the spot with another applicant. We will do our very best to accommodate your request, but cannot make any guarantees."[9] The Department of Psychiatry at Washington University also tries to accommodate applicants. "It typically takes several weeks to create a schedule for a particular day. Thus, you should call us as soon as you know that you need to make a change so that you have the best chance to get the date you want and we have the needed time to create your schedule. Cancelling with less than a two-week notice, unless for an emergency, is considered unprofessional and prevents other applicants from visiting us. We have been encouraged to report such occurrences to ERAS."[10] Below is a template that can be used to reschedule interviews.

Template for Rescheduling An Interview

Dear _____:

My name is _______ (AAMC ID #). I am writing to inform you that, unfortunately, I must reschedule my interview with you scheduled for _______. This is due to an unexpected scheduling conflict, and I sincerely apologize for any inconvenience that this may cause you.

I do remain very much interested in your program, and I hope that I can reschedule this interview for another day. From your original communication with me, I understand that _____ and _____ are several of your other interview dates. If there happens to be space on one of these days, would it be possible for you to accommodate me? If not, I am open to other dates for rescheduling.

Would you be able to call or e-mail me to let me know? I very much look forward to meeting you, and interviewing at _____.

Sincerely,

Name

Rule # 125 Avoid scheduling interviews on consecutive days if at all possible.

Scheduling interviews on consecutive days is not recommended for two main reasons:

- Interview fatigue

The interview season can be a long one, which is why it's important to schedule your interviews at a reasonable pace. If you crowd too many interviews into a short period of time, you'll become fatigued and stressed. This may affect your interview performance. One of the keys to successful interviewing is to interview when you're well-rested. You're more apt to come across as attentive, enthusiastic, and relaxed, which are precisely some of the personal qualities that residency programs seek.

- Delays associated with travel

Time between interviews also allows for the challenges of travel, as Dr. Mary Brandt, Senior Associate Dean for Student Affairs at the Baylor College of Medicine, indicates below:

Residency interviews happen during the winter months. If you are flying through or to the northern states, there is a real risk of flights being delayed or cancelled. Don't book tight connections and last minute arrivals. Many programs have a social event the night before the actual interview day. This is really important to attend...In order to make sure you arrive in time, try to book flights early in the day. If there are weather delays, you will usually still have some options that let you get there in time. If you make the early flight and arrive early – enjoy a new city that might be your home for the next 3-7 years! Find a good museum, have a great lunch, go for a walk in a local park.[11]

Tip # 86

Try to arrange interviews in a specific geographic region during a single trip. While this won't always be possible, it will save you time, energy, and money. As you're planning the trip, if you haven't heard from a program in the same region, then consider contacting them. Let the program know of your upcoming trip. This may spur the program to review your application and offer an interview invite.

Did you know?

In a survey of 2006 urology match applicants, respondents reported a median of 12 interviews, with total costs at a median level of $4,000. The median expense per interview was $330, with travel expenses and lodging accounting for 60% and 25% of total costs, respectively.[12]

Rule # 126 Consider the ramifications of any special requests.

Avoid making special requests if at all possible, with few exceptions. "What bothers me is when candidates ask if they can have their own interview date because our dates do not work with their schedule," writes one residency program coordinator.[13]

How Do Residency Programs View Special Requests Made by Interviewees?

Residency Program	Recommendation
Department of Surgery Virginia Commonwealth University	"Occasionally, we receive requests to schedule private interviews. Since all faculty in the Department of Surgery play a role in forming the rank list, it is an advantage to the applicant to attend one of the three scheduled interview dates. Therefore, we do not arrange interviews on days outside of our scheduled dates."[14]
Department of Surgery University of North Dakota	"All sessions of the interview process are considered to be important in assessing and evaluating applicants as well as giving each applicant the appropriate exposure to the UND Surgical Residency Program. Therefore, applicants that cannot attend all portions of the interview process will not be considered for NRMP ranking."[15]

Department of Anesthesiology University of California San Diego	"Much preparation goes into our Wednesday 'interview day,' and although we can make exceptions, we believe that both the applicants and the committee members are best served if we meet one another on the regularly scheduled day."[16]

Although special requests should be avoided, there are some situations in which such requests are reasonable. Is there a particular faculty member at the program you would like to meet? If so, contact the program well in advance of the interview to see if they can consider your request. As you can see, many programs are receptive to such requests:

- "If you are invited to interview and have an interest in a certain subspecialty (i.e., Hem/Onc, Cardiology, Gastroenterology, Rheumatology, etc.), please let us know when you call to set up your interview, and every effort will be made to have you meet a faculty member in that subspecialty," writes the Department of Medicine at Dartmouth Geisel School of Medicine."[17]

- "If you have a particular research interest, please advise Leslie Fowler of this and she can arrange an interview with clinical or basic science faculty that share this same interest," writes the Department of Anesthesia at the Medical University of South Carolina.[18]

- "Some candidates take advantage of the extra time to meet with additional faculty members of their choosing or residents with a particular background or characteristics that would make their perspective valuable to the applicant" writes the Department of Anesthesiology and Critical Care Medicine at the Johns Hopkins University.[19]

Rule # 127 An update with new information may help you secure an interview.

If you haven't heard from a program, or have been placed on the waitlist, you may update the program with new information. Have you won an award? Did you present at a national conference? Was a paper that you submitted for publication accepted or published? This is the type of information that may lead the program to extend an interview offer.

Did you know?

You can update a program with new information by sending an e-mail to both the program director and coordinator. You should also update your status in ERAS, save the updated profile, and then transmit it to all programs on your list.

> **Did you know?**
>
> Last-minute cancellations are common. You may be more likely to be considered for these vacated spots if you let the program coordinator know that your schedule allows you to travel even with just a few days' notice.

Rule # 128 Always confirm.

Approximately one to two weeks prior to your interview, call or e-mail the residency coordinator to confirm your scheduled interview. Confirming each interview can help avoid this scenario, as described by one applicant:

At a few places, the coordinator did not communicate a change in the schedules for the interview day that was sent prior to the visit. This was particularly distressing for applicants who had made travel plans based on the original itinerary."[20]

> **Tip # 87**
>
> Don't just ask directions to the program's physical address. You also need directions to guide you to the department's office once you reach the hospital or medical center. Applicants have been late because they've gotten lost in the hospital.

Rule # 129 If you must cancel an interview, do it the right way.

Cancelling an interview can be an uncomfortable process. Applicants worry about offending a program. They're also unsure of the proper way to cancel. Delaying the process, though, can be harmful to both parties.

Cancellations are common. In a survey of AOA students at the University of Washington, 93% reported cancelling at least one interview. Among the reasons cited were finances, sufficient number of interviews at more desirable programs, geographical location unsuitable for student or partner, scheduling conflict, and interview fatigue.[21] If you must cancel, do so in a professional manner. Our recommendations:

- Programs expect that some applicants will cancel interviews, and they don't hold it against you if you must cancel.
- If you must cancel, do it as early as possible so the program can fill your vacated spot. If possible, provide at least 2 weeks' notice (the more time you give the better). If you have this much time, it's not necessary to provide a reason for cancellation.
- Don't cancel an interview at the last moment (barring any emergency). If you have to, present a compelling reason.

- We recommend calling the program coordinator to cancel the interview, and leaving a cancellation message if the coordinator is unavailable. This communication should be followed by an e-mail.
- An e-mail should also be sent to the program director. Indicate that you must cancel the interview, but always express appreciation for the interview offer.
- Don't consider the matter closed until you receive confirmation from the program that they've received your message. Save all correspondence.

Did you know?

"A cancellation with less than a week's notice requires a minor miracle for someone on the wait list to a) still be available and b) able to arrange transportation to get here. A program in a larger city probably doesn't have that issue to the extent we do. My personal pet peeve is getting a short-notice cancellation that ends in platitudes about hoping that you aren't causing too much inconvenience and/or hoping someone else can fill the spot."[13]

Residency Program Coordinator (Student Doctor Network)

Did you know?

If you must cancel your interview, do it the right way. Above all, never be a no-show. While this seems obvious, every year programs have no-shows. These individuals are remembered for years, and this could hurt you in the future when you apply for fellowships or jobs. Program directors have been known to communicate with each other about poor behavior. In some cases, the applicant's medical school has been notified.

Template For Cancelling An Interview (> 2 weeks' notice)

Dear _____:

My name is _______ (AAMC ID #). I am scheduled to have an interview with you on ________. I am writing to inform you that, unfortunately, I must cancel my interview.

I sincerely apologize for any inconvenience that this may cause you. Please also convey my sincerest apologies to [Program Director].

I would like to thank you again for considering my application and inviting me for an interview.

Sincerely,

Name

References

[1]University of Missouri Department of Surgery. Available at: http://medicine.missouri.edu/surgery/general-res-apply.html. Accessed February 2, 2016.
[2]Brown University Department of Surgery. Available at: https://www.brown.edu/academics/medical/about/departments/surgery/application. Accessed February 2, 2016.
[3]Louisville University Department of Medicine. Available at: http://louisville.edu/medicine/departments/medicine/divisions/internalmedicine/residency/application. Accessed February 2, 2015.
[4]HealthLeaders Media. Available at: http://healthleadersmedia.com/page-1/TEC-320006/Medical-Residency-Interview-Scheduling-Automated. Accessed December 18, 2015.
[5]Otterstad D. The role of the residency coordinator. *Acad Radiol* 2003; 10(Suppl 1): S48-53.
[6]Ohio State University Department of Anesthesiology. Available at: http://anesthesiology.osu.edu/11429.cfm. Accessed December 18, 2015.
[7]Martin-Lee L, Park H, Overton D. Does interview date affect match list position in the emergency medicine national residency matching program match? *Acad Emerg Med* 2000; 7(9): 1022-1026.
[8]Wajda M, O'Neill D, Tepfenhardt L, Yook I, Kim J. Timing of applicants residency interview cannot predict if they will match your residency program. *Anesthesiology* 2006; 105: A167.
[9]Georgetown University Department of Medicine. Available at: https://medicine.georgetown.edu/residency/application/faqs. Accessed January 14, 2016.
[10]Washington University Department of Psychiatry. Available at: http://www.psychiatry.wustl.edu/Education/FAQ#Q3. Accessed March 3, 2016.
[11]Residency Interviews Part 2: The Flights. Available at: http://wellnessrounds.org/2012/09/28/residency-interviews-part-2-the-flights/. Accessed February 2, 2016.
[12]Kerfoot B, Asher K, McCullough D. Financial and educational costs of the residency interview process for urology applicants. *Urology* 2008; epub 990-994.
[13]Student Doctor Network. Available at: http://forums.studentdoctor.net/threads/ask-the-program-coordinator.1107601/page-3. Accessed February 2, 2016.
[14]Department of Surgery at Virginia Commonwealth University. Available at: http://www.surgery.vcu.edu/education/residency/gensurg/selection.html. Accessed February 2, 2016.
[15]Department of Surgery at University of North Dakota. Available at: http://www.med.und.edu/residency-programs/surgery/application-process.cfm. Accessed February 2, 2016.
[16]Department of Anesthesiology at University of California San Diego. Available at: http://anesthesia.ucsd.edu/education/residency-program/application/pages/default.aspx. Accessed February 2, 2016.

[17]Department of Medicine at Dartmouth Geisel School of Medicine. Available at: http://gme.dartmouth-hitchcock.org/im/about_interview_day.html. Accessed February 2, 2016.
[18]Department of Anesthesia at Medical University of South Carolina. Available at: http://clinicaldepartments.musc.edu/anesthesia/education/residency/residentinterviews.htm. Accessed February 2, 2016.
[19]Department of Anesthesiology at Johns Hopkins University. Available at: http://www.hopkinsmedicine.org/anesthesiology/Residency/apply/interview_day.shtml. Accessed February 2, 2016.
[20]Nawotniak R, Gray E. General surgery resident applicants perception of program coordinators. *Curr Surg* 2006; 63(6): 473-475.
[21]University of Washington School of Medicine AOA Chapter. Available at: http://www.uwmedicine.org/education/md-program/current-students/student-affairs/groups/alpha-omega-alpha. Accessed November 2, 2015.

Chapter 13

Before the Interview

An invitation to interview is a significant honor. During the screening process, the program has worked hard to whittle down a large applicant pool into an elite group. Contrary to common belief, the purpose of the interview is *not* to determine if you have the qualifications needed to be a resident at their institution. By granting you an interview, the program has already made that determination. Rather, the purpose of the interview is to assess fit. Are you the right fit for the program? Is the program the right fit for you?

Fortunately, or unfortunately, your work has just increased exponentially. Although the CV, personal statement, letters of recommendation, and other aspects of the application are all of great importance, there's no disputing the fact that the interview is possibly the most critical step of the residency application process. While the other elements of the application will help you get an interview, your interview performance will strongly influence your ranking. Surveys of program directors have shown that success in the interview is critical towards securing a position in the program.

Unfortunately, many otherwise qualified applicants lose any chance of matching into the program of their choice because of a poor interview. In a study of internal medicine residency applicants, 1/3 of the applicants were ranked less favorably following an interview.[1] In a study of EM programs, with data obtained from 3,800 individual interviews, a total of 14% of interviews resulted in unranked applicants.[2] The conclusion here is that the interview has the potential to destroy your chances. Preparation is critical.

A successful interview is one that moves you higher on the program's rank list, and to a position where you're likely to match. Successful interviewing requires a considerable amount of preparation. You need to know what to research before the interview, what to wear, what to say, how to conduct yourself, and what to do after the interview. In this chapter, we outline the steps to ensure that every one of your interviews will be a success.

Rule # 130 The interview is a critical factor in ranking applicants.

Over the years, many surveys of PDs have inquired about the importance of the interview in the selection process. These surveys have consistently found the interview to be a major factor used to rank applicants. In fact, the results of multiple studies indicate that the interview is *the most* valuable factor used in the ranking of applicants. In the 2014 NRMP Program Directors Survey, 93% of residency programs in 22 specialties cited "interactions with faculty during interview and visit" as a factor in ranking applicants. Programs rated this factor 4.8 in importance on a scale from 1 (not at all important) to 5 (very important).[3] The following table highlights the importance of the interview relative to other selection criteria. As you can see, the top 3 criteria used in ranking all have to do with the residency interview.

Top Criteria Used By Residency Programs To Rank Applicants

Criteria	% Programs Citing Factor	Mean Importance Rating
Interactions with faculty during interview and visit	93%	4.8
Interpersonal skills	93%	4.8
Interactions with house staff during interview and visit	88%	4.7
Feedback from current residents	82%	4.6
USMLE Step 1 / COMLEX Level 1 score	80%	4.1
Letter of recommendation	74%	4.1
USMLE Step 2 CK / COMLEX Level 2 CE score	71%	4.1

*Survey participants were asked to rank each item on a scale of 1 (not at all important) to 5 (very important).

Adapted from Results of the 2014 NRMP Program Director Survey. Available at: http://www.nrmp.org/wp-content/uploads/2014/09/PD-Survey-Report-2014.pdf.

Applicants are often surprised to learn about the importance that programs attach to the interview. However, several studies have shown poor correlation between academic performance during medical school and later performance during residency training. In one study of radiology residents, while honors or A grades in clinical rotations (medicine, surgery, pediatrics) and high USMLE scores were predictive of performance on the American Board of Radiology exam, they were not predictive of clinical performance as a resident.[4] In a study of obstetrics and gynecology residents, Bell found similar results.[5] USMLE scores did not correlate with faculty evaluations of resident performance.

Therefore, programs can't rely solely on objective data such as class rank and USMLE scores to make resident selection decisions. Behavioral and noncognitive skills have significant value in predicting resident performance, and programs recognize this fact. However, they're limited in how they can assess these skills, and therefore the interview takes on greater importance. The interview becomes the chief means by which programs can evaluate these noncognitive skills.

Did you know?

In a survey of junior medical students and PDs at the Medical College of Wisconsin, researchers sought to learn the importance of different residency selection criteria. PDs seemed to place more emphasis on personal characteristics, whereas knowledge and skills were rated most important by students.[6] Swanson wrote that "social skills and the level of development of professional behavior are more important than the sophistication of clinical skills and knowledge gained in medical school."[7]

The interview is never just a formality. It can absolutely make or break your chances of matching. In support of this is a study performed by Gong and colleagues, who determined the importance of the interview on the ranking of internal medicine residency applicants.[1] They found that following an interview:

- 1/3 of applicants were ranked more favorably
- 1/3 of applicants were ranked less favorably
- 1/3 of applicants had no change in their ranking

Another study found that "final student rankings correlated well with interview scores and poorly with initial applicant scores based solely on pre-interview information."[8]

> **Did you know?**
>
> A poor interview can destroy your chances. In a survey of emergency medicine programs, data was obtained from 3,800 individual interviews taking place at 44 programs.[2] It was learned that 14% of these interviews resulted in unranked applicants. In another survey of general surgery programs, 19% of interviewed applicants were not placed on the rank-order list.[9]

Rule # 131 What are the goals of the interviewer? A successful interview involves understanding these goals and responding to them.

In order to interview successfully, you need to understand the goals of the interviewer. The primary goal is to determine if you would be an outstanding resident at their program. An AOA applicant with a 250 USMLE score does not equate to an outstanding radiology resident. Interview questions are asked to learn more about noncognitive factors, including your communication skills, your interpersonal skills, your strengths, and your drive. Interview questions are also asked to determine "fit" with the program. Depending on the goals of the particular program, interview questions may also seek to determine your commitment to community service, your interest in translational research, or your commitment to career in academic medicine.

> **Did you know?**
>
> In describing the results of a survey of EM PDs, Crane wrote that "much concrete and personal information about the applicant's interactive skills and mannerisms can be obtained from the interview. Similarly, the interview provides the opportunity to obtain more information or clarify deficiencies in the interviewee's application. Some interviewers also use this time to test the interviewee's composure, asking a nontraditional question, or offering a simple clinical scenario. Finally, the interview affords the applicant the opportunity to express items not specifically mentioned in the application, including hobbies, interests, volunteer activities, and previous exposure to the medical field."[10]

> **Did you know?**
>
> Contrary to common belief, the purpose of the interview is not to determine if you have the qualifications needed to be a resident. By granting you an interview, the program has already made that determination. The purpose of the interview is to assess fit. Is the program the right fit for you? Are you the right fit for the program? In a survey of radiology PDs, 15 directors stated that the "fit" of the candidates in the program and a "gut feeling" were the most important criteria for deciding admission.[11] In another survey, PDs wrote that they sought to find applicants who were "people like us."[12]

An interviewer can't learn about your interpersonal skills from your application alone. He can't find out what drives or motivates you. He can't discover how well you handle pressure. Do you have the qualities that make someone a valued team member? Will you fit in and work well with others in the department? The only way an interviewer can learn any of these things is by speaking with you and asking questions. While the personal statement and letters of recommendation provide some information, the interview is the chief means by which programs can directly assess these noncognitive factors.

> **Did you know?**
>
> Having the cognitive skills needed to succeed during residency is important, but is not enough. PDs also want residents who are socially competent. Social competence is defined as "someone who knows how to manage his/her emotions and responds to others' emotions in a mature manner."[13] Socially competent individuals are said to be emotionally intelligent. Emotional intelligence has been widely researched in business, but less so in medicine. Since many of the skills required for success in the workplace are also the skills needed for success as a resident, many have hypothesized that emotional intelligence would correlate with residency performance. In one study looking at the relationship between patient satisfaction and physicians' emotional intelligence, a relationship, albeit limited, was found.[14] Future studies will likely shed additional light on this issue.

In a survey of PM&R PDs, DeLisa and colleagues found that compatibility with the program was one of the three most important candidate traits, along with the ability to articulate thoughts and work with others.[15]

Programs are also interested in assessing an applicant's communication skills. The interview is considered a reliable way to assess this skill.[12]

In a survey of PDs of American Osteopathic Association-approved primary care graduate training programs, the authors determined the relative importance of academic and nonacademic variables related to resident selection. Work habits were rated highest, followed by the ability to work with others and maturity.[16] The following table lists personal qualities that are valued by residency programs, and therefore are important qualities to convey during an interview.

Personal Qualities You Should Aim To Convey During An Interview		
Ability to work with a team	Professional competence	Responsibility
Ability to solve problems	Willingness to admit error	Poise
Ability to manage stress	Perseverance	Positive attitude
Enthusiasm	Initiative	Reliability
Energy	Intelligence	Honesty
Flexibility	Maturity	Dedication
Effective time management	Motivation	Compassion
Efficient problem-solving	Communication skills	Curiosity
Confidence without arrogance	Conscientiousness	Determination
Recognition of limits	Work ethic	

Did you know?

Dr. John Eck, Associate Residency Program Director in the Department of Anesthesiology at Duke University, believes that the interview is a means for the program to assess fit of the applicant, "weed out applicants who are a poor fit," and determine if the applicant is someone the program staff and residents would like to work with.[17]

Rule # 132 Research the program in advance. Always.

As interviewers, we continue to be amazed by how many applicants come to interviews unprepared, having done little research about the program or the faculty. Consider the following exchange between interviewer and applicant at the Baylor College of Medicine:

> "Welcome to Baylor. How has your visit with us been?"
>
> "Great. The Texas Medical Center is so amazing. I had always heard that, but you don't really get an idea of its size until you see it firsthand. I think it's great that Baylor residents have the chance to rotate through such well-regarded hospitals. When do residents rotate through MD Anderson?"
>
> "Our residents don't spend any time at MD Anderson since it's affiliated with the University of Texas-Houston Medical School."
>
> "Oh, that's right. Do residents do research?"
>
> "Yes, our residents are required to pursue a scholarly project."

This was an actual exchange that I had with an applicant soon after joining the Department of Medicine as a faculty member. Although we now have an affiliation with the MD Anderson Cancer Center, at the time of the interview, our residents were not rotating through the institution. Not only did this applicant reveal his lack of knowledge about affiliated institutions, he also asked a very basic question about research which was clearly addressed in the program website. By choosing this particular question, he came across as uninformed.

Another example:

> "What are you looking for in a residency program?" asked Dr. Smart.
>
> "I loved spending time in the operating room during my general surgery rotation, so I'm looking for a program that will allow me a great deal of time in the OR right from the get-go," replied Gwyn.
>
> "You do realize, though, that our surgical interns are required to spend most of their time on the floors and in the clinics taking care of patients on the surgical service. We believe that it's important, early on, for interns to be comfortable evaluating patients preoperatively and managing their care postoperatively. Then, in the second year, we have our residents scrub in on cases…"

Prior to your visit, familiarize yourself with all information received from the residency program. Become familiar with both the institution and program, so that you can get the most out of your visit. Gathering information about the program before, during, and after your visit will help you make an informed decision when ranking.

Ask thoughtful and specific questions, the type that demonstrate your interest in the training program. This is one of the easiest ways to create a favorable impression. Utilize the following sources of information when researching the program:

- Printed materials sent from the program
- Fellowship and Residency Interactive Database (FREIDA)
- Websites for the program and its affiliated hospitals
- Other residency applicants
- Residents and faculty from your own institution who have trained at the institution where you will be interviewing
- Graduates of your medical school who are currently training at the program you will be visiting
- PD, chairman, and faculty advisors at your own medical school's residency program
- Internet search using the name of the program and its affiliated hospitals

- Internet and literature search (www.pubmed.com) to learn about the faculty's recent publications.

Utilize these sources to learn about the program's history, mission, philosophy, focus, areas of excellence, and key faculty. Programs and departments often post their latest news on their website. Print key information to read and reread before the interview.

Tip # 88

Have you researched the program before your visit? If not, you're doing yourself a great disservice. Without proper research, you won't be able to ask thoughtful and insightful questions. These are the questions that impress interviewers.

Tip # 89

In addition to knowing basic information, try to obtain information about the financial health and other aspects of the program. Studies of program closure have found that financial woes are the major reason for closure.[18]

Did you know?

Interviewers consider applicants who fail to do research about their program as showing a lack of serious interest in the program. It also calls into question your ability to prepare appropriately for an important task.

Reading information about the program may also enlighten you about the type of house officer the program seeks. This is essential information that you can use to demonstrate to the program that you are precisely that type of person. For example, at the website for the obstetrics and gynecology residency program at the Maricopa Integrated Health System, "factors important in the resident selection process include the following:

- Academic qualifications
- Interpersonal and communication skills
- Dependability, responsibility, maturity, courtesy, confidence
- Leadership skills
- Dedication to women's health
- Sense of humor and work ethic"[19]

An applicant to this program would be best served by highlighting her skills and qualities in these areas. In doing so, she would be seen as a "good fit" for the program.

Rule # 133 Learn about the faculty who will be interviewing you.

Try to learn your interviewers' names prior to your visit. If any have names that are difficult to pronounce, master the correct pronunciation. With names in hand, you can start your research. Who are these individuals? Are they purely clinicians, researchers, or both? What are their areas of interest? Do their interests overlap in any way with yours? For example, have you referenced their work in one of your projects? Where did they train?

It takes time and effort to perform this research, but it's well worth it. Advance knowledge of your interviewers may help you feel more comfortable. You may establish a connection. For example, if you learn that you and your interviewer are graduates of the same university, you might mention this during the interview. This may establish an immediate connection, as long as you don't overdo it. The key is to use this approach with tact.

Tip # 90

Learn all that you can about the interviewers by exploring the program's website. Websites often have faculty bios. Read about their areas of interest and background. Perform an internet and literature search (www.pubmed.com) using the interviewer's name. Look for anything you might share in common (e.g., attended the same university, research interests, etc.).

Tip # 91

Faculty from your home institution may know your interviewers. They may be able to fill you in on some background information.

Rule # 134 Prepare for the standard questions.

It's the fear of many applicants: Will the interview be a grueling grill session in which the interviewer asks questions to gauge the applicant's knowledge base? Highly unlikely. Grill session interviewing is a thing of the past. Interviews today are mainly an exchange of information, usually starting off with the interviewer asking some basic questions. Questions to assess your medical competence are rare, and most questions are asked in an effort to learn more about you as individual. The interviewer is trying to ascertain your personal qualities to determine how you will function as a resident.

Tip # 92

If asked a yes-or-no question, always elaborate. This is especially true of questions such as "Do you have research interests?" or "Do you plan to pursue fellowship training?"

Tip # 93

Applicants are often asked "Why did you choose to apply to our program?" Too often, applicants first mention their attraction to the city, weather, or family in the area, rather than using the question as an opportunity to discuss appealing aspects of the program. A far better answer would focus on factors such as the program's unique training opportunities, areas of research emphasis, and other program attributes.

In most cases, you should be able to predict the questions and prepare for them accordingly. If you think you can wing it, you're mistaken. To be at your best, you should anticipate the questions and think about your responses. Begin by jotting down the key points you would like to convey for each question. Then rehearse your answers. In rehearing your responses, your goal isn't to deliver a canned response, but rather to ensure that your responses convey the correct message. Some applicants choose to memorize their answers, which we don't recommend. Your responses will sound canned, and if you forget a point, you can easily become flustered.

Possible Questions From Faculty Interviewers

Tell me about yourself.

Why are you going into this specialty?

What have you done to inform yourself about a career in this specialty?

What do you see as the positive features of this specialty?

What do you see as the negative features of this specialty?

What problems do you think the specialty faces?

What are your future plans?

What are your practice plans after finishing residency?

Do you have plans to pursue fellowship training?

Do you have any research experience?

Do you have any interest in research?

Tell me about your research.

Where do you see yourself 10 years from now?

What do you consider to be important in a training program?

What are you avoiding in a training program?

What are you looking for in a program?

What is your ideal program?

Why have you applied to this residency program?

What is your perception of the strengths of this program?

What is your perception of the weaknesses of this program?

What qualifications do you have that set you apart from other applicants?
Why should we choose you over the other highly qualified applicants?
How would you contribute to our residency?
Tell me three things that would make you especially valuable to our residency.
Where else have you interviewed?
How have you done in medical school?
What is the best experience you had in medical school?
What is the worst experience you had in medical school?
What were the major deficiencies in your medical school training?
What rotation gave you the most difficulty and why?
What was your most difficult situation in medical school?
Are you prepared for the rigors of residency?
What was the most interesting case you were involved in?
What are your strengths?
What are your weaknesses?
How would your friends describe you?
Have you always done the best work which you're capable of?
Of which accomplishments are you most proud?
How do you deal with conflict?
Whom do you depend on for support?
What do you do with your free time?
What are your interests and hobbies?
With what kinds of people do you have difficulties working?
With what types of patients do you have trouble dealing?
What was your most memorable patient encounter?
What other programs have you applied to?
Can you explain your grades/board scores/leave of absence?
What if you don't match?
Why have you chosen to interview in this part of the country?
Are you applying to any other specialty?
What do you think about what is happening …? (current event question)
How do you see the delivery of health care evolving?
What was the last book you read?
In your CV, there is a gap of one year. What did you do during this time?
Why are your USMLE scores so low?
Do you have any questions for us?
Can you think of anything else you would like to add?

Possible Questions for IMG Applicants from Faculty Interviewers

I see that you are an IMG. Why did you leave your country?

As an IMG, you are familiar with the health care delivery system in your country. How does this system differ from the one here in the United States?

I see that you are IMG. What you have you done to familiarize yourself with medicine as it is practiced in the United States?

Do you have an ECFMG certificate? What ECFMG requirements remain for you to complete?

I see that you are an IMG. How would you rate your oral communication skills? How would you rate your written communication skills?

I see that you are an IMG. How well do you see yourself adapting to the American health system?

Rule # 135 Prepare for both the traditional and behavioral interview.

The most common interview format is the traditional one-on-one interview. Typically, the interviewer will ask questions about your education, activities, and goals. Examples include:

- Tell me about yourself.
- What are your strengths and weaknesses?
- Why are you interested in our residency program?

Note that these are broadly based questions, as are the questions listed previously in Rule # 134. Contrast these with the following questions:

- Tell me about a time when you had to deal with a difficult attending physician.
- Tell me about a time when you showed initiative.
- Describe a situation in which you had to deal with an upset patient.

These more specific questions, which ask for an example, are features of behavioral interviews. By learning how an applicant handled or reacted to the situation in the past, the interviewer may determine how he might handle the situation in the future. Behavioral interviewing is based on the premise that future behavior is best predicted by past behavior.

The behavioral interview was introduced and developed by Dr. Tom Janz, an industrial psychologist. Research looking at its validity and accuracy has shown that behavioral interviewing is more accurate than traditional interviewing in predicting success.[20-21] While more popular in the business community, residency programs may also conduct behavioral interviews. Since each question calls for a specific example, those who do best are those who have prepared in advance by recalling specific past experiences and scenarios.

In answering these questions, begin by describing what happened, what you then did, what was the result of your actions, and what you learned from the experience. Use the acronym STAR to help you answer these questions:

S – Situation (Describe the situation in detail.)

T – Task (What was the task or obstacle?)

A – Action (What action did you take?)

R – Result (What was the result?)

Below is an example of an effective response to a behavioral interview question.

Question: Tell me about a time when you made a mistake and had to admit it to your resident or attending.

Answer: I remember a time when I was a junior medical student on the Medicine Wards. My resident asked me to perform an ECG on a 70-year old woman. After completing the ECG, I pulled an old tracing from the patient's chart for comparison. I was shocked to see some significant changes, and my concern for possible MI grew. As I was comparing the tracings, my attending arrived on the unit. I expressed my concern to him, and he asked to see the tracings. He sat down and began his analysis. That's when I realized that one of the ECGs belonged to another patient, and that's why they looked so different. I was mortified to make this error, and quickly informed the attending. I told my attending how thankful I was that my error didn't harm the patient. I also realized how easy it was to make such a mistake. We discussed why such errors occur, and what I needed to do differently. My attending was very understanding, and even shared with me some similar stories from his training. I was very appreciative of his overall approach. From that point forward, I began checking the name first on all tests. Sure enough, there have been other instances where I could have made similar mistakes had it not been for my vigilance. What I learned from this experience is the importance of disclosing your errors, the way in which such discussions should take place, and the process by which you can prevent such errors from happening again.

A list of behavioral questions can be found in the table on the next page.

Examples of Behavioral Questions

Tell me about a time when you worked effectively under a great deal of pressure.

Tell me about a particularly stressful situation you encountered in medical school and how you handled it.

Tell me about a time when you made a mistake and had to admit it to your resident or attending.

How would you deal with a fellow resident who is not doing his share of the work?

Tell me about a negative interaction you had with an attending or resident. How did the two of you deal with it?

Tell me about a time when you were really upset by the words or actions of an attending or resident.

Tell me about a patient from whom you learned something. How will this experience help you as a physician?

Describe a relationship with a patient that had a significant effect on you.

Tell me about a time when you had a personality conflict with another team member. How did you deal with it?

Your attending physician asks you a question and you are not sure of the answer. What do you say or do?

Your colleague is abusing alcohol or drugs. How would you handle this situation?

Tell me about a time when you were disappointed in your performance.

Tell me about a time when you disagreed with how an ethical situation was being handled.

Tell me about a situation in which you overcame adversity.

Describe a clinical situation you handled well.

Tell me about a clinical situation that didn't go as well as you would have liked.

Give me an example of a time when you had a difficult communication problem.

Tell me about a time you had to build a relationship with someone you didn't like.

Tell me about a problem you had with a classmate, faculty member or patient. How did you handle it?

Tell me about a time when you handled a stressful situation poorly.

Tell me about a time when you became really angry over a situation at work.

Discuss a particularly meaningful experience in your medical training.

Discuss a particularly difficult experience in your medical training.

Describe to me a situation in which you had to break someone's confidence.

Was there a time during rotations in which you didn't feel like part of the team? How did you handle the situation?

Tell me about a time when you witnessed unprofessional or unethical behavior on the part of a resident or attending. How did you handle it?

Tell me about the major challenges you have faced in your medical school career.

Tell me about a time you were able to successfully work with another person even when that person may not have personally liked you.

Tell me about a time when you were able to successfully work with another person even when you did not personally like that person.

Tell me about a time during rotations in which you went above and beyond.

Describe to me a time when you received an evaluation with which you disagreed.

Your senior resident insists on a treatment plan you feel may harm the patient. What do you do?

Avoid These Errors When Answering Behavioral Questions

- These questions call for an actual example, and it's important that you provide just that. Don't provide vague answers that include generalizations without any reference to a specific situation.
- Some applicants respond with theoretical answers. Your answer is theoretical if you are describing what you would do in that situation. Remember that the question is asking what you did do.
- Note that some questions require you to discuss potentially negative situations. Use tact and sensitivity when describing these situations and the individuals involved. It can be very easy to criticize others. Quite often such answers detract from the strength of your response.
- If you're unable to come up with an example, do the best that you can. If an example pops into your mind later during the interview, you can always come back to the question. When the interviewer asks, "Do you have any questions for me?" you can say, "Before I ask you a few questions, do you mind if I elaborate on one of my earlier answers?"

Rule # 136 Remember that you do have a fair amount of control over the interview.

Most applicants feel that in an interview, all of the power is in the hands of the interviewer. This assumption is wrong. The interview is essentially an exchange of information during which two parties are learning more about one another. As long as you remain an active participant during the interview, you'll have a fair amount of control over the direction of the interview.

As the interviewee, you control the content of the discussion. You control the message that is conveyed. Because of this fact, you should enter the interview knowing full well the items that you wish to convey about yourself. Only with this knowledge, and some degree of assertiveness, will you be able to sell yourself effectively.

Interviewer: "What have you enjoyed most about your medical school education?"

Applicant: "Spending time with my patients and educating them about their illness has been most enjoyable for me. I really enjoy teaching. I've also had the chance to tutor freshman and sophomore students in the basic sciences. During clinical rotations as a senior student, I've had opportunities to mentor and teach junior students. These experiences have been very rewarding and I would like to make teaching a major part of what I do as a physician. I know that, in your program, residents have tremendous opportunities to teach. I'm particularly excited about the workshops your program offers to help residents improve their teaching skills. After interviewing at a number of programs, I must tell you that your program is unique."

This question asked what the *applicant* enjoyed most about their medical school education. Instead of only focusing on the education, as some applicants might have done - "Our medical school was great" - this applicant was able to also effectively convey a message about her own strengths and abilities, and how these fit well with the program's strengths.

Tip # 94

In the article, "The Residency Interview," available at the Society of Academic Emergency Medicine website, Dr. Jamie Collings, former program director of the emergency medicine residency program at Northwestern University, emphasized the importance of having a Top 5 Plan for every interview. This plan would consist of five key things that you want a program to know about you. In an interview with Dr. Collings, we asked her how applicants can decide which things would be of most interest to interviewers:[22]

Again, this goes back to remembering that this is a job interview. Think about the qualities that make a successful resident and emergency physician and try to highlight those when you interview. You would be amazed at how many students focus entirely on figuring out if a program is right for them and forget that there is a clear element of "selling yourself" that is needed.

Rule # 137 Everything in your application is fair game for the interviewer. Revisit each experience in detail.

Remember that everything on your application is fair game. Because some applicants have been known to exaggerate their involvement in activities and organizations, some interviewers will go through a process of fact checking. We've seen that some interviewees have difficulty answering what would be considered basic questions about an experience. In most cases, it's due to the fact that many years have passed since the experience, and the applicant just can't recall the information. To avoid this very common pitfall, we recommend that, for each experience on the application, you ask yourself the basics:

- When did I do this [activity/organization]?
- Where did I do this [activity/organization]?
- Why did I get involved with this [activity/organization]?
- Who did I work with in this [activity/organization]?
- How did I get involved in this [activity/organization]?

Don't stop there, though. That's just the beginning. Also ask yourself:

- What skills or qualities did I develop through this experience?
- Why was this experience meaningful to me?
- What impact did I make through my involvement?
- How will this experience help me as a resident and physician in the specialty?

The answers to these deeper questions will allow you to develop rich content. This can then be incorporated into your interview responses.

Tip # 95

Review each item in your application. Think about the information you would like to convey if an interviewer asked you about it.

Rule # 138 Have a case ready to present.

On occasion, you may be asked to present an interesting case. "Tell me about the patient you learned the most from."

As with all interview questions, the goal of the question is to learn more about the applicant and not the case itself. You need not, and probably should not, choose the most difficult or challenging case you've encountered.

Choose a patient who made an impact on you. What challenges did the care of this patient present? What did you learn from the patient? Did your involvement in the patient's care change the way you practice? Did it lead you to see things differently, or help in your career choice, or highlight certain goals for you as a physician?

In asking this question, your interviewer is also hoping to learn how well you present clinical information. You must be able to present patient information clearly and concisely.

Prepare an approximately one to two-minute case presentation. Your goal is to be able to intelligently discuss all aspects of the case. You may want to consider preparing two cases. These cases should deal with topics in two different subspecialties. It's usually preferable to present a case that's outside of the interviewer's discipline. If your interviewer is a cardiologist, you may wish to present your endocrinology case. If you choose to, or must, present a case in the interviewer's discipline, make sure that you're well read on the current literature, as you may just be presenting to the world's foremost expert.

Rule # 139 Panel interviews may be used to gauge your composure and ability to deal with a stressful situation.

In a panel interview, you'll be interviewed by two or more interviewers simultaneously. Although not as common as the traditional one-on-one interview, panel interviews are utilized by programs in every specialty. In a survey of radiology PDs, it was learned that 6.5% of programs utilize panel interviews.[11]

Panel interviews allow the program to assess your composure, your ability to deal with stressful situations, and your interactions with different people. Through the use of panel interviews, programs can expose more members of their selection committee to applicants. This provides the program additional judgments on each interviewee. This can allow for a more productive discussion of each candidate at the resident selection committee meeting.

Although panel interviews may seem more intimidating, your preparation will essentially be the same as it would for a one-on-one interview. Don't let the fact that you're outnumbered affect your poise, confidence, and ability to sell yourself.

Recommendations for the Panel Interview

- Be clear on the interviewers' names and, from time to time, use them during the interview.
- Try to position yourself so that you can see all members of the panel without having to move your head from one side to another. Constant head movement can be stressful, and will appear distracting.
- Often, one of the panel members will take the lead in asking questions. The natural response may be to focus on this individual. However, your goal is to establish rapport with all interviewers.
- Direct your response initially to the interviewer who asked the question.
- As you delve further into your answer, make eye contact with the other interviewers. Remember that all panel members will have input in the group's assessment of your overall performance.
- Do not dart your eyes from one interviewer to another. Instead, make eye contact, pause briefly on each, and then move on to the next panel member.
- As you conclude your response, make eye contact once again with the interviewer who asked the question.
- Don't be alarmed if one or more interviewers show little or no expression or enthusiasm. Don't let their lack of emotion dampen the enthusiasm of your responses.
- Don't be surprised if one or more members of the panel take notes. It's common for panels to assign different roles, and note-taker may be one of them.
- Although it may seem difficult to do with a large panel, it's important to thank each member of the panel at the end of the interview.

Tip # 96

Panel interviews can be intimidating for all applicants, but may be especially difficult for shy candidates. Some applicants have a hard time relaxing in such situations. If so, we recommend that you arrange mock interviews where you have several friends or classmates interview you at the same time.

Rule # 140 The conversational interview can be quite dangerous.

"That didn't feel like an interview. It was just a normal conversation."

We've heard many applicants say something to this effect following an interview. If you leave an interview feeling this way, you've taken part in what is termed a conversational interview. In this type of interview, the interviewer does not have a list of prepared questions. The next question is often based on a point you just made.

Conversational interviews may be conducted by both trained and untrained interviewers. The goal of the former is to put you at ease and build rapport in an effort to learn more about you as a person. The trained interviewer has a certain agenda in mind, knows what information he seeks, and has decided that a conversational interview is the best way to elicit this information. The interview quickly becomes a chat. With this type of interview, you can't become too relaxed, or you may reveal things you wouldn't have in a traditional interview.

By contrast, the untrained interviewer has no plan. Direction and focus are lacking. The danger here is that if you are not proactive, you may leave the interview without sharing key experiences and strengths that demonstrate that you're a good fit for the program. If you sense that the interview is lacking focus, we recommend that you make efforts to redirect the conversation.

Tip # 97

While you can't control the type of interview you'll experience, you do have control over the content of your responses. Always enter an interview with an agenda. In advance of the interview, ask yourself what are the key experiences, skills, and strengths that you need to convey to the interviewer.

Tip # 98

If an interviewer runs out of questions well before the allotted time is over, you may wish to take some initiative. "Perhaps this would be a good time for me to share with you…" If the interviewer seems receptive, you can proceed from there.

Rule # 141 There are always two goals of all interviews. Don't forget the second one.

You must have a clear understanding of your goals for the interview. All of your goals can be summed up by the major two:

- You must have a successful interview so that the program will rank you highly.
- You must gather enough information about the program to make an informed decision regarding its place on your rank list.

In your desire to demonstrate compatibility with the program, you may lose sight of the second goal. While it may not always feel that way, remember that the interview process involves two parties selling themselves. While the program is trying to ascertain your strengths and weaknesses, you should be doing the same with respect to the program. You must use the short time that you have during your visit to learn as much as possible about the program. With every program you visit, ask yourself:

- How compatible am I with this program?
- Can I see myself working well with the program's faculty and residents?
- Will this program provide me with an environment in which I can thrive?
- How well will this program help me meet my future goals?

Rule # 142 Always prepare with a mock interview.

Practice, practice, practice. We cannot emphasize this rule enough. Unfortunately, we've sat through too many residency selection meetings in which strong applicants are unranked due to their interview. The message they sent during the interview was that they absolutely did not belong in this residency program. We believe that most of these applicants are completely unaware of the messages they send during the interview. Be it the inappropriate answers to interview questions, the mannerisms that overshadow the message, the affect that hides their true qualities, or the subtle findings that send a negative message, we believe that most of these applicants just didn't realize what message they were actually sending.

Interviewing is not a skill where you can just wing it. Too many students are overly confident about their abilities to convey their individuality, their strengths, and their fit for the program in one 15-minute session. Too often applicants prepare minimally for interviews. Such overconfidence has the potential to inflict serious damage. To interview successfully, you must anticipate the questions that will be asked, prepare your responses, and deliver them confidently.

In preparing, practicing both alone and with others is a must. With adequate practice, you can become comfortable with the interview process. Practice improves self-confidence. It also helps pinpoint deficiencies in your interviewing skills. You may not recognize your own tendency to twirl your hair, but an interviewer will find it distracting. Nervous habits, distracting mannerisms, poor grammar, a blunted affect, or a tendency to speak too softly may all be features that you're not likely to recognize in yourself.

Rehearsing your interview in front of a mirror may help you identify some problems. Note body language, as it sends a significant message. Do you smile? Do you keep your arms folded across your chest? Do you clench your hands?

Practice with a friend. Have him ask you interview questions, and respond as if you're at a real interview. Consider videotaping your performance. Together, you can review the interview, critique your performance, and use this information to make improvements in your verbal and nonverbal impressions.

One of the most useful methods of preparation, and one of the most underutilized, is to ask your advisor if they would feel comfortable helping you prepare by participating in a mock interview. Many advisors are members of residency selection committees, and they often have considerable experience in interviewing applicants.

The mock interview with your advisor can be designed to simulate the real interview. Ask your advisor to assume that he knows nothing about you but that which is found on your CV and personal statement. After the mock interview, you should meet with your advisor to evaluate your performance. Ask for specific feedback on:

- Content of your responses
- Your body language
- Your poise and level of confidence
- Whether he would select you based upon your performance

This type of feedback is invaluable, and should be utilized. If you're unable to set up a mock interview, check with your medical school. Some schools have developed workshops to help students with these skills.

Rule # 143 Every element of your residency application is up for discussion. Know it cold.

Prior to each interview, review each element of your residency application. Anything in your application is fair game for an interviewer. As you review each line of your CV, determine if an interviewer might ask about an item, why he might ask, what he might ask, and how you might respond. Do the same for the rest of your application. Such an approach will help avoid this unfortunate real-life scenario:

Jordana spoke eloquently about her research during her interview for internal medicine residency at a major university institution. She had performed this research between the first and second years of medical schools. In describing her role in the project, she spoke with great enthusiasm and energy. The interviewer asked, "Which journal was your work published in?" Jordana couldn't remember, stammering "I'm blanking on the journal but I believe I have it here somewhere." She fumbled through her portfolio, finally saying, "I think it was *Vaccine*."

Did you know?

Dr. Judith Amorosa, a faculty member in the radiology department at UMDNJ/Robert Wood Johnson Medical School, reminds applicants that they may be asked about anything in their application. "Make sure that whatever research or other experience you have had, you know it cold – otherwise you have lost your credibility. Be prepared to answer questions about yourself and other experiences."[23]

Tip # 99

Are there any areas of concern that might come up during the interview? A failing grade? A low USMLE score? Unfavorable clerkship evaluation comments in the Dean's letter? A leave of absence? If so, determine how you'll handle these queries well in advance of your interview.

Did you know?

In the article, "USMLE Scores, matching formulas, and more," Dr. Paul Jones, Associate Provost of Student Affairs at Rush Medical College, wrote that "in his experience, students who are unsuccessful in the residency match are unaware of how they measure up against other applicants. Students who have a red flag, but who also realize it and address it in their interviews, seem to do better."[24]

Rule # 144 Meet with residents or faculty in your own institution who trained at the institution where you will interview.

Before you visit a program, seek out all house officers and faculty at your own institution who've received any of their training at the institution where you will be interviewing. These individuals may be able to give you important information about the program. They can often discuss how the program compares to your home institution.

Tip # 100

Some medical schools ask their students to complete forms describing their interview experiences at other institutions. If so, you should read about their experience at the program you'll be visiting. Check with your student affairs office to see if your school does this.

Information obtained from someone "in the know" is often the most useful knowledge. Using this information, you can make powerful statements about your desire to become a resident in that program. As always, craft these statements carefully, and don't overdo it.

- "I've had a chance to speak with Dr. Lisa Sanders, who is a faculty member at my medical school. She is a graduate of your training program and had wonderful things to say about her residency experience. In particular, she spoke glowingly about morning report and how it…"

- "Our internal medicine chairman at Strong University, Dr. Grant, was invited by your program to be a visiting professor several years ago. Dr. Grant has always spoken very highly about your program. He was especially impressed with how your program encourages and supports residents to participate in research and scholarly activity."

- "While attending the ACP conference, I had the opportunity to meet with Dr. Chen, one of the faculty members in your department. We spoke at length about the residency program. From him, I learned a great deal about your program's strengths. What particularly piqued my interest was the unique mentorship program…"

Rule # 145 Prepare for a typical interview day.

The typical day will begin with the program director welcoming applicants, introducing the program, and providing an overview of the program. Following this, applicants are often invited to morning report, another conference, or rounds. One or more interviews will then take place with faculty and possibly residents. A tour of the institution and lunch with the residents are also common. The day may conclude with a wrap-up session, which at some places is one-on-one with the program director.

With so many programs, this schedule will understandably vary. You should review the interview materials to learn about the interview day. How will your day be structured? Knowing what to expect may allow you to feel more at ease. It may also help you prepare better for the interview. For example, if you'll be attending a conference, what will be the topic? While you won't be asked to participate, advance reading may allow you to ask insightful questions or participate in a meaningful discussion.

Rule # 146 Not all of your interviewers will have access to your file. Always arrive prepared with your own materials.

Applicants generally believe that interviewers will have read their applications prior to the interview. However, some programs don't allow interviewers to view a candidate's application. These interviews are called closed file interviews because the interviewer knows nothing about you. Interviewers may also be given some application information, but quantitative information such as grades and USMLE scores may be absent from the file (i.e., partially open file interviews). In other cases, interviewers have full access to your application, but haven't reviewed it yet, or haven't reviewed it thoroughly.

Programs that limit access to the full application file feel that an interviewer who has quantitative information at his disposal may develop preconceived notions about the strength of an applicant. For example, an interviewer may be quite impressed with an applicant's grades and USMLE scores. Colored by this information, the interviewer may approach the interview differently than if he had been blinded to this information.

Did you know?

In one study, Smilen found "a strong, striking, and statistically significant correlation between interview scores and board scores when their interviewers knew these grades, with no correlation when they did not. This finding should not be particularly surprising. The halo effect is a well-known phenomenon…in which a conclusion is reached about a job applicant within the first half minute of an encounter. After that point and during the remainder of the interview, the interviewer will subconsciously discount anything that does not fit the predetermined image of the candidate. By providing interviewers with the available performance markers, this effect can be established even in advance of interview."[25]

Did you know?

If you have strong grades, good board scores, or have been elected to AOA, you should convey this information to an interviewer who lacks access to your file. You may benefit from the halo effect. At the beginning of a closed file interview, you may offer the interviewer a copy of your CV and transcript. Make sure that your honors grades and board scores are on your CV.

Did you know?

In a survey of general surgery residency programs, 20% reported blinding their interviewers to parts of the residency application.[26]

Rule # 147 Don't ever be remembered for what you're wearing.

I've interviewed a few applicants that I can still, to this day, remember distinctly what they were wearing. I can't remember their scores or strengths, but I can remember the dangling, hypnotic earrings, the too-short skirt with the high heels, the long pinky nail, and so many more. In an interview, you never want to be remembered for what you were wearing. You want to be remembered for your strengths, your communication skills, your great scores, and your outstanding letters of recommendation, or any or all of these.

You should dress conservatively, with the goal of presenting yourself neatly and professionally. In choosing interview attire, select clothing in which you feel comfortable. Your clothing should not interfere with your ability to give a successful interview.

Interview Attire		
	Yes	**No**
Men	Suit (well-fitting, dark blue or gray) Shirt (ironed, long-sleeved) Tie (long, conservative) Shoes (clean, polished) Hairstyle (well-groomed, neat) Beard and mustache (neat, trimmed) Nails (clean, trimmed)	Earrings Visible body piercings Strongly scented cologne Strongly scented aftershave
Women	Suit or tailored dress (dark blue or gray) Shoes (clean, closed toe, dark or neutral color, low to moderate heels) Hosiery (conservative, at or near skin color) Hairstyle (well-groomed) Nails (clean, trimmed, if nail polish present – clean or conservative color)	Low neckline Excessive/ distracting jewelry Strongly scented perfume Distracting hair or make-up

Your appearance is of the utmost importance, since it's one of the first factors that telegraphs a message during an interview. If you are sloppily dressed or poorly groomed, your message is that you are not the highly professiona,l mature physician with compulsive attention to detail that the residency program seeks. Highly qualified applicants are sometimes, unfortunately, remembered more for their attire than for their qualifications.

Did you know?

In a survey of orthopedic residency PDs, directors were asked to rank the importance of 26 residency selection criteria. Personal appearance was ranked fifth.[27] In another study involving 54 residency applicants, ratings of neatness and grooming correlated positively with final interview ratings for women.[28]

Tip # 101

If you're flying to the interview, keep your interview outfit in your carry-on luggage.

References

[1]Gong H, Parker N, Apgar F, Shank C. Influence of the interview on ranking in the residency selection process. *Med Educ* 1984; 18(5): 366-369.
[2]Martin-Lee L, Park H, Overton D. Does interview date affect match list position in the emergency medicine national residency matching program match? *Acad Emerg Med* 2000; 7(9): 1022-1026.
[3]Results of the 2014 NRMP Program Director Survey. Available at: http://www.nrmp.org/wp-content/uploads/2014/09/PD-Survey-Report-2014.pdf. Accessed March 3, 2016.
[4]Boyse T, Patterson S, Cohan R, Korobkin M, Fitzgerald J, Oh M, Gross B, Quint D. Does medical school performance predict radiology resident performance? *Acad Radiol* 2002; 9(4): 437-445.
[5]Bell J, Kanellitsas I, Shaffer L, Selection of obstetrics and gynecology residents on the basis of medical school performance. *Am J Obstet Gynecol* 2002; 186(5): 1091-1094.
[6]Zagumny M, Rudolph J. Comparing medical students' and residency directors' ratings of criteria used to select residents. *Acad Med* 1992; 67(9): 613.
[7]Swanson W, Harris M, Master C, Gallagher P, Maruo A, Ludwig S. The impact of the interview in pediatric residency selection. *Amb Pediatr* 2005; 5(4): 216-220.
[8]Curtis D, Riordan D, Cruess D, Brower A. Selecting radiology resident candidates. *Invest Radiol* 1989; 24(4): 324-330.
[9]Dort J, Trickey A, Kallies K, Joshi A, Sidwell R, Jarman B. Applicant characteristics associated with selection for ranking at independent surgery residency programs. *J Surg Educ* 2015; 72(6): e123-129.
[10]Crane J, Ferraro C. Selection criteria for emergency medicine residency applicants. *Acad Emerg Med* 2000; 7(1): 54-60.
[11]Otero H, Erturk S, Ondategui-Parra S, Ros P. Key criteria for selection of radiology residents: results of a national survey. *Acad Radiol* 2006; 13: 1155-1164.
[12]Villanueva A, Kaye D, Abdelhak S, Morahan P. Comparing selection criteria for residency directors and physicians' employers. *Acad Med* 1995; 70(4): 261-271.
[13]Carson K, Carson P, Fontenot G, Burdin J. Structured interview questions for selecting productive emotionally mature and helpful employees. *Health Care Manag* 2005; 24(3): 209-215.
[14]Wagner P, Moseley G, Grant M, Gore J, Owens C. Physicians' emotional intelligence and patient satisfaction. *Fam Med* 2002; 34(10): 750-754.
[15]DeLisa J, Jain S, Campagnolo D. Factors used by physical medicine and rehabilitation residency training directors to select their residents. *Am J Phys Med Rehabil* 1994; 73: 152-156.
[16]Bates B. Selection criteria for applicants in primary care osteopathic graduate medical education. *J Am Osteopath Assoc* 1988; 88: 391-395.
[17]Duke University Department of Anesthesiology. Available at: http://anesthesiology.duke.edu/wp-content/uploads/2013/08/AIG-how-to-interview.pdf. Accessed February 4, 2016.

[18]Gonzalez E, Phillips R, Pugno P. A study of closure of family practice residency programs. *Fam Med* 2003; 35(10): 706-710.
[19]Department of Obstetrics and Gynecology at Maricopa Integrated Health System. Available at: http://mihs.org/medical-education/obstetrics-and-gynecology#residency. Accessed February 4, 2016.
[20]Motowildo S, Carter G, Dunnette M, et al. Studies of the structured behavioral interview. *J Appl Psychol* 1992; 77(5): 571-587.
[21]McDaniel M, Whetzel D, Schmidt F, Maurer S. The validity of employment interviews: a comprehensive review and meta-analysis. *J Appl Psychol* 1994; 79(4): 599-616.
[22]Getting into Emergency Medicine. Available at: http://studentdoctor.net/2010/08/the-successful-match-getting-into-emergency-medicine/. Accessed January 30, 2013.
[23]Amorosa J. How do I mentor medical students interested in radiology. *Acad Radiol* 2003; 10: 527-535,
[24]Get the residency you want: Tips and tools. Available at: http://www.medscape.com/viewarticle/548355_2. Accessed February 4, 2016.
[25]Smilen S, Funai E, Bianco A. Residency selection: should interviewers be given applicant's board scores. *Am J Obstet Gynecol* 2001; 184(3): 508-513.
[26]Kim R, Gilbert T, Suh S, Miller J, Eggerstedt J. General surgery residency interviews: are we following best practices? *Am J Surg* 2016; 211(2): 476-481.
[27]Bernstein A, Jazrawi L, Elbeshbeshy B, Della Valle C, Zuckerman J. Orthopedic resident-selection criteria. *J Bone Joint Surg Am* 2002; 84-A(11): 2090-2096.
[28]Boor M, Wartman S, Reuben D. Relationship of physical appearance and professional demeanor to interview evaluations and rankings of medical residency applicants. *J Psychol* 1983; 113: 61-65,

Chapter 14

The Interview Day

Rule # 148 **Your interview day begins long before you meet your interviewer.**

Your interview doesn't start when you sit down with your interviewer. It begins as soon as you enter the premises. Many applicants mistakenly assume they only need to "be on" during the interview. In reality, everything you say or do on the day of the interview may be noted and duly reported.

It's not unheard of for faculty to ask their secretaries and administrative staff for their opinions of the applicants. They may ask the secretary about a candidate's appearance or behavior. Our secretaries have commented on a host of negative behaviors. These range from the disinterested applicant leafing through the waiting room *Sports Illustrated* instead of program information, to the applicant with the arrogant, unfriendly demeanor, to the pesky applicant asking inappropriate questions, especially when the secretary is clearly busy.

Did you know?

Dr. Andrew Lee, Chairman of the Department of Ophthalmology at Houston Methodist Hospital, wrote that "many programs (including our own) use the informal feedback from the residency coordinator, the secretaries, and the other residents to obtain a more complete view of the applicant. Important sentinel behaviors both positive (e.g., politeness, altruism, helpfulness) and negative (e.g., condescension, arrogance, rudeness) may only manifest during applicant interactions with perceived subordinates (e.g., the appointment secretary)."[1]

Did you know?

Poor behavior reported by anyone before, during, or after your interview day has the potential to be communicated to a residency program. "We did not rank a candidate as they had a negative encounter at the airport announcing that they had interviewed for a position with us and if the gate agent ever needed their services they would refuse to treat them," wrote a residency coordinator at a major residency program. "The gate agent or someone affiliated with the airline tracked down the physician recruitment office to share what happened. The recruitment office in turn told us. The world is very, very small and word gets around quickly when you least expect it."[2]

Interviews often don't start on time. Applicants may wait as long as an hour or two. Since many interviewers are practicing physicians, patient care-related issues can arise at any point and require immediate tending. Some candidates lose their patience, and have been known to approach the secretary impatiently or rudely, demanding to know the reason for the delay. How you handle a situation of this type is very telling.

Tip # 102

Applicants should be on their best behavior, not just during the interview, but throughout the entire visit. Programs can gain much insight into your personal characteristics by observing your interactions with other applicants, program staff, residents, and others. The best rule of thumb is to conduct yourself as if there are hidden cameras watching your every move.

Tip # 103

Ask the receptionist where you can place your excess belongings (coat, umbrella, etc.). You don't want to walk into your interview bogged down with clutter.

Rule # 149 Be compulsive about bringing everything that you need for the interview.

Bring the following with you to your interview:

- Curriculum vitae (CV)
- Personal statement
- Application
- Board scores
- Medical school transcript
- Copies of any published articles
- Copies of submitted, accepted, or in press articles, with your advisors' permission
- All correspondence between you and the program
- Notepad portfolio with pen
- Money
- Parking ticket
- Personal items (dental floss, mint, etc.)

While the program is likely to have your application (including CV, personal statement, board scores), you should be prepared with copies in the event that an interviewer asks for one of these items. You may have a closed file interview, or a patient emergency may result in an interviewer substitution. The pen that you use should be a nice one. Specifically, bring a pen that has not been provided by a drug rep.

Did you know?

Research on publication misrepresentation among residency applicants has revealed that some applicants exaggerate their level of involvement in research or even fabricate publications. Some residency programs are requiring applicants to submit in advance or bring published articles to the interview for confirmation.

Rule # 150 Arrive early for the interview.

Start your interview day properly by arriving early. Aim to reach the city the day before the interview. Stay as close to the hospital as possible. If possible, make a trip to the hospital to gain familiarity with the interview destination. In the morning, plan to be at your destination an hour before the start time. This extra time will be useful when the unforeseen occurs – such as heavy traffic, inclement weather, or an accident. Running in at the last minute can affect your interview performance, as many applicants have learned the hard way.

Entering the designated interview location more than fifteen minutes before the start time can be just as bad. Arriving too early can make you seem anxious, and you may interrupt the staff as they set up for the interview day. When you do enter the reception area, introduce yourself to the residency program's secretary. "Good morning. My name is ________ and I have an interview today."

Even with meticulous planning, unforeseen circumstances may cause you to be late. Arriving late is one of the reasons that program directors cite for not ranking an applicant highly. It's possible to recover from this situation, but only if it's handled with great poise. If you'll be late, call the program to apprise them of the situation. When speaking on the phone, be polite no matter how flustered you are. Once you've arrived, take time to compose yourself before entering the room. Apologize and explain, at an appropriate time, what detained you. Never rush in complaining about what happened.

Tip # 104

Make sure you have the phone number of the program readily accessible in the event that you are running late. "We have had applicants email a few days before their interviews to request a phone number for somebody in the program – just in case they get lost or have any issues," writes Dr. Gopi Astik, former chief resident at UMKC. "This shows us they are prepared and want to keep us informed if anything comes up."[3]

Tip # 105

If you're driving, determine in advance the route you'll take. Plan an alternate route in case you encounter heavy traffic. If you're taking the train or bus, familiarize yourself with the bus or train line you'll be riding, including the times. What will you do if service is interrupted for some reason? Always have a back-up plan.

If You're Late...

- Contact the program as soon as possible to inform them of the circumstances.
- You don't have to wait until you're late to make this call. It's preferable to contact the program sooner rather than later if you're doubtful you'll make it on time. Calling a program to inform them of your tardiness after you're late is more irritating to the program. Calling ahead says something about your responsibility and accountability.
- Acknowledge your mistake, and apologize.
- Offer a reason for your tardiness but recognize that traffic, missed wake up call, or a malfunctioning alarm is not likely to appease the program. Hopefully, you have a good reason to offer.
- If you don't have a good reason, don't make something up or offer excuses. Be honest, straightforward, and apologetic. Don't go on and on with your explanation.
- After you apologize, move on. If you'll have any chance at this program, it will depend on your ability to regain your composure. If you dwell on being late, it's likely to affect the rest of your interview performance.

Rule # 151 Project self-confidence, not anxiety

It's common and completely natural to be nervous. However, you don't want to convey the message that you're an anxious, distracted, unqualified applicant. Your message should be that you're an extremely well qualified applicant, and therefore you are calm and confident. The first and best way to conquer anxiety is thorough preparation. Learning about the interview process, anticipating questions, preparing responses, rehearsing with friends, and performing a mock interview with an advisor are all important parts of interview preparation.

Despite extensive preparation, anxiety can remain a significant problem for some applicants. We have a few additional suggestions for the days before an interview:

- Utilize stress-reduction techniques. Many articles and books provide specifics on effective techniques utilized by actors, professional athletes, and public speakers. Such techniques include controlled breathing, progressive muscle relaxation, and visualization, among others.

- Channel your nervous energy into concrete, positive action. One example would be focusing on action items for interview preparation such as re-reading the program information or practicing some of your responses for anticipated questions.

- Direct your nervous energy into action that is unrelated to interview preparation. You've heard of the fight or flight response. Expend that extra adrenaline by heading to the gym or going for a run.

- Look over your CV to remind yourself of your accomplishments. The program would not be interviewing you if they weren't impressed with you. You have a great deal to offer a residency program, and you should be specific when reminding yourself of what you can bring to a program.

- Your career does not ride on your performance at one interview. Remind yourself of this fact. For most applicants, other interviews will follow.

Tip # 106

Although you'll be nervous, you don't want to convey the impression of an anxious, nervous applicant. Residency is inherently stressful. As such, interviewers seek residents who are able to think clearly in the most stressful of situations. Avoid comments that convey anxiety.

Did you know?

Some applicants are under the impression that interviewees shouldn't be nervous. That's not at all true. If you speak with accomplished individuals who are veterans of the interview experience, you'll realize that even the most experienced continue to feel nervous during interview situations. It's completely normal.

Did you know?

In evaluating interview performance, interviewers take note of both what you say and how you say it. High levels of anxiety have been shown to adversely affect a variety of factors, including eye contact, body language, voice level, and projected confidence.[4] In her article, "Anxiety patterns in employment interviews," Young wrote that "anxious individuals are less likely to be hired…possibly because interviewers perceive highly anxious people to be less trustworthy, less task-oriented…than low anxiety interviewees)."[5]

Rule # 152 Shake hands properly.

You'll have the opportunity to shake hands when you first meet the interviewer and again when you complete the interview. You must be ready for a handshake at these two points. Not all interviewers will offer to shake hands. In general, the interviewee should follow the lead of the interviewer. If she doesn't extend her hand, don't offer yours.

The initial handshake is an important component of a first impression. Be prepared to shake hands by keeping your right hand free at your side, as opposed to clutching your portfolio. If you suffer from hyperhidrosis and are prone to sweaty palms, be prepared to subtly wipe your palm. Your goal is to convey self-confidence, not anxiety. Shake hands using a firm grip, conveying an impression of confidence. Avoid a weak, limp, or crushing grip. Since it's difficult to evaluate the quality of your own handshake, you may need to solicit input from friends or colleagues.

Did you know?

In the *Lancet* article, "Getting a grip on handshakes," Larkin reported the results of a study by Chaplin in which the handshake characteristics of men and women were evaluated.[6-7] Larkin wrote that "a strong correlation was found between a firm handshake – as evidenced by strength, vigor, duration, completeness of grip, and eye contact – and a good first impression….Given the power of first impressions, the researchers advise that women as well as men try to make that first handshake a firm one."

Rule # 153 The first few minutes of an interview can be critical.

We've all heard the importance of the first impression in making hiring decisions outside of medicine. Is there any evidence to suggest that first impressions are also crucial in residency interviews? Researchers in the Department of Anesthesiology at the University of Kentucky applied the "Blink test" defined as "overall impression of a candidate within 30 seconds of meeting them" to over 400 applicants over a 3-year period. Interviewees were given a Blink score of 1 to 5 (5 = excellent). These quick judgments were found to correlate fairly well with the candidate's final position on the program's rank order list.[8] Why do some people make a better first impression than others? "I think a lot of it is a person's interpersonal communications, how they come across," said Dr. Regina Fragneto, lead author of the study. "Do they look you in the eye when they come in? Do they have a firm handshake? Things like that."[9]

As soon as you walk into the room, your interviewer will be sizing you up. Initial impressions may even dictate the course of the interview. A favorable first impression may lead to a more relaxed interview. An interviewer who perceives you to be disinterested or sloppy, though, may be more likely to grill you extensively to try to support or refute that impression.

Below are key guidelines to promoting a favorable impression within the first few minutes of an interview:

- Dress well and be impeccably groomed.
- Stand up and greet the interviewer with a firm handshake ("Hello, Dr. Smith, I'm Evan Chen. It's a pleasure to meet you.")
- Smile when meeting the interviewer.
- Walk into the room with confidence.
- Make eye contact.
- Pronounce the interviewer's name early ("How do you do, Dr. Smith?")
- Make small talk easily.

You must have a polished entrance, introduction, and opening. In my experience conducting mock interviews with residency applicants, I find that applicants focus almost exclusively on developing answers to questions. Few applicants give thought to the opening of an interview. Since we rarely receive feedback about the first impression we make on others, practice the opening of your interview through role play with others.

Tip # 107

After you're invited into the interviewing room, don't sit down until the interviewer offers you a seat. It's considered bad manners to be seated before the interviewer asks you to (or does so) herself.

Tip # 108

After introductions have been made, most interviewers will engage applicants in some small talk. You may be asked the following:

How was your trip here?
Did you have any problems finding our office?
What's the weather like in _______?

In answering these questions, avoid long statements. The interviewer doesn't want to hear about the "terrible traffic," how much you "hate the snow," or the problems you had finding the office. To start off on the right foot, answer these questions with brief, positive answers.

Tip # 109

"How has your day with us been so far?" is a commonly asked question at the beginning of an interview. You can use this opportunity to say something positive about the program. Talk about how happy the residents looked, how much you enjoyed morning report, or any other positive aspect of the program.

Did you know?

Dr. Roy Ziegelstein, Vice Dean for Education at Johns Hopkins University School of Medicine, states that "individuals who interview and judge others for a living (e.g., program directors) often form very strong first impressions. Typically, those individuals are flexible and those impressions are changeable, but those first impressions are nevertheless important."[10]

Rule # 154 Your nonverbal communication is a potent part of your message.

In all personal interactions, communication occurs in two fashions: verbal and nonverbal. So much focus is placed on what an applicant should say during the interview that they often neglect to focus on how they say it. However, nonverbal communication can be as important, and in some cases more important, than verbal communication. Body language cues can overcome the content of your interview answers, especially if your body language conveys hesitation, uncertainty, or a lack of conviction.

Interviewers do analyze body language, although most of the time this is done on a subconscious level. Any inconsistency between verbal and nonverbal communication may raise red flags. We've interviewed applicants who can't send a consistent message. While their self-proclaimed greatest strength is passion and dedication, they're slouched in their chair, leaning on the armrest, and looking a little bored. Others say the right things, but seem to lack sincerity. In response to a question on why a resident is switching fields: "I found that my passion lay not in spending hours in the operating room, but in spending time in an outpatient setting speaking with patients." Although the content of the answer was fine, the poor eye contact suggested insincerity.

Tip # 110

Are you aware of how you communicate nonverbally? Most applicants are not. When preparing for an interview, applicants focus most of their attention on verbal communication. Much less emphasis is placed on nonverbal communication or body language. In fact, many applicants don't even think about nonverbal communication. However, it's estimated that 65 to 90% of every conversation is interpreted through body language.[11] There are many qualified applicants who interview poorly because their nonverbal language is not congruent with the content of their answers. Participating in a mock interview is an excellent way to learn about how you communicate nonverbally.

It's difficult, and in some cases impossible, to evaluate your own body language. We've interviewed applicants who send strong, clear messages with their unconscious use of body language. The student who twirls her hair constantly. The applicant who rests his head on his hand during the interview. The other applicant who is slumped down in the chair. The student who can't seem to maintain eye contact, even when stating how much she loves your program. The applicant who keeps smiling and laughing, even when discussing a sad patient case, or the student who maintains such a blunted affect that it's difficult to tell if they're bored, tired, or just at baseline. You'd be surprised how often such cues can lead an interviewer to make snap judgments about a candidate's qualifications.

Your own evaluation of this type of communication should include a conscious awareness of several items. What are you doing with your hands? How is your posture? Are you maintaining eye contact? While you can perform a self-evaluation, mock interviews are critical in evaluating your nonverbal cues. Mock interviews can be staged with colleagues, advisors, or interview coaches, and feedback should cover your nonverbal communication skills. Mock interviews can be videotaped as well. Reviewing your performance can prove uncomfortable but enlightening.

Successful nonverbal communication includes adhering to the following rules:

- Stand and walk with erect posture and shoulders back.
- Shake hands firmly. Avoid a limp or crushing handshake.
- Your facial expressions should be relaxed. Avoid indicators of excessive anxiety, such as the furrowed brow or tense jaw.
- Maintain appropriate eye contact. Don't stare down your interviewer.
- Hand gestures should be appropriate, and not overdone.
- Avoid excess. While you should smile and nod occasionally, some applicants exhibit nervous laughter or excessive head bobbing.

Did you know?

Weiten, in his book *Psychology Applied to Modern Life: Adjustment in the 21st Century*, wrote (citing the work of Riggio) "it has been found that interviewees who emit positive nonverbal cues – leaning forward, smiling, and nodding, are rated higher than those who do not."[12]

Equally important is the avoidance of nervous and distracting habits. We could list endless examples, but here are a few of the most common:

- Looking down or glancing away
- Tapping the foot or drumming fingers on desk or chair
- Fiddling with jewelry or other accessories
- Twirling the hair
- Glancing often at the watch

Tip # 111

Failure to maintain eye contact while speaking may suggest a lack of confidence or even dishonesty. However, avoid prolonged eye contact. An interview is not a staring contest.

Body Language 101

What should I do with my hands?

Rest your hands in your lap. It's acceptable to clasp your hands together, but don't clasp too tightly or make a fist. Avoid folding your arms across your chest. This can create an impression of rigidity, unapproachability, disagreement, or even dishonesty. Do not cover your mouth or touch your face while you speak. Touching the face may give the impression of dishonesty. Avoid touching your tie, tugging at your collar, or straightening your clothing. Fidgeting, playing with hair, and adjusting clothing are signs suggestive of anxiety or uncertainty. We also recommend that you not hold your pen in your hand. Many applicants end up fiddling or tapping with it.

How should I sit?

Posture can weigh heavily in how others perceive you. Maintain an alert, straight posture while you sit, stand, and walk. Leaning forward slightly demonstrates interest. Applicants who slouch can appear lazy, unmotivated, or disinterested.

What should I do with my feet?

Keep your feet flat on the floor. You may cross your legs at your ankles. Do not rest your ankle on your opposite knee. Constant movement of the legs can be irritating to interviewers.

Tip # 112

With the mirroring technique, an individual makes subtle efforts to adopt the pose and position of those with whom they're speaking. It's based on the concept that people generally like those who are similar to them. In fact, in the book "Handbook of Cultural Psychology," Kitayama and Cohen reviewed the literature in this area and wrote that "people have more positive subjective experiences of rapport as a result of mirroring exhibited by interaction partners."[13]

Rule # 155 **You need to know how well you're doing in an interview. Pay close attention to the nonverbal cues of the interviewer.**

The interviewer's body language may be your only clue as to how well you're doing. Most interviewers won't interrupt to tell you that you're rambling. They won't share with you that your last response came across as very defensive. Better than words, their posture, movements, facial expressions, and tone of voice can indicate their reactions. This type of indicator can be useful if you make it a point to notice these nonverbal cues.

As we've stated before, interviews are stressful, and many applicants focus all of their attention on preparing their next response. In response to the simple "Tell me about yourself," one applicant went off on a five-minute monologue. She didn't notice the obvious impatience of my colleague and myself because she wasn't paying any attention to us. The interview is bilateral communication, and it's very important to monitor how well you're doing. In many cases, your only effective way to do so is by paying close attention to the nonverbal cues of the interviewer.

What You Can Learn From The Interviewer's Body Language

If the interviewer…	**It might mean…**
Is leaning forward and nodding at you Mirroring your body language Feet/shoulders/face facing you	The interviewer has interest in and is in agreement with what you're saying
Stops taking notes Picks up the pace of his questioning Repeatedly checks watch or clock	The interviewer may be bored.
Arms folded across chest Flared nostrils Feet/shoulders pointing towards the exit	The interviewer may be offended.
Raising eyebrows Smirking	The interviewer may be in disagreement or disbelief with what you're saying

Keep in mind that you can never be sure what the interviewer is thinking or feeling. The interviewer who picks up the pace of his questions may not be losing interest in you; he may be running short of time. There are also interviewers who purposefully stifle their body language, and appear serious or even disengaged. I can't tell you how often my mock interview clients have told me, "The interview went terribly. The interviewer never cracked a smile, and I couldn't form any type of connection with him" only to match with that very program.

Tip # 113

As a general rule, don't speak for longer than 1 ½ minutes. Running on and on is one of the most common mistakes applicants make during the residency interview. Remember that the interview is a dialogue rather than a monologue, and that every interviewer has an agenda. That agenda may include a set number of questions, and interviewees who talk too much may prevent the interviewer from accomplishing his goals.

Rule # 156 Pay attention.

It's extremely stressful to be seated in front of an interviewer anticipating the next question. Most applicants nervously focus on what they're going to say. Instead of focusing on their next answer, they should be focused on the interviewer. Listening carefully doesn't mean waiting for the chance to speak. It means concentrating on what the interviewer is saying and making it clear that your entire attention is focused on the interviewer. Your goal is to create an impression of poise and confidence. We've sat in interviews where applicants were obviously nervous and distracted. They misunderstood the question or provided an answer that didn't address the question. Some asked questions that were answered earlier in the interview.

Rule # 157 Plan what you'll do when you don't know how to answer the question.

Among an applicant's greatest fears is that of being asked a question to which she doesn't know the answer. While practice is the best defense against the unexpected, we do think that some reassurances and suggestions here are necessary. Remember that one subpar interview response is unlikely to torpedo the entire interview. Most important is that you maintain your confidence and focus.

If you're asked a difficult question or one that you're not sure how to answer, avoid stammering, stuttering, apologizing, or making something up. Don't rush into a disjointed and hurried answer. Pause for a few seconds to gather your thoughts. Or you can say, "That's an interesting question. Let me think about it for a moment." If the question is ambiguous, you can also ask the interviewer for clarification. Remind yourself that with many questions, there are simply no right or wrong answers. If you still can't come up with anything other than "I don't know" or "I'm not sure how to answer that question," say so.

Your recovery is likely much more important than your response to a single question. Maintain your composure and focus on the next question. If, at the end of the interview, you come up with an answer, then volunteer it. "I've been thinking about one of the questions you asked me earlier. Would you mind if I expand on my answer?"

When You Don't Know How To Answer The Question

- If your mind goes blank and you need a little time to think, remember to pause. A 5-10 second pause may seem like an eternity to you, but won't be viewed as such by the interviewer. If you're uncomfortable with pausing, you can consider saying:

  That's a really good question. May I have just a moment to gather my thoughts?

- If you're still unable to come up with answer, ask the interviewer if you can return to the question later:

  I don't have an answer for your question but I was wondering if I could return to this question later during the interview.

- If you're still unable to come up with an answer, don't worry about it.

Rule # 158 Learn how to handle silence.

Silence during an interview is a common occurrence. If inexperienced, the interviewer may not be able to come up with any more questions. At other times, a savvy interviewer may purposefully become silent after you've answered a question. She may simply stare at you without saying a word. The natural response is to wonder what you did wrong. "Did I say something inappropriate?" "Did she not like my answer?" The other natural response is to reword your answer, repeat a comment you made earlier, or even retract your answer. Applicants may assume that the reason for silence is that the interviewer doesn't agree with your answer. However, the silent response is often used as a tactic to gauge an interviewee's confidence in their response.

The best course of action is simply to remain silent without fidgeting or displaying signs of anxiety. Look at the interviewer with interest as you wait for the next question. In time, the interviewer will break the silence with the next question.

How can you tell if your interviewer is testing you or just can't come up with anything else to say? If her attention is focused on you, it's more likely that she's utilizing this stress tactic. If, on the other hand, the interviewer is fidgeting or isn't looking at you, she may be trying to come up with the next question. In this case, you could break the silence by asking some questions about the residency program.

Tip # 114

While most applicants are uncomfortable with silence, it does have the potential to elevate your interview performance. Nervous applicants often rush right into their answer, letting the words just pour out. A period of silence may be used to convey a more powerful and organized response. To become more comfortable pausing before you answer, practice this in your mock interviews.

Rule # 159 Convey enthusiasm.

Enthusiasm is contagious, even in the setting of an interview. It doesn't matter how well you've prepared the content of your interview answers. The manner in which that content is conveyed has a great deal to do with its reception. Your goal is to appear personable, sincere, and down-to-earth. You need to avoid appearing flat, blunted, tired, or robotic. It's easy to stiffen up, become too formal, or become so focused on what you're going to say that you fail to convey a personality. In all of these cases, you may fail to connect with your interviewer or even leave a frankly negative impression.

Your goal should be to appear enthusiastic about yourself, the specialty, and the residency program. This rule is especially applicable to interviews that occur late in the season. After your thirtieth conversation with an individual interviewer, you may find it difficult to muster the energy and enthusiasm that came so easily initially.

Did you know?

In his advice to students at the University of Florida College of Medicine, Dr. Patrick Duff, Associate Dean for Student Affairs, recommends that applicants keep their "energy level up throughout the day. When I reviewed the interview performance of over 200 students who applied for our ob-gyn training program in the last 5 years, the single biggest reason for a low interview score was 'did not appear interested, no spark.'"[14]

Did you know?

Dr. Alex Macario is the program director of the Stanford University Anesthesiology Residency Program, and a strong proponent of showing enthusiasm. "Show positivity/excitement about the specific residency. That energy will fuel a better evaluation." This may be particularly challenging for applicants who've completed a number of interviews. "Even though you may be fatigued because you are on your twelfth interview please look alive and interested during the presentation by the chair or program director or others."[15]

Rule # 160 Avoid phrases that suggest a lack of credibility.

Programs are on their guard against applicants who exaggerate their achievements, or outright lie. Therefore, you need to safeguard your own credibility. Avoid the following phrases:

- "I'm going to be honest with you…"
- "To tell you the truth…"
- "To be perfectly candid…"

Prefacing a statement with phrases such as these may raise red flags. Some people associate these phrases with dishonesty. The reason we specify these particular phrases is that many individuals who use them are unaware of their use, and are unaware of their connotations.

Rule # 161 You may be asked inappropriate or illegal questions. Plan in advance how to handle them.

Results of the 1996 AAMC Medical Student Graduation Questionnaire revealed that 45% of students were asked about marital status or family plans.[16] In a more recent survey of over 7,000 applicants applying to five specialties (internal medicine, general surgery, orthopedic surgery, obstetrics & gynecology, and emergency medicine), nearly 65% reported being asked at least one potentially illegal question.[17] Despite efforts to eradicate questionable interview practices, interviewers continue to ask applicants inappropriate, unethical, or outright illegal questions.

Federal and state civil rights acts make it unlawful for employers to discriminate on the basis of:

- Religion
- Age
- Gender
- Race
- Sexual preference
- Marital status/living situation
- Family planning
- Height
- Weight
- Military discharge status

Most of these questions are asked not out of malice, but out of simple ignorance. Naïve or less experienced interviewers may ask these questions simply to make conversation, not recognizing their inappropriateness.

Before you begin the interview process, develop an effective way to handle these types of questions. Some applicants, unprepared for such questions, have unfortunately reacted in an emotional manner. Some have refused to answer the question and some have even responded in a hostile manner: "That is a completely inappropriate question. I can't believe you would ask me that."

An outright refusal to answer an improper question is certainly your right. However, you will offend the interviewer and create a situation from which you may not be able to recover. It goes without saying that if the question is blatantly offensive, then you should choose this option (and later discuss with the program director or chairman).

If at all possible, however, you should try to answer the question as you would any other, with poise and confidence. There are several possible strategies to utilize. We describe two ways of handling these types of questions:

Answer the question directly

Some applicants will simply answer the question directly. If you're comfortable answering the question, then this may be the right approach for you. If the interviewer has asked the question just to make conversation, it's unlikely that your response would affect your chances of matching with that program. If the interviewer is deliberately asking the question, then your response may have a direct impact on your chances of matching.

"I see that you're a nontraditional student, already in your 30s. When do you plan on having children?"

> Examples of direct responses:
>
> "My husband and I hope to have children in the next few years."
>
> "My spouse and I have discussed it, and we'd like to delay until after residency, since it would be so challenging during residency."
>
> "We really haven't come to any decision yet on that issue."

Answer the intent or concern behind the question

Using this approach, you won't directly answer the question. Your goal is to address the interviewer's concern. The key is to try to understand why the question is being asked.

"I see that you're a nontraditional student, already in your 30s. When do you plan on having children?"

This applicant assumes that the question is asked to determine if she would continue to be an effective resident in the event that she were to have a young child at home during residency:

"Dr. Lowell, I understand that the residents at Seymour Hospital deal with a very high patient volume when on call. I can assure you that I have a strong work ethic and sense of responsibility, along with the ability to deal with a demanding patient case load. You'll find that my transcript and letters of recommendation attest to this fact."

> **Did you know?**
>
> In a survey of 230 urology residency applicants conducted in 1999, "being asked about marital status was recalled by 91% of male and 100% of female, if they had children by 25% of male and 62% of female, applicants, respectively."[18]

> **Did you know?**
>
> As offensive as some of these questions may be, please realize that most interviewers who ask these questions do so out of ignorance, rather than with any intent to discriminate. In my conversations with colleagues, I've found that these questions are often asked because of genuine interest in the applicant. Some interviewers are simply unaware of what is, or isn't, appropriate. Clearly we need more training to educate residency interviewers in this important area. This was echoed by Dr. H. Gene Hern, Program Director of the emergency medicine residency program at Alameda Health System, who wrote that "each program should, regularly and in the beginning of interview season, reeducate their interviewers about what constitute illegal and inappropriate questions. The problem is that interviewers often do not consider their discussions with candidates as part of the protected aspect of job interviews. Faculty may pursue certain lines of questions unaware that they are technically violating employment law because of the setting of the conversation."[19]

Rule # 162 **If the interviewer asks if you have any questions about the residency program, the correct answer is "Yes, ma'am, I do."**

Most interviewers will set aside some time, usually at the end of the interview, for your questions. The advantage of asking questions is twofold:

- You can gather information about the program in order to make an informed decision about the program's place on your rank list.
- You can demonstrate to the interviewer your interest in the program.

When the interviewer asks, "Do you have any questions about the residency program?" the right answer is "Yes, I do." One of the worst answers you can give is "No, I don't have any questions." This is akin to saying, "I have no interest in your program," which may or may not be true.

Often, applicants prepare a question or two, only to find that the questions are answered during the course of the interview day. Then, when asked if they have any questions, they're forced to respond "No, I believe you've answered all my questions." To avoid this, prepare at least five or six questions. Although you need to prepare your questions in advance, don't read them off a piece of paper. Be careful not to ask a question that has already been answered. Doing so will prompt the interviewer to question your listening skills.

Even if a previous interviewer has answered all of your questions, there's no reason why you can't ask a different interviewer the same set of questions. It's better to repeat the same questions than to say, "I believe my questions were all answered by the other interviewer."

Tip # 115

When the interviewer asks "Do you have any questions?" this generally signifies the closing phase of the interview. If you didn't have the opportunity to communicate important points earlier, you can use this opportunity to do so. "Before I ask my first question, I would like to take a moment to mention a few other points. Would you mind if I do so now?" Keep your comments concise, especially at this closing phase of the interview.

Did you know?

In his article offering advice to dermatology applicants, Heymann encourages applicants to "ask questions that are stimulating and try to learn as much about us as we are trying to find out about you. There is a tremendous difference between the applicant who takes the time and effort to learn about our program and faculty's expertise compared with the person who only applies to be near his girlfriend in Philadelphia."[20]

Did you know?

Dr. Fitzgibbons, Associate Program Director of the internal medicine residency program at Lehigh Valley Hospital, encourages applicants to "ask unique questions. Something that will make the interviewer remember you."[21]

Did you know?

Be ready to ask questions. Some of my mock interview clients have reported that their entire interview consisted of the interviewer asking, "Do you have any questions?" One University of Buffalo medical student recalled his interview experiences. "Some interviewers brought me into the room, and just wanted to know what questions I had for them. Be sure to have a list memorized, as I am sure this will happen to you! Ask the same questions over and over at each place, even if you already know the answer - make sure to have enough questions to avoid a 30 second interview and to reduce the number of 'awkward silence' moments because you didn't have anything to ask, and they didn't want to ask you anything."[22]

Rule # 163 **The questions that you ask an interviewer send a message. Don't ask the wrong questions.**

Don't ask questions to which you should already know the answers. If the answer is readily found in the program's brochure or website, the interviewer will assume that you didn't bother to read the material, and that you're clearly not all that interested in the program. Therefore, the first rule of asking the right questions is to research the program before you arrive. Read the brochure. Read the program information that's sent before the interview. Study the program's website. Read the profiles of the faculty members.

Also avoid asking faculty about issues pertaining to vacation, call schedule, salary, insurance, or benefits. The image you wish to portray is that of an individual who's hard working, even in the face of long, stressful hours. That's hard to do when you're focused on how much you'll be paid and how much time off you're going to get. This information should be available in the program information sent to you. If not, save these questions for the house staff.

There are other types of questions that may be perceived in a negative fashion:

- Don't get so personal that you make an interviewer uncomfortable. "Are you married?" "How many children do you have?" (Applicants have actually asked me this.)
- Do not reveal your biases. "Will I be working with a lot of HIV patients?"
- Do not exhibit a poor sense of taste or strange sense of humor.
- Don't ask questions that make you appear too aggressive. Be especially careful with "why" questions. "Why doesn't the program have a liver transplant program?"

Tip # 116

Don't ask faculty about vacation, call schedule, salary, insurance, or benefits.

Did you know?

On July 1, 2003, the Accreditation Council for Graduate Medical Education (ACGME) implemented common standards for resident work hours. The goals were to improve patient safety and resident well-being while maintaining the educational quality of the residency experience. Applicants are understandably interested in a program's compliance with work hour guidelines. However, realize that this is a sensitive area.

In a 2004 survey of obstetrics/gynecology residency directors, many felt that the changes have negatively impacted resident education, the acquisition of key skills during residency, and work ethic.[28] In a survey of otolaryngology program directors, most were opposed to work hour restrictions, with only 23.9% being in favor.[29] In a more recent survey of nearly 240 internal medicine program directors, 60% believed that resident education had worsened following further work hour changes adopted in 2011. Only a small percentage of respondents believed that quality (8%) or safety of patient care (11%) had improved.[30]

Asking Questions: Advice For Applicants From Residency Program Interviewers	
Residency Program	**Comments**
Dr. Karen Horvath Program Director Department of General Surgery University of Washington	"You WILL be asked 'What questions do you have for me?' numerous times, be prepared and thoughtful! You may have to guide your own interview...Do not ask questions about work hour violations...You may be asked about work hour restrictions, and should have a thoughtful opinion...You should be ready to explain what YOU would bring to the program, which would improve things for the program somehow."[23]
Dr. Roy Ziegelstein Executive Vice-Chairman Department of Medicine Johns Hopkins Bayview Medical Center	"To me, 'meaningful questions' are those that seem 'meaningful' to the applicant. Just be yourself. Don't ask questions because someone told you that those are the questions you should ask. Ask the questions that are important or relevant to you. Also, come prepared – read about the program before your interview and try not to ask a lot of questions whose answers should be known to you before you visit the program."[10]
Department of Medicine University of Washington	"Some interviewers may not have received your application until that day and won't have had time to read it. They'll depend on you to hold up the conversation, so know enough about the program to ask some good questions."[24]
Dr. John McConville Program Director Department of Medicine University of Chicago.	"Prepare for your interviews by learning about the program through the web or other information materials. Ask questions that reflect you've studied the program (i.e. do not ask questions that are easily answered by the website or program materials)."[25]
Amy Voet Senior Advisor American Society of Anesthesiologists – Medical Student Component.	"Inevitably you will be given the opportunity to ask questions, usually ad nauseum. I highly recommend writing down a minimum of 10 specific open-ended questions about each program. You can ask general questions about the program, education, clinical duties, research opportunities, teaching opportunities and mentoring programs are good places to start. It is definitely a red flag if you don't have any questions to ask."[26]
Dr. Michelle Knight Department of OB/GYN Abington Jefferson Health	"The most uncomfortable part of interviewing is when there is silence. If you have a bunch of generic questions in the back of your mind, then you will be able to quickly cover over any lulls in conversation. Try to make your questions level-specific, i.e. think about your audience. A chairman won't know specific details about the curriculum or call schedule. An MFM attending won't know about the surgical facilities. It can be a pain in the butt, but try your best to ask the right questions of the right people."[27]

Your goal is to ask intelligent, thoughtful, and specific questions. Too often, applicants ask general questions that could be asked of any program. In phrasing your question, consider making a reference to the program's website, informational material, or a point that was raised earlier in the interview day (see example in Chapter 15: Interview Questions). When using this approach, don't go overboard. In some cases, it's clear that an applicant could care less about the answer, and in flaunting their research they only appear insincere. "I happened to notice that your residents last year published 14 original research articles, 20 case reports, and 10 book chapters."

Finally, ask your questions in an appropriate fashion. If you're not careful with your language usage or tone of voice, your interviewers may feel that you're grilling, challenging, or confronting them. For example, rather than asking "What are your program's weaknesses?" Dr. Wiebe suggests modifying the question to "If you had unlimited resources as a program director, what would you improve in the program?"[31]

Tip # 117

While you're free to ask general questions about the program, specific questions that demonstrate that you've researched the program will have more of an impact.

Questions To Ask Faculty Interviewers

General

- What are the major strengths of the program?
- What are the main differences between this program and others in the area?
- If you could change one thing about your program, what would it be and why?
- What changes in the residency program are likely in the next few years?
- What qualities are you looking for in a residency applicant?

Education

- How does your program demonstrate its commitment to the residents' education?
- What percentage of attending or teaching rounds is spent at the bedside?
- Is attendance at a national conference encouraged? Does the program offer any funding?
- What resources are available to assist residents in the fellowship application process?
- What resources are available to assist residents in locating an academic position following residency?
- How does the program assist residents seeking private practice positions in the local area?
- Is there flexibility to do rotations at other institutions?

Clinical duties/responsibilities

- How autonomous would you say the residents are in the program?

Research opportunities?

- What research opportunities are available for residents?
- Is protected time available for research during residency?
- What type of research have the residents done in recent years?
- What research projects are currently ongoing?

Teaching opportunities/responsibilities

- What teaching responsibilities do residents have in regard to medical students?
- Are there resources for improving resident teaching, such as workshops?

Advising/mentoring

- Is there a formal advising/mentoring program for new residents? If so, how does this program work?
- How often are advisors and advisees expected to meet?

Specialty board examination

- How have your graduates performed on the specialty board exam?
- Is there a didactic series to help residents prepare for the boards?

Graduates

- Where are your graduates (private practice, academics, local area, etc.)?
- What percentage of your graduates successfully place in fellowships? Which fellowships do they get into? Where?
- What percentage of your graduates pursue private practice? Where?

You won't have unlimited time to ask questions. Therefore, use your judgment to decide when to ask your last question. Keep track of the time and pay close attention to your interviewer's body language. If you sense that your time is up, proceed to your closing statement.

Rule # 164 **You need to make a good first impression. You also need to leave the interviewer with a good final lasting impression.**

Earlier we discussed the importance of making a good first impression. You also need to leave the interviewer with a good final lasting impression. You can do so by telling the interviewer you were glad to meet her. Thank her for this opportunity to meet, and for considering you for one of their positions. Leave with a smile, direct eye contact, and a firm handshake (if the interviewer extends her hand to you).

Some applicants go a step further by expressing interest in the program:

Thank you very much for taking the time to interview me. I've really enjoyed my visit and have been quite impressed with your program. I would be very excited to be a resident here. Is there any other information I can provide you?

Tip # 118

Practice your closing statement so that you can deliver it smoothly.

Tip # 119

Although you'll have opinions about how the interview went, don't reveal emotions to the interviewer. We've seen candidates unfortunately end interviews with sighs of relief or disappointment. End your interview in a confident manner.

Rule # 165 Meet with house staff on your interview day.

Some of the most valuable and forthright information about a residency program will come from the interns and residents currently in training. They'll usually be honest about their experience and are usually willing to answer any questions.

As we've mentioned, certain types of questions are best asked of residents. Questions regarding call schedule, salary, vacation, and moonlighting are examples. However, when speaking to residents, be very careful about what you ask, how you ask, and when you ask. Program directors frequently ask the current residents for their impressions of the candidates. Your interactions with the residents are all up for later discussion. Meeting a resident for the first time, and then immediately jumping in with questions about benefits or salary, could lead one to wonder about your priorities and values. Save these questions for later in the discussion.

Since questions about programs often arise after the interview, ask several residents for their e-mail address. Follow up later if necessary.

During most interview days, applicants typically have an hour or so, perhaps at lunch, to meet with the house staff. This may not be enough time, especially if the ratio of applicants to residents is high. In your interactions with the residents, strive to find answers to the important questions:

- Are the residents happy?
- Would I fit in with the current group of house staff?
- Would I be happy as a resident in this program?

Did you know?

In survey after survey, among the most important factors affecting medical student ranking of programs was the perceived happiness of the current residents.

If you aren't offered an opportunity to meet with the residents, consider this a red flag. It's quite possible that the program is shielding you from their residents because they want to discourage a free exchange of candid information. If the program remains one in which you are seriously interested, be aggressive about contacting the residents at a later date.

Tip # 120

Because there's often insufficient time to spend with residents on the interview day, make it a point to attend all pre-interview dinners. Also, don't be afraid to contact residents to follow up on issues after your interview day.

Tip # 121

Don't just focus on the first year of residency, as many applicants do. Learn and ask questions about each year.

Questions To Ask Residents

General

What are the major strengths of the program?
What are the major weaknesses of the program?
Do you feel that you've received good training?
Are the residents happy?
What do residents like the most?
What do residents like the least?
What is an average day like?
What are the main differences between this program and others in the area?
What is the morale of residents? Faculty?
If you could change one thing about your program, what would it be and why?
What changes in the residency program are likely in the next few years?
What has changed since you came to the program?
Is the program responsive to suggestions for change?
Knowing what you now know, would you still train here?

Inpatient clinical duties/responsibilities

What is the patient load like? How does it vary from service to service?
Do you feel that the patient load is too much, too few, or just right?
How many residents/ interns are present on each service?
What is the call schedule like? What is the experience like?
When you are on call, which patients are you responsible for?
What are your on-call responsibilities?
What rotations are required during the first year of residency?
What rotations are required during the second and third years of residency?
How are the clinics organized? Are attending physicians present?

Do you feel that you have enough faculty supervision on the floors? What about the clinics?
Do you feel that you have enough autonomy?
What kind of attending backup support is available while on call?
What type of ancillary support (phlebotomy, physical therapy, respiratory therapy, social workers, and discharge planning) is available at each of the affiliated hospitals? How is it different on weekends?
How much time do you spend in the operating room?
When in the residency do you begin to operate?
What are the total number and variety of procedures/surgeries per resident?

Outpatient clinical duties/responsibilities

How much time is spent in the clinics? What about subspecialty clinics?
Are residents able to follow patients whom they've discharged from the hospital?
What is the teaching like in the clinics?

Patients

What is the nature of the patient population?
Are residents involved in the care of patients followed by private physicians? If so, what percentage of my patients will be private? With regard to private patients, who writes the patient orders?
Do private physicians take the time to discuss patient-related issues with residents?

Resident education

Can you fill me in on the conference schedule (lectures, grand rounds, morbidity and mortality, morning report, journal club, board review course)?
How many of the resident conferences are required?
Do you have time to attend conferences?
What is the quality of the conferences?
Who runs these conferences – faculty or residents?
Is there an appropriate balance between service obligations and the educational program?
Are there opportunities for research? Is research required?

Medical student teaching

Are there medical students on the team? If so, how many patients do they follow?
What are the expectations of the residents as teachers?

Radiology

Does the program offer any formal training in the reading of films, CT scans, other?
Is a radiologist available 24 hours a day?
Are there formal radiology rounds?
How difficult is it to schedule radiology tests and procedures after the regular work day?

Faculty

What is the relationship between residents and faculty?
How responsive and committed to the residents are the faculty?
How much teaching do they do?
How much supervision do you have?
Are there any known upcoming faculty changes?
Is the department stable?
How approachable are the faculty?
Are the program director and faculty open to suggestions about the program?
Is there a particular subspecialty lacking in either quality or quantity?

Residents

What do residents do in their free time?
Is it a collegial environment?

What is the level of camaraderie among the residents?
Have any residents left the program in the past few years? If so, why?
What is the function of the upper level residents on the team?
How well do senior residents relate to their junior colleagues?

Specialty Board Examination

Do you feel that the program prepares you well for boards?
Do you have enough time to read?

Graduates

Do residents have any difficulty finding jobs in private practice?
Do residents have any difficulty securing fellowship positions?
How does the program support residents who plan to pursue subspecialty training?
How many people get the fellowships they want?
How many people were unable to land a fellowship position last year?
Do any of the residents stay on as faculty?

Employment benefits

What is the starting salary?
What are the basic resident benefits?
Does the program pay for parking? Is it easily available?
How is the health/life insurance?
Is there a stipend for travel to conferences? If so, how much?
Can you moonlight during residency? If so, what are the rules? What opportunities are available locally?
Is there a resident union or association? Is membership mandatory? Does it cost anything to be a member?
What is the program's family leave policy? Do you have maternity/paternity leave?

Vacation/Time Off/Sick Leave

What is the vacation schedule?
Do you have any days off during a rotation?
Is the program in compliance with ACGME work hour guidelines?
Do you ever exceed the maximum work hours?

City

What is it like to live in this city?
Where do most of the residents live? What is the housing situation? What is the cost of housing?
What is the cost of living?
Is the area safe?

Rule # 166 During your interview visit, meet with faculty or house staff from your own institution.

During your interview visit, try to meet with faculty or house staff who trained at your own medical school. Seek out these individuals. They can be a valuable source of information. Because you share a common bond, they may be forthright with you about the strengths and weaknesses of the residency program you're considering. In addition, they can compare and contrast the program with the residency program you know best, the one at your medical school.

Not sure how to locate these individuals? Start with your student affairs office. Ask to see a list of senior medical students who've graduated over the past three to five years. Make a note of those who are now training at the institutions you'll be visiting. Call or e-mail them to schedule a time to speak over the phone. If you can't locate their e-mail address, write to them using the program's address. See if you can meet with them on the interview day.

Tip # 122

While on the interview trail, you'll meet students from a variety of schools. Discussions with these applicants can be informative, especially if they attend schools affiliated with programs to which you've applied.

Rule # 167 Grade the residency program immediately after your visit.

As soon as you have a chance, write down your impressions of the program. What did you like? What didn't you like? Do this as soon as possible, while the program is fresh in your mind. Be as specific as possible. After just a few interviews, it will be difficult to keep track of each program's details. Similarities and differences between programs will blur.

Prior to your first interview, make a list of characteristics that are important to you in a residency program. For an example, see the "Residency Program Evaluation Guide" in the publication *Strolling Through the Match* (available at the AAFP website).[32] After the interview, grade each program on a scale of 1 to 5 according to each criterion. After your last interview compare the grades, notes, and information from the various programs. This will help you create your rank list for the final decision process.

Did you know?

In their article "Impact of the interview in pediatric residency selection," Swanson and colleagues offered some insight into what happens following an interview at their institution.[33] At the conclusion of the interview, the interviewer completes a score form. The candidate is given a score from 1 to 6, with a 1 indicating "outstanding: a must have" and a 6 indicating "poor fit." The candidate is then presented to the selection committee by the interviewer at a meeting that takes place the day following the interview.

Tip # 123

As soon as you can, jot down some points discussed during the interview. This will help you personalize your thank-you notes.

Did you know?

In a survey of radiology PDs, it was learned that 76.5% of programs use residents and fellows as interviewers.[34] All members of the interviewing body vote in the ranking of candidates in 88.1% of the programs. 6.5% of the programs use panel interviews and 15 directors stated that the "fit" of the candidates in the program and a "gut feeling" were the most important criteria for deciding admission. The interviewing body is responsible for making the final ranking in 62.9% of the programs, while the PD has the final word in 33.8%.

Rule # 168 Grade yourself after the interview.

Some candidates leave an interview thinking they "aced it" while others feel like they "blew it." Such impressions are based on opinions that students form from the interviewer's disposition and bearing during the interview. Because interviewers won't usually share their thoughts about your performance, this type of thinking is not productive. In fact, there are many students who match into a program despite feeling as if they "blew it" during the interview. There are many examples of the opposite as well – applicants who were sure that they "aced" the interview but didn't match.

There are many more interviews to come. It's more productive to ask these questions after every interview:

- Did I make a good first impression?
- Did I answer each question appropriately and effectively?
- Were my answers supported by evidence whenever possible?
- Could I have answered some questions better?
- Did any of the questions surprise me? If so, which ones? Why did they surprise me?
- Was I able to establish rapport with the interviewer?
- Did I make a good final impression?
- How can I use this experience to better prepare for my next interview?

References

[1]The Successful Match: Getting into Ophthalmology. Available at: http://studentdoctor.net/2009/08/the-successful-match-interview-with-dr-andrew-lee-ophthalmology/. Accessed September 20, 2012.

[2]Student Doctor Network. Available at: http://forums.studentdoctor.net/threads/ask-the-program-coordinator.1107601/. Accessed February 22, 2016.

[3]Insights on residency training. Available at: http://blogs.jwatch.org/general-medicine/index.php/2011/12/be-all-that-you-and-the-program-want-you-to-be/. Accessed February 22, 2016.

[4]Freeman T, Sawyer C, Behnke R. Behavioral inhibition and the attribution of public speaking anxiety. *Communication Education* 1997; 46: 175-187.

[5]Young M, Behnke R, Mann Y. Anxiety patterns in employment interviews. *Communication Reports* 2004; 17(1): 49-57.

[6]Larkin M. Getting a grip on handshakes. *Lancet* 2000; 356: 227.

[7]Chaplin W, Phillips J, Brown J, Clanton N, Stein J. Handshaking, gender, personality, and first impressions. *Journal of Pers Soc Psychol* 2000; 79: 110-117.

[8]Blink Test Research presented at the 2011 International Anesthesia Research Society. Available at: http://www.iars.org/abstracts/11_Abstract_Supplement_FINAL.pdf. Accessed August 12, 2012.

[9]Gastroenterology and Endoscopy Reviews. Available at: http://www.gastroendonews.com/ViewArticle.aspx?d=In+the+News&d_id=187&i=December+2011&i_id=794&a_id=19879. Accessed August 21, 2012.

[10]The Successful Match: Interview with Dr. Roy Ziegelstein. Available at: http://studentdoctor.net/2009/06/the-successful-match-interview-with-dr-roy-ziegelstein/. Accessed September 5, 2012.

[11]Cole K. *The Complete Idiot's Guide to Clear Communication*. Published by Alpha Books in 2002.

[12]Weiten W, Lloyd M. *Psychology Applied to Modern Life: Adjustment in the 21st Century*. Thomas Wadsworth 2005.

[13]Kitayama S, Cohen D. *Handbook of Cultural Psychology*. Guildford Press; 2007.

[14]University of Florida College of Medicine. Available at: http://osa.med.ufl.edu/first-year-orientation/faq/student-advice/. Accessed February 20, 2016.

[15]Stanford University Department of Anesthesiology. Available at: http://askalex.stanford.edu/archives/applicant-questions/. Accessed August 18, 2012.

[16]AAMC Graduation Questionnaire – 1996. Available at: https://www.aamc.org/data/gq/. Accessed March 3, 2008.

[17]Hern H, Alter H, Wills C, Snoey E, Simon B. How prevalent are potentially illegal questions during residency interviews? *Acad Med* 2013; 88 (8): 1116-21.

[18]Teichman J, Anderson K, Dorough M, Stein C. Optenberg S, Thompson I. the urology residency matching program in practice. *J Urol* 2000; 163(6): 1878-1887.

[19]Hern H, Wills C. In reply to Clancy. *Acad Med* 2014; 89 (3): 371.
[20]Heymann W. Advice to the dermatology residency applicant. *Arch Dermatol* 2000; 136: 123-124.
[21]Kohli N. 411 on Acing the Residency Interview. *ACP Impact*; 2004: 10(4):
[22]State University of New York at Buffalo. Available at: http://www.smbs.buffalo.edu/polityorg/sig/files/SIG%20Applying%20For%20Surgery.doc. Accessed February 20m, 2016.
[23]University of Washington Surgery Interest Group. Available at: http://students.washington.edu/uwsig/resources/Surgery_Med_Student_Advice_%20Final.pdf. Accessed February 22, 2016.
[24]University of Washington Department of Medicine. Available at: http://depts.washington.edu/medclerk/drupal/pages/Internal-Medicine-Residency-Application-FAQ. Accessed September 15, 2012.
[25]University of Chicago Residency Process Guide. Available at: http://pritzker.uchicago.edu/current/students/ResidencyProcessGuide.pdf. Accessed September 3, 2012.
[26]American Society of Anesthesiologists. Available at: www.asahq.org/~/media/.../Optimize%20Your%20Match.ashx. Accessed on August 2, 2012.
[27]Jefferson Medical College. Available at: http://jeffline.jefferson.edu/Students/residency/pdf/Ob-Gyn.pdf. Accessed September 12, 2012.
[28]Nuthalapaty F, Carver A, Nuthalapaty E, Ramsey P. The perceived impact of duty hour restrictions on the residency environment: a survey of residency program directors. *Am J Obstetr Gynecol* 2006; 194(6): 1556-1562.
[29]Brunworth J, Sindwani R. Impact of duty hour restrictions on otolaryngology training: divergent resident and faculty perspectives. *Laryngoscope* 2006; 116: 1127-1130.
[30]Garg M, Drolet B, Tammaro D, Fischer S. Resident duty hours: a survey of internal medicine program directors. *J Gen Intern Med* 2014; 29(10): 1349-1354.
[31]Wiebe C. Face-to-face value. *New Physician* 1994; 43: 15-17.
[32]AAFP Strolling Through the Match. Available at: http://www.aafp.org/dam/AAFP/documents/medical_education_residency/the_match/strolling-match2015.pdf. Accessed February 2, 2016.
[33]Swanson W, Harris M, Master C, Gallagher P, Maruo A, Ludwig S. The impact of the interview in pediatric residency selection. *Amb Pediatr* 2005; 5(4): 216-220.
[34]Otero H, Erturk S, Ondategui-Parra S, Ros P. Key criteria for selection of radiology residents: results of a national survey. *Acad Radiol* 2006; 13: 1155-1164.

Chapter 15

Interview Questions

How are you today?

Did you have any trouble getting here?
How do you like the weather?
Did you have any trouble finding a place to park?
How do you like [our city]? Have you ever visited [our city] before?
Was there a lot of traffic on your way here from the airport (or hotel)?

The above questions, known as icebreaker or "small talk" questions, are usually asked at the beginning of an interview. While this portion of the interview may only last several minutes, its importance can't be overemphasized. If icebreaker questions are answered well, they can set a positive tone for the rest of the interview, and put both you and the interviewer at ease.

While these questions appear simple, many applicants handle them improperly. Generally, applicants prepare heavily for the deeper questions, but give no thought to these types of icebreaker questions. Savvy interviewers recognize this and purposefully engage applicants in small talk. In doing so, they hope to learn more about an applicant's true personality.

The key with this type of interaction is to reinforce your overall message, and therefore respond in a confident and positive manner. Answer "How are you today?" with an answer such as "I'm doing great. I'm really happy to be here today" rather than "OK," or "Tired." Unfortunately, we've interviewed many applicants who end up whining or complaining about one thing or another. You may hate the weather or dislike the city. You may have had difficulty finding the office or struggled with the commute. There's no reason to share this with your interviewer.

Do you have any questions?

Applicants expect this question will be asked at the end of the interview. However, this isn't always the case. Occasionally, an interviewer will open with this question. She may wish to test your composure and initiative. Or you may be dealing with an inexperienced interviewer. Have a list of questions ready.

Regardless of when asked, this is a very important question. In fact, some would argue that it is the most important question. Some interviewers consider the quality of the questions asked to be more important than answers given.

Many interviewers consider it a red flag when an applicant has no questions. The worst thing you can say is "No, I don't have any questions" or "My questions have already been answered." This is akin to saying that you have no interest in the program. Your interviewer may also wonder if you've actually prepared for the interview. Answering "no" also robs you of the opportunity to gain valuable knowledge about the program, the type of knowledge that would help you make an informed ranking decision.

Too often, applicants ask standard or basic questions that have been answered at the program's website or in their brochure; such questions imply poor preparation. Ask informed questions to learn more about the program. You should convey the fact that you are knowledgeable about the specialty, and your questions should convey the fact that you were interested enough in the program to research it in advance.

To ask the "right" questions, begin by researching the program in great depth. Learn all that you can about the program by using a variety of sources – the program's website, an internet search, the program brochure, your advisors and faculty, and so on. Savvy applicants begin their question with a reference to what they have learned. "On your website I learned about the importance the program places on developing resident teaching skills. I was excited to read about this because I've really enjoyed my teaching experiences as a medical student tutor. I understand that teaching workshops are offered several times a year. Can you tell me more about these workshops?" Note that in this example, the applicant starts by making a reference to the program's website. He then proceeds to ask a thoughtful and specific question tailored to the residency program. In doing so, he clearly conveys his experiences teaching as a medical student, his passion for it, and his desire to continue it as a resident. If the program is seeking dedicated teachers, this applicant has succeeded in matching his skills to the needs of the program.

Often the best questions are those derived from something the interviewer said earlier. "You mentioned that the program offers a unique lecture series to train residents as researchers. What topics are covered in this series?"

We've provided a full table of possible questions to ask faculty members in Chapter 14 "The Interview Day" (see Rule # 163).

Some other tips

- After making a list of questions, prioritize them. You usually won't have the chance to ask all of your questions. If you could only ask a single question, which one would it be?

- Use your best judgment regarding the number of questions to ask and when to ask them.

- Ask open-ended rather than yes/no questions.

- Keep the questions short.

- Avoid "Why" questions. These can sound critical.

- Be aware of the manner in which you ask your questions. If you are not careful with the language you choose or the tone of voice you use, your interviewer may feel that you are grilling, challenging, or confronting her.

- Take care in how you phrase a question. Avoid asking questions that suggest biases, such as "Will I have to work with a lot of private attendings?"

- Allow the interviewer to finish replying; do not interrupt.

- You are permitted to ask the same questions of different interviewers. Hearing the perspectives of multiple people at the program is very helpful.

- Never ask a faculty member about salary, vacation, or benefits.

Tell me about yourself

This question is typically asked at the start of an interview, either as the first question or the question that immediately follows icebreaker questions. Given its common use, you should prepare for this question in advance. Outline and rehearse your response.

In developing your response, include the type of information that the program wants to know about you. What is impressive about your qualities or achievements? What sets you apart from other candidates? Why should the program select you as a resident?

Too often, applicants give their entire life stories, beginning with when and where they were born. Don't interpret this question as one that is focused purely on your personal background. Rather, regard it as an opportunity for you to share your most important skills, experiences, and accomplishments. In developing your response, focus on what qualifies you to be a resident at their institution.

Think of your response as a positioning statement. The questions from the interviewer that follow will often be based on the information you provide.

Summarize your background in ninety seconds. Time yourself to make sure you don't exceed this amount of time. Avoid providing irrelevant details, since we can state from personal experience that many candidates tend to ramble needlessly.

Because this question can be interpreted in different ways, interviewers are also eager to learn about the approach that you take in answering it. What do you focus on? How do you organize the information? Your content and delivery provides the interviewer information about your composure and communication skills.

What are your weaknesses?

What is your worst quality?

If you could change one thing about your personality, what would it be?

What are your pet peeves?

What would your friends say is your biggest weakness?

What might your last resident or attending physician want to change about your work habits?

First of all, don't respond by saying you have no weaknesses. Some interviewers actually ask for several, so you should prepare three weaknesses to discuss.

You are not obliged to share your worst qualities with the interviewer. Unfortunately, many applicants do just that, usually because they're taken off guard. When choosing a weakness to discuss, avoid stating one that is damaging. If your weakness would interfere with your ability to function as a resident, then present a different one. Stating that you are often late or have trouble working with other people would be presenting damaging weaknesses. Avoid sharing a character flaw or a negative personality trait. These can be difficult, if not impossible, to change.

Classically, applicants have been advised to relate a potential strength as a weakness. One example of this approach is the classic "People tell me I'm a workaholic." Who wouldn't want a resident with a strong work ethic? Equally common is the "perfectionist" example. Who wouldn't want a resident who pays close attention to detail? "I expect too much of others" is another commonly used example. This suggests that you set high standards. Yet another example is "I try to be friends with everyone." This suggests that you would be a good team player. We caution you on these four examples. Because many applicants have used these weaknesses over the years, they have become trite and unoriginal, and interviewers are tired of hearing them.

One approach would be to present an area that needs improvement, preferably something that can be acquired through training. For example, you could discuss how you would like to become fluent in Spanish and how that would be beneficial to you as a resident physician. With this type of response, you would always include the steps taken to correct this weakness.

What are your strengths?

What sets you apart from the crowd?

What do you think your fellow medical students would say about you?

How would your friends describe you?

How would your teammates describe you?

How would you describe yourself?

Name three adjectives that describe you.

What are your key skills?

What attributes will make you a valued presence at our program?

Why are you a more attractive candidate than others?

What personal quality makes you perfect for a position in our residency program?
What are your greatest assets?

While these may seem like easy questions, too often applicants deliver a response that isn't as strong as it could have been. Your choice of which strengths to share should not be taken lightly. Too often, applicants choose to mention strengths that have little or no relevance to one's ability to excel as a resident. You should research and determine the qualities that are highly valued in your chosen specialty and at the specific program. Think about work strengths (e.g., organizational skills, problem solving) and personality traits. Cite those strengths that you have in common and that are most relevant to the position you are seeking. For example, the American Society of Anesthesiologists states that "an anesthesiologist has to be incredibly detail-oriented, skillful at procedures, calm in stressful situations, and warm and caring to ease patient's anxiety."[1]

Rather than providing a long list of strengths, pick three of your top strengths. Too many applicants end up rambling. Keep your response concise. Many applicants will name their strengths and then stop. The responses that make the deepest impressions are those that use examples to support the strengths. One example: "My ability to persevere has been central to my success. The pathology interest club that I wanted to set up at my medical school was initially applauded, but my cofounder and I hit many obstacles. Even though I started during first year, the club didn't come into existence until my third year, and it was my perseverance that kept me going and dealing with all the roadblocks."

Be careful when you answer the questions, "What sets you apart from the crowd? And "Why are you a more attractive candidate than others?" Don't speak negatively about the rest of the applicant field, as is easy to do. Respond by stating that you realize the other applicants are qualified, but that you are confident that your abilities and qualifications will make you an excellent resident. There's a fine line between self-confidence and arrogance, so tread carefully.

Why have you chosen this specialty?

How can you be sure that this specialty is the right career for you?
Why would you be particularly good in this specialty?

Be prepared to discuss the factors or reasons that led you to select the specialty. One approach would be to begin with whatever piqued your interest in the specialty. Was it a personal experience, a course, or an inspiring professor or mentor? From there, consider discussing how your interest was further solidified through rotation experiences, discussions with residents and faculty in the field, and the knowledge you've gained through your own research and reading.

In asking this question, your interviewer is trying to determine your interests and motivations, and your fit with the specialty and the program. Avoid discussing lifestyle or financial issues as motivating factors. Don't say that a family member in the field encouraged you to consider the specialty; you need to emphasize your own enthusiasm for the specialty. Your interviewer is also interested in learning the steps that you took to make this important decision. The way you describe your decision-making process will give the interviewer an idea of how you might approach other important decisions.

As you progress through the interview season, you will become tired of answering this question. Avoid giving the impression that you are bored and lacking in enthusiasm for the field. It is essential that you remain passionate about your chosen field, even at the end of a long interview season.

Why did you apply to this program?

What qualities are you looking for in a program?
What are you looking for in a program?
Describe your ideal residency program.
What do you believe our program would give you that another program would not?
What interests you the most about our program?
Tell me what you know about this program.
What have you learned about our program from others?
Why do you want to be a resident here?
How do you view our program?
What two or three items are most important to you in a residency program?

Questions like these are often asked in interviews. Be prepared with an outstanding response. The best response is one that demonstrates that you are perfect for the program, and that the program is perfect for you. After answering this question, your interviewer should be convinced that you really want to be a resident in their program.

Begin by researching the program thoroughly. What makes the program unique? What do you find particularly attractive about the program? This information will allow you to tailor your response to the program. In other words, if the program values research highly, you should discuss your experience and interest in research.

If a faculty member recommended the program, then by all means say so. Programs like to know that they are well regarded. Taking the time to speak with someone who has firsthand knowledge of the program also demonstrates that you have taken the time and initiative to learn as much as you can about the program. It demonstrates the seriousness of your interest in the program.

Be as specific as possible to confirm that your selection of their program as a possible residency choice was based on some thought and effort. Too often, applicants give a general answer. If you could give the exact same answer at another program, then your answer isn't good enough. "I first learned about your program through my faculty mentor. Dr. Garcia is a graduate of your program and she has always spoken glowingly of the training she received. As I researched your program, I learned about how many of your graduates have gone on to become academicians at medical schools across the country. As I look to the future, I too see myself as an academician and would like to go to a residency program that will prepare me for a career in academics. I have also developed an interest in healthcare management and was quite excited to learn that you offer residents the ability to obtain an MBA degree during residency. I know of no other program that can say that."

There are certain responses that you need to avoid at all costs. Avoid answers that confirm a disconnect between what you're seeking and what the program offers. Never put down another program. Lastly, while the geographic location of the program may be a major factor in your interest, avoid offering program location as the only or initial reason for applying to the program.

What will you contribute to this program?

In what specific ways will our program benefit from selecting you?

Make a list of your attributes and skills. Which of these would be highly valued by the program? While the skill set valued by programs is, in general, very similar, programs will often describe what they are specifically seeking in a resident. This information is typically available at the program's website. If it is, determine which skills or qualities you possess. Then prepare your response accordingly.

For example, at the website for the Department of Surgery at the Temple University School of Medicine, Dr. Goldberg, the chair, writes that "we achieve excellence in patient care and resident education by adhering to our departmental core values...They are quality, respect, safety, teamwork, trust, and integrity. These are the core values that our faculty, residents, and support staff will not compromise...We are looking for people who share our department's core values."[2]

Having read this, an applicant preparing for an interview at Temple may respond, "I know that your program highly values professionalism. In me, you'll find someone who shares the same values. I have been fortunate to work with many attendings who have demonstrated compassion, respect, and sensitivity in their interactions with patients and colleagues. These faculty members have been my role models. Recently, I was selected for membership in the Gold Humanism Honor Society chapter of my medical school. As a resident, I will continue to make this a top priority."

Why are you interested in training in this city/area?

Programs recognize that the geographic location of a program is a major factor influencing how candidates rank a residency program. In a survey of applicants to one emergency medicine residency program, program location was one of the five factors rated most important.[3] In a larger survey of over 7000 applicants applying to a variety of surgical and nonsurgical specialties, geographic location again was cited as a top factor influencing residency selection.[4]

Express your sincere interest in the city or area (and if you're applying there, you should have a sincere interest in living there for the next several years). If you're dealing with an unfamiliar geographic region, you'll have to do some research. What does the city have to offer? If you have family or friends in the area, feel free to mention that fact.

What do you do outside of medical school?

What is your favorite hobby?
What extracurricular activities do you participate in?
What are your leisure-time activities?

Programs are looking for applicants with outside interests, not those who are all work and no play. While the degree to which programs value outside interests and hobbies varies considerably, it's important to emphasize that you're interested in more than just work.

Stating that you have no time for hobbies or extracurricular activities may be viewed as a red flag. It would be better to state that although your free time is limited, you do enjoy ________.

Consider what your hobbies or interests reveal. Do they demonstrate your attention to detail or your ability to work as part of a team? These are qualities that are valued by residency programs. Savvy applicants use this question as an opportunity to highlight these types of qualities.

Unique interests or hobbies may also serve as a point of departure for further conversation or serve to increase rapport. They may also help faculty remember you more easily when it comes time to rank. I really liked the Meharry student who was an amateur entomologist.

Avoid the obvious negatives, such as activities or interests that are controversial or may be viewed negatively.

Did you know?

In a survey of otolaryngology PDs, personal or professional stress was the most common underlying problem in problematic residents.[5] Expect to be asked about your interests outside of work, and the ways in which you manage stress in your life.

Where do you see yourself in 10 years?

What are your long-term goals?
How much thought have you given to your future plans?
Are you planning to pursue a fellowship?
What are your plans after residency?

While these may seem to be innocent questions, the interviewer's intent may be to learn whether your professional goals are compatible with the overall philosophy of the program and the opportunities available there.

In answering this question, think about the program's mission. How does the mission align with your future plans? Does the program pride itself on the development of academicians? If so, telling the interviewer that you wish to enter private practice will clearly demonstrate that your goals are incompatible or unrelated to the program's mission.

Never lie about your future goals and plans. The pressure that many applicants feel to do so is real, and we acknowledge this fact. We discuss this issue further in Chapter 16. However, you do need to research and determine a program's mission before you start the application process. If their mission differs markedly from yours, then the program won't be the best place for you to reach your own goals.

There are several points we emphasize to applicants when preparing for this question. First, many students just aren't sure of their future plans at this stage in their career. Faculty recognize this fact. Therefore, avoid giving the impression that your plans are rigid. You may state that you are considering…as a future professional goal. While you may not be sure of your eventual goals, however, you should always provide evidence that substantiates your interest in, and potential for, achieving that goal. For example, if you state an interest in international health, then you should use this question as an opportunity to highlight your past experiences in the area.

Second, your answer should emphasize those aspects of your own application that would dovetail with the program's mission. If the program values the development of clinician-educators, then you should emphasize how much you enjoy teaching, how that is reflected in your prior employment and volunteer commitments, and how you plan to incorporate that goal in your future professional career.

Lastly, this question almost always refers to professional goals. We've had many applicants respond with the classic "I see myself as married and with children." Who doesn't? Your goal is to distinguish yourself with your answer, and to emphasize your personal and professional attributes that will lead to the development of an outstanding clinician.

What happens if you don't match?

Applicants applying to highly competitive specialties are most likely to be asked this question. International medical graduates applying to any field may also be asked about their future if they don't match. Don't be unnerved by this question. Some candidates mistakenly assume that if the interviewer asks this question, they are not a competitive candidate.

The interviewer asks this question hoping to learn about the depth of your commitment to the specialty. If you don't match, will you abandon your desire to enter the field? Or do you have a back-up plan that will allow you to reapply in one year? What does your back-up plan consist of? Will you do a transitional or preliminary year with the intent to reapply? Will you pursue a research fellowship in an effort to strengthen your application? A well thought out back-up plan that allows reapplication implies a deeper commitment to the specialty.

Where else are you interviewing? Where have you applied other than here?

According to the NRMP Match Communication Code of Conduct, programs are no longer allowed to ask these questions. "Applicants shall at all times be free to keep confidential the names or identities of programs to which they have or may apply."[6]

Unfortunately, many interviewers are not aware that these questions are prohibited. We continue to encounter many applicants every year who've been asked these questions. With that being the case, we encourage you to consider how you would handle such queries.

Most applicants would answer these questions in a straightforward and honest fashion. You may have applied to, or interviewed at, twenty programs, but you don't need to provide the entire list. It's acceptable to state, "I've applied to over twenty programs, including..."

In choosing which programs to name, consider your current interview location. Try to offer programs that are similar in caliber, philosophy, geographical location, and so forth. We've seen applicants try to impress interviewers by naming two or three top tier academic programs. This may not resonate well with an interviewer at a community-based program.

While you may not see the need to be honest in answering this question, remember that the community of program directors is a small one. Once you respond, your interviewer may ask for your impressions about other programs. Respond, but avoid negative comments.

Close your response effectively. After providing the names of some programs, restate your interest in the current program.

Did you know?

In the NRMP Match Communication Code of Conduct, it is clearly stated that programs should not ask applicants about other programs to which they have applied or interviewed.[6] This is a relatively new rule, and we've found that some interviewers are not aware of it. You don't have to answer these questions during the interview, but you should give serious thought as to what you would say. Be gentle in your approach, because it's not usually malice that leads interviewers to ask these questions. To avoid awkwardness, we've found that most applicants will answer this question. Consider a nonthreatening response such as, "I'm still working on scheduling interviews but I'm looking at programs mainly in the Midwest." Finally, in the event that this happens to you, you do have the right to notify the NRMP about this practice. Your notification will lead the NRMP to initiate a violation investigation.

Tell me about your research.

Tell me about _____.

Everything in your application is fair game, including your research experience. Prepare in advance to discuss your research experience succinctly and eloquently. Review your projects and rehearse your response. Be prepared to discuss your research at any possible level, since you may be discussing it with an expert in the field. This is more important if your project was done several years ago. A poor response to this question may suggest that you embellished or exaggerated your involvement in the work.

I see that you had some difficulty in _____ course/clerkship. Could you tell me what happened?

I understand that you passed your USMLE Step 1 exam on the second attempt. Can you tell me what happened?

What explains this D on your transcript?

No one has a perfect application. Some applicants have a blemish on their record that requires explanation. Since interviewers will often bring up these issues, you need to have a plan in place to field these difficult questions. We recommend that you discuss your approach with your advisors.

Of major concern to the interviewer is the possibility that your poor performance was related to a lack of commitment, dedication, or intellectual ability. The concern is that these problems may resurface during residency training.

To alleviate these concerns, provide an explanation of the circumstances. Was there a death or serious illness in the family? Were you sick at the time? Life presents everyone with challenges, and medical students are no exception. If a hardship of this sort caused academic difficulty during a short period of time, a brief explanation will generally suffice. Make sure you emphasize that you performed at a higher level outside of this time period. In other words, finish by pointing to your successes.

If poor grades or scores were the result of academic rather than nonacademic issues, you must take responsibility for your record. Acknowledge it. Don't make excuses and don't sound defensive. If you do, the interviewer may question your ability to handle criticism or your willingness to admit to mistakes. Apologizing is not a good idea because it may be viewed as an indicator of low self-confidence. Some candidates have tried to inject humor into their response, hoping to defuse a difficult situation. This is not a good approach. A serious question requires a serious answer.

Explain the situation, why it happened, what you learned, how you overcame it, and why it won't happen again. End by emphasizing that your performance since then is a far better indicator of your motivation and intellectual ability.

Addressing a disciplinary problem noted in the Dean's letter will be far more challenging. Issues such as falsifying information, failure to respect patient confidentiality, failure to fulfill responsibilities, inappropriate interactions with team members, arrogance, inability to handle criticism, and inadequate personal commitment to patients are examples that will raise red flags. In fact, some studies have shown that these types of problems in medical school are predictive of future disciplinary action by state medical boards. You'll need to discuss these issues with your advisors, and formulate a response that emphasizes the lessons you learned and why you wouldn't repeat the behavior.

Tip # 124

Residency programs are on alert for any red flags in the application. The concern is that the prior issues may resurface during residency. Programs worry about the effects such issues may have on patient safety, morale among staff, and program reputation. If you have an area of concern, it is imperative that you be ready to discuss the situation and provide the evidence needed to reassure programs.

Did you know?

In a survey of otolaryngology PDs, the most common deficiencies noted among problematic residents were the following, in descending order of frequency:

- Unprofessional behavior with colleagues and staff
- Insufficient medical knowledge
- Poor clinical judgment[5]

What type of people do you have difficulty working with?

"None. I get along with everyone." This response will be viewed with skepticism. Few people can honestly make this claim, so avoid this answer.

The question, obviously, is asked to determine how well you work with others. One way to respond would be to state that you work well with all types of people, but you have found it challenging to work with people who "..." Examples would include people who don't fulfill their responsibilities, complete their share of the work, or who complain incessantly.

Do you prefer working as a member of a team or would you rather work alone?

While carrying out the duties of a resident requires the ability to work well with others as part of a team, it is also essential that you have the ability to perform individually. The best answer is one that demonstrates to the interviewer that you work well in both settings.

What do you perceive as the negatives about this program?

No program is perfect. In your research, you will undoubtedly come across some negatives. Some may be significant, while others may be minor. Should you be asked for your opinion about a program's negatives, tread carefully. The interviewer is hoping to hear that you don't see any major negatives, and therefore remain very interested in training at the program. Therefore, convey minor negatives, and always end your response with a positive spin.

What was your least favorite course or clerkship in medical school? Why?
What rotation was your most difficult?

Don't mention a course or clerkship that is related in any way to your chosen specialty. Stating that pharmacology was your least favorite course would be a poor answer for an applicant to anesthesiology. If asked why, avoid saying anything negative about those with whom you worked. For example, "I would have to say neurology. I had really looked forward to the rotation, but of all my rotations, it was the least hands-on."

Why did you attend your medical school?

Through this question, the interviewer is trying to learn about the way in which you make decisions. Provide a specific answer that demonstrates that your choice was not a random one. For example, you might comment on a particularly appealing aspect of the curriculum which was not available elsewhere.

> **Note...**
>
> If you're seeking more interview preparation beyond the chapters in this book, we've created an online course to help guide you further on how to develop winning answers to residency interview questions. The course includes numerous sample answers to questions you will encounter during interviews. Visit TheSuccessfulMatch.com for course information.

References

[1]American Society of Anesthesiologists. Available at: http://www.asahq.org/career/faq.htm. Accessed December 4, 2015.
[2]Temple University Department of Surgery. Available at: https://medicine.temple.edu/departments-centers/clinical-departments/surgery/about. Accessed March 3, 2016.
[3]DeSantis M, Marco C. Emergency medicine residency selection: factors influencing candidate decisions. *Acad Emerg Med* 2005; 12 (6): 559-561.
[4]Nuthalapaty F, Jackson J, Owen J. The influence of quality-of-life, academic, and workplace factors on residency program selection. *Acad Med* 2004; 79 (5): 417-425.
[5]Bhatti N, Ahmed A, Stewart M, Miller R, Choi S. Remediation of problematic residents – A national survey. *Laryngoscope* 2015; Sep 22 (epub).
[6]NRMP Match Communication Code of Conduct. Available at: http://www.nrmp.org/code-of-conduct/. Accessed March 7, 2016.

Chapter 16

After the Interview

Post-interview communication is an important part of the residency selection process, and includes such practices as sending thank-you notes and letters, arranging for second looks, and responding to inquiries and communication from programs. You'll hear mixed opinions of the value of sending thank-you notes following interviews. Some advisors will vehemently urge you not to send notes, while others feel strongly that notes should be sent to every interviewer. Also heavily debated is the value of second look visits, a practice that adds considerable expense to a process that's already consumed thousands of dollars. In this chapter, we will present the evidence so that you can make an informed decision as to how to proceed in this important area.

Rule # 169 **Communicating with a residency program after the interview is an important aspect of the application process.**

Applicants can initiate post-interview communication in several ways. Most communicate with programs by sending letters, handwritten notes, or e-mail. Some candidates will even phone program directors or revisit institutions. There are many reasons that applicants communicate with programs following an interview:

- Common courtesy
- To thank the program
- To help the program remember them
- To demonstrate interest in the program
- To communicate their intent to rank the program highly
- To ask questions that come up after the interview day
- To request a "second look"
- For fear that not communicating will lower their place on the rank list
- To provide new information to the program about credentials ("update")

We review in more detail the three cornerstones of post-interview communication:

- Plan to thank every program for the opportunity to interview.

- Plan how to communicate and what to say to the top programs on your rank list.
- Plan how to respond to programs that initiate contact with you following the interview.

Did you know?

Following the interview, it is possible to move up the rank-order list. Updating the program with new information (award, publication, presentation, etc.) is one way to make this happen. "Candidates are subsequently re-evaluated based on the information in the file as well as additional information that becomes available," writes the Department of Orthopedic Surgery at Drexel University. "The program director and program chairman in consultation with members of the faculty and residents determine the final rank order that is submitted to the NRMP and GME offices."[1]

Rule # 170 **You should communicate with every program at which you interviewed.**

Unless a program specifically makes it known that it does not wish to be contacted, you must at the very least send a thank-you note. Not only is this common courtesy, but at *some* programs post-interview communication may serve as a selection factor, as we more fully describe below.

Note we specified "some" programs. We've talked to some faculty who don't care if they never receive any notes from applicants, and in fact find the flood of mail after an interview to be a hassle.

However, the opposite is true for many faculty members. "This applicant didn't even bother to send a thank you note. They must not be interested in our program. If they're not interested in coming here, they wouldn't be a good fit for us."

While some applicants recognize these facts and are diligent about communication with programs following the interview, not enough applicants do so. In one study, only 39% of applicants sent follow-up communication to every program with whom they interviewed. 55% communicated only with select programs.[2]

Did you know?

If a program informs you not to send a thank-you note, respect their wishes. Failure to do so may raise concerns about your ability to follow instructions. Understand that such policies don't mean that you can't communicate with these programs after the interview if you have questions or seek additional information. "We instruct applicants to not send 'thank-you' letters to interviewers and to not ask about their rank status before Match Day," writes the Department of Anesthesiology at the University of Miami. "We emphasize 'meaningful communication' with our applicants, specified as questions about our program, perspectives on living in our city, and contact information for current residents."[3]

Did you know?

"Some say (even some residency program directors say) that a thank-you note is not necessary after your interview," writes Dr. Terry Kind, Director of Pediatric Medical Student Education at George Washington University. "That it doesn't matter. That it neither enhances nor diminishes your chances of matching. I say, do send a thanks. Take a moment to compose a thoughtful thank you. Maybe mention something that occurred on or shortly after the interview day. Or convey something you meant to say during the interview. You can be brief. But be sincere. You could send it immediately, or take a few days if you are pressed for time. You can email, particularly if your interviewer gave you his/her email address (i.e. it was on his/her card or conveyed to you otherwise). Or you can send it the old fashioned way. Wouldn't text or tweet it, though."[4]

Tip # 125

Thank-you letters are not expected or desired at every program. In a survey of ophthalmology residency programs, only 14% wished to receive such letters.[5] Since you'll generally not know how a program views thank-you letters, our advice is to send these letters to each program (unless specifically instructed otherwise).

Rule # 171 **Your expressed interest in a program may impact their interest in you.**

Is there a chance that your communication with a program following the interview can influence your ranking? Absolutely. Not for every faculty member, and not for every program, but there is a chance that at some programs your expressed interest in the program may influence your ranking.

How would your interest in a program affect their interest in you? Your negative interest can provide a negative influence. For some faculty, the fact that an applicant didn't even bother to send a thank-you note sends the message that they're not interested in a particular program. Programs don't wish to rank applicants who have no interest in the program, because lack of interest can be an indicator of a poor fit.

A positive interest may have a positive influence. An applicant who ranks a program highly is likely to feel that the program would be a good fit for their interests and abilities, which is what a program seeks. An applicant who plans to rank a program highly would be thrilled to match there, and that hopefully translates to an enthusiastic, hard-working resident. It's also a point of pride for many programs to match those applicants at the top of their own rank list. In a study examining communication between programs and applicants, the authors wrote that "some program directors appear to construct their match lists with the goal of 'matching well' i.e., not having to go too far down their lists. To achieve this, knowing where applicants plan to rank them is a high priority."[6]

However, programs do differ widely in their beliefs on the value of post-interview communication. For some programs, what you say following the interview will have no effect whatsoever on the program's decision-making process. In a study of general surgery PDs, the authors found that they "were very skeptical of student ranking assurances, and were seldom influenced by such information."[2] In another study looking at recruitment behavior, the authors wrote that "program directors were very skeptical of student ranking assurances."[7]

However, the authors did feel that such assurances had an effect on ranking decisions at some programs. They felt that the impact of the rank order list was "limited to one third of programs."[7] Such information is clearly important to some programs, as shown in the following table.

Importance Of Post-Interview Contact By Specialty		
Specialty	**% Of Programs Citing Post-Interview Contact As A Factor In Ranking Applicants**	**Mean Importance Rating**
Anesthesiology	28%	3.7
Dermatology	22%	3.6
Emergency Medicine	36%	3.9
Family Medicine	43%	4.1
General Surgery	36%	4.1
Internal Medicine	21%	3.6
Med/Peds	26%	3.3
Neurosurgery	46%	4.2
Neurology	37%	4.0
Obstetrics & gynecology	35%	4.0
Orthopedic surgery	15%	3.9
Otolaryngology	20%	4.3
Pathology	40%	4.3
Pediatrics	27%	3.8
PM&R	30%	4.1
Psychiatry	30%	3.8
Radiation Oncology	25%	4.5
Radiology	38%	3.7
Results of the 2014 NRMP Program Director Survey. Available at: http://www.nrmp.org/wp-content/uploads/2014/09/PD-Survey-Report-2014.pdf.		

When Miller and colleagues surveyed graduating students at ten U.S. medical schools with respect to post-interview communication from programs <u>to</u> applicants, they found that 23% were asked how they planned to rank the program, and 21.7% were told that their level of interest would have bearing on their ranking (note that the NRMP states that programs are not allowed to ask applicants how they plan to rank programs).[6]

Surveys of PDs support this as well. In one study, emergency medicine PDs were asked to rate the importance of 20 items in the selection process. An applicant's expressed interest in the program was found to be a moderately important selection factor, although the standard deviation was noticeably high. In this study, it ranked of higher importance than the USMLE Step 1 score. The large standard deviation, however, indicates that there were significant differences in how PDs viewed this factor.[8] Other surveys indicate that programs commonly tell applicants to keep in touch if they have an interest in matching with their program, as outlined below.

Post-Interview Communication: Does It Help?

Study	Findings
Survey of emergency medicine program directors[8]	Respondents were asked to rate the importance of 20 items in the resident selection process on a scale of 1 to 5, with five being most important. An applicant's expressed interest in the program was found to be a moderately important selection factor with a mean score of 3.30 and a standard deviation of 1.19. of note, it was ranked of higher importance than the USMLE Step 1 score and nearly as high as the USMLE Step 2 score. The authors commented on the large standard deviation, emphasizing considerable differences between programs in the way they viewed post-interview communication.
Survey of fourth-year students at three medical schools[2]	Following the interview 57% were told by programs to keep in touch if they had an interest in matching there; 21.4% of PDs said that confirmatory rank-order statements from applicants had some positive effect; 2% of directors stated that such statements had a significant positive effect.
Survey of family practice program directors[7]	82% of programs told at least some of their applicants to keep in touch if they had an interest in matching with their program
Survey of urology program directors[9]	67% of programs told applicants to keep in touch if they had an interest in matching with their program.
Survey of obstetrics and gynecology program directors[10]	Approximately 30% of programs indicated that applicants who do not communicate following interviews were at a disadvantage.

Did you know?

"So many students are writing thank you notes that without a thank you note, you may be perceived as not interested in the program," writes Dr. John McConville, IM PD at the University of Chicago.[11]

Rule # 172 **The thank-you letter serves as another chance to emphasize your overall message, so don't send a generic one. Send a compelling and memorable thank you.**

The most effective thank-you letters contain the following information:

- Statement of appreciation for the opportunity to interview, and for the interviewer's time
- Statement indicating that you enjoyed meeting the interviewer
- Expression of appreciation for information shared with you
- Brief statement of why you are a good fit for the program (i.e., highlighting your ability to make a contribution to your program)
- Reference to a point raised or topic discussed during the interview (i.e., personalizing the note)
- Intent to rank the program highly (optional, as this must be truthful)
- Final statement of thanks

It's particularly important to emphasize how your qualities, skills, or strengths match the program's needs. What did you learn about the program that can help you explain more effectively why you are a good fit for the program? Few applicants take this additional step. Those that do so distinguish themselves from other candidates. The sample thank-you letter we've included in this chapter demonstrates how to emphasize your fit with a program.

Tip # 126

If the interviewer raised a concern about your application and you feel that you did not address it to the best of your ability, you may consider addressing it further in the thank you letter.

Tip # 127

If your thank-you notes are being sent early in the interview season, avoid communicating your intent to rank the program at the top of your list. Since you'll have other interviews, such a statement will cast doubts about your sincerity. Save statements about ranking until later in the interview season when you communicate again with a program to reiterate your interest.

Rule # 173 **Thank you letters may be sent in the form of a handwritten note, a typed letter, or an e-mail.**

All forms of thank-you correspondence are acceptable. While individual faculty members may have their own preference, it would be impossible for you to know that preference. The handwritten note implies a great deal of time and care in its production, and immediately sends a more personal message. However, the production of multiple handwritten notes is difficult, especially if you follow the norms of sending one to every single interviewer, and include sufficient information to personalize the note. While the typed letter can easily be expanded to include more information, it can give an impression of mass production, and therefore may not be as memorable. However, you can include sufficient detail to create a memorable letter and overcome this negative. The e-mail thank you may be seen as too informal and suggestive of a shortcut, particularly for more traditional faculty, but has the benefit of speed.

Our suggestion is to immediately send an e-mail thank-you letter to every interviewer, preferably within one day. This should be followed by either a typed letter or handwritten note. Either type should include specific details that refer back to the interview, and should include specific information that substantiates your fit for the program.

Note that these are not necessarily the norms of post-interview correspondence. Most students don't send immediate thank-you e-mails, and few of the thank-you letters we receive include the type of specific details that we suggest. Therefore, your utilization of these suggestions will aid in your goal of creating a memorable impression.

Did you know?

"After your interview, always send a thank you note by either snail mail or e-mail to thank your interviewers, program director and chairman," writes Dr. William McDade, Associate Professor of Anesthesiology at the University of Chicago Pritzker School of Medicine. "If the chief resident or other residents were especially helpful to you, thank them too. Do not be obsequious, but if you enjoyed yourself and see a place for your career development there, let them know it and why you would be a good fit for them. On rank list submission meeting day, all your comments have been kept and are brought out for discussion for final rankings in that department."[12]

Rule # 174 **As a general rule, thank you letters should follow the norms of a business letter.**

A typewritten thank-you letter that is to be mailed should follow the proper format. It should be considered a form of business correspondence and should follow the norms of a business letter. It should convey a professional message, and should be sent on professional stationery.

Proper Format of the Typewritten Thank-You Letter

Return address (your full name and address)

Date

Inside address (full name, including title/position, of interviewer and address)

Salutation ("Dear Dr. Smith:")

Body of letter

Closing ("Sincerely," or "Yours truly,")

Signature line (your signature above your typewritten full name)

AAMC ID #

Note that the above format is for typewritten letters that will be mailed. If you're planning on sending your letter by e-mail, the format will differ to some extent. Your e-mail message will begin with the salutation. You will then proceed to word the letter in the same way. Below your signature line, you should include your AAMC ID # so that your correspondence makes its way to your file. Before sending the e-mail, double check your subject line to make sure it's clear and concise. A subject line with "Thank you – residency interview (applicant name)" will ensure that your e-mail is not ignored or deleted as junk.

Rule # 175 A thank-you letter should be personalized.

Some applicants send a thank you letter to each interviewer, but fail to personalize their letters. A letter that's tailored to the individual faculty member is more effective and more memorable. If every applicant sends a generic thank-you letter, the impact of your generic letter can easily be lost. Unfortunately, after reading the fifth "Thank you for the opportunity to interview at Baylor. The strength of your faculty and the diversity of clinical experience were very impressive. I would be honored to train at such a program," the letters tend to blur into one. Use the thank you letter to further emphasize your message, and use it to help your interviewer remember you as an individual, not as one of many candidates. This can easily be done by mentioning items that were discussed in the interview. "I enjoyed hearing about your favorite restaurants in Chicago." This should be followed by a reminder of why you as a candidate are a perfect fit for the program, as we demonstrate later in this chapter.

Did you know?

"Most agree that form letters, however, are a waste of everyone's time," writes Dr. Jeff Gonzalez.[13]

Rule # 176 Send a thank you letter to each individual with whom you interviewed.

To whom should you send a thank-you letter? Our recommendation is to send a letter to each individual with whom you interviewed. Many applicants choose to send a letter only to the program director. These applicants fail to realize that the selection process varies markedly from program to program. While the PD may make ranking decisions at one program, at another ranking decisions may be made by all residency selection committee members. For example, at the general surgery residency program at the Medical University of South Carolina, Brothers wrote that "…all surgical faculty are given equal input, with individual members providing insight into applicants whom they interviewed."[14] Therefore, you should send a letter to each interviewer. We also recommend sending a letter to the program coordinator who has worked diligently and tirelessly to make sure your interview visit goes smoothly. They often don't get the credit they deserve.

Did you know?

"There is a controversy over whether notes are necessary after these interviews," writes Dr. Jeff Gonzalez. "At some institutions, for instance, they are NOT EVEN READ and may even be thrown out. However, many of us have stories of letters being written back to us, referencing these notes and assuming a level of interest/enthusiasm based on them. While they may not help, everyone agrees that they can't hurt."[13] "For most interviewers it's a trivial issue, but you have no idea who the one is that may actually pay attention." writes the Department of Medicine at the University of Washington.[15]

Rule # 177 Send notes early

Post-interview communication should be sent early. By early, we mean sending a thank-you e-mail or delivering a thank-you letter within hours after your interview. Why? To be most effective, your thank-you message should reach your interviewer before she completes her interview evaluation form or meets with the selection committee to discuss your candidacy. Therefore, time is of the essence. At some programs, interviewers are even asked to complete their evaluation form at the end of the interview day.

In our experience, few applicants send an e-mail within hours of an interview. A few have prepared notes or letters that are delivered to the clinic mailboxes the same day. However, the more common scenario is to receive an e-mail a few days later. For the postal mail, the thank you letter may take many days to arrive. In the university or hospital setting, there are often additional delays as mail is routed within the institution. As we mentioned, if you choose to send an immediate e-mail thank you, we recommend that you follow it with a more traditional, formal form of correspondence.

Rule # 178 A poorly written thank you can damage your candidacy.

Not bothering to send a thank you note can affect your chances of matching at a particular program. However, sending a poorly written note can prove more damaging. Avoid the following indicators of a poorly written thank you letter:

- Poor readability

  It's acceptable to send a handwritten letter but only if your handwriting is legible. If your penmanship leaves a lot to be desired, send a typewritten letter instead.

- Informal

  Your letter should be written in a formal manner, even if is sent by e-mail. Throughout your letter, your goal is to maintain the image of a professional and polished individual. Avoid "cutesy" stationery. Avoid the use of informal language, smiley faces and other emoticons, as well as internet lingo such as lol.

- Misspelled words/poor grammar/improper punctuation

  Your letter must be flawless. This means that it cannot contain any misspelled words, grammatical errors, or improper punctuation. Failure to correct these errors suggests a lack of attention to detail on your part.

- Making manual corrections to the letter

  If you catch a mistake, don't make manual corrections to your typewritten letter. This may seem obvious, but we've received such letters.

- Bragging or overassertive

  While you must feel comfortable writing about your strengths, take care with the words you use and the tone in which you write. You never want to appear as if you're bragging or overassertive.

- Focusing entirely on yourself

  Too often, thank you letters focus entirely on what the program can do for the applicant, rather than what the applicant can do for the program. Think about how you can make valuable contributions to the program and include specifics in your letter.

- Too much information

  To be effective, your thank you letter must be concise. Often, applicants write and write, cramming as much information as they can into the letter. Faculty members don't have the time to read through such letters.

> **Did you know?**
>
> "Be sure to spell check the note and make sure that the names/institutions are correct," writes Dr. John McConville, Internal Medicine Residency Program Director at the University of Chicago.[11]

Rule # 179 Plan what you'll do and say when you're contacted by a program following the interview.

Post-interview communication from programs to applicants occurs much more often than applicants would suspect. In a survey of obstetrics and gynecology PDs, 76.6% indicated that their programs contacted residency applicants following interviews.[16] Not only is it a common practice, but it can be a stressful one for applicants. Programs may contact you via e-mail, postal mail, or phone. The chairman, program director, or faculty member may send a simple e-mail stating how much they enjoyed meeting you during the interview. They may ask you to keep in touch if you're interested in their program. They may go further and make informal commitments to you. They may even ask how you plan to rank their program. They may even ask which program will be first on your rank list. Every applicant must plan well ahead of time how to handle these situations.

Did you know?

In a survey of graduating students at ten U.S. medical schools, the following was found with respect to post-interview communication from programs to applicants:[6]

41.7% of applicants received guarantees of the program's intent to rank them highly.
23% were asked how they planned to rank the program
21.7% were told that their level of interest would have bearing on their ranking
17% were asked which program would be first on their rank list

As a result of this communication, many applicants felt pressured to offer assurances to programs. Nearly 30% of respondents felt either very or moderately pressured. Communication by phone posed the most pressure.

Your strategy to handle these situations must be established well before you need it. A phone call from a PD calling to say how highly the program feels about your potential as a resident is a highly stressful situation, and is not the ideal time to be formulating a response. Your response must be one that does not jeopardize your chances of matching into the program, and must be one that in no way compromises your ethics.

The easiest response is when you know the program will be first on your rank list. There is no legal or ethical injunction against volunteering that the program will be first on your rank list. If the program won't be first on your list, or you're not sure, you can still honestly convey your interest in the program and admiration for it.

As we've emphasized throughout the book, always include specifics. When you're speaking to a PD, these specifics add credibility and emphasize that you're interested enough in the program to have done your research. The use of specifics also emphasizes that the program made a significant impression. You should have already created summary sheets for each of the programs at which you interviewed. These sheets, listing the strengths and weaknesses of each program, should be kept easily accessible. In the event of an email or phone call, you'll be able to honestly convey your impressions of the program.

"It would be a privilege to train at your program, especially because of my interest in…and the opportunities in…provided by Pickens University."

"I haven't finished interviewing yet, but I was very impressed by the program at Dow University. I'm most interested in obtaining strong clinical training, and the quality of the faculty, the subspecialty strengths, and the strong didactic program all support that."

"I'm so honored that you took the time to contact me and I'm so excited about the opportunity to train at Berkshire University. The…of the program, the…of the faculty, and the…are all reasons that I was so impressed with the residency training."

Tip # 128

Be prepared for a phone call, e-mail, or letter from a program informing you of their intent to rank you highly. Are you prepared to handle such a situation? Have your strategy in place before this occurs.

Did you know?

In a survey of students graduating from three medical schools, 13% of applicants were contacted by one or more programs who stated their intent to rank them number one.[2]

Did you know?

Lack of contact or communication from programs following your interview does not imply lack of interest in your candidacy. "Our program here at the University of Michigan has a policy of minimal to no communication with candidates after their interview day to avoid any potential impropriety or placing undue pressure on candidates to state their intentions," writes Dr. Diana Curran, Assistant Professor of Obstetrics and Gynecology at the University of Michigan.[17]

Did you know?

"Some programs routinely call their interviewees after they have interviewed," writes Dr. Elizabeth Thilo, Chair of the Pediatric Residency Selection Committee at University of Colorado. "Some programs call or contact only their top candidates. Some programs have a policy not to call or email at all. The bottom line is that you should not rely on any statements that you will be highly ranked. Nothing is final until the match lists are in and things can change. If you get a call or email it is OK to feel flattered but don't make any decisions based on that. It could be that the program that has a policy not to call you values you even more!"[18]

Did you know?

Some specialties have developed statements or guidelines governing post-interview communication. "Our program strictly adheres to the A.U.P.O. and O.M.P. policy that residency programs will not initiate contact after the interview with applicants," writes the Texas Tech University Department of Ophthalmology.[19] According to the American Council of Academic Plastic Surgeons Uniform Policy and Guidelines for Post Interview Communication, "there will be NO communication between faculty and applicants after the interview…"[20]

Did you know?

Every year, hundreds of applicants change their rank-order lists after receiving positive communication from programs. In these e-mails and letters are often phrases such as "ranked to match," "ranked highly," or "would fit well." Although these phrases suggest a high level of interest in the applicant, these statements should not be viewed as guarantees or assurances of a certain outcome. Applicants should also understand that these phrases mean different things to programs. In a recent policy statement developed by the Association of Program Directors in Internal Medicine, the organization urged its members to be precise in their choice of terminology:[21]

Terms such as "ranked to match" should only be used if a candidate is ranked in a position numbered less than the positions you are filling (a so-called "lock" position), or the meaning fully explained to the applicant. For example, if you use the term "ranked to match" to mean that you are ranking an applicant higher than your program historically fills, but not in a lock position, then that should be explained to the applicant.

The bottom line: don't alter your rank-order list because of communication you receive from programs.

Rule # 180 Don't lie.

"Although truthfulness and honesty have long been considered fundamental values within the medical profession, lying and deception have become standard practices within medicine's residency selection process."[22]

These were the words of Tara Young in her article, "Teaching medical students to lie." She also wrote that candidates must "lead their interviewers to believe that they are interested in the program they are being interviewed for, even if they have no intention of ranking it anywhere near the top of their list of choices." Although written after her experiences with the residency selection process in Canada, her discussion of the potential negative effects of the process is pertinent to the NRMP, San Francisco, and Urology matches.

We've touched upon this subject elsewhere, and yet feel compelled to review this rule in more depth. Lying and unethical practices are rampant in the residency application and residency selection process. These practices are shockingly common, as the literature demonstrates. In one survey of graduating medical students, 12.4% of respondents reported making misleading statements or assurances to programs.[6] Recognize that these were the students who actually admitted to such a practice. A review of PDs suggests that the numbers may be much higher. A survey of emergency medicine PDs found that 42% frequently felt that applicants had lied to them, while another 42% sometimes felt lied to by applicants.[23]

Many applicants believe that they must be dishonest with programs to avoid an unfavorable match outcome. They fear that being completely honest about their level of interest will harm their candidacy at programs. While some applicants report feeling uncomfortable, most would describe it as just playing along with "the game."

Such unethical practices are not limited to applicants. In Rule # 187, we describe how PDs may also make misleading statements or assurances to applicants. The bottom line is this: You must proactively plan how to navigate the complex application process, while being completely honest and without ever compromising your ethics.

Did you know?

Dr. Ziegelstein, Vice Chair for Education at Johns Hopkins University School of Medicine, wrote that you should not "tell a program director that you are ranking that program # 1 on your list if it is not true. The statement is not binding, but you do not want someone to develop bad feelings about you that could count against you later. Most physicians have good memories or they would not have passed anatomy."[24]

Rule # 181 The top programs on your rank list should be informed of this fact.

As detailed previously, your expressed interest in a program can, in some situations, impact their interest in you. Therefore, we recommend that you inform the top programs on your rank list of this fact. However, this can be a difficult area in which to proceed. *You must never lie.* We can't state it any more clearly than that. However, if you're certain that a program is your number one choice, and you rank that program number one on your rank list, you may legally and ethically let them know that fact. There is no NRMP rule against stating your interest in a program. The NRMP states that "you may volunteer information about...how you plan to rank programs." (www.nrmp.org).

Did you know?

As much as you would like to know your standing as a candidate following the interview, applicants are not permitted to make such inquiries with programs. To do so would be a violation of NRMP policy. Research indicates that this rule is often violated. In a survey of obstetrics and gynecology PDs, 84% of programs indicated that candidates had asked about ranking status. How do programs respond to these inquiries? Approximately 1% reported informing the candidate about his or her chances. 16% offered a vague reply. 60% told candidates that the ranking status could not be disclosed.[16]

While such ranking statements are not binding, we all know of applicants who've made such statements, only to be proven as liars after the match results are available. Medicine can be a surprisingly small world, and your reputation is one of your most important assets. There are too many opportunities to lose your moral compass during the residency application process. Maintain the highest ethical and moral standards now and throughout your career, and your reputation will reflect that fact.

There is a potential negative in informing the top programs on your rank list of that fact. The world of program directors can be a small one, and there is a small chance that your strong interest in a particular program may be conveyed to another program.

A more important consideration is that you may not be able to inform the top programs on your rank list, because you may not have identified those programs. One small study of 21 anesthesiology residents found that 76% made their final ranking choices within a week prior to the final submission date.[25] There's no point in informing programs at that late date, because most have submitted their own rank lists by that point. In order to take advantage of this rule, you would have to confirm your choices earlier in the process.

Tip # 129

At the end of the interview season, you'll have a better idea of where you will place programs on your rank-order list. This is the time to send programs one final communication. In this letter, you'll want to communicate your level of interest in the program. Include details on why the program is such a good fit for you, and convey the type of contributions you would like to make as a resident in their program. Don't wait until February to send this communication. Your goal is to have your letter or e-mail received before the selection committee meets to finalize their rank-order list. To be on the safe side, aim to have your communication in the program's hands during the third week of January (even earlier if you're participating in an early match).

Tip # 130

If you have any reason to believe that you won't be ranked high enough to match at one of your top programs, there are concrete steps that you can take following the interview that may improve your chances. First, communicate with the program following the interview to remind them of your interest in and enthusiasm for the program. Second, consider updating your file with new course/clerkship grades, USMLE Step 2 CK score, an additional letter of recommendation, or a recently received award (e.g., election to AOA). Third, consider a "second look" visit to programs. Finally, talk to one of your letter writers to see if she might call the program to rave about you. If you have a compelling reason to match at a certain program, you can let the program know that as well.

Tip # 131

Do you know a faculty member at your school who has a strong relationship with the PD or chairman at a program you covet? If so, consider asking the faculty member to make a call on your behalf. In a recent survey of obstetrics and gynecology PDs, 29% of respondents indicated that they would give consideration to ranking applicants higher if there was an expression of interest beyond a routine thank you.[10] One example offered was if a faculty advocate known to the program informed the program that the applicant intended to rank the program at the top of the rank-order list. Such calls can be made after the interview, and may be effective in elevating your position on the rank-order list. However, you should realize that disclosing your desire to attend another program could affect your chances at your own institution. If you decide to utilize this approach, your faculty advocate may ask you if the program you desire is your top choice. Because his reputation is at stake, he may be reluctant to advocate for you if it isn't your top choice.

Rule # 182 You do have the option of visiting a program again.

After completing your interviews, you'll review in detail the information that you've gathered. You'll use this information to create your rank list. As you may suspect, this is not an easy process. You'll be spending three or more years at the program where you match, and it can be difficult to make such an important decision based on a few hours spent at a program.

You do have the option of visiting a residency program after your interview. You would simply contact the program and ask if you can arrange for another visit, known as a "second look."

Although some programs are not receptive to such requests, most will accommodate you. In fact, some programs will strongly urge you to return for a second look, and will view your request as a serious sign of interest in their program. There is evidence to indicate that, at some programs, second look visits are an important part of the selection process. In the 2014 NRMP Program Director Survey, 26% of emergency medicine programs cited the second visit as a factor in ranking applicants.[26] "Asking for a 'second look' visit goes a long way in impressing a program," writes Dr. Todd Berger, PD of the emergency medicine residency program at Dell Medical School.[27] The importance of second look visits varies significantly from specialty to specialty, as shown in the following table.

Importance Of Second Look Visits By Specialty

Specialty	% Of Programs Citing Second Interview/Visit As A Factor In Ranking Applicants	Mean Importance Rating
Anesthesiology	16%	3.3
Dermatology	3%	2.0
Emergency Medicine	26%	3.4
Family Medicine	36%	3.8
General Surgery	23%	4.0
Internal Medicine	13%	3.0
Med/Peds	11%	2.8
Neurosurgery	31%	3.9
Neurology	22%	4.0
Obstetrics & gynecology	22%	3.5
Orthopedic surgery	12%	3.7
Otolaryngology	2%	5.0
Pathology	21%	3.9
Pediatrics	18%	3.5
PM&R	9%	3.3
Psychiatry	17%	3.6
Radiation Oncology	7%	4.3
Radiology	12%	3.8

Results of the 2014 NRMP Program Director Survey. Available at: http://www.nrmp.org/wp-content/uploads/2014/09/PD-Survey-Report-2014.pdf.

As you can see from the data, most programs don't cite second look visits as a factor in ranking decisions. Therefore, they shouldn't be considered routine. We recommend the following approach:

- If you truly feel the need to obtain more information and the program is open to a second look visit, then by all means you should feel comfortable scheduling another visit.
- Some programs make the importance of a second look visit clear on their website or during the interview. "We encourage all interested parties to come back for a second look," writes the Department of Neurology at Mt. Sinai Beth Israel. "Please contact our coordinator to arrange a date after your interview."[28] In such cases, you should consider scheduling another visit if you are interested in the program.
- The importance of the second look visit won't be clear at some programs. At these institutions, we recommend asking program personnel on the day of your visit. Residents are an excellent source of information in this regard.

Before your repeat visit, review all program information. Since the reason for your visit is to collect more information, start by formulating new questions. During this second visit, you may be able to spend a full day observing a resident as she fulfills her responsibilities. Take note of the interactions between faculty and residents, evaluate the hospital and program resources, participate in the didactic sessions, and ask your additional questions. You may gain valuable insight about the program, information that can help you assess whether the program is a good fit for you. An experience such as this can often put to rest any lingering doubts you may have about the program.

Your visit will essentially be an extended interview. While you're more fully evaluating the program, the program is evaluating you as well. If you perform well, this second visit may have the potential to improve your chances of matching with the program.

Tip # 132

Some programs do not recommend "second look" visits, making it clear to applicants that such opportunities are not available. Other programs may not be so explicit. Try to gain some insight into how a program views such a request on your interview day. Avoid making this request to any program that you feel might view it as an inconvenience. Dr. Judith Amorosa of the radiology department at UMDNJ/Robert Wood Johnson Medical School states that "a second look should be a sincere effort to clarify a specific aspect of the residency, not just one more hurdle the student thinks he needs to jump over to get higher on the match list."[29]

Did you know?

Dr. Amy Stier is the program director of the pediatrics residency program at the University of Iowa. She recommends second looks if:

- "You did not get to see an aspect of our program that is important to you.
- You have additional questions you'd like to ask or observe in person.
- You came early in the season and now your memories of the people or facilities are getting fuzzy."

"Second look interviews are intended to give the applicant more exposure to our residency program to determine if this is the program to best fit their needs," writes Dr. Stier.[30]

Did you know?

If you're unable to arrange a "second look" visit, you can still call or e-mail the program with questions. In fact, follow-up questions may demonstrate your continued interest in and enthusiasm for the program.

References

[1]Department of Orthopedic Surgery at Drexel University College of Medicine. Available at: http://www.drexel.edu/medicine/Academics/Residencies-and-Fellowships/Orthopaedic-Surgery-Residency/How-to-Apply/. Accessed February 22, 2016.
[2]Anderson K, Jacobs D. General surgery program directors' perceptions of the match. *Curr Surg* 2000; 57(5): 460-465.
[3]Banks S, Gaitan B, Katz J, Lewis M. Don't throw the baby out with the bathwater: Post-interview no-call policies may serve no one. Available at: http://www.asaabstracts.com/strands/asaabstracts/abstract.htm;jsessionid=1001546CE95795E4A9A2088CE335774C?year=2008&index=12&absnum=774. Accessed February 22, 2016.
[4]Children's National Health System. Available at: http://childrensnational.org/news-and-events/our-blogs/pediatric-career-blog/2014/november/tip-tuesday-thanking-the-residency-program-and-the-applicant. Accessed February 22, 2016.
[5]Nallasamy S, Uhler T, Nallasamy N, Tapino P, Volpe N. Ophthalmology resident selection: current trends in selection criteria and improving the process. *Ophthalmology* 2010; 117(5): 1041-1047.
[6]Miller J, Schaad D, Crittenden R, Oriol N, MacLaren C. Communication between programs and applicants during residency selection: effects of the match on medical students' professional development. *Acad Med* 2003; 78(4): 403-411.
[7]Carek P, Anderson K, Blue A, Mavis B. Recruitment behavior and program directors: how ethical are their perspectives about the match process? *Fam Med* 2000; 32(4): 258-260.
[8]Crane J, Ferraro C. Selection criteria for emergency medicine residency applicants. *Acad Emerg Med* 2000; 7(1): 54-60.
[9]Teichman J, Anderson K, Dorough M, Stein C, Optenberg S, Thompson I. The urology residency matching program in practice. *J Urol* 2000; 163(6): 1878-1887.
[10]Frishman G, Matteson K, Bienstock J, George K, Ogburn T, Rauk P, Schnatz P, Learman L. Postinterview communication with residency applicants: a call for clarity! *Am J Obstet Gynecol* 2014; 211(4): 344-350.
[11]University of Chicago Residency Process Guide. Available at: http://pritzker.uchicago.edu/current/students/ResidencyProcessGuide.pdf. Accessed September 3, 2012.
[12]American Medical Association. Available at: http://www.ama-assn.org/ama/pub/about-ama/our-people/member-groups-sections/minority-affairs-section/transitioning-residency/residency-programs-an-inside-look.page. Accessed August 18, 2012.
[13]The application process: A timetable for success. Available at: http://www.ama-assn.org/ama/pub/about-ama/our-people/member-groups-sections/minority-affairs-section/transitioning-residency/the-application-process-a-timetable-success.page%3F. Accessed February 2, 2015.
[14]Brothers T, Wetherholt S. Importance of the faculty interview during the resident application process. *J Surg Educ* 2007; 64(6): 378-385.

[15]University of Washington Department of Medicine. Available at: http://depts.washington.edu/medclerk/drupal/pages/Internal-Medicine-Residency-Application-FAQ. Accessed September 15, 2012.
[16]Curran D, Andreatta P, Xu X, Nugent C, Dewald S, Johnson T. Postinterview communication between obstetric and gynecology residency programs and candidates. *J Grad Med Educ* 2012; 4(2): 165-169.
[17]University of Michigan Health System. Available at: http://www.uofmhealth.org/news/medical-residency-training-practices. Accessed February 22, 2016.
[18]University of Colorado Department of Pediatrics. Available at: http://www.ucdenver.edu/academics/colleges/medicalschool/departments/pediatrics/meded/students/Electives/Documents/University%20of%20Colorado%20Pediatric%20Residency%20Preparation%20Manual.pdf. Accessed September 23, 2012.
[19]Texas Tech University Department of Ophthalmology. Available at: https://www.ttuhsc.edu/som/ophthalmology/residency/faq.aspx. Accessed February 22, 2016.
[20]ACAPS Uniform policy and guidelines for post interview communication. Available at: http://acaplasticsurgeons.org/multimedia/files/ACAPS-Uniform-Policy-on-Post-Interview-Communication.ppt. Accessed February 22, 2016.
[21]Guidelines for post-interview communication and second looks. Available at: http://connect.im.org/p/cm/ld/fid=802. Accessed February 22, 2016.
[22]Young T. Teaching medical students to lie – the disturbing contradiction: medical ideals and the resident-selection process. *CMAJ* 1997; 156(2): 2219-2222.
[23]Wolford R, Anderson K. Emergency medicine residency director perceptions of the resident selection process. *Acad Emerg Med* 2000; 7(10): 1170-1171.
[24]The Successful Match: Interview with Dr. Roy Ziegelstein. Available at: http://studentdoctor.net/2009/06/the-successful-match-interview-with-dr-roy-ziegelstein/. Accessed September 5, 2012.
[25]Lewis M, Banks S, Dollar B, Cobas M, Katz J. The residency selection process: The when and how of the match order list. *Anesthesiology* 2007; 107: A409.
[26]Results of the 2014 NRMP Program Director Survey. Available at: http://www.nrmp.org/wp-content/uploads/2014/09/PD-Survey-Report-2014.pdf.
[27]Emergency medicine residency: How to apply. Available at: http://dellmedschool.utexas.edu/residency/emergency-medicine/apply. Accessed February 22, 2016.
[28]Department of Neurology at Mt. Sinai Beth Israel. Available at: http://bethisraelgme.org/Neurology.asp. Accessed February 22, 2016.
[29]Amorosa J. How do I mentor medical students interested in radiology. *Acad Radiol* 2003; 10: 527-535,
[30]University of Iowa Department of Pediatrics. Available at: http://www.uihealthcare.org/GME/ResProgInsidePages.aspx?id=236518&taxid=225081. Accessed September 27, 2012.

Chapter 17

Ranking Residency Programs

The last step in the residency application process is the creation and submission of your rank order list. On the official rank list, you list those programs, in order of preference, which you would be willing to attend. Programs also submit their own rank lists, in the order in which they would extend offers. Sometime in February, the Match takes place. A computer matches each applicant to the highest ranked program on the applicant's list which has offered him a position. The results are announced throughout the country in mid-March on "Match Day."

For many, Match Day is the happy culmination of a very long, hard application process. Other applicants experience bitter disappointment. There are a whole host of reasons as to why match results may not be favorable. However, we've seen some students who do everything right, only to make critical errors when it comes time to create and submit their rank list. Errors at this final step in the process can undo all of your previous efforts.

Rule # 183 Always rank according to your own criteria.

After the interview season ends, the process of finalizing your rank list begins in earnest. The rank list is a list of the residency programs at which you interviewed, placed in your order of preference. This involves sorting through a great deal of data. Some students are tempted to rank based on reputation alone. "I'd like to attend the most prestigious program I can get into." Ranking programs is rarely that simple. You'll be spending a minimum of three years of your life at this program, and you need to take into account a whole host of other factors. A useful checklist for evaluating residency programs can be found in Strolling Through the Match, a publication produced by the American Academy of Family Physicians. It's accessible free to applicants at www.aafp.org. Consider also the following questions:

- Will the residency program provide me with strong clinical training?
- Will that training be broad-based, with exposure to all facets of the field?
- Will it provide some subspecialty training in my areas of interest?
- Will it provide training in additional areas important to me, such as research training?
- How did I feel when I visited the program?

- Would I be able to work with the people there?
- Could I live and work in this city for the next several years?
- What are the strengths and weaknesses of the program relative to others?
- Does the program offer an environment that will allow me to reach my full potential?

Tip # 133

Don't ignore your gut feeling about a program. A program may look outstanding on paper, but if your visit left you feeling that you would be miserable there, consider that an important data point. While objective information is obviously important in the ranking process, emotions can, and should, play an important role.

Rule # 184 Never rank a program that you wouldn't want to attend.

If you have serious doubts about a program, *do not* put that program on your rank list. If you place it on the rank list and you match, you are bound to accept it. In fact, in registering for the Match, the NRMP has applicants affix their passwords to the Match Participation Agreement. This agreement states that a "match between an applicant and a program creates a binding commitment to accept or offer a position. A decision not to honor that commitment is a breach of the Agreement and will be investigated by the NRMP."[1]

While applicants can be granted a waiver from their Match commitment, only the NRMP can grant this waiver. Programs are not allowed to grant waivers and must report all waiver requests to the NRMP. If the NRMP denies the waiver request, you will be expected to honor your commitment to the program. Failure to accept the position may lead the NRMP to prohibit you from acceptance into another NRMP-participating program for a period of one year following the decision.

While the NRMP has approved some waiver requests, others have been denied. Overall, it would be better to not match at all than to match at a program you have no desire to attend. In the event that you don't match, you still have additional opportunities to strengthen your application and apply again.

Tip # 134

Think long and hard before you rank any program where you feel you would be unhappy. You may ultimately match there.

Rule # 185 Rank every single program that you would consider attending.

You should place every program you would consider attending on your rank list. Submitting a longer list will not affect your chances of matching with those programs that are higher on your rank list. This is clearly explained in the information the NRMP provides to applicants regarding the Match.

Some students, for various and often misguided reasons, do not wish to rank every program that they would consider attending. Before you leave any programs off your list, factor in:

- Competitiveness of the specialty
- Your qualifications
- Competition for the specific programs being ranked

We have encountered students who create too short of a rank list because they feel confident of matching into one of their top choices. These students are devastated when they don't match at all. Don't let overconfidence ruin your chances.

Did you know?

Per the words of the San Francisco Matching Program:

"Pay attention to the bottom of your list! Each year some applicants tell us that they omitted a lower choice because they overestimated their chances elsewhere. They ended up unmatched because the omitted program turned out to be their only offer. The only reason not to list a program is that you would rather remain unmatched to explore other options after the match."[2]

This is echoed by the American Urological Association:

"Maximize your chances! Previous years' matches have demonstrated the need for applicants to include on their preference lists all of the programs they would be willing to attend. Some applicants who were not matched at all received offers from programs they did not list. If the applicants had listed all programs preferable, some of these 'misses' might have been avoided."[3]

Rule # 186 Don't wait until the last minute to certify your rank order list.

Candidates are allowed to modify their rank order lists as often as necessary until the posted deadline, which is usually in the middle of February. Before the deadline, you must certify your list; otherwise, the NRMP will not receive it. The following advice is offered by the NRMP:

"Participants are advised not to wait until the last minute to enter their Rank Order Lists so as to avoid any problems at the deadline."[1]

"If you make a change to your Rank Order List by moving or deleting a program, the change is saved and the previous rankings are deleted, and your old Rank Order List is NOT certified if previously certified. You must then certify your ROL again for it be used in the match."[1]

Tip # 135

You are free to modify your list as often as necessary. However, several days before the posted deadline, you must certify your list. The NRMP will not act on your list until you certify it.

Rule # 187 **Don't believe everything you're told. Not only are misunderstandings common, but some programs do engage in questionable ethical practices.**

Although the first match was run in 1952, it did not become known as the National Resident Matching Program (NRMP) until 1978. The system was designed to allow programs and applicants to confidentially rank one another and make selection decisions without pressure.

However, every year both parties try to influence selection decisions in their favor. While the NRMP expects that all match participants will conduct themselves in an above-board and ethical manner, in reality this may be compromised.

Programs may engage in questionable ethical practices, and this may be more common than one would think. Misunderstandings are also common. These practices include the following:

- Making informal commitments

  In a survey of fourth-year students at three schools, 43% felt that they had received informal commitments from at least one program.[4] A similar result was found in a survey of urology residency applicants.[5] In this study, 40% of applicants felt that they had received informal commitments.

- Dishonesty with applicants

  A survey of urology residency applicants found that over 50% of the informal commitments failed to result in an actual match. In this same survey, only about half of the PDs felt uncomfortable being dishonest with applicants.[5] Another study surveyed family medicine

PDs and learned that 94% felt pressured to be dishonest with applicants in an attempt to recruit coveted applicants.[6]

- Asking applicants how they planned to rank the program

Did you know?

In their Statement on Professionalism, the NRMP states that "although the Match Participation Agreement does not prohibit either an applicant or a program from volunteering how one plans to rank the other, it is a violation of the Match Participation Agreement to request such information."[1]

Tip # 136

You stand the best chance of matching into the residency program that you want if you rank it as your top choice. Do not create your rank list based upon where you think you will be accepted.

Rule # 188 You cannot naively believe comments made by program directors.

After interviewing at a program, you may receive a follow-up e-mail, letter or telephone call from the PD stating that the program plans on ranking you at the top of their list. You may be thrilled to hear such great news. Beware. Such a statement made by a program in no way serves as a guarantee that they will rank you highly. You cannot allow comments such as these to affect the order of your rank list.

Surveys have shown that students for the most part are skeptical about any assurances made by programs regarding their place on the program's rank list. They generally report that these assurances, including informal commitments, have little effect on their rank order list.

However, some applicants are in fact influenced by these types of statements. They may let a program's expression of interest change the way in which they rank programs on their list. They may even create too short of a rank list believing that they are an "in" or a "lock" at a certain program because they were told so. These students have been devastated when they learn they didn't match into any residency program.

At the NRMP website, it is clearly stated that applicants should not rely on statements made by programs when creating their rank order lists. As thrilling as it may be to hear "Our program plans to rank you high on our list," this isn't binding in any way. We know of multiple cases in which students have been given such assurances, only to subsequently <u>not</u> match at those programs.

Did you know?

In their Statement on Professionalism, the NRMP writes that each year it is "contacted by applicants who believe that an error has occurred in the Match because they did not match to programs whose directors had promised them positions (i.e., had promised to rank them high enough to ensure a match.) In every case, the NRMP has determined that the applicant did not match to the desired program because, contrary to the applicant's expectation, the program did not rank the applicant high enough on the program's rank order list for the applicant to match there."[1]

Tip # 137

While some programs will remain in contact with all applicants, some will only communicate with selected applicants. Other programs have a policy not to communicate whatsoever with any applicant. Don't let the lack of communication alter the position of the program on your rank list.

Tip # 138

A recent survey of nearly 1,200 residency applicants revealed that programs commonly called applicants in the post-interview period. 42% of respondents indicated that this contact was important in determining the program's place on their rank-order list.[7]

Rule # 189 Know what constitutes a match violation.

Applicants often seek an understanding of the Match policy, including what might constitute a violation, from their peers. This practice often leads to misinformation. In one study, nearly half of students perceived a violation that did not meet NRMP definition for a violation.[8]

To gain a solid understanding of the Match policy, attend all orientation and information sessions about the process at your school. Read the rules of the Match, which are often given to students by their schools and are also available at the NRMP website.

Tip # 139

Feel free to turn to your peers for information, but realize that they may not always be the ideal source of information. Always verify what you hear.

Myth or Fact?

- Programs that tell you where they're ranking you on their list are in violation of the NRMP guidelines.

  -Myth. Programs and applicants can volunteer how they plan to rank one another. However, the NRMP prohibits either party from asking one another.

- Programs are prohibited from asking applicants if they are applying to another specialty.

  -Myth. Programs are free to ask you if you are interviewing in more than one specialty.

- It is permissible for a program director to ask me where else I am applying.

  -Myth. Programs may not ask applicants for names of other programs the applicant has applied to or will be applying to.

- Programs may recommend applicants return for second visits or looks.

  -Myth. The NRMP Match Communication Code of Conduct prohibits program directors from requiring or implying that second looks are used to determine a candidate's place on the rank-order list.

- Programs are not allowed to contact you following the interview.

  -Myth. Programs are free to contact applicants following the interview, but they are not allowed to ask applicants how they plan to rank their program.

Tip # 140

A study found that 12% of general surgery PDs felt that it was ethically wrong to interview in more than one specialty.[4] In the same study 75% of directors reported that an applicant's forthright admission to multispecialty interviewing would have a negative effect on the applicant's rank order.

Rule # 190 Recognize if you're at risk for an unsuccessful match, and take steps to prepare for SOAP.

After you've finished ranking programs, there's one more question to ask yourself. Are you at risk for not matching? According to the AAMC, there are seven major reasons why U.S. allopathic seniors may fail to match:[9]

- Low USMLE scores
- USMLE exam failure
- Not competitive for chosen specialty
- Lack of backup specialty plan
- Failure to follow recommendations of Dean's office or faculty advisor
- Poor interviewing or interpersonal skills
- Ranking too few programs

If you believe that you're at risk for an unsuccessful match, we urge you to become familiar with the Match Week Supplemental Offer and Acceptance Program (SOAP). SOAP was established by the NRMP and serves as the process through which unmatched applicants apply for positions in unfilled residency programs. To maximize your chances of success during SOAP, there are a number of measures that can be taken. They do, however, require time. Please refer to Chapter 19 for more information.

References

[1]National Resident Matching Program. Available at: http://www.nrmp.org/faq-questions/what-do-i-do-if-an-applicant-who-has-a-binding-commitment-to-my-program-does-not-show-up-for-training/. Accessed March 2, 2011.
[2]San Francisco Matching Program. Available at: www.sfmatch.org. Accessed November 2, 2008.
[3]American Urological Association. Available at: www.auanet.org/residents/resmatch.cfm. Accessed November 2, 2008.
[4]Anderson K, Jacobs D. General surgery program directors' perceptions of the match. *Curr Surg* 2000; 57(5): 460-465.
[5]Teichman J, Anderson K, Dorough M, Stein C, Optenberg S, Thompson I. The urology residency matching program in practice. *J Urol* 2000; 163(6): 1878-1887.
[6]Carek P, Anderson K, Blue A, Mavis B. Recruitment behavior and program directors: how ethical are their perspectives about the match process? *Fam Med* 2000; 32(4): 258-260.
[7]Nagarkar P, Janis J. Fixing the match: a survey of resident behaviors. *Plast Reconstr Surg* 2013; 132 (3): 711-719.
[8]Phillips R, Phillips K, Chen F, Melillo. Exploring residency match violations in family practice. *Fam Med* 2003; 35(10): 717-720.
[9]American Medical Association. Available at: http://www.ama-assn.org/ama/ama-wire/post/arent-medical-students-matching-happens-next. Accessed March 22, 2016.

Chapter 18

Couples Match

Any two individuals participating in the NRMP Match can apply as a couple in an effort to match with programs in the same geographic region. You need not be married or engaged. You don't even need to be romantically involved. When it comes time to create your rank-order list, you'll simply do it together, listing pairs of programs. Using its algorithm, the NRMP will match you with the highest ranked pair of programs in which both of you have been accepted.

In 2015, 2,092 applicants participated in the Match as couples, shattering the previous record. Couples in the Match have typically fared well, matching at rates over 90% since 1984, the inaugural year for the Couples Match. In 2016, the match rate was 95.7%, higher than the 93.8% match rate for U.S. allopathic seniors applying alone.[1]

Rule # 191 **Many advisors are not as familiar with the Couples Match. It's therefore important that you seek out multiple sources of information.**

A strong working knowledge of the process is important to avoid common pitfalls. Fortunately, all medical schools have experience with couples participating in the Match. However, it can sometimes be difficult to find mentors and advisors with experience in this area. We recommend:

- Discussing your plans to participate in the Couples Match with your Dean of Student Affairs. It's likely that your Dean is an authority in this area, having counseled many couples before you.
- Seeking the advice and perspectives of faculty advisors in your chosen specialty, as well as your partner's, who have experience guiding couples.
- Consulting with residents who have matched as couples.
- Learning from the experiences of recently matched couples.

Did you know?

"One of the biggest stressors is just the lack of knowledge about the Couples Match. Most people don't really know what the process involves until they're in it, and advisors can be helpful but they don't always have as much experience with couples as single applicants."[2]

- Dr. Calvin Kagan, University of Vermont School of Medicine Graduate

Did you know?

If you or your partner are participating in different matches (e.g., NRMP and early match), then you won't be able to match as a couple. The exception to this rule is if the early match specialty (such as urology) requires initial training in another field (such as general surgery). If the other field participates in the NRMP Match, then you and your partner can participate in the couples match for this initial period of training.

Rule # 192 **Determine geographic regions of interest for residency training.**

At the earliest stages of the process, consider your geographic areas of interest, and ask your partner to do the same. Then compare notes. Are you interested in the same parts of the country? If not, don't worry. This is the time to have an open dialogue about your respective interests, and learn about areas that you may be unfamiliar with. Because larger metropolitan areas have more options in terms of residency programs, couples will generally focus more on these sites, and apply to multiple programs in the same area.

Did you know?

Once you've decided your geographic areas of interest and then identified desirable programs within these areas, you and your partner will apply separately to these programs.

Rule # 193 **Apply to a larger number of programs. You can always cancel interviews later.**

Couples generally apply to more programs. The number of programs to which you apply should be based on:

- Competitiveness of the specialties you and your partner are seeking
- Competitiveness of each partner's application for the specialty
- Geographic area of interest, and the competitiveness of programs within these areas
- Familiarity of your medical school to these programs
- Red flags in your (or your partner's) application

Another factor which requires consideration involves increasing competition for residency positions. This is due to rising medical student enrollment in existing medical schools and newly created schools. To ensure an adequate number of interviews, apply to a larger number of programs. If you and your partner are fortunate to be deluged with interviews, you can always cancel some.

Tip # 141

Although it's important for every applicant to apply early, it's even more so for couples. Doing so will give you the most flexibility in scheduling and coordinating interviews with your partner.

Tip # 142

If one half of the couple is academically weak, then both have to apply to a wider range of programs.

Rule # 194 Decide whether to disclose your intent to match as a couple to programs.

Although many couples disclose their intent to match as a couple to programs, there's no rule that indicates that you must do so. To match as a couple, you simply have to register as a couple on the NRMP website. Some couples do participate (as a couple) without ever informing programs. Unless you communicate your intent to match as a couple to programs, programs won't know this. In other words, the NRMP will not disclose this to programs.

However, most couples do opt to inform programs of their desire to participate in the couples match. You can inform programs of your intent at different points in the application process. On the ERAS application form, you are permitted to designate your status as a couple. If you're not ready to disclose this at the time of submission, or you decide later to participate as a couple, you can communicate this to the program via email or phone when scheduling interviews, during your interview visit, or through communication with programs following interviews.

Rule # 195 Decide to participate in the Couples Match sooner rather than later.

Although you may delay indicating your intentions to participate in the Couples Match, we believe that it's preferable, in most cases, to make your intentions known earlier in the process. Reasons include:

- Many residency programs are receptive to applicants applying as couples, because couples often make happy residents. Happy residents are less likely to become problem residents.

- Once programs are informed of your plans to participate in the Couples Match, it often becomes easier for you and your partner to coordinate interviews in the same institution or area.
- If you and your partner are applying to different specialties at the same institution, the departments can communicate with one another for your benefit. For example, if one department would like to interview you, then they may contact the other department to bring attention to your partner's application. Such efforts have been known to lead to interview offers.

Did you know?

"Residency is such a very intense time that I think a lot of program directors actually prefer people who are already in relationships because in some ways they are more stable. If you're in a relationship with someone who is in medicine, they understand what you are going through maybe a little bit better. Students have told us that when program directors found out that they were in a couples relationship, they were very positive about that."[3]

James M. Hill, Associate Dean for Student Affairs at New Jersey Medical School

Did you know?

If you and your partner are applying to the same specialty, you should realize that some programs, particularly those with smaller class sizes, may be hesitant to accept more than one student from a single school. Smaller programs may also be concerned about problems that could arise during residency. For example, if one partner is struggling, what effect will that have on the other partner and on the residency program? If one partner has to take time off for medical reasons, will the other partner have to do the same and how will the program cope with the absence of two residents? Smaller programs may also worry about relationship problems between partners, and how this may affect morale in the program. Larger programs may not have such concerns.

Tip # 143

The less competitive specialties often send interview invitations shortly after receipt of the ERAS application. In contrast, competitive specialties tend to wait until after October 15 when the MSPE is released nationally. If one partner begins receiving interviews well before the other, don't wait. Accept the invitation and schedule the interview. Secure the interview date, and then work towards receiving an interview invitation for the other partner. Remember that you can always cancel interviews later.

Did you know?

In a survey of nearly 6,000 medical students attending 176 M.D. and D.O. granting institutions in the U.S. and Canada, 15.8% of respondents identified themselves as sexual or gender minority students (sexual orientation other than heterosexual).[4] Approximately 30% did not disclose their sexual orientation during medical training. Researchers inquired about reasons for concealment, and nearly 37% cited concerns about future career options. Respondents were also invited to add comments on the survey questionnaire, and review of these comments revealed that students were particularly concerned about disclosure if they were considering careers in a surgical specialty or training in rural medicine.

"Medicine is such a hierarchical field that one person really has the power to wreck your career, so it makes a lot of sense [to hide sexual and gender identity], so why would anyone want to risk that?" said Dr. Mitchell Lunn, study investigator.[5] Same-sex couples understandably have concerns about discrimination during the residency selection process. Dr. Lee Jones, Associate Dean for Student Affairs at the University of California-Davis School of Medicine, encourages his students to assess programs during interview visits to determine how welcoming they are with respect to gender and sexual orientation. Some couples choose to reveal their status as a same-sex couple, as John Huddle and Matthew Zampella did when they applied for residency as Johns Hopkins medical students. "We didn't want to end up in a place where being gay would be an issue," said Huddle. "Being out on the application was kind of a way of filtering out those places that just wouldn't be a good fit for us."[6]

Rule # 196 Make efforts to visit programs in the same area together.

In a survey of fourth-year medical students in Texas during the 2012 – 2013 residency application season, the authors found that the average cost for applying and interviewing for residency positions was $4,783.[7] The costs to apply and interview for couples can easily exceed this figure. To significantly decrease this expense, many couples would like to travel to areas together, and share the costs associated with travel, including transportation, lodging, and meals. Fortunately, many programs are sensitive to the costs associated with interviewing, and work with couples to accommodate them. We recommend that you do the following:

- If you're offered an interview at a site before your partner, be proactive. In your email communication, inform or remind the program coordinator that you are applying as part of a couple. Include the name of your partner, AAMC ID #, and the program to which he or she has applied. With this information, the program may then reach out to the appropriate department, and advocate for your partner. This technique has allowed many couples to secure interviews in the same area during one trip. Although coordinators will make every effort to accommodate you, there will be times when interview dates are different. If so, you'll have to interview on different trips.

- If your partner has been offered an interview, and you haven't heard from the same institution yet, you may contact them. In your communication, indicate that you're matching as part of a couple and that your partner will be interviewing at another program in the hospital. This will often spur the program to take a closer look at your application, and may net you an interview on that same day.

- Keep in mind that coordinators can advocate for you or your partner at other institutions in the area. Coordinators in the same region often know each other very well.

Tip # 144

When one partner receives an interview invite, we encourage the other partner to contact their program of interest at the same institution. Simply inform them of the situation, reiterate your interest in the program, and politely ask the program if they'd be willing to review your application. The program may take a closer look at your application and then inform you of their decision, or you may be told that the program won't review applications until a later date.

Rule # 197 Avoid the disastrous and common mistakes made by couples in the ranking process.

This is arguably the most difficult part of the process. Unlike the single applicant, you and your partner will be ranking programs as pairs. Therefore, your rank list will be much longer. With some simple math, you'll quickly see that the number of permutations can be very large. For example, if you're ranking 12 programs and your partner 10 programs, then as a couple you will have 120 possible combinations for matching together. It can be laborious to determine and list this many combinations, but it's crucial that you list all combinations that are acceptable to you and your partner. Every year, there are couples who fail to match because they created too short of a rank-order list.

Tip # 145

Before meeting to discuss combinations of programs for the rank-order list, we recommend that partners create a list independently, from most to least desirable. Then you can share your thoughts with one another, and work to develop acceptable combinations.

Another common error has to do with the bottom of your rank-order list. At the end of the list, you must add combinations which will protect you in the event that you fail to match as a couple. Let's take the following example to highlight the importance of this strategy:

Scott decides to rank four programs: A, B, C, and D
Stephanie decides to rank four programs: 1, 2, 3, and 4

If Scott and Stephanie choose to rank all combinations of these programs, they will both enter 16 combinations on their rank-order lists [Co-author's note: This is like the SAT all over again!]. Let's assume that Scott and Stephanie decide to do just that. After discussion, they create the following rank-order list:

	Scott's Program	**Stephanie's Program**
Combination # 1	A	1
Combination # 2	A	2
Combination # 3	A	3
Combination # 4	A	4
Combination # 5	B	1
Combination # 6	B	2
Combination # 7	B	3
Combination # 8	B	4
Combination # 9	C	1
Combination # 10	C	2
Combination # 11	C	3
Combination # 12	C	4
Combination # 13	D	1
Combination # 14	D	2
Combination # 15	D	3
Combination # 16	D	4

A - 1 represents the combination of programs which they have ranked # 1. The last on this list, D – 4, is the pair that they have ranked last. In this scenario, if they fail to match as a couple, both partners will have to participate in the SOAP, previously known as the Scramble, to find positions in residency programs that did not fill completely during the Match. This outcome may be acceptable to the couple, if both partners would rather go unmatched than have one partner match.

If Scott and Stephanie had chosen to add combinations of programs at the end of their rank-order list which allowed one partner to go unmatched, the outcome could be very different. For example, the couple could have created the following list:

	Scott's Program	Stephanie's Program
Combination # 1	A	1
Combination # 2	A	2
Combination # 3	A	3
Combination # 4	A	4
Combination # 5	B	1
Combination # 6	B	2
Combination # 7	B	3
Combination # 8	B	4
Combination # 9	C	1
Combination # 10	C	2
Combination # 11	C	3
Combination # 12	C	4
Combination # 13	D	1
Combination # 14	D	2
Combination # 15	D	3
Combination # 16	D	4
Combination # 17	A	Unmatched
Combination # 18	Unmatched	1
Combination # 19	B	Unmatched
Combination # 20	Unmatched	2
Combination # 21	C	Unmatched
Combination # 22	Unmatched	3
Combination # 23	D	Unmatched
Combination # 24	Unmatched	4

The last 8 positions on their rank-order list include combinations where one partner is unmatched. If the couple did not match with any of their paired choices, then Scott could have matched at the A – unmatched combination (following D – 4). If this happened, Stephanie would be unmatched. She would have to scramble to find a position in an unfilled program. While it's not easy to secure a position in an unfilled program, this approach does ensure that at least one half of the couple matches successfully.

References

[1]Advance Data Tables: 2016 Main Residency Match. Available at: http://www.nrmp.org/match-data/main-residency-match-data/. Accessed April 23, 2016.
[2]American Medical Association. Available at: http://www.ama-assn.org/ama/ama-wire/post/its-like-experience-match-couple. Accessed January 2, 2015.
[3]Rutgers The State University of New York. Available at: http://news.rutgers.edu/feature/match-day-rutgers-produces-medical-residencies-and-two-marriage-proposals/20150320#.Vt39pvkrJhE. Accessed March 2, 2016.
[4]Mansh M, White W, Gee-Tong L, Lunn M, Obedin-Maliver J, Stewart L, Goldsmith E, Brenman S, Tran E, Wells M, Fetterman D, Garcia G. *Acad Med* 2015; 90(5): 634-644.
[5]Medscape Medical News. Available at: http://www.medscape.com/viewarticle/839934. Accessed January 14, 2016.
[6]Kaiser Health News. Available at: http://khn.org/news/some-medical-students-seek-a-match-for-two/. Accessed January 14, 2016.
[7]Guidry J, Greenberg S, Michael L. Costs of the residency match for fourth-year medical students. *Texas Medicine* 2014; 110(6): e1.

Chapter 19

Supplemental Offer and Acceptance Program (SOAP)

In 2012, the NRMP established the Match Week Supplemental Offer and Acceptance Program (SOAP) for unmatched applicants and unfilled residency programs. During SOAP, applicants apply to residency programs through ERAS. Programs interview applicants, usually by phone or Skype, and then create and submit preference lists. Through a series of rounds, positions are offered to applicants. The following are notable findings from the 2016 SOAP[1]:

- There were 13,920 applicants who were designated SOAP-eligible.
- Over 40% of participants were non-U.S. citizen IMGs.
- Over 25% of participants were U.S. citizen IMGs.
- Approximately 15% of participants were U.S. seniors.
- There were 513 unfilled programs, and most (454), but not all, chose to participate in SOAP.
- These programs made available 1,097 unfilled positions.
- 55% of the available positions were for PGY-1 spots, the bulk of which were preliminary surgery positions.
- The specialties with the largest numbers of unfilled positions were Family Medicine, Radiology, Anesthesiology, Internal Medicine, and Pathology.
- By the end of the SOAP process, nearly 93% of positions were filled. 65.1% of these positions were filled by U.S. seniors, 12.9% were filled by osteopathic students/graduates, and 16.8% were filled by IMGs.

The SOAP replaced a process known as the Scramble, an incredibly chaotic experience for both applicants and programs. During the Scramble, there was a flurry of emails, faxes, and phone calls from applicants to programs. Applicants often had friends, family, advisors, and consultants advocate on their behalf, and the process was overwhelming for all those involved. The creation of the SOAP brought order to the process, and established a set of rules to which both applicants and programs must adhere.

Commonly Asked Questions About SOAP

Allopathic, osteopathic, and international medical students and graduates may participate in SOAP, as long as eligibility requirements are met. These requirements include registering for the NRMP Main Residency Match, and being eligible to start residency training on July 1 of that year. Below we answer some common questions about SOAP participation:

I did not apply to any programs prior to SOAP. Can I still participate in SOAP?

Assuming that you are eligible to participate, you need not have applied earlier to participate in the SOAP process. However, you must register for the NRMP Match. The late registration deadline is in February.

I applied to one specialty prior to SOAP. Can I apply to other specialties?

Yes. You can apply to other specialties.

I didn't submit a rank order list. Am I still eligible to participate in SOAP?

Yes. You need not have ranked any programs to participate.

How do I know if I am eligible to participate in SOAP?

You will receive communication informing you of your eligibility to participate. If you're a U.S. medical student, you will be eligible for SOAP if your medical school indicates that you are on schedule to graduate before residency training begins on July 1. For international medical students and graduates, ECFMG is responsible for verifying successful completion of required examinations (USMLE Step 1, Step 2CK, Step 2CS). Following verification, IMG applicants are SOAP-eligible. Note that you don't have to be ECFMG certified to participate in SOAP. You simply have to be on schedule to graduate from your medical school by July 1 (but you must have ECFMG verification of exam completion).

Below we describe the timeline of events during the SOAP process, with specific recommendations to improve your odds of success.

ONE MONTH BEFORE MATCH WEEK

After being notified of an unsuccessful match on Monday of Match Week, applicants only have several hours to create, complete, and submit their applications for SOAP. To make the most of this very short period of time, application documents should be prepared well in advance for applicants who are at risk of not matching (and for those applicants who know they'll be participating in SOAP). Are there new letters of recommendation that need to be obtained for your specialty of choice? Do you need additional letters for back-up specialties? Will you need to write a personal statement for another specialty? Will you benefit from an updated transcript? Can the MSPE be updated to reflect all that's happened since it was prepared the past summer? These are important considerations that should take place well before Match Week. Once you determine what needs to be done, take appropriate steps to ensure these documents are available to you for the SOAP.

> **Tip # 146**
>
> If you're at risk of not matching, give some thought to your SOAP strategy well before Match Week. Will you apply to programs only in your chosen specialty, or will you also include back-up options (e.g., another specialty, preliminary year)?

FRIDAY (Before Match Week)

All applicants who are eligible to participate in SOAP will be notified of their eligibility on the Friday before Match week. Do not infer from this communication that you have failed to match. This communication is sent to all SOAP-eligible applicants.

MONDAY (Match Week)

11 AM EST

On Monday of Match Week at 11 AM EST, program directors and applicants learn the outcomes of the match process. One of three outcomes is possible for applicants:

- Complete match

  With a complete match, your work is complete. Congratulations!

- Incomplete or partial match

  An incomplete or partial match indicates that you are missing some component of your required training. If you've matched to an advanced position (starting at the PGY-2 level or higher), then you are lacking a preliminary PGY-1 position. If you've matched to a preliminary PGY-1 position, then you're lacking an advanced position to enter following completion of your PGY-1 year.

  Failure to match to an advanced or preliminary position does <u>not</u> negate your successful partial match. Per NRMP rules, you must attend the program to which you've matched, but you have to now secure a position for the training you lack. Most applicants in this situation will attempt to secure positions through participation in SOAP.

- Fully unmatched

Partially matched and fully unmatched applicants may participate in SOAP.

Tip # 147

If you are partially matched, your best course of action is to participate in SOAP. This will give you the best chance of securing a position in an unfilled program. Although there are usually some positions left unfilled after SOAP is completed, don't wait until after Match Week to begin your search.

What happens next?

Partially matched and unmatched applicants will gain access to the list of unfilled residency programs. If you're a U.S. medical student, contact your Dean's office as soon as you learn of your unmatched or partially matched status. Medical schools often have resources and personnel ready to help you with the SOAP process.

2 PM EST

You have one hour (from 2 PM to 3 PM EST) to work on your application, and then submit it. **Programs are not permitted to view applications until 3 PM EST**. Programs will receive hundreds of applications by 3 PM. They may never look at applications received at 3:30 PM. Aim to have your application submitted as early as possible. You can apply to up to 35 programs.

Tip # 148

Although you may be tempted to contact unfilled programs, please note that the NRMP prohibits applicants from communicating with programs. Applicants may only do so after programs initiate contact. Your advocates are also not permitted to initiate contact until after a program has communicated with you.

Did you know?

Don't be afraid to apply to programs which did not invite you for an interview when you applied earlier in the cycle. It's possible that they'll view the strength of your application differently during the SOAP process.

Did you know?

What is the SOAP process like for residency programs? In an article describing one program's experience with the SOAP in 2012, the authors conveyed the magnitude of the challenge facing them following submission of applications to their program[2]:

Over the next 48 hours, we received almost 1,900 new applications (2,900 when all was said and done by the end of the week), downloaded (or tried to) 30,000 files, made no less than 15 desperate calls to the NRMP with either process questions or computer 'issues,' talked with 20 candidates (before giving up on that tactic), reviewed about 200 files, spent A LOT of time with our GME director, and almost lost our residency coordinator to general freaking out.

What happens next?

At 3 PM EST, programs may view applications, and contact applicants. From this point until the end of SOAP on Thursday of Match Week, you must be readily available. You never know when a program may initiate contact, and you must be ready to respond to these communications by email or phone. Local programs may request an in-person interview. If you're scheduled for clinical work, inform your supervisors of your situation and free yourself from your responsibilities. If you fail to take a phone call or respond to email in a timely manner, the program will simply move to the next applicant. Use the time you have to become familiar with each program to which you've applied. In the event that a program contacts you, your research will allow you to make a favorable impression.

TUESDAY (Match Week)

11:30 AM EST

Programs create a SOAP preference list. In contrast to the NRMP Match (where both programs and applicants create rank order lists), in the SOAP only programs create and submit preference lists.

WEDNESDAY (Match Week)

The earliest that offers can be made is at Noon on Wednesday. Applicants who receive an offer have 2 hours to accept or reject the offer. If you receive an offer, we recommend that you take it, unless you have a compelling reason not to do so. You should not assume that a better offer is coming. If you reject an offer or let it expire, you will not receive an offer again from the same program. Once an offer is accepted, it becomes a binding agreement between you and the program. If no offer is extended, you will be given a list of programs that remain unfilled. SOAP allows you to send applications to as many as 10 new programs.

SOAP Schedule for Wednesday (Match Week)	
Time	**Activity/Deadline**
Noon	Applicants begin to receive offers for unfilled positions (Round 1).
2 PM EST	Applicants must accept or reject Round 1 offers by 2 PM.
3 PM EST	Applicants begin to receive offers for unfilled positions (Round 2).
5 PM EST	Applicants must accept or reject Round 2 offers by 5 PM.

THURSDAY (Match Week)

SOAP Schedule for Thursday (Match Week)	
Time	**Activity/Deadline**
9 AM EST	Applicants begin to receive offers for unfilled positions (Round 3).
11 AM EST	Applicants must accept or reject Round 3 offers by 11 AM.
Noon	Applicants begin to receive offers for unfilled positions (Round 4).
2 PM EST	Applicants must accept or reject Round 4 offers by 2 PM.
3 PM EST	Applicants begin to receive offers for unfilled positions (Round 5).
5 PM EST	Applicants must accept or reject Round 5 offers by 5 PM. SOAP ends.
6 PM EST	List of unfilled programs becomes accessible.

When the SOAP ends on Thursday afternoon, the list of unfilled programs will be made available.

This list will also include programs which did not participate in SOAP. You are free at this point to contact those programs.

References

[1]Advance Data Tables: 2016 Main Residency Match. Available at: http://www.nrmp.org/match-data/main-residency-match-data/. Accessed April 23, 2016.

[2]Detterline S, Ferguson R. In the SOAP: The Supplemental Offer and Acceptance Program (SOAP) from the perspective of a community hospital residency. *J Community Hosp Intern Med Perspect* 2012; 2(2).

Chapter 20

Osteopathic Students

Most osteopathic applicants secure residency positions through either the AOA or NRMP Match. Over the past five years, competition for positions in the AOA and NRMP Match has intensified. Although there has been a 22% increase in the number of available AOA-approved residency positions from 2010 to 2014, this growth has not kept pace with the rising number of osteopathic applicants. From 2010 to 2014, the number of applicants participating in the AOA Match increased by 44%: from 1,896 in 2010 to 2,743 in 2014, due to an influx of students from new colleges of osteopathic medicine, as well as expanding enrollment at established schools.[1]

In the 2014 AOA Match, 22% of participating applicants failed to match.[1] A similar percentage failed to secure positions through the NRMP Match.[2] A major reason for failure to match has to do with career aspirations. Since 2007, the American Association of Colleges of Osteopathic Medicine has annually surveyed fourth-year osteopathic medical students in an effort to identify specialties of interest. For the 2012-2013 academic year, only 32% of fourth-year students indicated plans to pursue careers in family medicine, general internal medicine, or general pediatrics.[3] It is clear that many osteopathic applicants wish to match with non-primary care specialties.

Unfortunately, most positions available in the AOA Match exist in primary care specialties. Specialties participating in the AOA Match can be divided into three groups – primary, secondary, and traditional internship. Primary specialties include family medicine, internal medicine, and pediatrics. 55% of available positions are in primary specialties. Secondary specialties are defined as all non-primary care specialties. 28% of all positions are in secondary specialties. 18% of all positions are in traditional rotating internships.[1]

With limited numbers of available positions, competition for positions in the non-primary care specialties is intense. Examination of AOA Match data in recent years has shown that there is a high fill rate for positions in non-primary care specialties, reflecting demand for training in these specialties. In contrast, many primary care positions go unfilled. Of the 599 unfilled positions in 2014, 90% represented positions in family medicine, internal medicine, and pediatrics. These positions went unfilled despite the fact that 679 applicants failed to match. It's likely that most of these applicants desired positions in non-primary care specialties. The competitiveness of specialties participating in the AOA Match is presented in the following table, in descending order based on the number of applicants per position.[1]

Competitiveness of Specialties Participating in the 2014 Osteopathic Match		
Specialty	**Applicants Per Position**	**% Applicants Matching to First-Choice Specialty**
Ophthalmology	2.41	36.6%
Otolaryngology & Facial Plastic Surgery	2.37	42.2%
Urological Surgery	2.00	50.0%
Orthopedic Surgery	1.80	53.5%
Anesthesiology	1.77	54.7%
Pediatrics	1.66	50.9%
Obstetrics & Gynecology	1.65	58.9%
Dermatology	1.60	56.9%
Physical Medicine & Rehabilitation	1.50	50.0%
Emergency Medicine	1.44	60.7%
General Surgery	1.31	66.5%
Neurological Surgery	1.19	63.2%
Psychiatry	1.18	55.9%
Family Medicine/Emergency Medicine	1.14	62.5%
Neurology	1.10	73.9%
Diagnostic Radiology	1.09	78.4%
Internal Medicine/Emergency Medicine	1.06	64.7%
Proctology	1.00	100%
Internal Medicine/Pediatrics	1.00	100%
Internal IM/NMM	1.00	100%
Neuromusculoskeletal Med/OMT	1.00	42.9%
Internal Medicine	0.77	81.7%
Family Medicine	0.66	82.9%
Traditional Internship	0.37	79.5%

Adapted from Osteopathic GME Match Report for the 2014 Match. Available at: http://www.aacom.org/reports-programs-initiatives/aacom-reports/special-reports/ogme-match-2014.

Osteopathic applicants may also apply to training positions offered through the NRMP Match. Unlike the AOA Match, where osteopathic applicants are competing among themselves, the NRMP Match also includes allopathic and international medical school applicants. Although the NRMP Match offers significantly more residency training positions in non-primary care specialties, history has shown that many of these specialties have traditionally admitted few osteopathic applicants.

2016 NMRP Match Results for DO Applicants Seeking Positions in Competitive Specialties	
Specialty	**# Matched DO Applicants/Total Candidates Matched**
Anesthesiology	208/1513
Dermatology	3/410
Emergency Medicine	224/1894
General Surgery	58/1239
Neurological Surgery	0/214
OB/GYN	128/1257
Orthopedic Surgery	4/717
Otolaryngology	1/302
PMR	114/383
Radiation Oncology	4/182
Radiology	108/1088

Adapted from Results and Data 2015 Main Residency Match. Available at: http://www.nrmp.org/wp-content/uploads/2015/05/Main-Match-Results-and-Data-2015_final.pdf.

The end result is that, while nearly 2,400 osteopathic applicants found success in the 2016 NRMP Match, 60% matched with residency programs in primary care specialties.[2] The non-primary care specialties where osteopathic applicants have found some success include anesthesiology, emergency medicine, obstetrics/gynecology, physical medicine & rehabilitation, and radiology.

What happens to osteopathic applicants who fail to match?

In the 2014 AOA Match, there were 679 unmatched applicants. What happened to these applicants? Some may have secured positions through the NRMP Match, which takes place after the AOA Match. Those who did not participate in or failed to secure positions through the NRMP Match may have obtained positions which were unfilled in the AOA or NRMP Match. It's also likely that a significant number accepted a traditional rotating internship position, with the intent to reapply the following year.

Below we answer important questions related to the AOA and NRMP Match.

How do I participate in the AOA Match?

The osteopathic or AOA Match is administered by National Matching Services (NMS). To participate in the AOA Match, you must register directly with NMS.

Can I participate in both the AOA and NRMP Match?

Some osteopathic applicants participate in both the AOA and NRMP Match. The AOA Match takes place one month before the NRMP Match, and applicants who are successful in the AOA Match will have to withdraw from the NRMP Match. This prevents a single applicant from matching in two different programs. There is an exception to this rule. If you secure **only** a one-year position (e.g., osteopathic traditional rotating internship) in the AOA Match, you may still participate in the NRMP Match, as long as you remove all programs on your NRMP rank-order list that include the first year of training (PGY-1). You may still list programs that begin in the PGY-2 year. If all of your programs begin with PGY-1 training, then you will have to withdraw from the NRMP Match altogether. Applicants who fail to match in an osteopathic program will continue forward with the NRMP Match if they have applied to allopathic programs.

Are there any other matching programs?

Most osteopathic applicants will participate in the AOA and/or NRMP Match. However, several other matching programs exist. These include the Military Match, San Francisco Match, and Urology Match. Although the San Francisco Match is open to allopathic and osteopathic applicants pursuing careers in ophthalmology, few osteopathic applicants have been successful in securing residency positions in these allopathic programs. The same can be said for the Urology Match, which is administered by the American Urological Association. The Military Match takes place before the AOA Match. Osteopathic applicants who are successful in the Military Match are not permitted to participate in the AOA Match. Those who fail to secure positions in the Military Match may move forward with the AOA Match.

Should I take the USMLE exams?

In recent years, an increasing number of osteopathic students have been applying to allopathic residency programs. While many allopathic residency programs accept the COMLEX, some may require or prefer you to take the USMLE exams. This is because it allows for easier comparison of board scores among allopathic and osteopathic candidates. At allopathic residency program websites, commonly encountered are the following types of statements:

- "We strongly encourage you to take the USMLE exams." – George Washington University Department of Emergency Medicine[4]
- "Doctor of Osteopathy (DO) applicants must take USMLE Step 1 to be considered for an interview. The COMLEX alone is not sufficient." – University of Rochester Department of Obstetrics & Gynecology[5]
- "We will accept applications from students who have only taken COMLEX exams, but do find it additionally helpful if you have taken

at least one of the USMLE exams." – Carolinas Medical Center Department of Medicine.[6]

Advisors are commonly asked if osteopathic students should take the USMLE exams. The reasons offered to not take the exams include the added time, effort, and expense associated with the process. Although these are important factors, we believe that a compelling case can be made to take the exam for many osteopathic applicants. Why? At the end of the basic science years, when students typically sit for the COMLEX Level 1 and USMLE Step 1 exams, few students know with 100% certainty the specialty they will choose to pursue as a career. Many students are also not sure whether they will seek residency training in osteopathic or allopathic programs. Taking both the COMLEX and USMLE allows students to keep their options open until their career choices become clear.

For some students, we recommend not taking the USMLE exam. These include:

- Osteopathic students who are **completely confident** that they will only be participating in the AOA Match.
- Osteopathic students who have **decided without question** to pursue specialty training in allopathic programs which do not require submission of USMLE scores.

To ascertain the viewpoints of osteopathic medical students regarding the USMLE, researchers surveyed students at nineteen osteopathic medical colleges.[7] Over 70% of the participants felt that osteopathic students should take the USMLE. Reasons cited by respondents for taking the USMLE are described in the table below.

Reasons Cited by Graduating Osteopathic Medical Students for Taking the USMLE

Main Reason Cited for Taking the USMLE	Percentage
I wanted to keep my options open.	46%
I wanted to enhance my chances of getting into an allopathic residency.	35.3%
I did not want to go to an osteopathic residency.	6.5%
There were no osteopathic programs in my desired geography.	5.7%
There were no osteopathic programs in my desired specialty.	1.6%
To improve my chances of getting into a fellowship after an osteopathic residency.	1.4%
Other	3.6%

From Hasty R, Snyder S, Suciu G, Moskow J. Graduating osteopathic medical students' perceptions and recommendations on the decision to take the United States Medical Licensing Examination. *J Am Osteop Assoc* 112; 83-89.

How do I apply to residency programs?

Most osteopathic and allopathic residency programs require applicants to submit applications through the Electronic Residency Application Service (ERAS). Through this service, applicants transmit applications, medical school transcripts, COMLEX/USMLE transcripts, the Medical Student Performance Evaluation (MSPE), letters of recommendation, and personal statements. You can begin working on your application on July 1. Please note that some programs do not participate in ERAS, and instructions for applying to these institutions will be found on program websites.

> **Did you know?**
>
> Registering for the AOA or NRMP Match does not register you for use of ERAS. You must register for ERAS separately.

When should I submit the application?

Residency programs will have differing deadlines for applications. However, we strongly recommend that you submit your application as soon as possible. Late-applying applicants, even those with strong credentials, may find it difficult to obtain interviews because interview slots fill quickly. Osteopathic residency programs may begin downloading applications on July 15. The first day applicants may submit applications to allopathic residency programs is September 15. Note that programs may not consider your application until they receive letters of recommendation. Avoid delays in the processing of your application by requesting LORs in a timely manner.

I've heard that it is more difficult to be licensed in some states as an osteopathic graduate. Is that true?

There are five states (Florida, Michigan, Oklahoma, Pennsylvania, West Virginia) that have additional requirements for the licensing of osteopathic graduates. These requirements pertain to graduates who complete training in ACGME–accredited residency programs. If you wish to practice in one of these states, understand that licensing boards in these states will make additional requests of you. You can meet their requirements by working with the AOA to receive AOA recognition of ACGME training. This will often meet the needs of the licensing boards in Florida, Michigan, Oklahoma, and Pennsylvania. West Virginia requires osteopathic graduates who have trained in ACGME residency programs to complete CME in osteopathic medicine with osteopathic manipulative treatment.

Residency Match Timeline for Osteopathic Applicants (AOA Match)	
Month	**Key Events**
June	Osteopathic applicants may register for AOA Match.
July	MyERAS (access requires ERAS token ID supplied by your school) website opens for osteopathic students, and work can now begin on the residency application. Osteopathic applicants may begin applying to AOA-accredited residency programs. Osteopathic residency programs may start downloading ERAS applications.
September	Registration for NRMP Match begins Osteopathic applicants may begin applying to ACGME-accredited residency programs. Allopathic residency programs may start downloading ERAS applications.
October	MSPE (Dean's Letter) released to residency programs
November	Deadline for registration for the AOA Match Deadline for registration for the NRMP Match (late fee applies after this date) Osteopathic applicants may begin ranking programs for the AOA Match.
December	Military Match takes place
January	Deadline for AOA Match rank-order list submission Osteopathic applicants may begin entering NRMP rank-order list Urology Match takes place
February	AOA Match takes place Deadline for NRMP Match rank-order list submission Deadline for withdrawal from NRMP Match
March	NRMP Match takes place followed by Supplemental Offer and Acceptance (SOAP) process for unmatched applicants

Some residency programs are dually accredited by the ACGME and AOA. What does that mean?

Thirty years ago, the AOA permitted residency training programs to become dually accredited by both the ACGME and AOA. The impetus for this was the desire to boost the number of residency training positions available to osteopathic graduates. In 2002, an AOA/ACGME Collaboration Task Force found that most osteopathic students prefer training in a dually accredited program because of the belief that such training is superior to that offered by AOA only-approved programs.[8-9] At the end of training, osteopathic residents in dual programs will receive AOA credit for their training. They may also receive ACGME credit. Following training, these residents can become board certified by the AOA, American Board of Medical Specialties, or both. For programs, dual accreditation is a means to attract osteopathic applicants.

What is the future of the AOA Match?

In 2013, the AOA, ACGME, and American Association of Colleges of Osteopathic Medicine (AACOM) announced their plan to move forward with a single graduate medical education system for residency and fellowship programs. It is the intent of these governing bodies to consolidate the NRMP and AOA Match into a single match. It is not clear when this change will take place.

ANESTHESIOLOGY

Osteopathic students and graduates may secure residency positions in anesthesiology programs through either the NRMP or AOA Match:

- NRMP Match

  There are 133 anesthesiology residency programs that fill their positions through the NRMP Match.[10] It can be difficult for osteopathic applicants to secure these positions. The NRMP classifies osteopathic applicants as independent applicants. In 2015, approximately 30% of independent applicants failed to match. Despite this, nearly 200 osteopathic applicants found success in the NRMP Match.[2]

- AOA Match

  There are 13 AOA-approved anesthesiology residency programs offering 31 positions. These programs are located in California, Florida, Michigan, Missouri, Ohio, Oklahoma, and Pennsylvania. Nearly half of the programs are in Michigan or Ohio.[11] In the 2014

AOA Match, there were 53 applicants vying for approximately 30 positions.[12]

Competition for anesthesiology residency positions has intensified in recent years, and applicants with higher board scores are at an advantage. In 2014, the mean COMLEX scores for matched applicants were 523 and 550 for the Level 1 and 2 exams, respectively.[12] "We only look at students whose COMLEX or USMLE scores are in the top 10% or top 15% nationally," says Dr. Dennis Kane, Program Director of the AOA-approved anesthesiology residency program at South Pointe Hospital in Warrensville Heights, Ohio.[13]

Should osteopathic applicants interested in allopathic anesthesiology residency programs take the USMLE? Allopathic anesthesiology programs have differing policies on accepting COMLEX scores in lieu of USMLE scores, as shown in the following table.

COMLEX Policy At Some Allopathic Anesthesiology Residency Programs	
Residency Program	**COMLEX Policy**
University of Pittsburgh	"We accept COMLEX scores for applications, but USMLE scores are required, even for graduates of osteopathic schools."[14]
University of Arkansas	"COMLEX Scores of 550 or above accepted in lieu of USMLE."[15]
Mayo Clinic	"Mayo has had several residents (and even faculty members) with D.O. degrees. We consider each applicant based on all merits. It's beneficial, although not mandatory, if you take the USMLE exams."[16]
University of Missouri	"COMLEX scores are accepted. We like to see them in the 600 range."[17]
University of Kentucky	"Although we do accept COMLEX scores as part of the application, we do encourage osteopathic candidates to also provide USMLE scores."[18]
University of Utah	"DO Students must take USMLE Step 1."[19]

We concur with Dr. George Mychiaskiw, former chairman at Drexel, who cautions osteopathic applicants. "Many of the more than 130 ACGME-accredited anesthesiology programs do not accept the COMLEX-USA..."[13] Therefore, if you seek to train in allopathic programs, taking the USMLE is highly recommended.

Some programs make it clear that an audition rotation is necessary or strongly recommended for matching. Several osteopathic programs are in this group.

Osteopathic Residency Program	Views on Audition Elective
NSUCOM/Largo Medical Center	"Interested medical students should complete a visiting student rotation during their 4th year for serious consideration of their application."
Des Peres Hospital	"Applicants to this program must complete a rotation in Anesthesiology at Des Peres Hospital (minimum 2 weeks)."
OUCOM/Grandview Hospital & Medical Center	"Applicant rotation at the base hospital is recommended."
Data from American Osteopathic Association. Available at: http://opportunities.osteopathic.org/index.htm. Accessed March 3, 2016.	

Dermatology

Osteopathic students and graduates may secure residency positions in dermatology programs through either the NRMP or AOA Match:

- NRMP Match

  Although there are 114 dermatology residency programs that fill their positions through the NRMP Match, very few of these positions are awarded to osteopathic applicants. To give you an idea of the difficulty involved with matching into allopathic programs, only 0.7% of all residents training in these programs are osteopathic graduates.[10] In the 2016 NRMP Match, 3 osteopathic applicants matched.[2]

- AOA Match

  There are 32 AOA-approved dermatology residency programs open to only osteopathic applicants, and offering approximately 50 positions. These programs are located in 15 states. Nearly half of the programs are in Michigan, Ohio, or Florida.[11]

Competition for dermatology residency positions in the AOA Match is intense, with more applicants than positions available. In 2014, there were 1.6 applicants for every available position. In 2014, the mean COMLEX scores for matched applicants were 602 for the Level 1 and 590 for the Level 2 exam.[12] To match into osteopathic dermatology, you must complete a traditional rotating internship. Only those applicants who are currently in or have completed such an internship are eligible to apply for osteopathic dermatology residency training.

Tips to Maximize Chances of a Successful Match in Osteopathic Dermatology

- Build a strong academic record. Because of the deep interest in the field, osteopathic dermatology residency programs have the luxury of selecting trainees among a large group of academically qualified applicants.
- Bolster your credentials outside of the classroom through your involvement in extracurricular activities, community service, and research.
- Seize opportunities to make important contributions as a leader.
- Contact current residents in osteopathic dermatology programs to seek their advice on the residency selection process. What was their overall strategy? What did they find particularly effective? What are different programs looking for?
- Plan your schedule so that you are able to complete as many dermatology electives as possible at institutions with osteopathic dermatology residency training programs.
- Take care in how you decide where to perform away electives. Select programs where you stand a good chance of securing an interview.
- Letters of recommendation are particularly important in the process. Find ways to work closely with program leaders. Letters written by program directors, clerkship directors, and chairmen carry considerable weight.
- Complete your internship at an institution which has a dermatology residency. Your proximity to the program will allow you to take an active role in the department, and become well known to the key decision-makers.
- Attend local, regional, and national dermatology meetings. The American Osteopathic College of Dermatology holds several meetings throughout the year during which students can interact and network with residents and practicing dermatologists.

Diagnostic Radiology

Osteopathic students and graduates may secure residency positions in radiology residency programs through either the NRMP or AOA Match:

- NRMP Match

  There are over 1,100 radiology residency positions available in the NRMP Match.[10] In the 2016 NRMP Match, over 100 osteopathic graduates matched.[2] Although osteopathic applicants have found success matching with allopathic programs, 30% of independent applicants (osteopathic and international medical graduates) failed to match in 2014.[20]

- AOA Match

  There are 13 AOA-approved diagnostic radiology residency programs offering approximately 30 positions.[11] "The number of applicants vary from year to year with most programs receiving anywhere between 60 to 100 applicants," writes the American College of Osteopathic Radiology (ACOR).[21] In 2014, the mean COMLEX scores for matched applicants were 548 for the Level 1 and 571 for the Level 2 exam.[12] Joining the ACOR is an excellent way to demonstrate interest in the specialty, and offers you the opportunity to network with residents and attending physicians. Applicants should find ways to become known to residency programs. The most common way is to complete rotations at the programs of interest. Many programs have 2- or 4-week rotations. If you're unable to secure an away elective at a coveted program, consider rotating in a different department. This will allow you exposure to the radiology staff, opportunities to meet with key decision-makers, and chances to spend time in the department before and after your workday.

Emergency Medicine

Osteopathic students and graduates may secure residency positions in emergency medicine programs through either the NRMP or AOA Match:

- NRMP Match

  There are over 160 emergency medicine residency programs that fill their positions through the NRMP Match.[10] In recent years, approximately 10% of positions have been awarded to osteopathic applicants. In the 2016 NRMP Match, 224 osteopathic applicants matched.[2]

- AOA Match

  There are 62 AOA-approved emergency medicine residency programs offering approximately 300 positions. These programs are located in 16 states. Nearly 70% of the programs are in Michigan, New York, Ohio, Oklahoma, and Pennsylvania.[11] In the 2015 AOA Match, there were only 8 unfilled positions. [1]

Competition for emergency medicine residency positions in the AOA Match is intense, with more applicants than positions available. In 2014, there were 1.5

applicants for every available position.[12] Dr. Otto Sabando is the program director of the emergency medicine residency program at St. Joseph's Regional Medical Center. He reports that the program receives 250 to 300 applications a year for six positions. "We look first at applicants with scores in the 600s for COMLEX Level 1 and Level 2 and work our way down from there."[22] In a recent report, applicants matching into osteopathic emergency medicine programs had mean COMLEX Level 1 and 2 CE scores of 513 and 543, respectively.[12]

Should osteopathic applicants interested in allopathic emergency medicine residency programs take the USMLE? In an interview with Dr. Jamie Collings, former program director of the emergency medicine residency program at Northwestern University, we asked her to address this important issue. Below is her answer.

Question: Of the total number of residents training in allopathic programs, 9.0% are osteopathic graduates. For osteopathic medical students interested in training at an allopathic residency program, a difficult issue is whether to take the USMLE in addition to the COMLEX examination. Do allopathic EM residency program directors prefer that osteopathic students take the USMLE? If so, is Step 1 sufficient or should students plan to take both the step 1 and 2 exams?

Answer: I think it is important for osteopathic students to take both Step 1 and Step 2 of the USMLE if they plan to apply to an allopathic residency program. Most programs understand what those scores mean and it really is the only way we have to objectively compare knowledge across the board.[23]

In further support of this recommendation was a survey of allopathic emergency medicine residency programs. 77% of PDs considered taking the USMLE extremely or somewhat important for osteopathic students.[24] From this data, it is clear that the osteopathic applicant who wishes to be considered at all programs will have to take the USMLE. Of note, programs that accept COMLEX scores may also encourage osteopathic applicants to take the USMLE. "We do accept COMLEX scores, but prefer you also take the USMLE to help better compare you with the larger applicant pool of MD candidates," writes the Department of Emergency Medicine at the Oregon Health Sciences University.[25]

Osteopathic applicants seeking a career in emergency medicine should create a strategy to make their application as competitive as possible. Between July and September of the senior year, complete away electives in emergency medicine. If you're interested in training in an allopathic program, you should target electives at institutions which have been known to be DO friendly. Even better are rotations at programs where there are DO graduates from your school. How many rotations should you complete in emergency medicine? If possible, we recommend that you perform at least two rotations before October so that you can secure EM standardized letters of recommendation (SLOR). During your rotations, arrange to work closely with key decision-makers at the program, including clerkship director, program director, and chairman.

Did you know?

There are also two osteopathic residency programs that offer combined training in Family Medicine and Emergency Medicine. In the 2015 AOA Match, there were a total of seven positions. One position went unfilled. There are also five osteopathic residency programs that offer combined training in Internal Medicine and Emergency Medicine. In the 2015 AOA Match, there were a total of 11 positions. Two positions went unfilled.[1]

Family Medicine

Osteopathic students and graduates may secure residency positions in family medicine programs through either the NRMP or AOA Match:

- NRMP Match

  In the 2016 NRMP Match, there were a total of 3,238 family medicine residency positions. Approximately 12% of these positions were filled by osteopathic applicants.[2] Of note, in recent years, approximately 95% of available positions have been filled through the match. This represents a significant increase over the 82.4% fill rate reported in 2005. Although interest in family medicine among allopathic students has increased slightly over the past ten years, the rise in fill rate is largely due to independent applicants, including osteopathic students. There has been a concerted effort among family medicine residency programs to build stronger ties with the osteopathic community to combat the relative lack of interest in family medicine among allopathic students. In recent years, an increasing number of ACGME-accredited family medicine residency programs have sought out AOA accreditation in an effort to become more attractive to osteopathic applicants.

- AOA Match

  Family medicine is one of the least competitive specialties in the AOA Match with 0.8 applicants per position. In the 2015 AOA Match, 362 positions went unfilled.[1] Many of these positions are ultimately filled by osteopathic graduates who fail to secure positions through the AOA or NRMP Matches. In a recent report, applicants matching into osteopathic family medicine residency programs had mean COMLEX Level 1 and 2 CE scores of 473 and 499, respectively.[12] The table below offers recommendations on how to explore the 260 available osteopathic family medicine residency programs offering approximately 900 positions.[11]

Learning About Osteopathic Family Medicine Residency Programs

- Join the ACOFP Student Chapter at your medical school. Program directors have visited chapters to speak about their residency programs. Some chapters invite residents to serve on a "resident panel." During these Q & A sessions, you can learn about life as a resident, the paths these residents took to reach their goals, and tips for success during the residency selection process.
- Review program websites.
- Attend the ACOFP Convention Residency Fair. At the spring convention of the ACOFP, students can take part in the annual residency fair. This is an excellent opportunity to speak to program personnel, and meet key decision-makers.
- Participate in Medical School Hospital Days. Many osteopathic schools have "hospital days" during which residency programs set up booths to facilitate interaction between the program and interested students.
- Complete Medical Student Electives. An elective at the institution is an excellent way to determine your level of compatibility with the program. Of course, such rotations are essentially an extended interview, allowing the program to better assess your fit with their program.

General Surgery

Osteopathic students and graduates may secure residency positions in general surgery residency programs through either the NRMP or AOA Match:

- NRMP Match

  In the 2016 NRMP Match, there were a total of 1,239 general surgery residency positions. 58 of these positions were filled by osteopathic applicants.[2] Securing residency positions is particularly difficult for osteopathic and international medical graduates. The NRMP designates these two groups as independent applicants. In 2014, 58.2% of independent applicants failed to match.[20]

- AOA Match

  General surgery is one of the more competitive specialties in the AOA Match with 1.3 applicants per position.[12] In the 2015 AOA Match, only five positions went unfilled.[1] In a recent report, applicants matching into osteopathic general surgery residency programs had mean COMLEX Level 1 and 2 CE scores of 531 and

550, respectively.[12] The table below offers recommendations on how to explore the 61 available osteopathic general surgery residency programs offering approximately 150 positions.[11]

Learning About Osteopathic General Surgery Residency Programs

- Join the Student Osteopathic Surgery Association (SOSA) Community. This will allow you to apply for student membership in the American College of Osteopathic Surgery.
- Attend SOSA conventions where you can learn more about the specialty, and network with residents and surgeons. The annual conference offers students the opportunity to participate in residency mock interviews, and visit with programs during the residency fair. Many surgery program directors and faculty are present at the residency fair.
- SOSA members can participate in the "Mentor Match" program which links students with surgical mentors.
- Consider serving as a SOSA leader either locally or nationally.
- Review program websites.
- Complete Medical Student Electives. An elective at the institution is an excellent way to determine your level of compatibility with the program. Of course, such rotations are essentially an extended interview, allowing the program to better assess your fit with their program.

Did you know?

General surgery residents training in osteopathic programs take the American Osteopathic Board of Surgery In-Training Examination (AOBSITE). In a retrospective study, AOBSITE performance was examined for all programs from 2008 to 2012 to determine if the size of the program has bearing on performance. Researchers found that larger general surgery residency training programs outperform smaller programs.[26]

Internal Medicine

Osteopathic students and graduates may secure residency positions in internal medicine programs through either the NRMP or AOA Match:

- NRMP Match

  In the 2016 NRMP Match, there were a total of 7,024 internal medicine residency positions. Approximately 500 of these positions were filled by osteopathic applicants.[2] Securing positions in internal medicine residency programs is considerably more difficult for osteopathic and international medical graduates. The NRMP designates these two groups as independent applicants. In 2014, 41.4% of independent applicants were unable to land positions in the field.[20]

- AOA Match

Internal medicine is one of the least competitive specialties in the AOA Match with 0.7 applicants per position.[12] In the 2015 AOA Match, there were 683 positions, but 186 of these positions went unfilled.[1] Although not all positions are filled in the Match, many of the positions that remain are ultimately filled by osteopathic graduates who fail to secure positions through the AOA or NRMP Matches. In a recent report, applicants matching into osteopathic internal medicine residency programs had mean COMLEX Level 1 and 2 CE scores of 484 and 507, respectively.[12] The table offers recommendations on how to explore the 146 available osteopathic internal medicine residency programs offering approximately 700 positions.[11]

Learning About Osteopathic Internal Medicine Residency Programs

- Join the Student Osteopathic Internal Medicine Association (SOIMA) Chapter at your medical school to learn more about the field.
- Consider serving as a leader in your SOIMA chapter.
- Review program websites.
- Student members of the American College of Osteopathic Internists (ACOI) may participate in the ACOI Mentoring Program. Program goals include increasing the percentage of osteopathic students entering the profession and completing training in osteopathic internal medicine residency programs.
- ACOI student members may participate in the Research Abstract Poster Contest. Cash awards are given for the top research posters, and winners are allowed to present their work at the ACOI Convention. There is also a category for interesting case presentations, and these winners are also given cash awards.
- Complete Medical Student Electives. An elective at the institution is an excellent way to determine your level of compatibility with the program. Of course, such rotations are essentially an extended interview, allowing the program to better assess your fit with their program.

Did you know?

In a recent article, Dr. Scott Girard, a member of the ACOI Board of Directors, encouraged osteopathic applicants to make inquiries with residency programs about their intent to maintain their "Osteopathic Focus."[27]

With the agreement by the AOA and the ACGME to have only one system of GME accreditation by 2020, internship and residency programs are now in the process of deciding if they are going to pursue "Osteopathic Focus." We assume that programs that have been traditionally Osteopathic in the past will pursue this designation, but this should not be taken for granted...As Osteopathic medical school graduates, you have the opportunity to hone and put your Osteopathic skills and treatment traditions into clinical use during your residency. Only a program with Osteopathic Focus will have a clear cut, Osteopathic curriculum in place for your postgraduate education. Even more important will be asking this question of program directors of internships/residencies that have been traditionally dually-accredited by both AOA and the ACGME. Will they continue to offer the Osteopathic skills education when the new system is in place?

Neurological Surgery

In 2012 – 2013, there were 1,272 total residents training in a total of 104 allopathic neurosurgery residency programs. Unfortunately, only 0.5% of these residents were osteopathic graduates.[10] In the 2016 NRMP Match, no osteopathic applicants landed positions in neurosurgery. With these odds, it's no surprise that most osteopathic applicants focus their efforts on osteopathic neurological surgery residency programs. Unfortunately, there are far more applicants interested in the field than positions available in the 11 osteopathic training programs. In the 2014 AOA Match, there were 1.3 applicants per position. In 2011, the average COMLEX Level 1 and 2 scores among students who matched was 577 and 608, respectively.[12] Involvement outside of the classroom through extracurricular activities, volunteer work, and research is also valued. Students interested in the field are encouraged to complete their core and elective rotations at institutions with neurological surgery residency programs. This will allow the student the opportunity to build connections with faculty and residents, shadow, and take part in departmental activities when other commitments do not interfere with such activities. It is essential to complete away rotations for consideration at most programs. At the Doctor's Hospital, where the neurological surgery program receives typically 20 applications for two positions, only applicants who have rotated through the department are considered. "This is the only way you can judge somebody's potential to become a neurosurgeon," says Dr. Louis Jacobs of Garden City Hospital. "You have to see how they react to people and how they look in the operating room."[28]

Neurology

Osteopathic students and graduates may secure residency positions in neurology residency programs through either the NRMP or AOA Match:

- NRMP Match

  In the 2016 NRMP Match, there were nearly 750 total positions at both the PGY1 and PGY2 levels. 70 of these positions were filled with osteopathic graduates.[2] Independent applicants (osteopathic and international medical graduates) find it more difficult to land positions. In 2014, 42.2% of independent applicants were unable to land positions in the field.[20]

- AOA Match

  Neurology is one of the less competitive specialties in the AOA Match with 1.0 applicant per position. In the 2015 AOA Match, 7 of the 22 available positions went unfilled. In a recent report, applicants matching into osteopathic neurology residency programs had mean COMLEX Level 1 and 2 CE scores of 502 and 533, respectively.[12]

Obstetrics & Gynecology

Osteopathic students and graduates may secure residency positions in obstetrics & gynecology residency programs through either the NRMP or AOA Match:

- NRMP Match

  In the 2016 NRMP Match, there were a total of 1,257 obstetrics & gynecology residency positions. Nearly 130 of these positions were filled by osteopathic applicants.[2] Securing residency positions is particularly difficult for osteopathic and international medical graduates. The NRMP designates these two groups as independent applicants. In 2014, 44% of independent applicants failed to match.[20]

- AOA Match

  Obstetrics & gynecology is one of the more competitive specialties in the AOA Match with 1.7 applicants per position.[12] In the 2015 AOA Match, there were 80 positions. Only six positions went unfilled.[1] "When we started our obstetrics and gynecology residency in 2006, we had four applicants for one or two slots," says Craig S. Glines, DO, the director of the AOA-approved program at Oakwood Southshore Medical Center in Trenton, Mich. "Last year, I had 85 applicants for one opening."[29] In a recent report, applicants matching into osteopathic obstetrics & gynecology residency programs had

> mean COMLEX Level 1 and 2 CE scores of 493 and 525, respectively. "I want someone who will make us proud in five years when they take their board certification exam, someone who will glow amongst others in the profession," says Dr. Hamid Sanjaghsaz, former program director of the obstetrics and gynecology residency program at Garden City Hospital. "I won't take someone who, for example, has not passed COMLEX Level 2 twice."[29]

Should osteopathic applicants interested in allopathic obstetrics and gynecology residency programs take the USMLE? In a survey of allopathic programs, 79% indicated that they do use COMLEX Level 1 scores when considering which applicants to interview.[30] Although you may find this reassuring, a significant number of these programs also prefer that osteopathic applicants take the USMLE exams. "You are not required to take USMLE," writes the Department of Obstetrics & Gynecology at the University of Cincinnati. "USMLE is preferred as it can be difficult to compare COMLEX and USMLE scores."[31] "A USMLE score is not required for osteopathic candidates, but will enhance your application," writes the Department of Obstetrics and Gynecology at Reading Hospital. To be considered at all programs, it is clear that the osteopathic applicant will have to take the USMLE.[32]

Ophthalmology

Osteopathic applicants interested in pursuing residency training in allopathic programs should realize that few applicants are successful. In 2012 – 2013, there were 1,323 total residents training in a total of 116 ophthalmology residency programs. Only 1.7% of these residents were osteopathic graduates.[10] Because of these odds, most interested applicants pursue training positions in the AOA Match. Unfortunately, the competition for these spots is intense because of the limited number of positions offered by the 15 available training programs. In the 2014 AOA Match, there were 2.4 applicants per position, making ophthalmology the most competitive specialty along with otolaryngology.[12] Because the number of applicants far exceeds the available positions, osteopathic residency programs have the luxury of selecting trainees with strong COMLEX scores. According to Dr. Carlo J. DiMarco, CEO for the American Osteopathic Colleges of Ophthalmology and Otolaryngology-Head and Neck Surgery, applicants with scores below the 90th percentile are not considered at many programs.[33] In a recent report, applicants matching into osteopathic ophthalmology residency programs had mean COMLEX Level 1 and 2 CE scores of 571 and 582, respectively.[12] Osteopathic ophthalmology programs also tend to prefer applicants who have rotated in their programs, and interested students are highly urged to complete multiple electives.

Orthopedic Surgery

The odds are against success in the NRMP Match for osteopathic applicants seeking training in allopathic orthopedic surgery residency programs. In the 2016 NRMP Match, only 4 osteopathic applicants secured a position.[2] For this reason, most osteopathic applicants pursue training in osteopathic orthopedic surgery residency programs. Although there are 44 programs, as you might expect, there are more applicants than available positions. In fact, in the 2014 AOA Match, there were 1.8 applicants per position, making orthopedic surgery the fourth most competitive specialty.[12] In the 2015 AOA Match, there were 111 positions. Only three positions went unfilled.[1] The Department of Orthopedic Surgery at Botsford Hospital receives over 100 applications for its three annual positions. According to Dr. Lee Vander Lugt, Executive Director of the American Osteopathic Academy of Orthopedics, some programs will only consider applicants in the top 10% of the class and with COMLEX scores at least in the 90th percentile.[34] In a recent report, applicants matching into osteopathic orthopedic surgery residency programs had mean COMLEX Level 1 and 2 CE scores of 598 and 621, respectively.[12] Although scores and numbers are an important part of the selection process, non-cognitive skills and qualities are important to many programs. "Of course we want someone who is bright," says Dr. Drouillard of Garden City Hospital. "But a willingness to learn is more important to us than superb scores." Although letters of recommendation are a way for programs to assess these important qualities, orthopedic surgery residency programs place a high premium on rotations performed at their institution. "Over the years, 80 to 90% of the residents we've taken on have been people who've rotated with us," says Dr. Linard of Botsford Hospital.[34]

Otolaryngology-Facial Plastic Surgery

Although the NRMP Match offers many more training positions in otolaryngology than the AOA Match, few osteopathic applicants are successful in securing allopathic positions. In 2012-2013, only 0.3% of the 1,454 residents training in allopathic programs were osteopathic graduates.[10] These steep odds lead many osteopathic applicants to devote their efforts to the AOA Match. Although there are 20 programs, there are far more applicants than available positions. In the 2014 AOA Match, there were 2.4 applicants per position, making otolaryngology the most competitive specialty along with ophthalmology.[12] In the 2015 AOA Match, there were no unfilled positions.[1] According to Dr. Wayne Robbins, Program Director of the AOA-approved ENT residency at Genesys Regional Medical Center, it is typical for AOA-approved programs to receive 40-50 applicants for every position.[35] With such intense competition, programs have the luxury of choosing among an applicant pool with exceptional board scores. In a recent report, applicants matching into osteopathic otolaryngology residency programs had mean COMLEX Level 1 and 2 CE scores of 630 and 664, respectively.[12] Many programs favor applicants who have rotated at their institution. "It is rare that we would accept a student who didn't rotate through our clinical services," says Dr. Richard Scharf, Program Director of the AOA-approved ENT program at St. Barnabas Medical Center. "And the same holds true for the vast majority of programs in otolaryngology and facial plastic surgery."[35] Manual dexterity is understandably important to these programs, and some programs evaluate dexterity through computer simulation models, knot tying, and sculpting.

Pediatrics

Osteopathic students and graduates may secure residency positions in pediatric residency programs through either the NRMP or AOA Match:

- NRMP Match

  In the 2016 NRMP Match, there were a total of 2,689 positions in pediatric training programs. Over 350 of these positions were awarded to osteopathic graduates.[2] Independent applicants (osteopathic and international medical graduates) find it more difficult to land positions. In 2014, 42.2% of independent applicants were unable to land positions in the field.[20]

- AOA Match

  Pediatrics is one of the more competitive specialties in the AOA Match with 1.7 applicants per position.[12] In the 2015 AOA Match, there were 63 positions offered in sixteen residency programs. Twelve positions went unfilled.[1] In a recent report, applicants matching into osteopathic pediatric residency programs had mean COMLEX Level 1 and 2 CE scores of 476 and 494, respectively.[12]

Did you know?

The American Academy of Pediatrics Section on Osteopathic Physicians has nearly 2,500 members. For osteopathic students, membership is an excellent way to become more informed of the specialty, and network with key decision-makers in the field. Another organization worth joining as a student member is the American College of Osteopathic Pediatricians.

Physical Medicine & Rehabilitation

Although osteopathic students may secure positions in physical medicine & rehabilitation through either the AOA or NRMP Match, there are only 6 AOA-approved residency programs.[11] As you may expect, these programs are quite competitive. Fortunately, many allopathic residency programs are receptive to DO applicants. In the 2016 NRMP Match, 114 osteopathic applicants secured positions in the specialty.[2] In 2012-2013, 28.4% of total residents training in 77 physical medicine & rehabilitation residency programs were osteopathic graduates.[10] While some osteopathic applicants find success in the NRMP Match, many fail to match. Osteopathic and international medical graduate applicants are designated independent applicants by the NRMP. In 2014, 47% of independent applicants failed to match.[20] To maximize the chances of success, osteopathic applicants are encouraged to apply to both osteopathic and allopathic training programs.

Tips for Match Success for Osteopathic Applicants Interested in PM&R

- Join your school's chapter of the American Osteopathic College of Physical Medicine & Rehabilitation (AOCPMR). Chapters often hold a variety of events to expose students to the field, including workshops in which students can participate in PM&R diagnostic techniques.
- Consider serving as a leader in your school's AOCPMR chapter.
- There are also student leadership opportunities for the AOCPMR national organization. Although you can serve as President, Vice President, Secretary, or Treasurer, there are also positions available on the website, student conference, education, research, public relations, bylaws, mentorship, and membership committees.
- Student members of AOCPMR may participate in the Student Mentorship Program. Through this program, students are linked with resident or attending mentors.
- At the AOCPMR Mid-Year meeting, student members have opportunities to network with program directors, key faculty, and residents. Expert advice for match success may be offered by PM&R residency program directors and residents.
- Look for ways to contribute to organizations that provide services to people with disabilities. Students can raise funds, or serve as counselors for children and adults with physical or developmental disabilities.
- Since PM&R residents have to complete a scholarly project, programs look favorably on applicants who have gained research experience. Search for opportunities to perform research in the field. Note that the AOCPMR lists research opportunities for medical students on their website.
- Student members of AOCPMR may submit abstracts for display at the AOCPMR Mid-Year Meeting.
- Osteopathic students are also encouraged to attend the AAPMR Annual Assembly Residency Fair.
- Complete PM&R elective rotations. Dr. Wieting, former program director of the Michigan State University's dually accredited PM&R residency program, recommends completing at least one, but preferably two, such rotations. If your schedule permits it, he recommends doing more.

Psychiatry

Osteopathic students and graduates may secure residency positions in psychiatry residency programs through either the NRMP or AOA Match:

- NRMP Match

In the 2016 NRMP Match, there were nearly 1,400 positions. Many positions in psychiatry are filled with osteopathic and international medical graduate applicants. In 2016, there were nearly 200 osteopathic applicants who found success.[2]

- AOA Match

Psychiatry is one of the less competitive specialties in the AOA Match with 1.2 applicants per position. In the 2015 AOA Match, there were 55 positions offered in 18 residency programs. 14 positions went unfilled.[1] In a recent report, applicants matching into osteopathic psychiatry residency programs had mean COMLEX Level 1 and 2 CE scores of 440 and 461, respectively.[12]

Urological Surgery

Osteopathic students and graduates may secure residency positions in urology programs through either the American Urological Association (AUA) or AOA Match:

- AUA Match

In 2012 – 2013, there were 1,189 total residents training in a total of 123 urology residency programs. 94% were U.S. MDs, 4.6% were international medical graduates, and 1.3% were osteopathic graduates.[10] Given the small numbers of osteopathic graduates training in allopathic urology programs, nearly all osteopathic applicants will also apply for positions in the AOA Match.

- AOA Match

Urology is the third most competitive specialty in the AOA Match with 2.0 applicants per position.[12] In the 2015 AOA Match, there were 20 positions offered in 10 residency programs. There were no unfilled positions.[1] In a recent report, applicants matching into osteopathic urology residency programs had mean COMLEX Level 1 and 2 CE scores of 605 and 647, respectively.[12]

Audition rotations in urology are very important in the selection process for both allopathic and osteopathic residency programs.

References

[1]National Matching Services. Available at: https://www.natmatch.com/aoairp/. Accessed March 22, 2016.
[2]Advance Data Tables: 2016 Main Residency Match. Available at: http://www.nrmp.org/match-data/main-residency-match-data/. Accessed April 23, 2016.
[3]AACOM Reports. Available at: http://www.aacom.org/reports-programs-initiatives/aacom-reports/entering-and-graduating-class-surveys. Accessed March 2, 2016.
[4]George Washington University Department of Emergency Medicine. Available at: https://smhs.gwu.edu/emed/education-training/residency/apply. Accessed March 22, 2016.
[5]University of Rochester Department of Obstetrics & Gynecology. Available at: https://www.urmc.rochester.edu/education/graduate-medical-education/prospective-residents/obgyn/applicant-information/faq.aspx. Accessed March 22, 2016.
[6]Carolinas Medical Center Department of Medicine. Available at: http://www.carolinashealthcare.org/internal-medicine-application-information-medical-education. Accessed March 22, 2016.
[7]Hasty R, Snyder S, Suciu G, Moskow J. Graduating osteopathic medical students' perceptions and recommendations on the decision to take the United States Medical Licensing Examination. *J Am Osteop Assoc* 112; 83-89.
[8]Terry R. Dually accredited family practice residencies: wave of the future. *JAOA* 2003; 103(8): 367-70.
[9]Pecora A. Factors influencing osteopathic physicians' decisions to enroll in allopathic residency programs. *J Am Osteopath Assoc* 1990; 90(6): 527-33.
[10]Brotherton S, Etzel S. Graduate Medical Education, 2014-2015. *JAMA* 2015; 314(22): 2436-54.
[11]AOA approved residencies. Available at: http://opportunities.osteopathic.org/index.htm. Accessed March 3, 2016.
[12]Osteopathic GME Match Report (2014). Available at: file:///C:/Users/labme/Downloads/DO_GME_match_2014.pdf. Accessed March 3, 2014.
[13]The DO. Available at: http://thedo.osteopathic.org/2012/03/anesthesiologys-allure-high-pay-flexibility-intellectual-stimulation/2/. Accessed March 22, 2016.
[14]University of Pittsburgh Department of Anesthesiology. Available at: http://www.anes.upmc.edu/education/residency_program/application.aspx. Accessed January 28, 2013.
[15]University of Arkansas Department of Anesthesiology. Available at: http://anesthesiology.uams.edu/uamsanesthresidents. Accessed January 28, 2013.
[16]Mayo Clinic Department of Anesthesiology. Available at: http://www.mayo.edu/msgme/residencies-fellowships/anesthesiology/anesthesiology-residency-minnesota/frequently-asked-questions. Accessed January 28, 2013.

[17]University of Missouri Department of Anesthesiology. Available at: http://medicine.missouri.edu/anest/residency-apply.html. Accessed January 28, 2013.
[18]University of Kentucky Department of Anesthesiology. Available at: http://www.wildcatanesthesia.com/index.php?option=com_content&view=article&id=232&Itemid=329. Accessed January 28, 2013.
[19]AAMC Visiting Student Application Service. Available at: https://services.aamc.org/20/vsas/public/school/instID/177. Accessed January 28, 2013.
[20]Charting Outcomes in the Match (2014). Available at: http://www.nrmp.org/wp-content/uploads/2014/09/Charting-Outcomes-2014-Final.pdf. Accessed March 3, 2014.
[21]American College of Osteopathic Radiology. Available at: http://www.aocr.org/?page=StudentFAQ. Accessed March 3, 2016.
[22]DO Online. Available at: http://www.do-online.org/TheDO/?p=106851&page=2. Accessed January 30, 2013.
[23]Getting into Emergency Medicine. Available at: http://studentdoctor.net/2010/08/the-successful-match-getting-into-emergency-medicine/. Accessed January 30, 2013.
182014 NRMP PD
[24]Weizberg M, Kass D, Hussains A, Cohen J, Hahn B. Should osteopathic students applying to allopathic emergency medicine programs take the USMLE exam? *West J Emerg Med* 2014; 15(1): 101-106.
[25]Oregon Health Science University Department of Emergency Medicine. Available at: http://www.ohsu.edu/emergency/education/residency/faqs.cfm. Accessed April 20, 2016.
[26]Falcone J, Rosen M. The importance of residency program size and location on American Osteopathic Board of Surgery In-Training Examination outcomes. *J Surg res* 2013; 184 (1): 61-5.
[27]American College of Osteopathic Internists. Available at: https://www.acoi.org/. Accessed December 2, 2015.
[28]The DO. Available at: http://thedo.osteopathic.org/2013/10/how-to-become-a-neurosurgeon/. Accessed March 2, 2016.
[29]The DO. Available at: http://thedo.osteopathic.org/2012/10/despite-challenges-ob-gyns-revere-their-specialty/. Accessed March 2, 2016.
[30]Results of the 2014 NRMP Program Director Survey. Available at: http://www.nrmp.org/wp-content/uploads/2014/09/PD-Survey-Report-2014.pdf. Accessed March 3, 2015.
[31]University of Cincinnati Department of Obstetrics and Gynecology. Available at: http://med2.uc.edu/obgyn/education/residency/apply.aspx. Accessed March 3, 2016.
[32]Reading Hospital Department of Obstetrics and Gynecology. Available at: https://www.readinghealth.org/education-and-research/academic-affairs/residencies/obgyn/applicant-information/. Accessed March 3, 2016.
[33]The DO. Available at: http://thedo.osteopathic.org/2013/04/love-at-first-sight-ophthalmology-seduces-with-variety-hours-outcomes/. Accessed March 3, 2016.

[34]The DO. Available at: http://thedo.osteopathic.org/2013/03/work-ethic-elite-scores-dexterity-key-to-becoming-an-orthopedic-surgeon/. Accessed March 3, 2016.
[35]The DO. Available at: http://thedo.osteopathic.org/2013/07/procedural-diversity-satisfying-outcomes-draw-dos-to-otolaryngology/. Accessed March 3, 2016.

Chapter 21

U.S. Citizen International Medical Graduates

Over the past two decades, there's been a tremendous increase in the number of U.S. citizen graduates of international medical schools. In 1995, 527 U.S. citizen IMGs achieved ECFMG certification, representing 9% of all such certifications. By 2013, the number had increased nearly six-fold, and these 2,963 ECFMG-certified graduates accounted for 30% of all certifications.[1] U.S. citizen IMGs make up nearly 15% of the total residency applicant pool.

There's been a remarkable change in the countries where U.S. citizens have trained. Up until the mid-1970s, Americans seeking medical education abroad sought training primarily in Europe, in countries such as Belgium, France, Italy, Spain, and Switzerland. As European schools placed more of an emphasis on the education of their own citizens, Americans began to look elsewhere. Offshore schools in the Caribbean were first established in the late 1970s. Growth of these schools continued in the 1980s but then declined, only to accelerate again after the turn of the century. 40% of Caribbean medical schools were founded after 2000.[2]

U.S. citizen IMGs have made important contributions to medicine in such areas as patient care, teaching, and research. At a time when the U.S. is facing a growing shortage of primary care physicians, U.S. citizen IMGs are doing their part to fulfill the nation's primary care manpower needs. Over 50% of Caribbean-educated physicians involved in direct patient care are practicing primary care.[3] The primary care physician workforce shortage is felt most deeply in rural areas. Over 60 million Americans lack access to primary care, and there's evidence to indicate that IMGs are filling these gaps in many states.[4] Many IMGs are performing high quality research at institutions across the U.S. The number of full-time IMG faculty doubled from 1984 to 2004. In 2004, there were over 17,000 IMGs serving as faculty members. In 2004, 21.3% of full-time faculty identified as principal investigators on NIH research grants were IMGs.[5]

To make such an impact in the United States as licensed physicians, U.S. citizen IMGs must face and overcome significant obstacles. In a survey of 125 general surgery PDs, respondents were asked to indicate their level of agreement with the following statement:[6]

In reality, all things being equal, our program would rather offer positions to USMGs than to IMGs.

87% strongly agreed or agreed with the statement. Nearly 20% of PDs reported having experienced pressure to rank U.S. medical school applicants higher than more accomplished and qualified IMGs. Over 70% believed that there was discrimination against IMGs in the residency selection process.

For U.S. citizen IMGs, failure to obtain a residency position can be economically devastating. There is also the risk of emotional distress associated with failure to match or even a match that results in a position in an unfulfilling career. As an advisor and consultant to IMG applicants, I've been privy to some heartbreaking stories. In working with applicants over a period of many years, I've been able to identify the factors that prevent success in the residency match. In this chapter, I discuss these factors, and offer recommendations to navigate this complex process.

Rule # 198 Understand the challenges of matching in the U.S.

In the 2016 NRMP Match, 5,323 U.S. citizen IMGs participated, hoping to secure residency positions in the U.S. Unfortunately, 46.1% of these applicants failed to match.[7]

2016 NRMP Success Rate for Different Applicant Groups	
Applicant Type	**Success Rate in NRMP Match**
U.S. seniors (allopathic medical schools)	94%
Students/Graduates of U.S. osteopathic schools	80%
US citizen IMGs	54%
Non-U.S. citizen IMGs	50%
Adapted from Advance Data Tables: 2016 Main Residency Match. Available at: http://www.nrmp.org/match-data/main-residency-match-data/. Accessed April 23, 2016.	

For IMGs, there's concern that these numbers may worsen. To meet the needs of an anticipated physician manpower shortage, U.S. medical schools have expanded enrollment considerably over the past five years. Unfortunately, because of governmental funding issues, there has not been a corresponding rise in the number of residency positions. As more and more graduates have entered the Match, I've seen the competition for available residency positions intensify. Unless funding for more positions is secured, the coming years will likely be very difficult for all residency applicants, and especially so for IMG applicants.

Rule # 199 Research the competitiveness of your chosen specialty, and factor that into your decision-making process.

Certain specialties are far more competitive than others. Specialties such as ophthalmology, otolaryngology, radiation oncology, dermatology, urology, plastic surgery, and orthopedic surgery are highly competitive. There are many more U.S. applicants who wish to enter these fields than positions available. Consequently, a significant number of U.S. applicants fail to match. As you might expect, U.S. citizen IMGs find these specialties the most difficult to enter. Specialties with the highest numbers of U.S. citizen IMG trainees include family medicine, internal medicine, pediatrics, and psychiatry.

Percentage of U.S. citizen IMGs Who Failed to Match in 2014 by Specialty

Specialty	Number of U.S. citizen IMGs who applied	% Failing to Match
Anesthesiology	160	41%
Emergency Medicine	190	72%
Family Medicine	1,233	57%
General Surgery	308	49%
Internal Medicine	1,594	47%
Neurology	103	43%
Obstetrics & Gynecology	177	56%
Pathology	115	60%
Pediatrics	347	44%
Physical Medicine & Rehabilitation	83	52%
Psychiatry	459	56%
Radiology	102	46%

Adapted from Charting Outcomes in the Match: International Medical Graduates. Available at: http://www.ecfmg.org/resources/NRMP-ECFMG-Charting-Outcomes-in-the-Match-International-Medical-Graduates-2014.pdf. Accessed June 23, 2015.

I'm often asked if it's possible for U.S. citizen IMGs to match into the most competitive specialties. It's definitely possible, and I've enjoyed helping these applicants reach their professional goals. However, while U.S. citizen IMGs have successfully matched into highly competitive specialties, it requires a well thought out application strategy, and it's far from easy.

Because of the large numbers of IMG applicants matching into less competitive specialties such as psychiatry and family medicine, IMGs often believe that it's easy to match into these fields. As you can see from the data, over 50% of applicants fail to match in these specialties. Regardless of your chosen specialty, the key to a successful match hinges on the development of a carefully developed strategy.

Rule # 200 **As competition for residency positions has increased, the USMLE has taken on more importance than ever before.**

Although U.S. residency programs seek to accurately assess the quality of an applicant's medical education, it's impossible for programs to become familiar with each and every international medical school. Instead, programs place considerable emphasis on a tool they're intimately familiar with – the USMLE exams. These exams have made it easier for programs to assess the medical knowledge of IMG applicants. Since all applicants are required to take these, programs are readily able to compare scores of one applicant with another.

According to the NRMP, the mean USMLE Step 1 score among matched U.S. IMG applicants in 2014 was 217.[8] In an interview with Dr. Su-Ting Li, Program Director of the University of California Davis Pediatrics Residency Program, we asked her about the importance of the USMLE for IMG applicants:[9]

IMGs need to pass USMLE 1, 2 and CS on their first attempt, preferably with scores higher than 220, and need to complete all steps of USMLE in as short a time frame as possible. IMGs are being compared with other applicants who took the exams while still in medical school, without the luxury of months preparing for each examination. In addition, passage of the USMLEs needs to be done as soon as possible – the chances of matching go down with each successive year away from clinical care.

Below are the mean USMLE Step 1 and Step 2 CK scores for matched and unmatched U.S. citizen IMG applicants by specialty.

Mean USMLE Step 1 Scores for Matched Vs Unmatched U.S. citizen IMGs by Specialty (2014)

Specialty	Mean Step 1 Score for Matched Applicants	Mean Step 1 Score for Unmatched Applicants
Anesthesiology	234	210
Emergency Medicine	225	215
Family Medicine	206	198
General Surgery	227	216
Internal Medicine	221	205
Neurology	216	203
Obstetrics & Gynecology	221	207
Pathology	224	204
Pediatrics	216	201
Physical Medicine & Rehabilitation	223	207
Psychiatry	205	198
Radiology	237	223

Adapted from Charting Outcomes in the Match: International Medical Graduates. Available at: http://www.ecfmg.org/resources/NRMP-ECFMG-Charting-Outcomes-in-the-Match-International-Medical-Graduates-2014.pdf. Accessed June 23, 2015.

Mean USMLE Step 2 CK Scores for Matched Vs Unmatched U.S. citizen IMGs by Specialty (2014)		
Specialty	**Mean Step 2 CK Score for Matched Applicants**	**Mean Step 2 CK Score for Unmatched Applicants**
Anesthesiology	239	212
Emergency Medicine	235	223
Family Medicine	213	203
General Surgery	234	216
Internal Medicine	228	210
Neurology	222	206
Obstetrics & Gynecology	232	213
Pathology	226	205
Pediatrics	224	208
Physical Medicine & Rehabilitation	231	212
Psychiatry	211	202
Radiology	241	223

Adapted from Charting Outcomes in the Match: International Medical Graduates. Available at: http://www.ecfmg.org/resources/NRMP-ECFMG-Charting-Outcomes-in-the-Match-International-Medical-Graduates-2014.pdf. Accessed June 23, 2015.

Rule # 201 **As a preclinical student, your first priority is to do well in your courses and score high on the USMLE Step 1 exam. Be sure to also improve your credentials outside the classroom.**

During the preclinical years, you'll put forth tremendous effort to do well in your classes and score high on the USMLE Step 1 exam. While this should be your focus, a compelling argument can be made for involvement in activities outside of the classroom.

Extracurricular activities

With long days, many lectures, and vast amounts of information to absorb, preclinical students often wonder if it's even feasible to participate in extracurricular activities. Despite demanding schedules, many preclinical students are able to do just that, provided they make participation a priority. Your involvement has the potential to provide a boost to your residency application. Extracurricular activities are a significant nonacademic factor in the residency selection process. In a recent NRMP survey of approximately 1,800 PDs representing the 23 largest medical specialties, 54% of respondents cited volunteer/extracurricular experiences as a factor in selecting applicants to interview.[10] Extracurricular activities "might provide evidence for non-cognitive attributes that predict success," writes Dr. Andrew Lee, Chairman of the Department of Ophthalmology at The Methodist Hospital. "The first priority of a residency selection committee is insuring that the applicant does not wash out or cause trouble during their time in the program. This is sometimes referred to generically as 'fit.' Everyone wants a team player who is unselfish and working towards a common goal."[11] Your involvement in extracurricular activities can highlight these important qualities.

7 Benefits of Extracurricular Activities for Residency Applicants

- You further develop skills that are directly applicable to success as a physician. A few examples of vital skills in the daily life of a doctor are teamwork, self-discipline, time management, and leadership.
- Involvement in organizations is a way to develop and strengthen bonds with classmates.
- Since student organizations often have a faculty advisor or sponsor, students have extraordinary opportunities to work closely with faculty members.
- Extracurricular activities are a significant nonacademic factor in the residency selection process.
- Once accepted for a residency interview, the depth and breadth of your involvement in extracurricular activities can help you stand out in a sea of academically qualified applicants.
- Residency programs look closely at extracurricular activities to gain some insight into an applicant's potential to be a leader in the field.
- Some residency programs believe that activities chosen as a student may predict involvement during residency. An applicant who served on a medical school committee may have an interest in serving on a residency committee.

Did you know?

In evaluating extracurricular activities, residency programs will look at the depth of a student's involvement. While some students believe there's strength in numbers, residency programs value the quality of involvement. Programs are interested in learning whether a student excelled in one or two activities. Did you demonstrate serious commitment to an organization? Were you able to make meaningful contributions? When comparing residency applicants of equal academic ability, factors such as depth and breadth of extracurricular activities may help one student stand out.

Community Service

Although community service clearly benefits others, students themselves gain tremendous benefits from their involvement and participation. Community service is good for the psyche. Research has shown that volunteering increases positive feelings, improves mental health, reduces the risk of depression, and lowers stress levels. Community service involvement can serve as a draw for residency programs. In a recent NRMP survey of 1,840 PDs representing the 19 largest medical specialties, 56% cited community service as a factor in selecting applicants to interview.[12] Is there a relationship between community service involvement and performance in medical school and residency? One study suggested just that. In research done to determine if there is a relationship between students' volunteer community service hours and medical school academic and residency performance, students in the highest service group were found to have significantly better grade point averages, USMLE Step 2 scores, and residency director assessments, as compared to students having no community service hours.[13]

Leadership

As a member of an organization, you have the power to make meaningful contributions through active involvement. This can take different forms. A student can serve in a leadership capacity, such as president or vice-president. Since many groups host events, students can volunteer to spearhead or coordinate an event. Students can also head committees within the group. Such demonstration of leadership ability is another way to strengthen your application. In the aforementioned NRMP survey of PDs, 63% of respondents cited leadership qualities as a factor in selecting applicants to interview.[10] When asked to rate the importance of this factor on a scale of 1 (not at all important) to 5 (very important), PDs gave it an average rating of 4.0. There is evidence to suggest that leadership qualities may make for better residents. A survey of emergency medicine PDs revealed that having a "distinctive factor," such as being a medical school officer, was one of three factors more predictive of residency performance.[14]

Research

In a recent survey of PDs conducted by the NRMP, 43% of respondents cited demonstrated involvement and interest in research as a factor in selecting applicants to interview.[10] While research experience is not highly valued relative to other academic selection criteria, the most competitive specialties do place greater importance on research experience. In evaluating research experience during medical school, programs will look closely at the level of your involvement. Did you merely collect data? Or were you involved through all phases of the project, including design, data collection, interpretation and analysis of data, and preparation of the manuscript. Programs also assess your productivity. Did your work result in a tangible measure, such as an abstract, manuscript, or presentation at a meeting?

Did you know?

Although you seek to publish or present your research, all is not lost if you don't reach these goals. Research experience that doesn't lead to publication can still be an invaluable addition to your application. It demonstrates your dedication to the field, may result in stronger LORs, and provides a topic of discussion in interviews.

No matter which activity or activities you choose, your involvement and accomplishments can bolster the strength of your application. In the event that you receive a low USMLE score, your success outside of the classroom may help you secure interviews at programs where your score alone would not be competitive. I've found that low-scoring applicants with an established area of non-academic excellence have an easier time attracting the interest of programs when compared to low-scoring colleagues with bare applications.

Rule # 202 Awards are available for IMGs. Seize these opportunities.

International medical students and graduates are making important contributions in patient care, research, teaching, advocacy, and leadership, and may be recognized for these efforts. Awards can provide a significant boost to the strength of the residency application, and distinguish an applicant from his peers. In a survey of PDs, Green found that awards were tenth in importance among a group of 14 residency selection criteria.[15] Although not as important as UMSLE Step 1 scores and LORs, awards were ranked higher than such factors as preclinical grades, research while in medical school, and published medical school research.

I recently wrote the book, *Medical School Scholarships, Grants, & Awards: Insider Advice for Winning Scholarships*. Through this process, I've become familiar with grants and awards open to both U.S. medical students and IMGs. While it's true that many awards are only open to U.S. medical students, a surprising number are also available to international medical students and graduates. As competition for residency positions intensifies, applicants who've won awards will stand out from their peers. In 2015, I wrote an article describing 10 awards that can enhance the credentials of IMG applicants (originally published at StudentDoc.com). It is reproduced here.

10 Awards Available to International Medical Students/Graduates

ACP National Abstract Competition

Students enrolled in international medical schools may become members of the American College of Physicians (ACP) free of charge. Membership allows students to submit abstracts for the ACP National Abstract Competition. Abstracts can be submitted in the categories of basic research, clinical research, quality improvement/patient safety, high value cost conscious care, and clinical vignette. The first author of any winning abstract is asked to prepare an oral or poster presentation at the ACP Internal Medicine Meeting. In 2014, Eleah Porter, a medical student at the American University of the Caribbean School of Medicine, presented a poster entitled "A Rare Cause of Massive Hematuria: Renal Artery Aneurysm Rupture," at the ACP National Conference. The research was based on a patient encounter during her surgery core clerkship at

The Brooklyn Hospital Center. It was selected as a National Winner in the Student Clinical Vignette division.

ACP State Chapter Competition

State ACP Chapters also hold these competitions, and international students may be eligible to enter. In 2013, Namrata Kohli, a student at the American University of Antigua, won first place at the ACP South Carolina Annual Conference for her research on the Broken Heart Syndrome.

Society of Hospital Medicine Scientific Abstract and Poster Competition

International medical students and graduates may submit abstracts to the Society of Hospital Medicine (SHM). SHM holds the Scientific Abstract and Poster Competition, also known as "Research, Innovations, and Clinical Vignettes," at the SHM Annual Meeting. In recent years, there have been over 1,100 applicants competing for approximately 700 poster spots. To be eligible, the first author should be a member of the society. If the first author is unable to present the poster at the meeting, he can designate another author to do so, including international medical students or graduates. International medical students/graduates can join SHM and register for the meeting as an affiliate member.

Society of General Internal Medicine Clinical Vignette Competition

The Society of General Internal Medicine (SGIM) allows international medical students and graduates to submit vignettes for the Clinical Vignette Competition held at the SGIM Annual Meeting. Vignettes may also be submitted for competitions at regional meetings (Midwest, California-Hawaii, Northwest, Southern, Mid-Atlantic, New England).

AMA Research Symposium

IMGs who are ECFMG-certified and awaiting residency can join the American Medical Association. Members can submit abstracts of their scientific research for consideration of poster presentation at the AMA Research Symposium. A small number of abstracts will be selected for the Oral Presentation Competition. Every year, the AMA names winners for podium and poster presentation from the AMA IMG Section.

Excellence in Emergency Medicine Award

International medical students are encouraged to make inquiries with their medical school about their eligibility for the Excellence in Emergency Medicine Award bestowed by the Society for Academic Emergency Medicine. Although the award has traditionally been given to U.S. or Canadian medical students, a number of St. George's University graduates have been recipients of this prestigious honor.

Society for Public Health Education

Many IMGs seeking residency positions in the U.S. pursue MPH degrees. For graduate students in these programs, there are opportunities to win awards, scholarships, and fellowships through the Society for Public Health Education (SOPHE). Award opportunities are available for students interested in patient engagement, injury prevention, attendance at the SOPHE Annual Meeting, and research.

Dr. James A. Ferguson Emerging Infectious Diseases Fellowship

The Dr. James A. Ferguson Emerging Infectious Diseases Fellowship is a 9-week fellowship program funded by the Centers for Disease Control and Prevention. Fellows have opportunities to participate in public health research in the area of infectious diseases and health disparities. Full-time students in medical or public health graduate programs are eligible to apply. U.S. Citizens, U.S. Nationals, and Permanent Residents may apply for the fellowship (although international students with F1 or K1 visas are not eligible). Applicants who are members of underrepresented groups are particularly encouraged to apply.

Paul Ambrose Scholars Program

Medical (allopathic and osteopathic) and public health students may apply for the Paul Ambrose Scholars Program. Scholars learn how to address population health challenges at the national and community level. Participants complete online public health knowledge assessments, attend a leadership symposium, and plan and implement a local community health project.

American Psychiatric Association Poster Competition

The Annual Meeting of the Institute of Psychiatric Services of the American Psychiatric Association offers an opportunity for international medical students and graduates to present posters. At a recent meeting, Adam Hines, a medical student at the Ross University School of Medicine, presented "Meningioma and Psychiatric Symptoms: A Case Report and Review." The poster was based on a patient encounter he had during a rotation at St. John's Episcopal Hospital in Far Rockaway, NY. "The poster presentation was a really great experience," said Hines in an article posted on the Ross University School of Medicine website. "I was able to present to prestigious people and to discuss the case with them."[16] He later wrote an article that was accepted for publication.

Did you know?

For international medical students and graduates, the benefits of entering these competitions extend well beyond recognition. The process of applying for these awards leads to deeper relationships with research mentors, presentations at meetings, and opportunities to network with key decision-makers at residency programs across the country. It can certainly provide a significant boost to the residency application, and is well worth the effort.

Rule # 203 **Your core clerkship performance may either limit or expand your future career options.**

The skills and traits reflected in core clerkship grades are considered so important to future success as a resident that residency programs use these grades as a major factor in the selection process. Although programs look closely at clerkship grades and performance, it can be challenging to determine the significance and meaning of reported grades. This holds true for both U.S. medical school and IMG applicants. In a review of the clerkship grading practices at U.S. medical schools, researchers noted eight different grading systems in effect at 119 accredited schools. The percentage of students receiving the top grade varied tremendously, ranging from 2% to 93%.[17] This variability in grading makes it difficult to compare performance from one applicant to another. As difficult as it is for programs to decipher the meaning of grades for U.S. medical students, it's even more challenging to unravel the mysteries of grading at foreign medical schools. You may have achieved the top grade in internal medicine, pediatrics, and surgery during rotations performed in another country, but programs struggle to understand how that will translate to performance here. The key question programs seek to answer is whether you have the skills and qualities to be successful as a resident in the United States. That's why we agree with the recommendations of Dr. Su-Ting Li:[9]

International medical graduates (IMGs) are at a disadvantage when applying to pediatric residency programs because of the difficulty programs have in assessing their potential for success during residency and beyond. In large part, this is due to difficulty programs have in assessing prior clinical performance of IMGs. Ideally, IMGs should demonstrate their readiness to begin training by participating in a clinical rotation at a U.S. medical school and obtaining strong letters of recommendation from established faculty members.

For U.S. citizen IMGs, I recommend the following:

- If your life situation and school permits it, we recommend that you arrange your core clinical rotations in the U.S. If you're unable to complete your core clinical rotations in the U.S., arrange for electives in the U.S.
- Complete your rotations at institutions with accredited residency programs. Such rotations are viewed by residency programs as being of higher caliber and offering more structured learning.
- Rotations taking place at academic institutions (university or community hospitals with residency training programs) are received well by selection committees.
- Letters of recommendation written by academic faculty carry more weight than community-based physicians lacking academic appointments yet another reason to seek out rotation experiences at teaching hospitals.
- In selecting rotations, ask about the number of students on the services. Too many students with few patients may limit opportunities to learn. Such environments may also prevent attending physicians from developing the stronger relationships with students necessary for the production of the best LORs.
- If you must rotate with a private or community-based physician, select attending physicians with faculty appointments. Many physicians in the community hold clinical faculty positions with nearby medical schools, and letters written on your behalf by these physicians will include their title.

Did you know?

"I do not think I have ever taken somebody sight unseen who has not rotated at our institution," writes Dr. Michael, Program Director of a general surgery residency program in the South. "Because of the variability of their clinical experience, different from a United States medical school graduate, I found that you really need to see how they function at your institution and with the resident team."[18]

Rule # 204 Avoid errors in scheduling electives at U.S. medical schools.

If you're currently enrolled in a foreign medical school, you should realize that it's easier to secure and complete **hands-on** rotations in the U.S. while you remain a medical student. Once you graduate, it becomes much more difficult to do so. To begin with, I encourage you to visit the AAMC website (www.aamc.org), where you'll find the Online Extramural Electives Compendium. Using this database, you can easily find U.S. medical schools offering elective opportunities for international medical students. The resource also includes contact information for rotation coordinators, application procedures, earliest date of acceptance for applications, earliest start dates, maximum number of weeks permitted in electives, and fees. Links are also provided to medical school websites where additional information can be found. Of note, this resource only presents opportunities at hospitals affiliated with U.S. medical schools. For similar opportunities at other hospitals, you'll have to contact each institution for information.

Common Errors U.S. Citizen IMGs Make in Scheduling Electives

- Start early. Your goal is to submit your application on the earliest date the institution begins accepting applications. Many hospitals ask applicants to submit applications nine months in advance.
- Choose and apply for electives at programs that have IMGs on their resident roster. Your chances of matching at a program are even better at IMG-friendly programs that have a history of taking students from your school.
- The application can be extensive, and includes such documents as immunization history, medical history, background check, transcript, HIPAA training, and TOEFL test results. It obviously takes time to complete these documents, and delays in doing so often prevent applicants from securing these elective experiences.
- Institutions also require the Dean of your school or designated official to complete paperwork (such as a letter of good standing). Notify your school as soon as possible of such requests so that the paperwork will be available when you're ready to apply.

Did you know?

In a survey of 73 U.S. medical schools, 58% reported allowing international medical students to complete electives or clerkships at their institutions. Fluency in English was required by 90% of schools, and 45% requested proof of completion of the Test of English as a Foreign Language (TOEFL). Schools accepting international medical students for rotations reported having students from Europe, Canada, Asia, Australia and New Zealand, Africa, South America, and Central America.[19]

Rule # 205 Embrace the power of networking.

At the recent National Arab American Medical Association Meeting, I had the opportunity to speak to a group of international medical students and graduates as part of a panel. I spoke about the importance of networking for applicants seeking residency positions in the U.S. In the Q & A that followed, a number of established physicians in the Arab American community spoke passionately about mentors who were influential in helping them secure residency training positions. Although I've seen amazing things happen when applicants embrace the power of networking, many applicants are uncomfortable with the process, and these fears prevent them from establishing the relationships that can open important doors. As the residency match becomes more competitive, networking has become even more important. Networking has been defined by the AAMC as "connecting and developing relationships with physicians and other health care professionals to use as a resource in your career."[20]

Networking Recommendations for U.S. Citizen IMGs

- Consider the people whom you already know. These may be family members, friends, advisors, and colleagues. Include acquaintances as well. After you've identified those within your network, you're ready to talk with them about your career plans and goals.
- Your established network may be able to provide you with names and contact information of people who can help you reach your professional goals.
- Your network should include graduates of your medical school who are practicing in the U.S. Some schools will provide you with names and contact information, and we've even heard of schools arranging phone appointments with alumni. If your school does not have a list of alumni practicing in the U.S, you can harness the power of the Internet to locate these individuals.
- Build your network by initiating relationships with U.S. citizen IMG physician graduates of other schools. Although you have not attended the same medical school, you still share a common bond with these physicians. It's likely that you're facing the same struggles that they faced when they went through the process, and you'll find that many will be receptive to your inquiries.
- You can also expand your network by joining professional associations. Organizations like the American Academy of Family Physicians and American Medical Association hold annual meetings with formal networking events.
- Ethnic physician organizations are yet another opportunity to expand your network.
- Although you may be initially uncomfortable approaching new people, remember that every person you encounter will have had people in their lives who played important roles in getting them to where they are today.
- To refine your approach, we recommend initially contacting residents and practicing physicians in the U.S. who have completed their education at your school. You may be more comfortable starting your efforts with this group, and then branching out to others.

Rule # 206 Be prepared to discuss sensitive issues during the interview.

As an IMG applicant, you'll encounter many of the same interview questions asked of allopathic and osteopathic applicants. However, some questions will be specific to your background and training as an IMG. Your reasons for pursuing your medical education abroad will be of great interest to programs. For some applicants, the decision to choose medicine as a profession came late in college, and this led them to enroll in overseas medical schools. A significant number of U.S. citizen IMGs complete training abroad because they change careers later in life, and prefer to not go through the lengthy U.S. medical school admissions process. For these two groups of applicants, the choice to attend a foreign medical school may be purely a personal choice. However, many U.S. citizen IMGs pursue their education abroad when attempts to gain entrance into U.S. medical schools fail, largely because of low GPA and/or MCAT scores. Program directors wonder about the factors that prevented these applicants from achieving better grades and higher scores, and may ask applicants "Why did you choose to leave the U.S. for medical school?" In the following table, we present the concerns of PDs with respect to these two factors. We encourage you to think about the evidence that you can provide to reassure PDs that any past difficulties would not resurface during residency.

Reason	Concerns of Program Directors
Low GPA	Was the undergraduate academic performance the result of a lack of focus or maturity, poor study habits, excessive involvement in extracurricular activities, relationship issues, or something else? What is the likelihood that such factors will impact performance as a resident?
Low or borderline MCAT	Multiple studies have shown that past standardized exam scores are predictors of future performance on standardized exams, including the specialty board certification exam. Low MCAT and USMLE scores lead to concerns about an applicant's ability to pass the specialty board exam. Failure to pass the specialty board exam has repercussions for the program. "Failure to pass the pediatric boards reflects poorly on our program and may cause problems with our residency review committee," said Dr. Daniel West, Program Director of the Pediatrics Residency Program at UCSF.[21]

Programs are also concerned about resident attrition. In one study, annual attrition rates in internal medicine, pediatrics, family medicine, general surgery, and psychiatry were 2.7%, 2.9%, 4.7%, 5.1%, and 7.9%, respectively.[22] Studies have shown higher attrition rates among IMG residents. When a resident leaves a program, it increases the workload for the remaining residents and faculty, makes it more difficult for the program to comply with duty hour guidelines, and affects morale. Although attrition may be due to poor resident performance, research indicates that it's often voluntary.[23] Among the reasons that trainees cite for leaving programs is the desire to enter another specialty. With that being the case, you can expect that interviewers will ask for your motivations in pursuing a career in the specialty. Think very carefully about your reasons, be able to express them with enthusiasm, and don't give programs a reason to doubt your desire for the field.

Yet another challenge facing programs in their evaluation of U.S. citizen IMGs is questions regarding the quality of education provided by the applicant's medical school. One PD described the challenge:[18]

[IMGs] tend to be far more diverse geographically, racially, and ethnically, have greater variation in their undergraduate grades and Medical College Admission Test (MCAT) scores, and most have been "rejected" at least once by accredited schools. The rejection toughens the resolve of the student to become a doctor and strengthens their motivation. Many offshore students are among the hardest working students I have ever taught…The big question facing program directors…regards the quality of the education received by offshore graduates they are considering.

Some schools have been in existence for decades with graduates well established in the U.S. PDs may be more familiar with these schools, especially if they've had former residents who were graduates of these schools. However, many schools are new, with smaller class sizes. If you are a student or graduate of a less established or recognized school, be prepared to discuss in depth your school's curriculum, resources, selection processes, and performance of students. You should be ready to provide indicators of quality.

Rule # 207 **If you fail to match, seek the expertise of an advisor with considerable experience assessing the strengths and weaknesses of IMG applicants, and develop a plan to overcome obstacles.**

An unsuccessful residency match can be the result of one or more factors. In my experience advising U.S. citizen IMGs, one thing is certain – applicants are not the best judge of their strengths and weaknesses. Is it just the USMLE score that's preventing you from reaching your goals? Or is it something in your ERAS application? Do you have the right combination of recommendation letters? Is your personal statement lacking in some respect? I regularly conduct Strategy for Success Sessions arranged through our website TheSuccessfulMatch.com. These sessions involve a careful analysis of all application materials, accurate assessment of strengths and weaknesses, and a detailed discussion focusing on strategy development. My goal is to provide every applicant with a strong plan moving forward that will enhance the chances of a successful match. Make sure your advisor does the same.

References

[1]ECFMG. Available at: http://www.ecfmg.org/resources/ECFMG-2013-annual-report.pdf. Accessed March, 2, 2016.
[2]Johnson K, Hagopian A, Veninga C, Hart G. The changing geography of Americans graduating from foreign medical schools. *Acad Med* 2006; 81(2): 179-184.
[3]van Zanten M, Boulet J. Medical education in the Caribbean: quantifying the contribution of Caribbean-educated physicians to the primary care workforce in the United States. *Acad Med* 2013; 88(2): 276-281.
[4]Thompson M, Hagopian A, Fordyce M, Hart L. Do international medical graduates (IMGs) "fill the gap" in rural primary care in the United States? A national study. *J Rural Health* 2009; 25(2): 124-34.
[5]Alexander H, Heinig S, Fang D, Dickler H, Korn D. Contributions of international medical graduates to US biomedical research: The experience of US medical schools. *J Investig Med* 2007; 55(8): 410-414.
[6]Moore R, Rhodenbaugh E. The unkindest cut of all: Are international medical school graduates subjected to discrimination by general surgery residency programs? *Curr Surg* 2002; 59: 228-236.
[7]Advance Data Tables: 2016 Main Residency Match. Available at: http://www.nrmp.org/match-data/main-residency-match-data/. Accessed April 23, 2016.
[8]Charting Outcomes in the Match: International Medical Graduates. Available at: http://www.ecfmg.org/resources/NRMP-ECFMG-Charting-Outcomes-in-the-Match-International-Medical-Graduates-2014.pdf. Accessed June 23, 2015.
[9]The Successful Match: Getting into Pediatrics. Available at: http://studentdoctor.net/2011/05/the-successful-match-getting-into-pediatrics/. Accessed September 2, 2012.
[10]Results of the 2014 NRMP Program Director Survey. Available at: http://www.nrmp.org/wp-content/uploads/2014/09/PD-Survey-Report-2014.pdf. Accessed March 3, 2015.
[11]The Successful Match: Getting into Ophthalmology. Available at: http://studentdoctor.net/2009/08/the-successful-match-interview-with-dr-andrew-lee-ophthalmology/. Accessed September 20, 2012.
[12]Results of the 2010 NRMP Program Director Survey. Available at: http://www.nrmp.org/wp-content/uploads/2013/08/programresultsbyspecialty2010v3.pdf. Accessed March 2, 2016.
[13]Blue A, Geesey M, Sheridan M, Basco W. Performance outcomes associated with medical school community service. *Acad Med* 2006; 81(10 Suppl): S79-82.
[14]Hayden S, Hayden M, Garnst A. What characteristics of applicants to emergency medicine residency programs predicts future success as an emergency medicine resident? *Acad Emerg Med* 2005; 12(3): 206-210.
[15]Green M, Jones P, Thomas J. Selection criteria for residency: results of a national program director survey. *Acad Med* 2009; 84(3): 362-7.
[16]Ross University School of Medicine. Available at: http://www.rossu.edu/medical-school/blog/12/458. Accessed March 3, 2016.

[17]Alexander E, Osman N, Walling J, Mitchell V. Variation and imprecision of clerkship grading in U.S. medical schools. *Acad Med* 2012; 87(8): 1-7.
[18]Friedell M, Nelson L, Marano M. A primer on Caribbean medical schools and students: APDS surgery panel session. *J Surg Educ* 2011; 68(4): 328-332.
[19]Mueller P, McConahey L, Orvidas L, Lee M, Bowen J, Beckan T, Kasten M. Visting medical student elective and clerkship programs: a survey of US and Puerto Rico allopathic medical schools. *BMC Medical Education* 2010; 10: 41.
[20]AAMC. Available at: https://www.aamc.org/cim/career/professionaldevelopment/. Accessed May 2, 2016.
[21]A Guide to the Perplexed: Residency Advice. Available at secure/ucdmc.ucdavis.edu/gme/ppts/residency_advice_1.pps. Accessed on July 26, 2010.
[22]Kennedy K, Brennan M, Rayburn W, Brotherton S. Attrition rates between residents in obstetrics and gynecology and other clinical specialties, 2000-2009. J Grad Med Educ 2013; 5(2): 267-271.
[23]Yaghoubian A, Galante J, Kaji A, et al. General surgery resident remediation and attrition: a multi-institutional study. Arch Surg. 2012; 147(9): 829-833.

Chapter 22

Non-U.S. Citizen International Medical Graduates

There are over 900,000 physicians in the United States. A substantial number of these physicians are international medical graduates (IMGs). According to the AMA, 228,665 are IMG physicians, representing 25.3% of the total physician population.[1]

Since most are involved in direct patient care, IMGs have had a vital role in meeting the medical manpower needs of the United States. IMGs have also made valuable contributions to medical education, furthered biomedical and health services research, and held leadership positions in academic medicine. In fact, 17% and 10% of department chairs in the basic sciences and clinical sciences at U.S. medical schools, respectively, are IMGs.[2]

The Educational Commission for Foreign Medical Graduates (ECFMG) is responsible for certifying the readiness of IMG physicians for entry into U.S. residency training. As you can see from the following table, the ECFMG has certified hundreds of thousands of IMGs (from a number of countries) in its 50 plus years of existence.

Top Countries by Country of Origin ECFMG Certificates Issued, 1958 – 2005

Citizenship at entry to medical school	Issued 1958-2005: No.	(%)	Issued 1996-2005: No.	(%)	Issued 2001-2005: No.	(%)
India	54,292	(18.9)	17,378	(20.8)	8,710	(22.8)
United States	40,051	(13.9)	13,476	(16.1)	7,917	(20.8)
Philippines	19,870	(6.9)	2,519	(3.0)	1,081	(2.8)
Pakistan	13,706	(4.8)	4,930	(5.9)	2,394	(6.3)
United Kingdom	7,534	(2.6)	1,183	(1.4)	467	(1.2)
China	7,072	(2.5)	3,791	(4.5)	1,214	(3.2)
Germany	6,863	(2.4)	1,862	(2.2)	539	(1.4)
USSR	6,171	(2.2)	3,282	(3.9)	1,201	(3.2)
Iran	6,169	(2.2)	1,956	(2.3)	870	(2.3)
Egypt	6,006	(2.1)	1,883	(2.3)	516	(1.4)
Korea	5,995	(2.1)	820	(1.0)	415	(1.1)
Syria	4,292	(1.5)	1,473	(1.8)	677	(1.8)
Nigeria	4,016	(1.4)	1,858	(2.2)	812	(2.1)
Australia	3,819	(1.3)	666	(0.8)	182	(0.5)
Taiwan	3,763	(1.3)	240	(0.3)	55	(0.1)
Lebanon	3,481	(1.2)	1,269	(1.5)	588	(1.5)
Total certificates	287,382	(100)	83,476	(100)	38,142	(100)

Hallock J, Kostis J. Celebrating 50 years of experience: an ECFMG perspective. *Acad Med* 2006; 81 (12): S7-16.

Although the sheer number of IMGs receiving ECFMG certification is impressive, these numbers tell you nothing of the difficulties these IMGs have experienced in their efforts to secure a position in a U.S. residency program. While gaining a desired residency position is difficult for U.S. medical students, it's much more so for IMGs.

IMGs often have to deal with adapting to a new culture in a foreign land, often without friends or family close by for support. For many IMGs, the lack of understanding of the criteria which programs find important makes the residency application process extremely stressful and difficult. In working with IMGs, I've come to realize that misperceptions abound, with IMGs frequently overestimating or underestimating certain residency application criteria. These misperceptions may result in a failure to match.

In this chapter my goal is to provide you with evidence-based advice from the literature on resident selection as it pertains to IMGs. In addition, I seek to deliver information from those individuals who are directly involved in the selection process – namely program directors and other members of the residency selection committee. What do programs value the most? How important are letters of recommendation? Why do programs prefer applicants with U.S. medical experience? How can IMGs secure U.S. clinical experience? What are common interview pitfalls? These are some of the questions I answer in my effort to help you develop an application strategy that will lead to match success.

Rule # 208 Research the competitiveness of your chosen specialty.

Certain specialties are far more competitive than others. Specialties such as ophthalmology, otolaryngology, radiation oncology, dermatology, urology, plastic surgery, and orthopedic surgery are highly competitive. There are many more U.S. applicants who wish to enter these fields than positions available. Consequently, a significant number of U.S. applicants fail to match every year.

As you might expect, IMGs find these specialties the most difficult to enter. For example, 97% of residents training in orthopedic surgery residency programs are graduates of U.S. allopathic medical schools. Of the 3,581 resident physicians in orthopedic surgery, only 1.8% were IMGs.[3] Contrast this with family medicine, internal medicine, and psychiatry. In these specialties, IMGs account for over 30% of all resident physicians.

While IMG applicants have successfully matched into highly competitive specialties, it requires a well thought out application strategy. Because of the large numbers of IMG applicants matching into less competitive specialties such as internal medicine and family medicine, IMGs often believe that it's easy to match into these fields. Statistics from the 2014 and 2015 Match results shown below debunk this common misconception.[4-5]

Key Statistics from the 2015 Match Results...

10,060 non-U.S. citizen IMG applicants participated in the 2015 Match.

898 (8.9%) withdrew.

1,796 (17.9%) did not submit a rank-order list.

Of the remaining 7,366 non-U.S. citizen IMG applicants, 3,725, or 50.6% failed to match.

Key Statistics from the 2014 Match Results...

72% of non-U.S. citizen IMG applicants failed to match into family medicine.

52% of non-U.S. citizen IMG applicants failed to match into internal medicine.

As you can see from this data, thousands of IMGs fail to match every year. Failure to match can be distressing. Those who fail to match often report feeling shocked, depressed, or embarrassed. "I couldn't believe it," said one applicant. "I've never failed anything before."

The financial effects of not matching are also significant. The financial cost of the residency application process for IMGs is substantial. IMG applicants incur significant costs every step of the way. Leon and Aranha described these costs in more detail.[6]

Economic constraints impede many competitive FMGs from applying because of the prohibitive fees requested, when analyzed in the context of average foreign wages. To begin with, international medical schools charge very high fees to issue all documents necessary to apply, including medical school transcripts...Several educational courses are available to FMGs to prepare for the USMLE tests. These courses often have prohibitive costs...For a 4-month period, some courses charge about U.S. $9,000...Testing costs by themselves are equivalent to average annual gross income in many countries.

These costs are just the start. Another area of high expense is that of travel, including travel to the United States and the costs incurred during the interviewing process. In one survey, the median expense per interview was $330.[7]

Regardless of your chosen specialty, the key to a successful match hinges on the development of a well-thought-out strategy. Such an approach will significantly increase your chances of a successful match.

Percentage Of Resident Physicians Who Are IMGs By Specialty			
Specialty	**Total number of residents***	**Number of IMG residents**	**Percentage**
Anesthesiology	5,668	671	11.8
Dermatology	1,184	51	4.3
Emergency Medicine	5,631	330	5.9
Family Medicine	10,077	3,467	34.4
General Surgery	7,890	1,312	16.6
Internal Medicine	22,971	9,514	41.4
Neurology	2,207	822	37.2
Neurosurgery	1,272	114	9.0
Obstetrics & Gynecology	4,942	670	13.6
Ophthalmology	1,323	77	5.8
Orthopedic Surgery	3,529	72	2.0
Otolaryngology	1,45	22	1.5
Pathology	2,276	810	35.6
Pediatrics	8,529	1,867	21.9
Physical Medicine & Rehabilitation	1,162	222	19.1
Plastic Surgery	377	58	15.4
Psychiatry	4,917	1,581	32.2
Radiation Oncology	686	15	2.2
Radiology	4,471	358	8.0
Urology	1,189	55	4.6

*Includes resident physicians on duty as of December 31, 2013.

Brotherton S, Etzel S. Graduate Medical Education, 2013-2014. *JAMA* 2014; 312 (22): 2427-2445.

Percentage of non-U.S. citizen IMGs Who Failed to Match in 2014 by Specialty		
Specialty	**Number of non-U.S. citizen IMGs who applied**	**% Failing to Match**
Anesthesiology	163	52%
Emergency Medicine	84	63%
Family Medicine	909	68%
General Surgery	308	49%
Internal Medicine	3,546	52%
Neurology	297	50%
Obstetrics & Gynecology	182	66%
Pathology	287	47%
Pediatrics	660	58%
Physical Medicine & Rehabilitation	47	55%
Psychiatry	440	63%
Radiology	129	49%

Charting Outcomes in the Match: International Medical Graduates. Available at: http://www.ecfmg.org/resources/NRMP-ECFMG-Charting-Outcomes-in-the-Match-International-Medical-Graduates-2014.pdf. Accessed June 23, 2015.

Rule # 209 **Becoming ECFMG certified is key.**

To begin residency training in an accredited U.S. residency program, IMGs must be certified by the ECFMG. The ECFMG, which came into existence in 1956, is responsible for certifying the readiness of IMGs for entry into U.S. residency training. To be eligible for ECFMG certification, an international medical graduate must:

- Submit an application for ECFMG certification.
- Take and pass the USMLE Step 1, Step 2 Clinical Knowledge (CK), and Step 2 Clinical Skills (CS) exams.
- Fulfill medical education credential requirements
- Be a graduate of a medical school listed in the International Medical Education Directory (IMED) which is available at http://imed.ecfmg.org. The graduation year must also be listed in the directory.
- Provide evidence that all requirements for the final medical diploma have been satisfied. Copies of the final medical school transcript must be submitted to the ECFMG.

Did you know?

There are time limits for completing the USMLE exams for ECFMG certification. Refer to the ECFMG website for more information.

It's to your advantage to be ECFMG certified prior to the submission of your application. Some programs do screen IMG applicants for ECFMG certification, and may not consider those who are not yet certified. Programs may be concerned about allocating interview positions to candidates who are not certified, since there are no guarantees that these candidates will become certified prior to starting residency training in the U.S.

Tip # 149

Before applying, IMG applicants who are not ECFMG-certified should inquire about each residency program's selection process with respect to ECFMG certification. Two questions are particularly important:

- Does the program require ECFMG certification before extending an interview invitation to an applicant?
- Does the program require ECFMG certification before placing an applicant on the rank-order list?

Applicants who are not certified can avoid applying to programs with these departmental policies, thus saving considerable expense.

Fortunately, many residency programs will consider and rank IMG applicants who are not certified, as long as the results of required examinations are available.

> **Did you know?**
>
> The ECFMG notifies the NRMP if you have passed the required examinations (USMLE Step 1, Step 2 CK, and Step 2 CS). Applicants who have not passed these examinations will be withdrawn from the Match shortly after the Rank Order List Deadline.

Rule # 210 Learn the selection criteria that are most important to residency program directors.

Every two years, the NRMP publishes its Program Director Survey. In 2014, over 1,800 PDs representing 22 specialties participated in the study.[8] The information allows applicants to gain a better understanding of the factors that PDs use to select applicants to interview and then rank. While this detailed document is a wonderful resource for all applicants, it does have some limitations. For example, the document reveals that 99% of anesthesiology PDs cite the USMLE Step 1 exam as a factor in selecting applicants to interview. We also know that 85% of programs have a target score. What we don't know is whether there are any differences in the target score between U.S. medical students and IMGs. For LORs, we know that 81% of programs cite letters as a factor in selecting applicants to interview. However, the document does not indicate how foreign LORs are viewed. In other words, the survey is not IMG specific.

Therefore, we have to rely on other sources of information. An older study sheds light on IMG-specific practices. In this survey of 102 internal medicine PDs, directors were asked to rate the importance of 22 selection criteria that best predicted the performances of foreign-born medical graduates during internal medicine residencies.[9] Criteria rated highest included performance on the NBME (precursor to the USMLE), interview performance, and postgraduate clinical experience in the U.S. Of note, LORs from foreign countries was ranked last in importance. The criteria are presented in descending order of importance on the next page.

> **Did you know?**
>
> Another publication packed with important information for IMGs is "Charting Outcomes in the Match: International Medical Graduates." This document is available at the ECFMG (www.ecfmg.org) and NRMP websites (www.nrmp.org).

Importance of 22 Residency Selection Criteria for IMG Applicants

Criteria	Rating[1]
Score on NBME II[2]	4.34
Fluency in English as determined during interview	4.30
Number of attempts on NBME II[2]	4.30
Postgraduate clinical experience in U.S.	4.20
Number of attempts on NBME 1[2]	4.10
Score on NBME I[2]	4.07
Interview performance on nonmedical issues (e.g., personality)	4.02
Medical school (if known to program director)	3.98
Year of graduation (recent graduates perform better)	3.84
Performance during interview with medical questions (e.g., quiz, case presentation)	3.65
Country of medical education	3.64
Score on FLEX	3.54
Rank order in medical school class	3.35
Age (younger graduates performing better respective to graduation date)	3.33
Letter of recommendation from the U.S.	3.27
Postgraduate clinical experience in foreign country	3.12
Passing FLEX before applying for residency	3.12
Duration of living in U.S.	3.03
Medical school grades (transcript)	2.94
Nonclinical graduate work in the U.S. (e.g., basic science graduate studies, research)	2.74
Dean's letter	2.32
Other letters of recommendation from foreign country	1.93

[1]Directors were asked to rate the importance of each criterion on a scale of 1 (least important) to 5 (most important).
[2]NBME I and II exams were the immediate precursors of the USMLE Step 1 and 2 CK exams, respectively

Gayed N. Residency directors' assessments of which selection criteria best predict the performances of foreign born medical graduates during internal medicine residencies. *Acad Med* 1991; 66 (11): 699-701.

Did you know?

Your year of graduation is important to programs. Some programs prefer recent graduates because they believe these applicants will do better during residency training. These programs may even screen out applications from IMGs who have graduated "too far in the past." Others evaluate such applicants on a case by case basis. As Rao stated, these applicants "may have gained valuable life and career experiences through professional work since graduation from medical school. They may have obtained additional postgraduate medical qualifications and administrative or research experience or may have worked in various cultures."[10] In Gayed's survey, while 27% of program directors agreed that "IMGs straight out of medical school performed better than those who had done clinical work in a foreign country," 33% disagreed and 40% were neutral.[9]

Rule # 211 The USMLE is important. Very important.

As discussed, to become certified by the ECFMG, you must take and pass the United States Medical Licensing Examinations (USMLE). These include the USMLE Step 1, USMLE Step 2 Clinical Knowledge (CK), and USMLE Step 2 Clinical Skills (CS) exams. The USMLE Step 1 and 2 CK exams were developed to assess medical knowledge. The Step 2 CS exam was designed to evaluate communication and interpersonal skills.

While the USMLE exams were not developed to be used as residency selection tools, scores have taken on significant importance in the residency selection process. This is true for both U.S. and IMG applicants, but even more so for the latter. According to 2006 data supplied by the ECFMG, nearly 300,000 IMGs from over 200 countries had received certification since the organization's inception. It is difficult for U.S. residency programs to accurately assess the quality of medical education in 200 plus countries, let alone the quality of each of the 1500 plus medical schools operating throughout the world.

While you may have been an outstanding medical student" or physician in your native country, your past performance will have little bearing on your chances of securing a residency position in the U.S. PDs will simply not be familiar with the quality of your medical education. Instead, programs place considerable emphasis on a tool with which they are intimately familiar – the USMLE exams. These exams have made it easier for programs to assess the medical knowledge of IMG applicants. Since all applicants are required to take these exams, programs are readily able to compare scores of one applicant with another.

The reality of the situation is this: the higher your USMLE scores, the better your chances of matching with a program in your chosen specialty. The following points deserve emphasis:

- The USMLE Step 1 and 2 CK exams are difficult. In 2006, Boulet and colleagues reported the USMLE first attempt pass rates (i.e., what percent of test-takers passed the exam on their first try) for IMGs who sought ECFMG certification between 1995 and 2004. The results are shown in the following table.

USMLE First Attempt Pass Rates for International Medical Graduates

	First Attempt Pass Rate for U.S. IMGs	First Attempt Pass Rate for non-U.S. IMGs
USMLE Step 1	60.5%	64.3%
USMLE Step 2 CK	70.4%	66.1%
USMLE Step 2 CS	91.6%	84.2%

Boulet J, Swanson D, Cooper R, Norcini J, McKinley D. A comparison of the characteristics and examination performances of U.S. and non-U.S. citizen international medical graduates who sought Educational Commission for Foreign Medical Graduates certification: 1995 – 2004. *Acad Med* 2006; 81 (10 Suppl): S116-119.

Since that study, first attempt pass rates have improved to some extent. In 2014, 78% of the 15,149 IMGs who took the USMLE Step 1 exam passed on their first attempt. The percentage was even better for first time takers of the USMLE Step 2 CK exam. 80% of the 12,713 IMGs passed.[11]

Many programs will not consider applications from IMGs who do not pass on the first attempt. Given the importance of these exams in the selection process, and the relatively high first-time fail rates, you must prepare extensively for these exams.

- With the exception of the USMLE Step 2 CS exams, the USMLE exams are not pass/fail exams. However, if you pass, you cannot take the exam again, and you cannot try to get a better score. In other words, once you pass, that score will be the score used by residency programs in their decision-making process.

Did you know?

The USMLE Step CS exam is important to residency programs. In the 2014 NRMP Program Director Survey, 81% of family medicine programs, 75% of internal medicine programs, and 82% of psychiatry programs cited a passing CS score as a factor in selecting applicants to interview. Respondents rated this factor 4.0 – 4.3 on a scale of 1 (not at all important) to 5 (very important).[8]

- Some residency programs will not consider applications from IMGs until the results of USMLE Step 1, 2 CK, and 2 CS exams are all available. Other programs will extend interview invitations to IMG applicants who have completed either the USMLE Step 1 or Step 2 CK exam.

- Many programs have score cutoffs for IMG applicants. Applicants who are at or above this threshold will be considered for an interview. Those with scores below this threshold will not be considered further. At times, this information is made available to applicants at program websites.

- IMG applicants are not required to take the USMLE Step 1 exam prior to taking the USMLE Step 2 CK exam. In other words, you're free to choose the order in which you would like to take these exams. The Step 1 exam is essentially a basic science exam, while the focus of the Step 2 CK exam is on the clinical sciences. If you're closer to the latter, consider taking the Step 2 CK exam first.

- The USMLE Step 3 exam is not a major factor used by programs in the residency selection process. Many IMG applicants, however, take the exam, since it's not possible to secure a H1-B visa without passing the Step 3 exam. In 2014, of the 9,403 IMGs who took the exam, 13% failed.[11]

While low USMLE scores or a failed attempt won't eliminate you from securing a residency position in the U.S., it does make it much harder. To overcome low scores, you'll need to strengthen every aspect of the residency application.

While high USMLE scores increase the likelihood of a successful match, every year IMGs with high scores fail to match. In the 2014 Match, 385 of the 1,272 non-U.S. citizen IMG applicants with Step 1 scores > 230 failed to match to any specialty (30%).[5] Clearly, attention needs to be given to every aspect of the application in order to maximize your chances of a successful match, even for applicants with competitive scores.

Did you know?

With completion of residency training, physicians are eligible to take the specialty board exam. Passing this exam makes the physician "board certified." Having the ability to pass the specialty board examination is important to programs because "specialty board certification has a demonstrated relationship with clinical outcomes and other measures of physician competence."[12] Failing the specialty board exam may also impact the program's ability to recruit residents, since some specialties require programs to make public the average pass rate. For these reasons, programs try to identify applicants who might be at higher risk of failing these exams. In several studies, USMLE test scores have been found to predict board passage.[13-15]

Mean USMLE Step 1 Scores for Matched Vs Unmatched non-U.S. citizen IMGs by Specialty

Specialty	Mean USMLE Step 1 Score for Matched Applicants	Mean USMLE Step 1 Score for Unmatched Applicants
Anesthesiology	226	219
Emergency Medicine	226	217
Family Medicine	213	204
General Surgery	233	221
Internal Medicine	231	217
Neurology	230	214
Obstetrics & Gynecology	226	215
Pathology	226	214
Pediatrics	223	211
Physical Medicine & Rehabilitation	220	211
Psychiatry	214	205
Radiology	232	219

Adapted from Charting Outcomes in the Match International Medical Graduates. Available at: http://www.ecfmg.org/resources/NRMP-ECFMG-Charting-Outcomes-in-the-Match-International-Medical-Graduates-2014.pdf. Accessed March 13, 2016.

Mean USMLE Step 2 CK Scores for Matched Vs Unmatched non-U.S. citizen IMGs by Specialty		
Specialty	**Mean Step 2 CK Score for Matched Applicants**	**Mean Step 2 CK Score for Unmatched Applicants**
Anesthesiology	234	221
Emergency Medicine	231	220
Family Medicine	219	210
General Surgery	240	224
Internal Medicine	236	221
Neurology	236	217
Obstetrics & Gynecology	234	221
Pathology	228	216
Pediatrics	231	217
Physical Medicine & Rehabilitation	225	210
Psychiatry	219	208
Radiology	238	220
Adapted from Charting Outcomes in the Match International Medical Graduates. Available at: http://www.ecfmg.org/resources/NRMP-ECFMG-Charting-Outcomes-in-the-Match-International-Medical-Graduates-2014.pdf. Accessed March 13, 2016.		

Number of non-U.S. Citizen IMGs who Matched with ≥ 2 USMLE Step 1 Attempts	
Specialty	**Number of Applicants Matching with ≥ 2 attempts**
Anesthesiology	8
Emergency Medicine	1
Family Medicine	29
General Surgery	5
Internal Medicine	39
Neurology	6
Obstetrics & Gynecology	1
Pathology	36
Pediatrics	12
Physical Medicine & Rehabilitation	2
Psychiatry	26
Radiology	1
Adapted from Charting Outcomes in the Match International Medical Graduates. Available at: http://www.ecfmg.org/resources/NRMP-ECFMG-Charting-Outcomes-in-the-Match-International-Medical-Graduates-2014.pdf. Accessed March 13, 2016.	

Rule # 212 Understand the concerns of program directors with respect to IMG applicants.

Residency programs seek to select applicants who will be successful residents. However, performance as a resident can be difficult to predict. While this holds true for both U.S. medical graduates and IMGs, PDs have a more difficult time assessing the potential of IMG applicants.

A major goal for PDs is to avoid selecting applicants who may become problem residents. The problem resident is defined as a "trainee who demonstrates a significant enough problem that requires intervention by someone of authority, usually the program director or chief resident."[16]

In a survey of 298 internal medicine PDs, Yao and Wright found that the mean point prevalence of problem residents was 6.9% for the academic year 1998 – 1999.[17] According to the American Board of Internal Medicine, 8% to 15% of residents have significant areas of learner difficulty, and 94% of internal medicine residency programs reported having one or more problem residents during the academic year 1998 – 1999.[17] While U.S. medical graduates and IMGs can become problem residents, in this study PDs felt that IMGs were more likely to be identified as problem residents.

Problem residents can negatively impact a program by compromising patient care and increasing the workload of their resident colleagues. In addition, to remediate the problem, considerable time, support, and guidance is required from the faculty. When a disproportionate amount of a program's resources are spent on one or two problem residents, less time may be available for the rest of the residents. The end result of this is often a lowering of the entire residency program's morale.

Also of concern to programs is whether a resident, once selected, will complete residency training. Several studies have examined resident attrition rates:

- In a study examining resident attrition rates from family practice residencies, a significantly higher attrition rate (18.5% vs. 7.8%) was found for IMGs than for U.S. medical graduates.[18]
- In another study, while the overall rates were found to be lower, the attrition rate of IMGs (3.7% vs. 1.4%) was higher than U.S. medical graduates.[19]
- A higher attrition rate (3.6% vs. 2.5%) for IMGs was also found in another study.[20]

From these studies, it's apparent that IMGs are less likely to complete residency training. While the attrition rate in the latter two studies seems small, the loss of even a single resident has significant effects on a residency program. Therefore, programs make it a priority to accurately identify applicants at higher risk of becoming problem residents, as well as those that are less likely to complete training.

In a study by Yao and Wright, apparent deficiencies in problem residents were identified.[21] These are listed below in descending order of frequency:

- Insufficient medical knowledge
- Poor clinical judgment
- Inefficient use of time
- Inappropriate interaction with colleagues or staff
- Provision of poor or inadequate medical care to patients
- Unsatisfactory clinical skills

- Unsatisfactory humanistic behavior with patients
- Excessive and unexplained tardiness or absences
- Unacceptable moral or ethical behaviors

Insufficient medical knowledge is at the top of this list. As discussed earlier, programs assess knowledge attainment mainly from an applicant's performance on the USMLE exams. To determine if an applicant is likely to become a problem resident for other reasons, such as inefficient use of time or inappropriate interaction with colleagues or staff, residency programs will rely on other components of the application. These other components include letters of recommendation and U.S. medical experience.

Rule # 213 Don't underestimate the importance of letters of recommendation (LORs).

While you may have been a highly competent physician in your home country, will you be one in the United States? How strong are your clinical skills? How readily and easily will you adapt to medicine as it is practiced in the U.S? How will you relate to U.S. patients? How well do you work with others? Do you have the written and oral communication skills needed to succeed? These are among the many questions that residency programs are trying to answer as they consider your application.

Programs wish to determine if you have both the professional and personal qualities to succeed as a resident and, later, as a practicing physician. To make this determination, programs rely heavily on LORs. In contrast to your USMLE scores, recommendation letters supply programs with qualitative, rather than quantitative, information about your cognitive and non-cognitive characteristics. A number of studies have shown that behavior, attitude, and other non-cognitive skills are important predictors of resident success. As such, programs place importance on these letters in evaluating your application.

IMGs often underestimate the importance of these letters, but these letters are crucial. I am often asked if it's acceptable to submit recommendation letters written by non-U.S. faculty members or physicians. While it's possible to match without having a single letter written by a U.S. faculty member, you will significantly strengthen your application and improve the chances of a favorable match outcome if you're able to submit letters from a U.S. faculty member. In a survey of 102 directors of internal medicine residency programs, directors were asked to rate the importance of 22 selection criteria.[9] Rated lowest were LORs from a foreign country: "Only 7% of the program directors disagreed with the statement that such letters are useless." In other words, 93% of program directors felt that letters of recommendation from a foreign country were useless.

In further support of this were the results of a survey of psychiatry PDs.[22] Less importance was attached to LORs written by foreign faculty. The authors wrote that "letters from abroad may be superficial and filled with generalities, addressing qualities that are more important in the applicant's culture of origin. For example, many reference letters from India mention loyalty, good behavior, and the devotion of an applicant as contrasted with articulateness, assertiveness, clinical competence, and ability to think independently.

The following points deserve emphasis:

- LORs written by non-U.S. faculty members or physicians carry very little weight in the residency selection process. In contrast, letters written by U.S. faculty members are highly valued because these physicians are familiar with the cognitive and non-cognitive skills and traits essential for success during residency. There are also cultural differences in the way in which letters are written, and letters written by non-U.S. physicians may not be as effusive, even when the letter writer is a strong proponent of the applicant.

- Can IMGs match without any U.S. LORs? Yes, but it's much more difficult. Many IMGs contact us after failing to match, wondering what went wrong. In many cases, these applicants had strong applications, including high USMLE scores, but were lacking LORs written by U.S. faculty members. I encourage these applicants to obtain these letters and reapply. The effects of doing so can be dramatic. Following submission of these letters, I've seen many of these applicants receive significantly more interview invitations.

- When considering IMG applicants of the same caliber, programs will offer an interview invitation to the applicant having LORs written by U.S. faculty members.

- Aim to obtain three or four recommendation letters from U.S. faculty. If this is not possible, then obviously one letter is better than no letter.

- IMGs often ask their friends or family members for LORs. However, these letters are useless, even if the writer is in the medical field. LORs should be written by physicians who have worked with you in a clinical capacity. Chapter 6: Letters of Recommendation outlines in comprehensive detail what factors make for a powerful LOR. Letters written by medical friends or family members who have not worked with you in a clinical capacity will be filled with generalities and superficial information. These types of letters can actually work to weaken your application.

Did you know?

In a study of IMG ophthalmology applicants, researchers analyzed the applications of successful and unsuccessful applicants. Having 3 LORs written by U.S. ophthalmologists was the strongest predictor of matching, and raised the odds of matching 6-fold.[23]

Did you know?

Several years ago, the ECFMG posted an announcement on their website regarding fraudulent LORs after investigating a dozen cases in which applicants had fabricated their letters. These letters were brought to ECFMG attention mainly by PDs after attempts to verify their authenticity raised suspicion. In this announcement, the ECFMG reminded applicants that submission of these letters was considered a form of irregular behavior, the consequences of which can be devastating. If irregular behavior is confirmed, the ECFMG may place a permanent annotation in the applicant's ECFMG Status Report. The behavior may also be reported to directors of graduate medical education programs, the Federation of State Medical Boards, and state medical licensing authorities. In 11/12 cases, the ECFMG revoked the applicant's standard ECFMG certificate.[24]

Tip # 150

When is a letter written by a foreign physician acceptable? If you have not worked with a sufficient number of U.S. physicians to generate 3-4 LORs, then you'll obviously need letters written by foreign physicians who are familiar with your clinical skills. In some cases, a foreign LOR may be to your advantage at certain residency programs. If the letter writer previously served on the faculty at a U.S. residency program and is known to the program, then a letter written by that individual may carry significant weight at that particular program.

Tip # 151

Be sure to have your letter writers submit current LORs. I've seen some letters that are several years old. Residency selection committees value letters that have been written recently. IMG applicants are urged to contact letter writers, and have the letters updated. Be ready to provide writers with your CV.

Tip # 152

If you plan to submit a letter from a physician who has served as your research supervisor, try to also find ways to work with him or her in a clinical capacity. Residency programs are most interested in your clinical skills, and a letter that combines your skills in research and clinical practice will serve you best.

Tip # 153

Often, IMGs must apply to multiple specialties to maximize their chances of success. For this reason, IMGs ask letter writers to refrain from including the specialty within the body of the letter. However, this isn't ideal. Since change of specialty is the most common reason residents leave programs, it's important that your letter writers convey your interest for the field and describe the attributes that would make you a desirable candidate for the specialty. Ask your letter writers for two versions of the letter – one for your specialty of interest, and the other for use in the event that you don't match.

Rule # 214 **To secure strong letters of recommendation, you must perform well, and you must do so during rotations in the United States.**

As we've emphasized, LORs from U.S. faculty members can significantly strengthen your application. To secure a strong letter from a U.S. faculty member, you must work with that physician in a capacity that allows him or her to evaluate you in the same way that they would evaluate a third- or fourth-year U.S. medical student.

During the third year of U.S. medical school, students generally rotate through their core rotations in internal medicine, family medicine, psychiatry, general surgery, pediatrics, and obstetrics/gynecology. These rotations typically offer students a "hands-on experience" taking care of patients. Students learn how to take histories, perform physical exams, analyze test results, make diagnoses from the available information, formulate a treatment plan, and follow their patients throughout the hospitalization until discharge. Students are also asked to write progress notes and present their patients daily to the rest of the team, which typically consists of the faculty preceptor, resident, and intern. Through these interactions, faculty preceptors are able to assess students' medical knowledge, clinical judgment, initiative, work ethic, ability to receive constructive feedback, quality of medical care provided, clinical skills, interpersonal skills, punctuality, and professionalism. Letters written by faculty preceptors often comment on these skills and traits.

For IMGs, participating in rotations allows preceptors the chance to evaluate their skills and qualities in the same manner. This can result in a letter containing the type of information that PDs seek. Rotations also offer IMGs a chance to gain familiarity with the U.S. medical system. Because most IMGs have never worked in a U.S. hospital or medical center, gaining such experience will help ease the transition from foreign training to U.S. residency training, leading to fewer professional adjustment problems.

Following are some important points about U.S. medical experience:

- IMGs often underestimate the importance of U.S. medical experience to residency programs.
- Some programs will not consider you as a candidate unless you have U.S. medical experience.
- Programs that do not have U.S. medical experience requirements per se will still favor applicants who have such experience. When two applicants with similar credentials and qualifications are compared, programs will most certainly favor the applicant with U.S. medical experience.
- Is it possible to match without any U.S. medical experience? It can and does happen, but you should realize that many IMG applicants have failed to match despite having competitive USMLE scores.
- The duration of the experience required varies from program to program. Some programs will require at least one year of experience, while others simply state that several months is sufficient. I'm often asked whether a few days or weeks are sufficient. Since one of your goals is to secure a strong LOR from the faculty member with whom you work, a short duration of experience may not result in the type of letter you truly need to strengthen your application. However, if your time is limited, some experience is better than none.
- Ideally, the rotation should be in your chosen specialty. Letters written by faculty in your field are valued more highly. However, at some programs, gaining U.S. medical experience in other fields may meet their application requirements.
- IMGs often participate in observerships. The American Medical Association (AMA) defines an observership as a "structured opportunity for an IMG to observe clinical practice in a variety of health care settings under the guidance of a physician mentor and to learn about the general structure, characteristics, and financing of health care delivery in the U.S."[25] While this type of rotation might satisfy some programs, others require "hands-on" experience. Rotations that offer hands-on experience are commonly referred to as externships.
- Obtaining a position as an observer or extern is difficult. In a survey of 33 IMG residents in an internal medicine residency program, 18 voiced frustration over the difficulties they experienced in finding such positions.[26]
- Opportunities to do externships are limited, especially for IMGs who have graduated from medical school. It is considerably easier to

arrange an externship while still in medical school, because you remain eligible for student group malpractice insurance rates.

- In the survey by Woods, one respondent stated that "a lot of programs request clinical experience in the U.S. from IMGs. This is even more difficult because a lot of residency programs do not give IMGs the opportunity for an externship." Another commented that "no one would give me an opportunity to prove myself."[26] For those who were successful in arranging these rotations, some reported that without the assistance of family or friends, it would have been much more difficult to secure a position.

- Externships are more highly valued because faculty preceptors are able to assess your skills while you are involved in hands-on care of patients. Since no clinical contact is allowed during observerships, these do not allow preceptors to accurately gauge key skills. LORs written by observership preceptors are limited in what they can say about your skills.

- The advantage of rotations is that you have the chance to make a strong impression on those with whom you work. This can be particularly helpful in gaining an interview at that particular program.

- Many IMGs have found rotation experience valuable in their preparation for the USMLE Step 2 CS exam.

- Impressing faculty preceptors during these rotations can be difficult for IMGs. Most IMGs are unfamiliar with the U.S. medical education system, usual expectations of U.S. physician supervisors, and the qualities which these supervisors value most. Bates wrote that "the usual style of North American Medical Education is a Socratic method in which trainees attempt to support their decisions to their supervising physicians and defend their actions. However, many IMGs come from cultures and training programs where deference to authority is the norm and questioning a professor's opinion is unthinkable. Unfortunately, in North America, the IMG's silence may be interpreted as lack of knowledge, lack of interest, or lack of confidence."[27]

To make the most of your rotation experiences, you need to be well informed of the qualities, skills, and behaviors that are highly valued. We wrote the book *Success on the Wards: 250 Rules for Clerkship Success* to help U.S. medical students excel on the wards. Feedback we've received from IMGs indicates that this book has also been useful for observerships and externships.

Rule # 215 Create a powerful personal statement.

While individual specialties, residency programs, and application reviewers assign varying degrees of importance to the personal statement, there is data showing that the personal statement is of major importance to the specialties that IMGs are most likely to pursue.

Importance of Personal Statement in the Residency Selection Process

Specialty	% Citing Personal Statement as a Factor in Selecting Applicants to Interview	Mean Importance
Anesthesiology	78%	3.4
Emergency Medicine	67%	3.0
Family Medicine	87%	3.9
General Surgery	72%	3.5
Internal Medicine	66%	3.3
Neurology	71%	3.7
Obstetrics & Gynecology	81%	3.5
Pathology	83%	3.8
Pediatrics	70%	3.4
Physical Medicine & Rehabilitation	79%	3.9
Psychiatry	92%	4.1
Radiology	74%	3.3

*Survey participants were asked to rank each item on a scale of 1 (not at all important) to 5 (very important).

Adapted from Results of the 2014 NRMP Program Director Survey. Available at: http://www.nrmp.org/wp-content/uploads/2014/09/PD-Survey-Report-2014.pdf.

As you can see, family medicine and psychiatry programs place considerable emphasis on the personal statement. Dr. Rao, Chair of the Department of Psychiatry and Behavior Sciences at Nassau University Medical Center, wrote that the personal statement "has proven to be a very useful method of assessing IMG applicants at the preinterview stage."[22] IMGs should also heed the words of the Department of Psychiatry at Stony Brook University School of Medicine:[28]

Writing skills are an essential component of medical record keeping, particularly in psychiatry...The Selection Committee will evaluate the preparation of the application and in particular the Personal Statement for evidence of writing skills...Applicants with poorly written essays, e.g., multiple spelling and grammatical errors will not be invited for an interview.

Rule # 216 The interview is extremely important.

In Gayed's survey of internal medicine PDs, the interview was found to be of major importance in the residency selection process.[9] Most important in the interview process were fluency in the English language, personality, and medical knowledge.

- Determination of the candidate's fluency in the English language

  Having the ability to understand and communicate with English-speaking patients is essential to delivering quality medical care and understandably important to program directors. For IMGs coming from English-speaking countries, this may pose little difficulty. However, for those who have practiced medicine in their native country using their mother tongue, this can be extremely challenging. Poor command of the English language can make it difficult for physicians to interview patients effectively, establish rapport, and interact with other healthcare professionals.

  Difficulties exist even for IMGs who are trained in English. Husain wrote that "variations in pronunciation, rhythm, and voice inflection may combine to produce a foreign accent that interferes with efficient transmission of the desired message, and this problem may occur despite excellent grammar and vocabulary use."[29]

  To determine your level of English language proficiency, programs will initially rely on the results of your USMLE Step 2 CS test. While passage of this exam is a measure of your communication skills, the interview will be the chief means by which your overall proficiency is assessed. Rao stated that "of primary importance for the interviewer is an assessment of the applicant's communication skills with respect to the pronunciation, grammar, grasp of idiom, and vocabulary…In listening to the applicant's responses to questions, the interviewer can assess the applicant's ability to express and understand abstract thought."[10]

- Assessment of personality

  During the interview, your interviewer will learn more about your non-cognitive traits, including your communication skills, your interpersonal skills, your strengths, and your drive. Interview questions are also asked to determine "fit" with the program.

  An interviewer can't learn about your interpersonal skills from your application alone. He can't learn about your strengths or weaknesses. He can't find out what drives or motivates you. He can't discover how well you handle pressure. Do you have the qualities that make someone a valued team member? Will you fit in and work well with others in the department? The only way an interviewer can learn any of these things is by speaking with you and asking questions. While the personal statement and LORs provide some information, the interview is the chief means by which programs can directly assess these non-cognitive factors.

- Assessment of medical knowledge

  In contrast to U.S. applicants, IMGs are more likely to be asked questions that gauge their medical knowledge. One IMG commented on this experience. They "would ask you medical questions and give you patient scenarios and…they made me examine and talk to a patient…it was awful. They asked all kinds of questions and gave you labs…it's like an exam. It was horrible."[26]

Other issues are shown in the following table.

Issues Which May Be Addressed During The Residency Interview	
Issue	**Concerns of Program**
Social support	Social support is essential for well-being during residency training. Many IMGs are separated from friends and family by long distances. Even when present, friends and family may not be able to understand the challenges faced by IMGs during the training period.
Familiarity with healthcare system	In one survey of IMG residents and PDs, researchers inquired about issues that were particularly difficult for IMG trainees. Among the IMGs surveyed, most frequently cited was knowledge of the healthcare system.[30]
Finances	Having left family behind in their home countries, many IMGs seek to provide their families with financial support. These obligations may be a source of stress during residency training.
Reasons for pursuing training in the U.S.	IMGs leave their home country for a variety of reasons. Commonly cited reasons include economic conditions, political environments, professional advancement and quality of life.
Embracing technology	Advanced technologies, such as CT or MRI, may not be readily available in other countries. The emphasis may be on clinical skills, and some IMGs are unfamiliar with investigational tools.

Working in multi-professional teams	Delivering high quality care in the U.S. is very much a collaborative effort with the involvement of a diverse group of health care professionals. Lack of familiarity with the roles and responsibilities of non-physician professionals can be challenging for IMGs.
Ability to handle constructive criticism	Constructive feedback is an important part of the educational process in the U.S., but some IMGs have a hard time receiving such feedback, viewing it as a "personal deficiency" or "academic failure."
Actively participating during rounds or conferences	IMGs educated in certain countries do not question or speak to supervising physicians unless addressed. "Many of the IMGs will never doubt the judgment of the attending, and you should," said Dr. Vijay Rajput. "When I grew up, it was 'Yes, sir,' 'No, sir,' 'Thank you.' I think that's a pretty big change." In the U.S., team members are expected to be active participants.[31]
Familiarity with electronic medical record	With the electronic medical record (EMR) in use at most teaching hospitals, PDs are understandably interested in knowing whether IMGs have gained experience working with the EMR. Among the concerns PDs may have about IMG trainees is their ability to type. In a study assessing the typing proficiency of residents in the U.S., the typing speed of non-U.S. citizen IMGs was found to be significantly slower than those of U.S. medical graduates. The concern with slower typing speeds has to do with the added time needed for documentation.[32]
Transitioning from physician-centered to patient-centered care	Many IMGs have trained in countries where patients simply follow physician recommendations without question. In these cultures and societies, physicians are revered, and sometimes given God-like status. "Patient-centered interviewing, ethical issues, empathy… sometimes are lost in other countries because of the fact that health care is just practiced at a very, very different level," said one internist, an IMG graduate from South Asia.[33] Adjusting to the patient-centered care of the U.S can be very difficult.
Educating patients	Patient education tends to be minimal in some countries, but not so in the U.S., where it is a major part of every physician-patient encounter. Patients tend to be more educated and informed in the U.S. Many IMGs are not used to being questioned or challenged, and expect that patients will cooperate with all recommendations. Sharing power with patients, seeking the input of patients in the decision-making process, and setting aside time to provide explanations may be frustrating to IMGs.

Rule # 217 **Understand immigration and visa issues as they relate to residency training.**

Without obtaining the legal authority to work in the U.S., you will be unable to begin residency training. For foreign-born IMGs who are naturalized U.S. citizens or holders of a permanent resident (immigrant) visa, this poses no difficulty. For IMGs who do not fit into these two groups, options generally include obtaining either a J-1 Exchange visitor visa or a H-1 B Temporary Professional Worker visa.

The ECFMG is authorized to sponsor IMGs for J-1 visas. To qualify for this visa, the IMG must show proof of acceptance into an accredited residency training program. In addition, a statement of need is also necessary. This statement is essentially a letter from the ministry of health of the country of nationality or last legal permanent residence, stating that a need exists in that country for physicians with the skills that IMGs are hoping to acquire through residency training.

The J-1 visa is an "exchange visitor" program that allows an IMG to reside in the U.S. while completing residency training. After completing training, the IMG must return to his or her country for a minimum of two years. After this period of time, the IMG becomes eligible for a change in visa status, permitting him or her to return to the U.S.

Since many IMGs prefer to stay in the U.S. permanently following completion of residency training, this requirement of the J-1 visa makes this visa unattractive. To avoid returning home, IMGs often explore ways to avoid fulfilling this requirement. One option is the receipt of the J-1 waiver from the U.S. government. IMGs who receive a waiver have to practice in a medically underserved area for at least three years.

Did you know?

States participating in the J-1 Visa Waiver Program are allocated a certain number of visa waiver slots on a yearly basis. The decision to grant waivers rests with the authority of each state's health department.

Because there is no "2-year home requirement," many IMGs prefer to train on a H-1 B visa. However, the H-1 B visa has traditionally been harder to obtain. To be eligible for this visa, you must pass the USMLE Step 3 exam, which can be challenging. In 2015, of the 7,637 IMGs who took the exam (first attempt), 11% failed.[34]

In addition, the process is more involved, sometimes requiring the assistance and efforts of an attorney. Furthermore, the H-1 B visa is not sponsored by the ECFMG but rather by the residency training program. Because of the effort and expense involved, fewer programs have traditionally offered the H-1 B visa. Recent data, however, suggests that this is changing. In 2014, 19.6% of IMG resident physicians were found to be on H visas (which include H-1B), a significant rise over the 6.5% reported in 2000.[3]

References

[1]American Medical Association. Available at: http://www.ama-assn.org/ama1/pub/upload/mm/18/img-workforce-paper.pdf. Accessed November 2, 2008.
[2]Alexander H, Lang J. Full-time faculty at U.S. medical schools with MD or equivalent degree: IMGs compared to U.S./Canadian graduates. Research Brief RB06-5. Washington, DC: Association of American Medical Colleges; April 2006.
[3]Brotherton S, Etzel S. Graduate Medical Education, 2014-2015. *JAMA* 2015; 314(22): 2436-2454.
[4]Results of 2015 NRMP Match. Available at: http://www.nrmp.org/press-release-nrmp-releases-results-and-data-2015-residency-match-record-number-of-positions-filled/. Accessed March 22, 2016.
[5]Results of 2014 NRMP Match. Available at: http://www.nrmp.org/2014-nrmp-main-residency-match-results/. Accessed March 22, 2016.
[6]Leon L, Aranha G. The journey of a foreign-trained physician to a United States residency. *J Am Coll Surg* 2006; 204 (3): 486-493.
[7]Kerfoot B, Asher K, McCullough D. Financial and educational costs of the residency interview process for urology applicants. *Urology* 2008; epub 990-994.
[8]Results of the 2014 NRMP Program Director Survey. Available at: http://www.nrmp.org/wp-content/uploads/2014/09/PD-Survey-Report-2014.pdf. Accessed March 3, 2015.
[9]Gayed N. Residency directors' assessments of which selection criteria best predict the performances of foreign-born foreign medical graduates during internal medicine residencies. *Acad Med* 1991; 66 (11): 699-701.
[10]Rao N, Meinzer A, Berman S. Perspectives on screening and interviewing international medical graduates for psychiatric residency training programs. *Acad Psychiatry* 1994; 18(4); 178-188.
[11]United States Medical Licensing Examination. Available at: http://www.usmle.org/performance-data/. Accessed March 2, 2015.
[12]Norcini J, Boulet J, Whelan G, McKinley D. Specialty board-certification among U.S. Citizen and non-U.S. citizen graduates of international medical schools. *Acad Med* 2005; 80(10): S42-S45.
[13]Sosenko J, Stekel K, Soto R, Belbard M. NBME examination part 1 as a predictor of clinical and ABIM certifying examination performance. *J Gen Intern Med* 1993; 8: 86-88.
[14]Case S, Swanson D. Validity of NBME part I and part II scores for selection of residents in orhopaedic surgery, dermatology and preventive medicine. *Acad Med* 1993; 68 (suppl): S51-S56.
[15]Fish D, Radfar-Baublitz L, Choi H, Felsenthal G. Correlation of standardized testing results with success son the 2001 American Board of Physical Medicine and Rehabilitation part 1 board certificate examination. *Am J Phys Med Rehabil* 2003; 82: 686-691.
[16]American Board of Internal Medicine. Association of Program Directors in Internal Medicine (APDIM) Chief Residents' Workshop on Problem Residents; 1999.

17Yao D, Wright S. National survey of internal medicine residency program directors regarding problem residents. *JAMA* 2000; 284(9): 1099-1104.

[18]Laufenburg H, Turkal N, Baumgardner D. Resident attrition from family practice residencies: United States versus international medical graduates. *Fam Med* 1994; 26: 614-617.

[19]Baldwin D, Roley B, Daugherty S, Bay C. Withdrawal and extended leave during residency training: results of a national survey. *Acad Med* 1995; 70: 1117-1124.

[20]van Zanten M, Boulet J, McKinley D, Whelan G. Attrition rates of residents in postgraduate training programs. *Teach Learn Med* 2002; 14 (3): 175-177.

[21]Yao D, Wright S. The challenge of problem residents. *J Gen Intern Med* 2001; 16(7): 486-492.

[22]Rao N, Meinzer A, Primavera L, Augustine A. Psychiatry residency selection criteria for American and foreign medical graduates. *Acad Psychiatry* 1991; 15(2): 69-79.

[23]Driver T, Loh A, Joseph D, Keenan J, Naseri A. Predictors of matching in ophthalmology residency for international medical graduates. *Ophthalmology* 2014; 121(4): 974-975.

[24]Educational Commission for Foreign Medical Graduates. Available at: http://www.ecfmg.org/reporter/2007/iss166.html. Accessed November 2, 2008.

[25]American Medical Association. Available at: http://www.ama-assn.org/ama. Accessed May 2, 2009.

[26]Woods S, Harju A, Rao S, Koo J, Kini D. Perceived biases and prejudices experienced by international medical graduates in the U.S. post-graduate medical education system. *Med Educ Online* 2006; 11: 20.

[27]Bates J, Andrew R. Untangling the roots of some IMGs' poor academic performance. *Acad Med* 2001; 76(1): 43-46.

[28]Stony Brook Department of Psychiatry. Available at: http://www.hsc.stronybrook.edu/som/psychiatry/selection_processes.cfm. Accessed March 2, 2015.

[29]Husain S, Munoz R, Balon R. International medical graduates in psychiatry in the United States: challenges and opportunities. *American Psychiatric Press* 1997.

[30]Zulla R, Baerlocher M, Verma S. International medical graduates (IMGs) needs assessment study: comparison between current IMG trainees and program directors. *BMC Medical Education* 2008.

[31]ACP Hospitalist. Available at: http://www.acphospitalist.org/archives/2010/07/img.htm. Accessed March 22, 2016.

[32]Kalaya A, Ravindranath S, Bronshteyn I, Munial R, Schianodicola J, Yarmush J. Typing skills of physicians in training. *J Grad Med Educ* 2014; 6(1): 155-157.

[33]Chen P, Curry L, Bernheim S, Berg D, Gozu A, Nunez-Smith M. Professional challenges of non-U.S. born international medical graduates and recommendations for support during residency training. *Acad Med* 2011; 86(11): 1383-1388.

[34]United States Medical Licensing Examination. Available at: http://www.usmle.org/performance-data/default.aspx#2015_step-3. Accessed March 2, 2016.

Chapter 23

Anesthesiology

How competitive is the specialty?

The attractiveness of anesthesiology as a career choice for U.S. senior medical students has fluctuated widely over the years. The number of students pursuing anesthesiology reached a low point in 1995 when only 36% of residency positions were filled by U.S. medical students. Since then, however, there has been growing interest in the field. In the 2016 NRMP Match, U.S. allopathic medical students filled 69% and 60% of the PGY-1 and PGY-2 residency spots, respectively.[1]

Did you know?

"Matching and matriculating in an anesthesiology residency in the United States has become much more competitive than 5 years ago," writes Dr. Gildasio de Oliveira, Assistant Professor of Anesthesiology at the Northwestern University Feinberg School of Medicine.[2]

Osteopathic and international medical graduate applicants are classified as independent applicants by the NRMP, and do not fare as well. In 2014, approximately 30% of independent applicants failed to match into anesthesiology.[3]

Highlights of the 2016 NRMP Anesthesiology Match[1]

- There were a total of 1,608 positions (PGY-1 and PGY-2 levels).
- Most positions were filled with allopathic medical student applicants (1,064).
- 208 osteopathic applicants matched.
- 114 U.S. IMG applicants matched.
- 80 non-U.S. IMG applicants matched.
- 47 U.S. graduates matched.
- 95 positions went unfilled.

How many years of training are required to become an anesthesiologist?

Four years of residency training are required to become an anesthesiologist. Training begins with either a transitional or preliminary year followed by three years of training in clinical anesthesia. There are two types of anesthesiology programs:

- Categorical four-year program

  The first year in these programs is considered the internship or clinical base year.

- Advanced three-year program

  These programs require a separate internship. Applicants applying to these programs must also apply to preliminary (medicine, surgery, pediatrics) or transitional year programs.

What percentage of available positions is filled by U.S. seniors? What about other applicants?

In 2013 – 2014, there were 5,686 total residents training in a total of 133 anesthesiology residency programs.[4] Of these, 78% were U.S. MDs, 11.9% were IMGs, and 10.3% were osteopathic graduates. As shown in the following table, the percentage of positions filled by international medical graduates has declined over the past five years.

Residents Training in U.S. Anesthesiology Residency Programs[4-5]					
Year	**Residency Programs**	**Total # residents**	**% US MDs**	**% IMGs**	**% DO**
2013-2014	133	5686	77.8%	11.9%	10.3%
2007-2008	131	5208	77.1%	13.1%	8.9%

Did you know?

Osteopathic applicants may also apply to 13 AOA-approved anesthesiology residency programs. In 2014, the mean COMLEX scores for matched applicants was 523 for Level 1 and 550 for Level 2.[6]

How do programs select residents?

Every few years, the NRMP conducts a survey of program directors. In 2014, the NRMP surveyed 67 anesthesiology residency program directors to determine the factors that are important in selecting applicants to interview.[7] The top five factors are USMLE Step 1/COMLEX Level 1 score, MSPE, graduate of U.S. allopathic medical school, USMLE Step 2 CK/COMLEX Level 2 CE score, and letters of recommendation in specialty. Factors are categorized in tiers of importance in the table on the next page.

Factors Identified as Important in Selecting Applicants to Interview by Anesthesiology Residency Program Directors	
Top Tier Factors (Cited by 70-99% of programs)	USMLE Step 1/COMLEX Level 1 score MSPE U.S. allopathic graduate USMLE Step 2 CK/COMLEX Level 2 score LORs in the specialty Class rank Personal statement Clinical clerkship honors Gaps in medical education Personal prior knowledge of the applicant Audition elective within your department Professionalism and ethics
Middle Tier Factors (Cited by 40-69% of programs)	Grades in required clerkships Perceived commitment to specialty Leadership qualities Honors in clerkship in desired specialty Grades in clerkship in desired specialty AOA membership Pass USMLE Step 2 CS / COMLEX Level PE Perceived interest in program Consistency of grades Volunteer/extracurricular experiences Graduate of well-regarded U.S. med school Involvement and interest in research Visa status Honors in basic sciences
Lowest Tier Factors (Cited by < 40% of programs)	Interest in academic career Gold Society membership Away rotation in specialty at another institution Fluency in language spoken by your patient population USMLE Step 3 / COMLEX Step 3 score
Adapted from Results of the 2014 NRMP Program Director Survey. Available at: http://www.nrmp.org/wp-content/uploads/2014/09/PD-Survey-Report-2014.pdf.	

% of Anesthesia Programs Citing Factors Used to Select Applicants to Interview (Comparison of 2008 and 2014 Data)[7-8]		
Factor	**2008**	**2014**
USMLE Step 1 score / COMLEX Level 1 score	81%	99%
MSPE	76%	87%
Graduate of U.S. allopathic medical school	65%	85%
USMLE Step 2 CK / COMLEX Level CE score	70%	82%
Letters of recommendation in the specialty	66%	81%
Personal Statement	66%	78%
Honors in clinical clerkships	59%	75%

How important are letters of recommendation?

Letters of recommendation are important to anesthesiology residency programs, cited by 81% as a factor in selecting an applicant to interview.[7] Programs generally ask applicants to submit 3 or 4 letters. Most programs request that 1 or 2 of these letters be written by academic anesthesiologists. Researching program requirements in advance will allow you to plan accordingly. Dr. William McDade, Professor of Anesthesiology and Critical Care at the Pritzker School of Medicine, recommends that applicants obtain letters of recommendation from anesthesiologists who are well-known in the field. For applicants who don't have this option, he recommends selecting anesthesiologists "who know you well and think highly of you."[9] Surgeons and internists who know you well should also be considered as potential letter writers. Dr. Kimberly Gimenez, former program director at the University of California-Irvine, feels that letters should ideally be written by faculty members in the departments of anesthesiology, critical care and surgery.[10] "At least two should be from anesthesiologists, and perhaps a surgeon you worked with extensively (the attributes of a good surgery resident tend to be quite similar to those which make for a good anesthesiology resident)" writes the Department of Anesthesiology at the University of Minnesota.[11] Please note that some programs may ask for a Chair's Letter.

How important is AOA?

The NRMP reports that 10.6% of U.S. seniors who matched to anesthesiology in 2014 were members of AOA.[3] This represents an increase over the 2007 percentage of 7.5.[12]

How important is the USMLE?

The mean USMLE Step 1 score for 2014 U.S. senior applicants who matched was 230.[3] Dr. Peter Moore, Chair of the Department of Anesthesiology at the University of California-Davis, states that "Step 1 is important as basic sciences particularly physiology, biochemistry, and pharmacology are the foundations of anesthesiology practice."[13] Of note, 30 of the 145 applicants with Step 1 scores ≤ 210 failed to match.[3] Applicants with low USMLE Step 1 scores can strengthen their application by showing improvement on the Step 2 CK exam. In 2014, the mean USMLE Step 2 CK score for matched applicants was 241.[3]

Did you know?

Although USMLE scores are not predictive of clinical performance during residency, scores have been found to be moderate to strong predictors of performance on the residency in-training and written board exams for anesthesiology.

When should I take the USMLE Step 2 CK?

A 2012 NRMP survey of 45 anesthesiology residency programs revealed that 11.1% of programs required passage of Step 2 CK for granting interviews. A much higher percentage (40%) required passage for placement on the rank-order list.[14]

Should osteopathic students interested in allopathic anesthesiology residency programs take the USMLE?

In "Optimize Your Match" published by the American Society of Anesthesiology, advice was offered to the osteopathic medical school applicant. "Osteopathic medical students have the option to apply for both osteopathic and allopathic residency programs. It is highly recommended that you take USMLE Step 1 to be competitive at the allopathic programs. Some programs will accept COMLEX but in my experience most of them prefer to have USMLE because it allows them a better comparison between candidates."[15]

Dr. George Mychiaskiw, former chairman of the Department of Anesthesiology at Drexel, echoes this advice. "Many of the more than 130 ACGME-accredited anesthesiology programs do not accept the COMLEX-USA…"[16]

Is it necessary to do an audition elective?

While it's not necessary to do an audition elective, Dr. Gimenez writes that "if the program has direct knowledge of the student they have a better chance of being accepted into the program."[10] This assumes that the applicant performs at a high level. The Mayo Clinic Department of Anesthesiology echoes this viewpoint. "Although a rotation with us is not necessary either for applying to the program or to eventually match into the program (all other factors being equal), we strongly believe that personal and professional interactions with potential candidates makes it much easier for our faculty to evaluate you beyond 'the numbers.'"[17]

Recommendations for Anesthesiology Audition Electives	
Anesthesiology Program	**Comments / Thoughts**
John Sullivan, M.D. Program Director Northwestern University	In deciding between possible audition electives, Dr. Sullivan believes that you should weigh your overall competitiveness against the reputation of the program that you are targeting. "This requires a very honest appraisal of their qualifications with their advisor and program director. For example, a 3rd quartile M4 with USMLE scores at or below national mean (but within at least 1 SD below the mean) will very likely need to audition to increase their desirability for a given program."[18]
Drexel University	Geography is another consideration in the decision-making process. "Away rotations are desirable, particularly for students seeking programs in geographically competitive areas (e.g., California), but are not mandatory."[19]
Catherine Kuhn, M.D. Program Director Duke University	"IF it is critical that you end up in a particular city, for family reasons, or whatever reason, then it might be a good idea to try to do an elective there. However, realize that away rotations can be good or bad...I've had visiting students really kill their chances for matching because of poor attitude, behavior, etc., that showed up in the month and might not have shown up during a one-day interview."[20]
Mayo Clinic	When should you do the away elective? The Mayo Clinic believes that August through November are ideal. "July is not the best time, as we have new trainees that we are orienting to the operating rooms. If you can do a fourth-year elective in May or June prior to starting your fourth year, you'll probably find even more learning opportunities."[17]

What are programs looking for in the personal statement?

Anesthesiology residency programs differ on the importance and role of the personal statement in the residency selection process. However, you have no way of knowing how the statement will be used. Therefore, plan to prepare a well-written, compelling statement that strengthens your overall application. "Believe it or not, every personal statement is read by several committee members," writes Dr. Marian Sherman, Program Director of Anesthesiology at The George Washington University.[21]

Recommendations for Anesthesiology Personal Statement	
Anesthesiology Program	**Comments**
University of Washington	"Should include your reasons for choosing anesthesia as a specialty. This statement affords you the opportunity to provide us with a personal profile and to point out any unusual features of your application."[22]
Gordon Willard, M.D. Program Director University of Minnesota	"It must be sincere, honest, and help the program understand your unique attributes."[23] He recommends that applicants address why they have chosen the specialty and the reasons why they would make a good anesthesiologist. Additional recommendations include substantiating any claims you make with concrete examples and showing how your values and interests match those of practicing anesthesiologists.
Society for Education in Anesthesia	"Your personal statement should be unique and leave a lasting and favorable impression of you."[24] The Society encourages making a list of your own special strengths, interests, accomplishments and experiences. "Compare the items on your list with your idea of what might make a 'perfect' resident in Anesthesiology. Select attributes from your list which resemble or support the characteristics of the "ideal" resident and incorporate these as the focus of your Personal Statement."
University of Pittsburgh	Areas of significant weakness in your application can be addressed in your personal statement. The Department of Anesthesiology at the University of Pittsburgh advocates this approach. "For instance, if you have failed a medical school course, you should briefly discuss in your personal statement any extenuating circumstances that may have contributed to the situation."[25] Before adopting this approach, it's best to discuss this with your faculty advisor.
Oregon Health & Science University	"Your personal statement should be a brief autobiography, your expectations of a residency program and a statement of your future goals."[26]
Robert Johnstone, M.D. Professor of Anesthesiology West Virginia University	"Most applicants enriched their statements with personal histories, usually as preambles or asides. These biographical anecdotes helped explain their backgrounds, qualities and styles, often making me want to meet them, with questions in mind…Their anecdotes were humanizing and intriguing, and sparked more interest in meeting them than their presumed required answers to desired program attributes and career goals."[27]

Anesthesiology Personal Statement: Common Features

A review of 670 personal statements to a single anesthesiology residency program provided insight as to the features commonly present in these statements.[28] The findings are summarized below.

1 Interest in physiology and pharmacology was mentioned in 60%.

2 Nearly 56% wrote about the enjoyment they received from intense patient interactions or their desire to comfort anxious patients.

3 Approximately 52% described enjoyment of anesthesiology because of its hands-on nature.

4 Enjoyment of acute care situations was discussed in nearly 44%.

5 In over 30% of statements, applicants discussed a particular case from medical school.

6 A desire to care for a diverse patient population was also commonly stated (31.5%).

7 Approximately 1/5 of applicants wrote about their intent for a career in academic anesthesiology.

8 Just over 20% of applicants indicated a desire to pursue fellowship training following residency.

9 The desire to care for one patient at a time was communicated in about 13% of statements.

10 Discussion of family/friend or personal illness was found in 11.1% and 6.1% of statements, respectively.

11 Approximately 6% of applicants wrote about their reasons for changing their specialty from surgery to anesthesiology.

12 Just over 4% of applicants wrote about their reasons for changing specialty from internal medicine to anesthesiology.

Features associated with higher ratings for originality included passion for physiology and pharmacology, case from medical school, enjoyment of acute care situations, desire to care for one patient at a time, desire to comfort anxious patients, and discussion of a family or friend's illness. Only 2 features present in statements were correlated with an invitation to interview – interest in physiology and pharmacology and desire to pursue a career in academic anesthesiology. In their conclusion, the authors made note of the similarities between applicant essays, and how this may represent a lost opportunity to impress programs. "We feel that the personal statement may be a missed opportunity for an applicant to show their unique qualities and distinguish themselves from other candidates."

Anesthesiology Personal Statement: How Is The Statement Evaluated?

A survey of 70 anesthesiology residency program directors revealed the role and importance of the personal statement in the selection process.[28]

1 Approximately 95% of program directors indicated that the personal statement was always or sometimes used in making decisions regarding interview invitations.

2 Less than half (41%) considered the personal statement somewhat or very important in deciding whom to interview.

3 Formal scoring of the statement was uncommon, reported by only 16% of program directors.

4 Over 90% reported that the applicant's use of English was somewhat or very important. "The data showed that applicants whose essays received high marks for grammar, word usage, and good overall organization, were more likely to receive an invitation for interview," wrote the authors.

5 The personal statement plays a major role on the interview day. 88% of program directors indicated that the statement was used to engage in discussion with the applicant.

Anesthesiology Personal Statement: Plagiarism

In a study of nearly 5,000 personal statements submitted to five residency programs (internal medicine, obstetrics & gynecology, general surgery, emergency medicine, and anesthesiology) at one academic medical center, researchers used specialized software to analyze and detect statements that were plagiarized from the Internet, published works, and previously submitted essays[29]The key findings pertaining to the anesthesiology statements are described below.

- 675 personal statements were examined.
- 534 were written by U.S. citizens.
- 141 were written by non-U.S. citizens.
- 4.4% of all statements had evidence of plagiarism.
- Evidence of plagiarism was found in 3.0% of U.S. citizen and 9.9% of non-U.S. citizen personal statements.

Anesthesiology Personal Statement: Observations of a Seasoned Residency Application Reviewer

As a faculty member in the Department of Anesthesiology at West Virginia University, Dr. Robert Johnstone has served on the residency selection committee for many years. He analyzed the personal statements of 65 applicants who received an interview invitation in 2010.[27] His findings may offer some guidance on the writing of your statement. Below, we've summarized his observations.

1 Applicants commonly write about personal experiences with anesthesiologists that spurred an interest in the specialty. 10 of the 65 statements described personal experiences that occurred before clinical rotations. 18 statements communicated personal experiences during clinical rotations.

2 Many applicants wrote about how they were awed by the skill and competence of anesthesiologists.

3 Positive statements about performing procedures were found in 22 of the 65 statements.

4 Communication and interaction with patients was a source of satisfaction for many applicants. Applicants pointed to examples of how compassionate anesthesiologists alleviated patient fear and anxiety before surgery.

5 Other common reasons why applicants expressed a desire to become an anesthesiologist included "the need to make decisions rapidly, their life-or-death importance, teamwork, the operating room environment with its attention to protocols and details, breadth of the specialty, and basic science foundation."

6 Most applicants provided brief insight into the factors important to them in a program. Often, no more than one sentence was devoted to this area.

7 Many applicants began their essay with an attention-grabbing opening but Dr. Johnstone often found this to be "contrived, unrelated, or weird." He recommends that applicants only try this approach if they are recognized for their writing ability.

8 He discourages the use of quotes, and finds statements beginning with bits of personal history more captivating.

9 Avoid overuse of I – in one statement, he counted the pronoun 39 times in 43 sentences. Overly flattering or heroic descriptions of anesthesiologists were not received well.

10 He also reminds applicants to take care with the last statement which are "commonly read during quick reviews." Dr. Johnstone prefers a positive ending which leaves him feeling positively inclined towards the applicant.

Did you know?

During the 2013-2014 application cycle, researchers at one anesthesiology residency program screened the personal statements of over 460 applicants for plagiarism using plagiarism software. 82% of statements were found to contain unoriginal content of at least 8 consecutive words. Plagiarized material was found in 13.6% and 4.0% of international medical and U.S. medical school graduates, respectively.[30]

How important is research experience?

In 2006, Dr. Marianne Green, Associate Dean for Medical Education and Competency Achievement at the Northwestern University Feinberg School of Medicine, surveyed anesthesiology residency program directors about the residency selection process. Program directors were asked to rate the importance of 16 criteria on a scale of 1 (unimportant) to 5 (critical). Among 16 academic criteria, Green found that published medical school research was last in importance.[31] Research experience is not required in order to match: among 2014 applicants, 99 of 109 applicants reporting no prior research experience matched.[3] Dr. Susan Luehr, former program director at the University of Texas-Houston, writes that "although not necessary, research experience is viewed very positively and encouraged for those applying to our specialty."[32]

How important is the interview?

Dr. Moore feels that an applicant's performance during the interview "is the deal breaker/maker."[13] In support of this is data from the 2014 NRMP Program Director Survey. "Interactions with faculty during the interview" and "interpersonal skills" were the two most important factors used by anesthesiology programs for ranking applicants. On a scale of 1 (not at all important) to 5 (very important), these factors received a mean rating of 4.8.[7]

References

[1]Advance Data Tables: 2016 Main Residency Match. Available at: http://www.nrmp.org/match-data/main-residency-match-data/. Accessed April 23, 2016.
[2]de Oliveira G, Akikwala T. Kendall M, Fitzgerald P, Sullivan J, Zell C, McCarthy R. Factors affecting admission to anesthesiology residency in the United States. *Anesthesiology* 2012; 117 (2): 243-251.
[3]Charting Outcomes in the Match (2014). Available at: http://www.nrmp.org/wp-content/uploads/2014/09/Charting-Outcomes-2014-Final.pdf. Accessed March 3, 2014.
[4]Brotherton S, Etzel S. Graduate Medical Education, 2014-2015. *JAMA* 2015; 314 (22): 2436-54.
[5]Brotherton S, Etzel S. Graduate Medical Education, 2008-2009. *JAMA* 2009; 302 (12): 1357-72.
[6]Osteopathic GME Match Report (2014). Available at: file:///C:/Users/labme/Downloads/DO_GME_match_2014.pdf. Accessed March 3, 2014.
[7]Results of the 2014 NRMP Program Director Survey. Available at: http://www.nrmp.org/wp-content/uploads/2014/09/PD-Survey-Report-2014.pdf. Accessed March 3, 2014.
[8]Results of the 2008 NRMP Program Director Survey. Available at: http://www.nrmp.org/wp-content/uploads/2013/08/programresultsbyspecialty.pdf. Accessed March 3, 2014.
[9]McDade W. Residency programs: an inside look. Available at: www.ama-assn.org. Accessed March 3, 2014.
[10]Gimenez K. Residency selection handbook: anesthesiology. Available at: www.ucihus.uci.edu. Accessed December 4, 2008.
[11]University of Minnesota Department of Anesthesiology. Available at: http://www.anesthesiology.umn.edu/residency/prospective/application/home.html. Accessed January 28, 2013.
[12]Charting Outcomes in the Match (2007). Available at: http://www.nrmp.org/wp-content/uploads/2013/08/chartingoutcomes2007.pdf. Accessed March 3, 2014.
[13]Moore P. A guide to the perplexed: residency guide. Available at www.ucdmc.ucdavis.edu. Accessed December 4, 2008.
[14]Program Requirements around Passage of USMLE Step 2 CK and USMLE Step 2 CS. Available at: http://www.student.med.umn.edu/osr/wp-content/uploads/2012/09/Program-Requirements-around-Passage-of-USMLE-Step-2CK-and-USMLE-Step-2CS-11.pdf. Accessed March, 3, 2014.
[15]American Society of Anesthesiology. Available at: www.asahq.org/For-Students/~/.../Optimize%20Your%20Match.ashx. Accessed January 28, 2013.
[16]The DO. Available at: http://www.do-online.org/TheDO/?p=88571&page=2. Accessed January 28, 2013.
[17]Mayo Clinic Department of Anesthesiology. Available at: http://www.mayo.edu/msgme/residencies-fellowships/anesthesiology/anesthesiology-residency-minnesota/frequently-asked-questions. Accessed March 3, 2014.
[18]Northwestern University Department of Anesthesiology. Available at: http://www.feinberg.northwestern.edu/education/current-students/career-development-residency/career-development-program/career-advising-specialties/anesthesiology.html. Accessed January 28, 2013.
[19]Drexel University Department of Anesthesiology. Available at: http://webcampus.drexelmed.edu/cdc/medSpecialtyAnesthesiology.asp. Accessed January 28, 2013.
[20]Duke University Department of Anesthesiology. Available at: http://anesthesiology.duke.edu/modules/anes_mse_aig/index.php?id=4. Accessed January 28, 2013.

[21]George Washington University Department of Anesthesiology. Available at: http://gwumc.edu/edu/anes/.../Anesthesiology-Newsletter-Spring.2011.pdf. Accessed April 2, 2012.
[22]University of Washington Department of Anesthesiology. Available at: http://depts.washington.edu/anesth/education/residents/apply.shtml. Accessed February 2, 2012.
[23]University of Minnesota Department of Anesthesiology. Available at: http://www.anesthesiology.umn.edu/residency/prospective/application/home.html. Accessed February 3, 2012.
[24]Society for Education in Anesthesia Medical Student Guide to Anesthesiology. Available at: www.studentorg.vcu.edu/soaig/SEAMedicalStudentGuide2009.pdf. Accessed February 5, 2012.
[25]University of Pittsburgh Department of Anesthesiology. Available at: http://www.anes.upmc.edu/education/residency_program/application.aspx. Accessed February 12, 2012.
[26]Oregon Health & Sciences University. Available at: http://www.ohsu.edu/xd/education/schools/school-of-medicine/departments/clinical-departments/anesthesiology/education/residency/prospective-residents.cfm. Accessed February 6, 2012.
[27]Johnstone R. Describing oneself: what anesthesiology residency applicants write in their personal statements. *Anesth Analg* 2011; 113 (2): 421-4.
[28]Max B, Gelfand B, Brooks M, Beckerly R, Segal S. Have personal statements become impersonal? An evaluation of personal statements in anesthesiology residency applications. *J Clin Anesth* 2010; 22(5): 346-51.
[29]Segal S, Gelfand B, Hurwitz S, Berkowitz L, Ashley S, Nadel E, Katz J. Plagiarism in residency application essays. *Ann Intern Med* 2010; 153: 112-20.
[30]Parks L, Sizemore D, Johnstone R. Plagiarism in personal statements of anesthesiology residency applicants. *AA Case Rep* 2015.
[31]Green M, Jones P, Thomas J. Selection criteria for residency: results of a national program director survey. *Acad Med* 2009; 84 (3): 362-7.
[32]Leuhr S. Career counseling: anesthesiology. Available at: http://www.uth.tmc.edu/med/administration/student/ms4/2003CCC.htm. Accessed March 3, 2014.

Chapter 24

Dermatology

How competitive is the specialty?

Dermatology is tremendously competitive, with many more applicants than available positions. 24% of U.S. allopathic seniors failed to match in 2014.[1] Dr. Christopher Shea, Section Chief of Dermatology at the University of Chicago, writes that their program "is extremely competitive. This year we had 530 applications for 4 slots, and interviewed about 36 applicants."[2]

Highlights of the 2016 NRMP Dermatology Match[3]

- There were a total of 420 positions.
- Most positions were filled with U.S. allopathic medical students (86%).
- 3 osteopathic applicants matched.
- 5 U.S. IMG applicants matched.
- 9 non-U.S. IMG applicants matched.
- 31 U.S. medical school graduates matched.
- Only 10 positions went unfilled.

Osteopathic and international medical graduate applicants are classified as independent applicants by the NRMP, as are graduates of allopathic medical schools. Independent applicants do not fare well. In 2014, approximately 61% of independent applicants failed to match into dermatology.[1]

Did you know?

Osteopathic applicants may also apply to 28 AOA-approved dermatology residency programs. In 2014, the mean COMLEX scores for matched applicants was 602 for Level 1 and 590 for Level 2.[4]

How many years of training are required to become a dermatologist?

To become a dermatologist, 4 years of residency training are required. Training begins with either a transitional or preliminary year, followed by 3 years of training in dermatology. Of note, a handful of programs offer combined medicine – dermatology training, which extends training to 5 years.

What percentage of available positions is filled by U.S. seniors? What about other applicants?

In 2013 – 2014, there were 1,212 total residents training in a total of 117 dermatology residency programs.[5] 95% were U.S. MDs, 3.3% were IMGs, and 1.0% were osteopathic graduates.

Residents Training in U.S. Dermatology Residency Programs[5-6]					
Year	**Residency Programs**	**Total # residents**	**% US MDs**	**% IMGs**	**% DO**
2013-2014	117	1212	95.7%	3.3%	1.0%
2007-2008	111	1069	94.3%	4.0%	1.6%

How do programs select residents?

Every few years, the NRMP conducts a survey of program directors. In 2014, the NRMP surveyed 59 dermatology residency program directors to determine the factors that are important in selecting applicants to interview and ranking. The results are available at www.nrmp.org.[7]

In a study published in 2014, researchers at the University of California Davis and Mayo Clinic sent surveys to 114 dermatology residency programs to determine the importance of criteria used in the selection process. In contrast to the 2014 NRMP Program Directors Survey, this study had a far better response rate (83.3% versus 53%). Programs were asked to rate 25 criteria on a scale of 1 (not at all important) to 10 (extremely important). Criteria were then subdivided into 4 groups based on the rating. The top 5 criteria in descending order of importance were residency interview, letters of recommendation, USMLE Step 1 score, medical school transcripts, and rotation at the PD's institution.[8] The findings are presented in the table on the following page.

How important are audition electives?

In a study of 2003 applicants, Dr. Jennie Clarke of Penn State University found that 53% of applicants matched at a program where they had had prior experience.[9] More recent studies continue to highlight the importance of audition electives. In the 2014 NRMP Program Director Survey, 64% cited "audition elective/rotation within your department" as a factor used to select applicants for interview. Respondents rated the audition elective 4.4 on a scale of 1 (not at all important) to 5 (very important).[7] Audition electives are clearly important in this highly competitive specialty.

Did you know?

In a recent study of dermatology residency selection criteria, researchers offered reasons why audition or away electives are so highly valued. "Away rotations may be of greater significance in the dermatology application review process as compared to other larger specialties considering that dermatology programs have a limited number of residency slots and therefore any personality conflicts may have a larger impact on the overall cohesiveness of a relatively smaller cohort of residents."[8]

Factors Identified as Important in the Dermatology Residency Selection Process

Importance	Criteria
Very Important (Rating 8-10)	Interview Letter of recommendation
Fairly Important (Rating 5-8)	USMLE Step 1 score Medical school transcript Rotation in PD's institution Personal statement USMLE Step 2 CK score Interest in academics Number of publications Extracurricular activities Dean's letter AOA membership Reputation of medical school Personal appearance Oral or poster presentation
Somewhat Important (Rating 2-4)	Prior unsuccessful attempt(s) to match Clinical fellowship Phone call made for candidate Ph.D. degrees Research fellowship M.P.H., M.B.A., and M.S. degrees Completing other residencies Reputation of undergraduate institution Age
Not Important (Rating 1-2)	Gender

Gorouhi F, Alikhan A, Rezaei A, Fazel N. Dermatology residency selection criteria with an emphasis on program characteristics: a national program director survey. *Dermatol Res Pract* 2014; 692760.

Tip # 154

"Most applicants arrange to take at least two months of dermatology electives," writes Dr. Aisha Shethi, Program Director at the University of Chicago. "We recommend going to away rotations in August – September of your MS4 year."[10] If your schedule allows you to complete rotations late in your third year (April – June), this might be advantageous for several reasons. At this time of the year, there are generally fewer medical students rotating through the department. This may make it easier for you to build relationships with residents and faculty.

Tip # 155

A rotation at your own medical school is always recommended before venturing off to complete away electives. "You might want to start with a program at your home school so that you will excel when you visit an outside program," writes the Department of Dermatology at the University of Texas Southwestern.[11]

Tip # 156

Choose your away electives carefully. Consider the following questions. Have students from your school matched with the program in the past? Does your school's dermatology faculty have well-established relationships with faculty at the program? Are the residents graduates of schools similar in caliber or reputation to your medical school? Will you have the opportunity to work closely with the program's key decision-makers? Is the program compatible with your interests in the field (i.e., research)? Speak with mentors, advisors, other faculty members, and dermatology residents. Ask your faculty for suggestions for away electives based on the competitiveness of your application.

Did you know?

Given how difficult it is to match in the field, applicants are understandably concerned about making a strong impression. Dr. Ali Alikhan, a faculty member at the University of California Davis, offers valuable advice for students. "Show genuine enthusiasm and interest without being overly aggressive or annoying…you can shine mainly through your presentations – by being able to accurately describe lesions, formulate appropriate differentials, and show evidence of nightly reading. Because patient turnover in dermatology clinics is high, being able to work at a reasonably quick pace is important as well."[12]

Did you know?

In an interview with Dr. William James, Chairman of the Department of Dermatology at the University of Pennsylvania, we asked Dr. James, "What sets apart students who shine during these rotations from those that are average?"[13]

First of all, enthusiasm. There are students, believe it or not, who show up and look a little bored. I think enthusiasm for the work and the subject is very important. The way students interact with others is certainly a key. You can have all the brains in the world, but if you can't get along with people, that doesn't say much for your ability to work on a team or work with patients. Sometimes students can be a little too aggressive in their interactions, probably because they're trying to either come across as enthusiastic or they're trying to show off their smarts. There is a fine line regarding what is appropriate for the level of training. At the same time, I think faculty members do take into account that students are trying to make a good impression, so I think there is some leeway there.

Hopefully, there will be opportunities to demonstrate their knowledge base or get involved with a project. If you find that the dermatologists are getting excited about a case and saying "I haven't seen this before" or "I don't really know what is a good treatment for this condition; let's go look it up", this would a great opportunity for the student to follow up by reporting "This is a case that I learned something from; I looked it up, I thought about it, and I'd like to pursue it a little further."

Who should be asked to write letters of recommendation?

Academic dermatology is a small community. As such, faculty members tend to know one another quite well. Strong LORs from senior faculty who are well known to the program carry great weight. In Gorouhi's survey of dermatology residency PDs, the source of the letter was very important.[8] The authors rated the source of letters on a scale of 1 (not at all important) to 10 (extremely important) as follows:

Someone PD knows (8.30) > LOR from chair or PD (7.78) > Well-known dermatologist (7.04) > Well-known expert in another specialty (5.58)

Dr. Jeffrey Miller, Professor and Chair of the Department of Dermatology at Penn State, encourages applicants to "think carefully about letters of recommendation. These letters usually come from colleagues we know in the field. Most of us also know your chairperson or residency program director. One of your letters should come from one of them. That letter should be strong and personal. Letters of recommendation can separate you from other applicants."[14] Dr. Adelaide Hebert, Professor of Dermatology at the University of Texas-Houston, states that "we also look for letters from the chairman of the dermatology program where the student trained."[15] Note that some programs require one or more letters from physicians outside the specialty. Researching program requirements well in advance will allow you to plan accordingly.

Did you know?

During our interview with Dr. William James, Chairman of the Department of Dermatology at the University of Pennsylvania, he offered important advice for applicants with respect to letters of recommendation:[13]

It should be from someone with whom you've worked and who knows you in some meaningful way. That would usually mean at least working in a clinic with the letter-writer. Specifically, not just observing in clinic but actually interacting with patients and discussing diseases. It may involve rounding with the inpatient team and presenting patients in follow-up. It could be writing or participating in a project, such as a clinical project or a case report. There should be some meaningful interaction. There needs to be information about how the applicant works, what kind of ideas they have, and how they interact with patients and the team. That really is the key: being able to get to know your letter-writer long enough so that they can take examples and then detail how an applicant would be a good person to have in the residency program. For the people reading the letters, they're going to be looking for some meaningful pieces of information that are based on personal observation.

Did you know?

It is acceptable to obtain and submit letters from dermatologists with whom you conducted research. However, you must also have letters from clinical supervisors. The University of Wisconsin requests "a minimum of two from physicians who clinically supervised your work."[16] Dr. Ali Alikhan of the Department of Dermatology at the Mayo Clinic offers this advice. "When deciding which letters to send to which programs, several factors may be of import. These include: 1) How well a particular letter writer knows you 2) The connections that a letter writer may have at a particular program 3) The emphasis of particular programs - clinical versus research."[17]

How important is AOA?

The NRMP reports that 50.8% of U.S. seniors who matched to dermatology in 2014 were members of AOA.[1] This represents an increase over the 2007 percentage (47%).[18] Of note, being an AOA member does not guarantee admission. In 2014, 20% of unmatched U.S. seniors were AOA members.

How important is the USMLE?

The mean USMLE Step 1 score for 2014 U.S. senior applicants who matched was 247.[1] Several years ago, Dr. Charles Ellis, Associate Chair of the Department of Dermatology at the University of Michigan wrote that "more than 100 of our applicants had achieved the top percentile on the United States Medical Licensing Examination."[19] Of note, the mean score among U.S. senior applicants who did not match was 239. Only 14 of 32 applicants with scores < 220 successfully matched. "The high level of competition for dermatology residency positions necessitates a standardized, objective measure, such as the USMLE Step 1, with which to compare applicants," writes Dr. Matthew Zirwas, Program Director at The Ohio State University. "Although USMLE scores have been shown to correlate poorly with overall residency performance, the reason for placing emphasis on Step 1 scores is that they tend to correlate with ITE scores and board passage."[20]

Is research experience required?

Among 2014 applicants, approximately 97% of applicants claimed at least one abstract, publication, or presentation.[1] In fact, most reported at least 4 such works. The Southern Illinois Department of Dermatology states that "exposure to research and participating in research are preferable. More importantly is attempt at publication and experience in scientific writing."[21] Dr. Shea encourages applicants, to "publish something (ideally in dermatology, but any publication is valuable, showing your ability to think, write, act independently, and follow through on project)."[2] Of note, being published is no guarantee of a residency position. Among 2014 applicants, 58 of 297 applicants claiming ≥ 5 abstracts, publications, or presentations failed to match.[1]

Did you know?

In a study of dermatology residency PDs, researchers determined that peer reviewed publications (7.04) were much more valued than oral presentations (5.97), poster presentations (5.72), and abstracts (5.64).[7]

Did you know?

In a study of all personal statements submitted to a single dermatology residency program in 2012, researchers identified the characteristics and themes of content in statements. Themes that were more prominent in matched applicants compared to unmatched applicants included: studying the cutaneous manifestations of systemic disease, contributing to the literature gap, and studying the pathophysiology of skin diseases.[22]

What recommendations do you have for the personal statement?

With so many well-qualified applicants, dermatology residency programs place great importance on the personal statement. "In a sea of applications, particularly in areas such as dermatology, the personal statement may truly make the candidate shine," says Dr. Jennifer Swearingen.[23]

Recommendations for Dermatology Personal Statement	
Dermatology Program	**Comments**
William James, M.D. Chairman of Dermatology University of Pennsylvania	"…one of the main things that bothers me with personal statements is reading about that first I did this, and then I did that, and I wrote this paper, and I did this research, and I published it in this journal, and I did this volunteer work. It's all in the CV already and the whole statement becomes 'I, I, I.' But while the personal statement is just that – personal – if it's all going to be about delineating accomplishments that are covered in other places, then that simply isn't helpful. What is helpful is to draw a picture of yourself that can't be obtained from anywhere else in the application. It should be personal - this is who you are, this is what makes you excited, these are your special interests. Sometimes it may be outside of medicine, sometimes it may be a volunteer experience that is expanded upon, or it could be a personal connection that stimulated the applicant to want to do something more, such as a specific part of Dermatology down the line. You might express your future goal, as that is something that wouldn't be revealed in other parts of the application. It certainly has to be sincere. If everyone just says at the end of their statement 'I want to be an academic dermatologist' and there's nothing else in the application that tells a reason for this, it's not believable."[13]
Russell Hall, M.D. Chair of Dermatology Duke University	Although more labor-intensive, applicants may wish to develop multiple statements. This approach allows for personalization of the statement for a particular program. "If appropriate it is also helpful to learn if there is a special reason you are interested in our particular program. Is there a connection to the area? Are you interested in the work of one of our faculty members? Have you known other residents from our program that were important in your career? If issues like these are important then we would like to know before we get to the interview stage."[23]
Jeffrey Miller, M.D. Chair of Dermatology Penn State University	He makes note of some common personal statement themes: Being a visual person / Dermatology offering opportunity to care for wide range of patients, including those of all ages / Ability to do procedures. Miller encourages applicants to think beyond these reasons to make the statement unique. "The bottom line is to balance why you are interested in the field with who you are, weighing more heavily on 'who you are.'"[14]

What recommendations do you have regarding an interview?

The interview is the most important factor used by programs to rank applicants. Study after study has shown that it is the top factor. We present advice offered by several academic dermatologists in the table below.

Dermatology applicants are also advised to consider how they would respond to communication initiated by program directors following the interview. In one study, researchers determined if program directors violated NRMP rules regarding post-interview communication. The following were notable findings:

- 14% of respondents were asked to reveal how they intended to rank a program before match day.
- 32% felt pressured to reveal their rank-order list intentions.
- 90% were asked about interviews at other programs[24]

Advice for the Dermatology Interview	
Warren Heymann, M.D. Head of Dermatology Cooper Medical School	Heymann encourages applicants to be themselves. "Honesty and integrity are of paramount importance; insincerity easily shines through. I am trying to learn if you will be a good 'fit' for our program." He stresses the importance of asking stimulating questions to learn as much as possible about the program. "There is a tremendous difference between the applicant who takes the time and effort to learn about our program and faculty's expertise compared with the person who only applies to be near his girlfriend in Philadelphia."[25]
Jeffrey Miller, M.D. Chair of Dermatology Penn State University	Miller offers similar advice. "We tell them to answer every question from their heart – not give the answer they think the interviewer expects or wants. If you earned an interview, you made the final cut and that is the time to find out if you are a 'fit' for the program. The only way that can be determined is by being yourself."[14]
James Twede, M.D. Southern Colorado Dermatology	Twede relates a story from his interview days. "The interviewer…cautioned me about using the phrase 'I'm a visual person' during future interviews. He commented that some academic dermatologists find the phrase trite, vague, and overused and therefore it might not enhance my application."[26]
Christopher Shea, M.D. Section Chief of Dermatology University of Chicago	Shea states that, "If granted an interview, run a Medline search of the faculty's publications. Get some notion of who your interviewers are likely to be, and what their program emphasizes…If asked why you are interested in a particular program, do not say that it's for geographic reasons (your home town, pleasant climate, etc.). Give a thoughtful, professional interview."[2]

Advice for the Dermatology Re-applicant

For applicants who have already graduated from medical school, what determines a successful dermatology match? In one study, researchers found that certain factors strongly correlated with matching, including:

- USMLE Step 2 score
- Submission of letters written by dermatologists from institutions that train dermatology residents
- Completion of preliminary medicine internship rather than transitional or other internship type
- Listing of research experience
- Publishing of medical manuscripts
- Completion of non-ACGME dermatology fellowships

The authors also noted that successful applicants limited personal statements to no more than one page, and refrained from discussing the prior unsuccessful match.[27]

References

[1]Charting Outcomes in the Match (2014). Available at: http://www.nrmp.org/wp-content/uploads/2014/09/Charting-Outcomes-2014-Final.pdf. Accessed March 3, 2014.
[2]Shea C. Pritzker residency process guide: dermatology. Available at http://pritzker.uchicago.edu/current/students/ResidencyProcessGuide.pdf. Accessed December 4, 2008.
[3]Advance Data Tables: 2016 Main Residency Match. Available at: http://www.nrmp.org/match-data/main-residency-match-data/. Accessed April 23, 2016.
[4]Osteopathic GME Match Report (2014). Available at: file:///C:/Users/labme/Downloads/DO_GME_match_2014.pdf. Accessed March 3, 2014.
[5]Brotherton S, Etzel S. Graduate Medical Education, 2014-2015. *JAMA* 2015; 314 (22): 2436-2454.
[6]Brotherton S, Etzel S. Graduate Medical Education, 2008-2009. *JAMA* 2009; 302 (12): 1357-1372.
[7]Results of the 2014 NRMP Program Director Survey. Available at: http://www.nrmp.org/wp-content/uploads/2014/09/PD-Survey-Report-2014.pdf. Accessed March 3, 2014.
[8]Gorouhi F, Alikhan A, Rezaei A, Fazel N. Dermatology residency selection criteria with an emphasis on program characteristics: a national program director survey. *Dermatol Res Pract* 2014; 692760.
[9]Clarke J, Miller J, Sceppa J, Goldsmith L, Long E. Success in the dermatology resident match in 2003: perceptions and importance of home institutions and away rotations. *Arch Dermatol* 2006; 142 (7): 930-2.
[10]University of Chicago Department of Dermatology. Available at: http://pritzker.uchicago.edu/current/students/ResidencyProcessGuide.pdf. Accessed April 16, 2012.
[11]University of Texas Southwestern Medical School. Available at: http://www.utsouthwestern.edu/utsw/cda/dept25717/files/169141.html. Accessed April 16, 2012.
[12]Alikhan A, Sivamani R, Mutizwa M, Aldabagh B. Advice for medical students interested in dermatology: perspectives from fourth year students who matched. *Dermatology Online Journal* 15 (7): 4.
[13]The Successful Match: Getting into Dermatology. Available at: http://studentdoctor.net/2009/10/the-successful-match-getting-into-dermatology/. Accessed April 30, 2012.
[14]Miller J, Miller O, Freedbert I. Dear dermatology applicant. *Arch Dermatol* 2004; 140: 884.
[15]Hebert A. Career counseling: dermatology. Available at: http://www.uth.tmc.edu/med/administration/student/ms4/2003CCC.htm. Accessed December 4, 2008.
[16]University of Wisconsin Department of Dermatology. Available at: http://www2.medicine.wisc.edu/home/housestaff/hsmeddermapply. Accessed April 12, 2012.
[17]Alikhan A, Sivamani R, Mutizwa M, Felsten L. Advice for fourth year medical students beginning the dermatology residency application process: Perspectives from interns who matched. *Dermatol Online Journal* 15(10): 3.
[18]Charting Outcomes in the Match (2007). Available at: http://www.nrmp.org/wp-content/uploads/2013/08/chartingoutcomes2007.pdf. Accessed March 3, 2014.
[19]Kia K, Gielczyk R, Ellis C. Academia is the life for me, I'm sure. *Arch Dermatol* 2006; 142; 911-13.
[20]Fening K, Vander Horst A, Zirwas M. Correlation of USMLE Step 1 scores with performance on dermatology in-training examinations. *J Am Acad Dermatol* 2011; 64(1): 102-6.

[21]Southern Illinois Department of Dermatology. Available at: http://edaff.siumed.edu/Year4/SurveyResults_041102.pdf. Accessed December 8, 2008.
[22]Olazagasti J, Gorouhi F, Fazel N. A critical review of personal statements submitted by dermatology residency applicants. *Dermatol Res Pract* 2014; Sep 14 Epub.
[23]Dermatology Interest Group Association. Available at: http://www.derminterest.org/phpbb3/viewtopic.php?f=8&t=355. Accessed April 30, 2012.
[24]Sbicca J, Gorell E, Peng D, Lane A. A follow-up survey of the integrity of the dermatology National Resident Matching Program. *J Am Acad Dermatol* 2012; 67 (3): 429-35.
[25]Heymann W. Advice to the dermatology residency applicant. *Arch Dermatol* 2000; 136 (1): 123-4.
[26]Twede J. Being a visual person. *Arch Dermatol* 2006; 242: 1357-8.
[27]Stratman E, Ness R. Factors associated with successful matching to dermatology residency programs by reapplicants and other applicants who previously graduated from medical school. *Arch Dermatol* 2011; 147 (2): 196-202.

Chapter 25

Emergency Medicine

How competitive is the specialty?

In the 2016 NRMP Match, there were 2,476 emergency medicine (EM) residency applicants, far more than the number of available residency positions (1,895).[1] Most of these positions were filled with U.S. allopathic seniors. The numbers are not as encouraging for osteopathic and international medical graduates. These groups are considered independent applicants. According to the NRMP, 41% of independent applicants failed to match.[2]

> **Did you know?**
>
> It can be very difficult to match with a highly coveted program. Dr. Ginger Wilhelm, former PD at the University of Texas-Houston, states that their program receives approximately 500 applications for 10 resident positions. From this group, interviews are offered to about 80 applicants.[3]

> **Highlights of the 2016 NRMP Emergency Medicine Match[1]**
>
> - There were a total of 1,895 positions.
> - Most positions were filled with allopathic medical student applicants (1,486).
> - 224 osteopathic applicants matched.
> - 87 U.S. IMG applicants matched.
> - 23 non-U.S. IMG applicants matched.
> - 73 U.S. graduates matched.
> - Only 1 position went unfilled.

> **Did you know?**
>
> Osteopathic applicants may also apply to 62 AOA-approved EM residency programs. In 2014, the mean COMLEX scores for matched applicants was 513 for Level 1 and 543 for Level 2.[4]

What percentage of available positions is filled by U.S. seniors? What about other applicants?

In 2013 – 2014, there were 5,731 total residents training in a total of 167 EM residency programs.[5] 83% were U.S. MDs, 11.0% were osteopathic graduates, and 5.7% were IMGs.

Residents Training in U.S. Emergency Medicine Residency Programs[5-6]					
Year	**Residency Programs**	**Total # residents**	**% US MDs**	**% IMGs**	**% DO**
2013-2014	167	5731	83.2%	5.7%	11.0%
2007-2008	149	4750	82.9%	6.4%	10.6%

How many years of training are required to become an emergency medicine physician?

To become an EM physician, a minimum of 3 years of residency training is required. There are two major types of EM residency programs:

- Three-year programs

  These programs, commonly referred to as 1-2-3 programs, provide three years of EM training following graduation from medical school. Over 75% of current training programs utilize this model.

- Four-year programs

  Four-year training programs can be divided further into two types. There are 1-2-3-4 programs which provide four years of EM training following graduation from medical school. The 2-3-4 programs require applicants to complete an internship in another field. After completing this year (internal medicine, surgery, or transitional year), residents begin the EM residency program as a PGY-2.

Did you know?

There are sharp divisions in the EM community about three versus four-year training programs. Those in favor of 48 months of training argue that the field is so broad that three years is simply an insufficient amount of time to gain proficiency in so many areas. Supporters of 36 months of training maintain that there is no evidence that an extra year of training results in more competent clinicians. In support of their position are ABEM In-Training Exam scores that show no difference in scores between trainees.

Pros and Cons of EM Residency Training Formats	
Format	**Pros and Cons**
1-2-3 Format	Offers trainees financial advantage of completing residency in a shorter period of time. Supporters of four-year training programs question whether graduates of three-year programs have the confidence and clinical acumen to deliver high-quality care. May restrict job prospects of physicians seeking academic positions at four-year institutions. Less elective time may make future career decisions more difficult. Faster pace of learning can be demanding, causing some trainees to experience greater stress.
1-2-3-4 Format	Proponents of three-year training programs have dubbed the extra fourth year as "the $250,000 mistake," referring to the lost income from not entering the workforce. Additional year of training may pose an advantage when applying for jobs. For those people with academic aspirations, there is more time to initiate and complete research projects. Fourth year allows senior residents to hone skills in supervision.
2-3-4 Format	Prior to starting, trainees have to complete an internship (internal medicine, surgery, or transitional year). Exposure to EM during internship may be limited. Like 1-2-3 format, trainees only have three years to learn EM core content. Trainees often have to move from one institution to another after completing internship (can be a pro or con depending upon trainee's life situation)

How do programs select residents?

Every few years, the NRMP conducts a survey of program directors. In 2014, the NRMP surveyed 101 EM residency program directors to determine the factors that are important in selecting applicants to interview. The top three factors are letters of recommendation in the specialty, USMLE Step 1/COMLEX Level 1 score, and USMLE Step 2 CK/COMLEX Level 2 CE score. Factors are categorized in tiers of importance in the table on the next page.[7]

Factors Identified as Important in Selecting Applicants to Interview by Emergency Medicine Residency Program Directors	
Top Tier Factors (Cited by 70-99% of programs)	LORs in the specialty USMLE Step 1/COMLEX Level 1 score USMLE Step 2 CK/COMLEX Level 2 score MSPE U.S. allopathic graduate Grades in required clerkships Class rank Clinical clerkship honors Gaps in medical education Honors in clinical clerkships Perceived commitment to specialty Audition elective within your department Leadership qualities Honors in clerkship in desired specialty Grades in clerkship in desired specialty AOA membership Away rotation in your specialty at another institution Professionalism and ethics
Middle Tier Factors (Cited by 40-69% of programs)	Personal statement Personal prior knowledge of the applicant Pass USMLE Step 2 CS Pass COMLEX Level PE Perceived interest in program Consistency of grades Volunteer/extracurricular experiences Graduate of well-regarded U.S. med school Involvement and interest in research
Lowest Tier Factors (Cited by < 40% of programs)	Visa status Honors in basic sciences Interest in academic career Gold Society membership Fluency in language spoken by your patient population USMLE Step 3 score COMLEX Step 3 score
Adapted from Results of the 2014 NRMP Program Director Survey. Available at: http://www.nrmp.org/wp-content/uploads/2014/09/PD-Survey-Report-2014.pdf.	

How important are audition electives?

According to the NRMP, 87% of EM residency PDs cited audition elective/rotation within the department as a factor in selecting applicants to interview.[7] Respondents rated the audition elective 4.4 on a scale of 1 (not at all important) to 5 (very important). "First of all, away electives are popular, and doing a rotation in your specialty at another institution is recommended in order to give programs a sense of perspective," writes Dr. Todd Berger, Program Director of the Dell Medical School Emergency Medicine Residency Program. "There are three big reasons to do them: to do something impressive at a big-name place, to 'audition' at a top choice program, or genuine interest."[8] Meet with your faculty advisor to develop an approach suited to your background and credentials. "Students should consult with their specialty advisor when deciding where to apply for away rotations, as there is a bit of strategy involved depending upon the applicant's competitiveness and the region of the country where they would like to train," writes Dr. Gregory Garra, Program Director at Stonybrook.[9]

Tip # 157

We encourage EM applicants to complete away electives by October if possible. Your goal is to present a complete application to programs before interview slots are fully taken. If you're seeking LORs from these electives, completing rotations sooner rather than later ensures timely consideration of your application. However, if your main goal in completing the away rotation is to impress that particular program, then a rotation in November or December is reasonable.

Tip # 158

Start early to secure away rotation spots. "Heavily subscribed student electives may fill their quota of students accepted into the rotation by spring of the academic year preceding the planned elective," writes Dr. Adrienne Birnbaum, Professor of Clinical Emergency Medicine at Albert Einstein College of Medicine. "To avoid being closed out of such rotations, start investigating options early. A student who has special interest in performing an elective at a particular institution that has filled its quota should speak directly to the preceptor of the rotation to express their specific interest in the program."[10]

Did you know?

There are some potential negatives to doing an away rotation. Dr. Suzanne Bryce from the Department of Emergency Medicine at Vanderbilt University writes: "If you rub any faculty member (or resident, for that matter) the wrong way, that could negatively influence your chances of matching to that program. It can be stressful adjusting to a new setting; finding the parking garage, locating the cafeteria, and figuring out how to log into the system may seem simple until you try to do them while simultaneously impressing your attending! By the time you get settled, your month-long rotation may practically be over."[11]

How important are letters of recommendation?

Letters of recommendation were ranked first in importance in the 2014 NRMP survey of PDs.[7] The Society of Academic Emergency Medicine encourages applicants to obtain one or more letters from academic emergency medicine faculty. Dr. Jennifer Oman, former program director at the University of California Irvine, states that applicants should obtain letters from faculty members in the departments of emergency medicine, critical care, surgery, and medicine.[12] Dr. Wilhelm states that "letters are probably the most carefully read portion of the application" and emphasizes the importance of obtaining letters from emergency physicians with academic ranks. "The positions of chairman, residency director, and assistant residency director or medical student coordinator are recognizable to other directors even if the names of those individuals are not."[3]

Dr. Lotfipour and colleagues in the Departments of Emergency Medicine at the University of California Irvine School of Medicine and University of California San Diego School of Medicine authored an excellent article entitled "Becoming an emergency medicine resident: A practical guide for medical students." The authors wrote that "an exceptional letter from a respected faculty member may sway residency program directors to offer an applicant with non-competitive scores and evaluations an interview due to the importance programs place on clinical abilities. Therefore, it is valuable for a student to orchestrate time to work with a well-known EM faculty member, such as program director or assistant program director, clerkship director, research director, or Chief/Chair. Opportunities include tag-alongs, research, or educational and leadership positions in an EMIG (emergency medicine interest group]"[13]

In contrast to other specialties, EM has developed a standardized letter of recommendation (SLOR). Generally, departments designate a particular faculty member to write the SLOR. Try to determine who that person is at your institution and then work with that attending as much as possible. If you don't have the opportunity to work directly with him, he will write your letter based on information from other faculty and residents.

The writer of the SLOR is asked to provide a bottom-line match recommendation. The choices available include "guaranteed match," which is the best superlative the applicant can receive. In a review of SLORs, 23% of applicants received this designation.[14] In another study, Girzadas found that the following factors were important in securing the "guaranteed match" rating:

- Having extended contact with the letter writer. Working with the writer for an extended period of time (defined as more than 10 hours of contact in the emergency department) increased the chance of receiving the rating twofold over those who had less contact.
- Working with the writer in other capacities. Applicants who worked with the writer in other settings, such as research, increased their chances of receiving the rating.

- Having a staff physician write the letter rather than a senior physician such as the chair or PD. The authors hypothesized that staff physicians may have more direct contact with applicants, making them feel more comfortable in giving the rating. Also postulated was the tendency of senior physicians to be more selective in giving applicants the highest rating.
- Doing as well as possible in the rotation. The EM rotation grade was the strongest predictor of the rating.
- Demonstrating an outstanding work ethic and ability for differential diagnosis were also positively associated with the highest rating.[15]

Did you know?

In one study, applicants who had SLORs written by less experienced faculty writers were more likely to have Global Assessment Score (GAS) of "Outstanding" and a "Likelihood of Matching Assessment" of "Very Competitive." Applicants who knew their letter writers for more than one year were also more likely to receive these designations when compared to applicants who had known their letter writers for less than one year.[16]

Did you know?

In a study done to assess how the SLOR is used by residency programs, researchers found that 61% of programs require one or more SLORs for interview consideration. Nearly 37% of programs recommend that applicants submit the SLOR but do not require it for interview. PDs indicated that the top two factors used to make interview decisions were the SLOR and EM rotation grades.[17]

Did you know?

In a multicenter study designed to determine how often applicants waived their rights to view LORs, researchers found that 7% did not waive their rights. Interestingly, applicants who did not waive their rights were more likely to receive an Outstanding Assessment on the SLOR.[18]

Tip # 159

Request LORs as soon as possible, as faculty often take considerable time to write these letters. "Solicit letters as early as possible, as they tend to be de-prioritized by the people who write them," writes Dr. Todd Berger. "Since many residencies won't look at your file unless it is complete, a tactful nudge is in order. If 'Thanks again for writing me a letter' elicits a confession, it is a license for you to remind the laggard. If when you check the ERAS system you still see a delinquent letter, asking, 'Did you have any trouble with the ERAS system?' may be an appropriate way to remind them again."[19]

Tip # 160

Dr. David Overton is Professor of Emergency Medicine at the Michigan State University/Kalamazoo Center for Medical Studies. He urges applicants to obtain letters from all EM rotations. "You clearly need to cover all emergency medicine rotations that you have completed with a letter. So, if you did an EM month early in your fourth year at your own school, and then did an away elective, you need a letter from both."[20] Why? Dr. Shahram Lotfipour, Professor of Emergency Medicine and Associate Dean for Clinical Sciences Education at the University of California Irvine, offers his reasoning. "The student must decide if this externship letter will enhance his application; its absence will likely raise a red flag with some program directors."[13]

Tip # 161

Should you obtain a LOR from your research supervisor? Dr. Gus Garmel, former program director of the Stanford/Kaiser Permanente Emergency Medicine Residency Program, offers some thoughts. "This is a great addition to your application if you have had a productive relationship with a research director and you have done an exemplary job. This letter might have additional importance for residency programs that consider research a strong point for an applicant, or for programs with designated research time…the research director should be able to discuss personal attributes that might make you successful during your residency training."[21]

How important is AOA?

The NRMP reports 12.0% of U.S. seniors who matched to EM in 2014 were members of AOA.[2] There has been no significant change in this percentage when compared to 2007 data.

How important is the USMLE?

The mean USMLE Step 1 score for 2014 U.S. senior applicants who matched was 230.[2] Dr. Molly Fling, Program Director at University of California Davis, states that "high board scores certainly help, but most EM programs focus on the 'whole package.' Very low board scores hurt most applicants."[22] Additional recommendations include "for those whose Step 1 score falls below the mean, it is recommended to take Step 2 before submitting the EM application."[11] The mean Step 2 CK score among matched applicants in 2014 was 243.[2]

Did you know?

Osteopathic students applying to allopathic programs frequently ask whether they should take the USMLE. In one study, 77% of PDs reported that it was extremely or somewhat important for osteopathic students to take the USMLE.[23]

When should I take the USMLE Step 2 CK?

A 2012 NRMP survey of over 70 EM programs revealed that 14.8% of programs required passage of Step 2 CK for granting interviews. A much higher percentage (42.6%) required passage for placement on the rank-order list.[24]

What are residency programs looking for in the personal statement?

Dr. Loftipour states that the statement "should pique the reader's curiosity through a story or personal anecdote, such as a patient encounter, leadership experience, or special accomplishment. Because the readers are emergency physicians well acquainted with the specialty, the statement should not describe what EM is, but rather how the specialty suits the student."[13] Additional recommendations are presented in the table on the following page.

How important is research experience?

Among 2014 applicants, 162/175 claiming no research experience matched.[2] Per the Society for Academic Emergency Medicine: "Research experience helps, but it is not necessary. It will strengthen an applicant's position. The research involved does not necessarily have to be in emergency medicine. Mostly, it denotes a student who goes above and beyond the expected. There may be volunteer work or other ways to show this."[25]

How important is the interview?

The interview is clearly an important selection factor. According to the NRMP, interactions with EM faculty and house staff during the interview day are two of the three most important factors used in ranking residency applicants.[7] Dr. Loftipour states that "some common pitfalls include emphasizing geography rather than program strengths, a lack of meaningful questions, and unfamiliarity with previous research projects."[13]

Did you know?

In a survey of all applicants to an academic EM residency during the 2006-2007 interview cycle, 89% of respondents reported being contacted by a program after their interview but before rank lists were due. Although email was most often used for communication, 55% indicated that they were contacted by phone. 58% reported feeling "happy" but a significant percentage of applicants felt "put on the spot" (21%) or "uncomfortable" (17%).[26]

Recommendations for Emergency Medicine Personal Statement	
EM Program	**Comments**
Jamie Collings. M.D. Former Program Director Northwestern University	"One of the things I hate most when reading a personal statement is when the student spends the whole time telling me why they like EM. I hate this because they all sound the same and they really don't tell me much. I recommend to students that they write their personal statement from the perspective of a job applicant (sometimes the students forget that this is what they are). Sit down and think about your strengths and how they will fit into EM and then start writing. Your personal statement should tell me about your experiences and accomplishments and how they will make you a successful EM physician. For instance, leadership positions taught you how to work with a variety of people and successfully accomplish your goals. This is extremely important in EM because you will be leading a team in the department and these skills are invaluable."[27]
Christine Babcock, M.D. Program Director University of Chicago	"...your personal statement should cover the following topics: • What experiences have informed you in your decision to become an emergency physician? • The personality characteristics that you possess that will allow you to be a successful emergency physician. • What you plan to do with your training – think lofty thoughts!"[28]
Department of EM Florida Hospital	Grammatical and spelling errors can definitely hurt you. Reasons for ineligibility include the "quality of the personal statement (content, typographical, and grammatical errors)," writes the Department of Emergency Medicine at the Florida Hospital. Be sure to have your statement read by several people, including your advisor.[29]
Jennifer Oman, M.D. Former Program Director UC Irvine	"However, it is not appropriate to make excuses for past mistakes or actions. If you feel you have a flaw on your application that absolutely needs explaining, simply acknowledge the experience, state what you have gained from it and move on. Many times, the problem that you believe is obvious on your application only becomes one when you focus on it in the PS...These are sensitive issues that may need consultation with your advisor, attendings or dean."[21]

References

[1]Advance Data Tables: 2016 Main Residency Match. Available at: http://www.nrmp.org/match-data/main-residency-match-data/. Accessed April 23, 2016.
[2]Charting Outcomes in the Match (2014). Available at: http://www.nrmp.org/wp-content/uploads/2014/09/Charting-Outcomes-2014-Final.pdf. Accessed March 3, 2014.
[3]Wilhelm G. Career counseling: emergency medicine. Available at: http://www.uth.tmc.edu/med/administration/student/ms4/2003CCC.htm. Accessed December 8, 2008.
[4]Osteopathic GME Match Report (2014). Available at: file:///C:/Users/labme/Downloads/DO_GME_match_2014.pdf. Accessed March 3, 2014.
[5]Brotherton S, Etzel S. Graduate Medical Education, 2014-2015. *JAMA* 2015; 314 (22): 2436-2454.
[6]Brotherton S, Etzel S. Graduate Medical Education, 2008-2009. *JAMA* 2009; 302 (12): 1357-1372.
[7]Results of the 2014 NRMP Program Director Survey. Available at: http://www.nrmp.org/wp-content/uploads/2014/09/PD-Survey-Report-2014.pdf. Accessed March 3, 2014.
[8]Department of Emergency Medicine at Dell Medical School. Available at: http://www.austingme.com/residency-programs/emergency-medicine/how-to-apply/application-advice. Accessed March 4, 2015.
[9]StonyBrook Medicine. Available at: http://medicine.stonybrookmedicine.edu/system/files/neofiles/Career%20Counseling%20Manual%20for%20Advisors%202014.pdf. Accessed May 4, 2015.
[10]Society of Academic Emergency Medicine. Available at: http://www.saem.org/docs/students/your_em_rotation.pdf?sfvrsn=2. Accessed January 30, 2013.
[11]Emergency Medicine Residents' Association. Available at: http://www.emra.org/content.aspx?id=595. Accessed January 30, 2013.
[12]Oman J. Residency selection handbook: emergency medicine. Available at: http://www.ucihs.uci.edu. Accessed December 8, 2008.
[13]Lotfipour S, Luu R, Hayden S, Vaca F, Hoonpongsimanont W, Langdorf M. Becoming an emergency medicine resident: a practical guide for medical students. *J Emerg Med* 2008; Jun 10 (epub).
[14]Girzadas D, Harwood R, Dearie J, Garrett S. A comparison of standardized and narrative letters of recommendation. *Acad Emerg Med* 2000; 7(8): 963.
[15]Girzadas D, Harwood R, Delis S, Stevison K, Keng G, Cipparrone N, Carlson A, Tsonis G. Emergency medicine standardized letter of recommendation: predictors of guaranteed match. *Acad Emerg Med* 2001; 8 (6): 648-53.
[16]Beskind D, Hiller K, Stolz U, Bradshaw H, Berkman M, Stoneking L, Fiorello A, Min A, Viscusi C, Grall J. Does the experience of the writer affect the evaluative components of the standardized letter of recommendation in emergency medicine. *J Emerg Med* 2014; 46 (4): 544-50.
[17]Love J, Smith J, Weizberg M, Doty C, Garra G, Avegno J, Howell J. Council of Emergency Medicine Residency Directors' standardized letter of recommendation: the program director's perspective. *Acad Emerg Med* 2014; 21 (6): 680-7.
[18]Diab J, Riley S, Downes A, Gaeta T, Hern H, Hwang E, Kass L, Kelly M, Luber S, Martel M, Minns A, Patterson L, Pazderka P, Sayan O, Thurman J, Vallee P, Overton D. A multicenter study of the family educational rights and privacy act and the standardized letter of recommendation: impact on emergency medicine residency applicant and faculty behaviors. *J Grad Med Educ* 2014; 6 (2): 292-5.
[19]UT Southwestern – Austin Emergency Medicine Residency Program. Available at: http://www.austingme.com/residency-programs/emergency-medicine/how-to-apply/application-advice. Accessed January 30, 2013.

[20]Department of Emergency Medicine at Michigan State University/Kalamazoo Center for Medical Studies. Available at: http://med.wmich.edu/node/103. Michigan State University/Kalamazoo Center for Medical Studies

[21]American Academy of Emergency Medicine Resident Section. Available at: http://www.aaemrsa.org/pdf/rulesoftheroad_students.pdf. Accessed January 30, 2013.

[22]Fling M. A guide to the perplexed: residency guide. Available at: http://www.ucdmc.ucdavis.edu. Accessed December 8, 2008.

[23]Weizberg M, Kass D, Hussains A, Cohen J, Hahn B. Should osteopathic students applying to allopathic emergency medicine programs take the USMLE exam? *West J Emerg Med* 2014; 15 (1): 101-6.

[24]Program Requirements around Passage of USMLE Step 2 CK and USMLE Step 2 CS. Available at: http://www.student.med.umn.edu/osr/wp-content/uploads/2012/09/Program-Requirements-around-Passage-of-USMLE-Step-2CK-and-USMLE-Step-2CS-11.pdf. Accessed March, 3, 2014.

[25]Society for Academic Emergency Medicine. Available at: https://www.saem.org/. Accessed September 1, 2014.

[26]Yarris L, Deiorio N, Gaines S. Emergency medicine residency applicants' perceptions about being contacted after interview day. *West J Emerg Med* 2010; 11 (5): 474-8.

[27]Getting into Emergency Medicine. Available at: http://studentdoctor.net/2010/08/the-successful-match-getting-into-emergency-medicine/. Accessed January 30, 2013.

[28]University of Chicago Department of Emergency Medicine. Available at: http://pritzker.uchicago.edu/current/students/ResidencyProcessGuide.pdf. Accessed February 2, 2013.

[29]Florida Hospital Department of Emergency Medicine. Available at: http://www.fhgme.com/EmergencyMed/EM%20Program%20Manual.pdf. Accessed February 2, 2013.

Chapter 26

Family Medicine

How competitive is the specialty?

For U.S. allopathic medical students, family medicine is not considered a competitive specialty. In the 2014 NRMP Match, only 3.6% of allopathic students failed to match. Securing positions in family medicine residency programs is considerably more difficult for osteopathic and international medical graduates. The NRMP designates these two groups as independent applicants. In 2014, nearly 50% of independent applicants failed to match to family medicine.[1]

Did you know?

Osteopathic applicants may also apply to 245 AOA-approved family medicine residency programs. In the 2014 AOA Match, 880 residency positions were available in family medicine.[2]

Highlights of the 2016 NRMP Family Medicine Match[3]

- There were a total of 3,238 positions.
- 45% of positions were filled with allopathic medical student applicants.
- 381 osteopathic applicants matched .
- 727 U.S. IMG applicants matched.
- 382 non-U.S. IMG applicants matched.
- 125 U.S. graduates matched.
- 155 positions went unfilled.

How many years of training are required to become a family medicine physician?

To become a family medicine physician, a minimum of three years of residency training is required. Of note, there are programs in which you can combine family medicine residency training with another specialty (family medicine/psychiatry, family medicine/preventative medicine, emergency medicine/family medicine).

What percentage of available positions is filled by U.S. seniors? What about other applicants?

In 2013 – 2014, there were 10,119 total residents training in a total of 483 family medicine residency programs.[4] 47% were U.S. MDs, 33.1% were international medical graduates, and 19.6% were osteopathic graduates.

Residents Training in U.S. Family Medicine Residency Programs[4-5]					
Year	**Residency Programs**	**Total # residents**	**% US MDs**	**% IMGs**	**% DO**
2013-2014	483	10,119	47.3%	33.1%	19.6%
2007-2008	457	9353	44.8%	40.4%	14.7%

How do programs select residents?

Every few years, the NRMP conducts a survey of program directors. In 2014, the NRMP surveyed 227 family medicine PDs to determine the factors that are important in selecting applicants to interview.[6] The top three factors are USMLE Step 1/COMLEX Level 1 score, personal statement, and USMLE Step 2 CK/COMLEX Level 2 CE score. Factors are categorized in tiers of importance in the table on the next page.

How important is the personal statement?

Among factors used to make interview decisions, the NRMP found that the personal statement was the second most cited factor used in selecting applicants to interview. 87% of family medicine residency programs cited it as a factor, trailing only the USMLE Step 1/COMLEX Level 1 score.[6] The Department of Family Medicine at the University of Chicago states that "we weigh these fairly significantly. It is a great opportunity to express your unique strengths and interests. Describe how you developed your interest in the field of family medicine, and why you feel family medicine is the specialty for you."[7] The Department of Family Medicine at the University of Washington also places great emphasis on the personal statement. "The best personal statements are memorable. They paint a picture in the mind of the reader and tell a story about who you are, how you got here, and where you want to go. The personal statement is vitally important because it is frequently used to help determine who gets interviewed and ranked."[8]

How important are letters of recommendation?

Applicants are advised to obtain at least one letter from a family medicine physician. Also highly valued are letters from other primary care faculty, including internists, pediatricians, and obstetrician/gynecologists.

Factors Identified as Important in Selecting Applicants to Interview by Family Medicine Residency Program Directors	
Top Tier Factors (Cited by 70-99% of programs)	USMLE Step 1/COMLEX Level 1 score Personal Statement USMLE Step 2 CK/COMLEX Level 2 score LORs in the specialty MSPE U.S. allopathic graduate Gaps in medical education Perceived commitment to specialty Professionalism and ethics Audition elective within your department Pass USMLE Step 2 CS / COMLEX Level PE
Middle Tier Factors (Cited by 40-69% of programs)	Grades in required clerkships Class rank Honors in clinical clerkships Leadership qualities Honors in clerkship in desired specialty Grades in clerkship in desired specialty AOA membership Visa status Fluency in language spoken by your patient population Personal prior knowledge of the applicant Perceived interest in program Consistency of grades Volunteer/extracurricular experiences Graduate of well-regarded U.S. med school
Lowest Tier Factors (Cited by < 40% of programs)	Involvement and interest in research Honors in basic sciences Interest in academic career Gold Society membership Away rotation in your specialty at another institution USMLE Step 3 score COMLEX Step 3 score
Adapted from Results of the 2014 NRMP Program Director Survey. Available at: http://www.nrmp.org/wp-content/uploads/2014/09/PD-Survey-Report-2014.pdf.	

How important are audition electives?

Audition electives are generally not necessary for resident selection. However, you have to consider the strength of your application. For example, if you have a red flag in your application, performing at a high level during an audition elective may alleviate concerns. Audition electives also allow applicants the opportunity to assess their fit for a particular program. "Doing an away rotation in family medicine can be a good way to help you see how family medicine differs across the country," writes Dr. Donna Meltzer, Program Director at Stony Brook University Hospital. "Family Medicine experiences can be different in different communities and different practice settings (i.e. academic, community, rural)."[9]

How important is AOA?

AOA membership is not an important factor in the family medicine residency selection process. The NRMP reports that 8% of U.S. seniors who matched to family medicine in 2014 were members of AOA.[1]

How important is the USMLE?

The mean USMLE Step 1 score (2014 U.S. senior applicants who matched) was 218.[1] Dr. Kay Nelsen, Program Director at the University of California-Davis, states that their program "gives no systematic weight to USMLE Step 1, but if it's low this could be a red flag to other evidences of academic difficulties which, collectively, might drop a student from contention."[10] However, family medicine as a specialty tends to take a comprehensive view of the entire application. For applicants who have failed or scored poorly on the USMLE, it is possible to overcome this obstacle with a well-developed and compelling application. "Your test scores are important," writes the Department of Family Medicine at the University of Arkansas for Medical Sciences. "Keep in mind that competition is fierce. If you have failed Step 1, Step 2, or Clinical Skills – you are at a disadvantage, and you will need to have something else to offer to make your application competitive."[11]

When should I take the USMLE Step 2 CK?

A 2012 NRMP survey of nearly 200 family medicine residency programs revealed that 35.6% of programs required passage of Step 2 CK for granting interviews. A much higher percentage (77%) required passage for placement on the rank-order list.[12]

What if I have a low USMLE score?

The Department of Family Medicine at the University of Colorado offers some important advice to U.S. medical students applying to the specialty. "Family Medicine programs are becoming more competitive but unless your scores are barely passing most programs will still consider you competitively if the rest of your application is positive."[13] Having one or more failed attempts is much more concerning to programs. That said, according to the NRMP, 35% of family medicine residency programs reported often considering applicants who failed Step 1 on the first attempt.[6]

How important is research experience?

In general, research experience is not necessary to secure a residency position. In 2006, Dr. Marianne Green, Associate Dean for Medical Education and Competency Achievement at the Northwestern University Feinberg School of Medicine, surveyed family medicine PDs about the residency selection process. PDs were asked to rate the importance of 16 criteria on a scale of 1 (unimportant) to 5 (critical). Among 16 residency selection criteria, Green found that published medical school research was last in importance.[14]

How important is the interview?

According to the NRMP, the interview is the most important factor used to place applicants on the program's rank-order list.[6] "Be ready to tell us what makes you stand out in a pool of 2,000 applicants," writes the Department of Family Medicine at the University of Arkansas for Medical Sciences.[11] The Department of Family Medicine at the University of Chicago recommends having "three times as many questions as you think you'll need, and you'll probably end up asking them all."[7]

References

[1]Charting Outcomes in the Match (2014). Available at: http://www.nrmp.org/wp-content/uploads/2014/09/Charting-Outcomes-2014-Final.pdf. Accessed March 3, 2014.
[2]National Matching Services. Available at: https://natmatch.com/aoairp/stats/2014prgstats.html. Accessed May 2, 2015.
[3]Advance Data Tables: 2016 Main Residency Match. Available at: http://www.nrmp.org/match-data/main-residency-match-data/. Accessed April 23, 2016.
[4]Brotherton S, Etzel S. Graduate Medical Education, 2014-2015. *JAMA* 2015; 314 (22): 2436-2454.
[5]Brotherton S, Etzel S. Graduate Medical Education, 2008-2009. *JAMA* 2009; 302 (12): 1357-1372.
[6]Results of the 2014 NRMP Program Director Survey. Available at: http://www.nrmp.org/wp-content/uploads/2014/09/PD-Survey-Report-2014.pdf. Accessed March 3, 2015.
[7]Hern T, Hickner J. Ewigman B. Pritzker residency process guide: family medicine. Available at http://pritzker.uchicago.edu/current/students/ResidencyProcessGuide.pdf. Accessed December 8, 2008.
[8]Department of Family Medicine at the University of Washington School of Medicine. Available at: http://depts.washington.edu/fammed/education/programs/advising/apply/impress/personal-statement. Accessed March 5, 2015.
[9]StonyBrook Medicine. Available at: http://medicine.stonybrookmedicine.edu/system/files/neofiles/Career%20Counseling%20Manual%20for%20Advisors%202014.pdf. Accessed May 4, 2015.
[10]Nelsen K. A guide to the perplexed: residency guide. Available at: http://www.ucdmc.ucdavis.edu. Accessed December 3, 2008.
[11]Department of Family Medicine at University of Arkansas for Medical Sciences. Available at: http://familymedicine.uams.edu/residency-program/frequently-asked-questions-family-medicine-residency-program/. Accessed March 5, 2015.
[12]Program Requirements around Passage of USMLE Step 2 CK and USMLE Step 2 CS. Available at: http://www.student.med.umn.edu/osr/wp-content/uploads/2012/09/Program-Requirements-around-Passage-of-USMLE-Step-2CK-and-USMLE-Step-2CS-11.pdf. Accessed March, 3, 2014.
[13]Department of Family Medicine at the University of Colorado School of Medicine. Available at: http://www.ucdenver.edu/academics/colleges/medicalschool/departments/familymed/education/predoc/Advising/Pages/FAQs---Information-for-Applying-to-Residencies.aspx. Accessed March 5, 2015.
[14]Green M, Jones P, Thomas J. Selection criteria for residency: results of a national program director survey. *Acad Med* 2009; 84 (3): 362-7.

Chapter 27

General Surgery

How competitive is the specialty?

General surgery is one of the more competitive specialties. In the 2014 NRMP Match, there were 1,833 applicants competing for 1,205 categorical positions.[1] Approximately 15% of U.S. allopathic medical students failed to match. It can be very difficult to match with a highly coveted program. "Each year we receive over 1,100 applications and interview between 70 and 80 candidates," writes the General Surgery Residency Program at Carolina HealthCare System.[2] Securing residency positions is particularly difficult for osteopathic and international medical graduates. The NRMP designates these two groups as independent applicants. In 2014, 68.2% of independent applicants failed to match.[1]

Did you know?

Osteopathic applicants may also apply to 59 AOA-approved general surgery residency programs. In 2014, the mean COMLEX scores for matched applicants was 530 for Level 1 and 550 for Level 2.[3]

Highlights of the 2016 NRMP General Surgery Match[4]

- There were a total of 1,241 positions.
- 76% of positions were filled with allopathic medical student applicants.
- 58 osteopathic applicants matched.
- 82 U.S. IMG applicants matched.
- 57 non-U.S. IMG applicants matched.
- 93 U.S. graduates matched.
- 2 positions went unfilled.

How many years of training are required to become a general surgeon?

To become a general surgeon, a minimum of 5 years of residency training is required. Applicants seeking one-year of general surgery training can apply to preliminary general surgery residency programs.

What percentage of available positions is filled by U.S. seniors? What about other applicants?

In 2013 – 2014, there were 8,053 total residents training in a total of 257 general surgery residency programs.[5] 81% were U.S. MDs, 16.6% were international medical graduates, and 3.3% were osteopathic graduates.

Residents Training in U.S. General Surgery Residency Programs[5-6]					
Year	**Residency Programs**	**Total # residents**	**% US MDs**	**% IMGs**	**% DO**
2013-2014	257	8053	80.1%	16.6%	3.3%
2007-2008	250	7712	78.6%	18.6%	2.7%

How do programs select residents?

Every few years, the NRMP conducts a survey of PDs. In 2014, the NRMP surveyed 115 general surgery PDs to determine the factors that are important in selecting applicants to interview.[7] The top three factors are USMLE Step 1/COMLEX Level 1 score, LORs in the specialty, and USMLE Step 2 CK/COMLEX Level 2 CE score. The findings are shown in the table on the following page.

How important are audition electives?

Several older studies have shown that audition electives in general surgery are not necessary for matching, and surgical faculty members often point to these studies when queried by students about the importance of audition electives in the field. "Most general surgery programs do not require that you do a surgery elective at program sites that you are interested in (sometimes referred to as audition electives)," writes the American College of Surgeons.[8] In a more recent study performed at a single general surgery residency program, however, researchers found that the match rate for students who completed away electives at the host institution was significantly better than for those who did not complete these electives (1:18 versus 1:237).[9] Although this data conflicts with the results of older studies, it remains to be seen whether this would hold true at other institutions. Until more data becomes available to guide decision-making, you are encouraged to discuss your away elective strategy with an advisor familiar with your credentials. If you do decide to perform an away elective in the field, the entire experience should be viewed as an extended interview. "This can be an invaluable step to make them competitive for the program as long as their application looks good and they perform well during the rotation," writes the Department of Surgery at Texas Tech University."[10] Although away electives may not be necessary for most allopathic students, these electives can be particularly helpful for osteopathic students and IMGs.

Did you know?

In one study, one-quarter of categorical general surgery slots were found to be filled with home program graduates. The authors wrote that "states with fewer medical schools are more likely to fill general surgery slots with home program graduates than states with more medical schools."[11]

Factors Identified as Important in Selecting Applicants to Interview by General Surgery Residency Program Directors	
Top Tier Factors (Cited by 70-99% of programs)	USMLE Step 1/COMLEX Level 1 score LORs in the specialty USMLE Step 2 CK/COMLEX Level 2 score MSPE U.S. allopathic graduate Grades in required clerkships Personal statement Class rank Honors in clinical clerkships Honors in clerkship in desired specialty AOA membership
Middle Tier Factors (Cited by 40-69% of programs)	Grades in clerkship in desired specialty Gaps in medical education Perceived commitment to specialty Audition elective within your department Leadership qualities Professionalism and ethics Personal prior knowledge of the applicant Pass USMLE Step 2 CS / COMLEX Level PE Perceived interest in program Volunteer/extracurricular experiences Graduate of well-regarded U.S. med school Involvement and interest in research Visa status
Lowest Tier Factors (Cited by < 40% of programs)	Consistency of grades Honors in basic sciences Interest in academic career Gold Society membership Away rotation in your specialty at another institution Fluency in language spoken by your patient population USMLE Step 3 score COMLEX Step 3 score
Adapted from Results of the 2014 NRMP Program Director Survey. Available at: http://www.nrmp.org/wp-content/uploads/2014/09/PD-Survey-Report-2014.pdf.	

Did you know?

In one study of general surgery and surgical subspecialty residency programs, 17% reported visiting social networking (SN) websites to gain more information about an applicant during the selection process. This led 33.3% of programs to rank an applicant lower.[12]

How important are letters of recommendation?

LORs are important, with the most desirable letters coming from academic surgeons who know the applicant well. If possible, applicants should work closely with leaders in their department of surgery. Such letters are particularly valued, but only if the letters reflect a real understanding of the applicant. No matter whom you select, make it as easy as possible for the writer to develop a strong LOR. "Over the years it has been apparent to me when there is only superficial involvement and shallow interest in the individual who is referenced," writes Dr. Frederick Greene, Chairman of the Department of Surgery at the Carolinas Medical Center. "It is also apparent when the essayist has not taken the time to meet with the reference to find out some special interests, characteristics or situations that would make both the letter and the applicant special."[13]

Did you know?

Strong letters written by senior faculty or surgeons holding important leadership positions in the department are highly valued. In an AMSA survey of approximately 140 general surgery residency programs, PDs believed that it was "very important to have strong letters only from surgeons, especially program directors, clerkship directors, chairmen, senior faculty, or from surgeons that the admissions committee know."[14] Note that some general surgery residency programs may request a letter from the Chairman of your Department of Surgery.

Tip # 162

How many of your letters should be written by surgeons? Some programs prefer that all letters be written by surgery faculty. The Department of Surgery at Washington University requires "three letters of recommendation from American Board of Surgery certified surgeons who are familiar with your work."[15] In general, the more surgical letters you have, the better. "Do not use a letter from a non-surgical person if it can be avoided," writes the Department of Surgery at the University of Washington.[16]

Did you know?

General surgery residency programs prefer letters written by surgeons because they believe that such letters will include more meaningful information. "As a surgery residency program director, I find it hard to evaluate an applicant's manipulative skills because the recommendations tend to cover other attributes like intellectual and clinical ability," writes Dr. John Herrman, Chair of the Division of Surgical Education at the University of Massachusetts. "I look for a student who plays a two-handed musical instrument, ties fishing flies, or does woodworking, and I explore the third-year surgical clerkship experience in relation to tying knots and using instruments."[17]

How important is AOA?

Most U.S. seniors who match are not members of AOA. The NRMP reports that 15% of U.S. seniors who matched to general surgery in 2014 were members of AOA.[1] That said, being an AOA member will provide a significant boost to the strength of the residency application.

Did you know?

In one study designed to determine the modern attributes of top-ranked applicants to 22 general surgery residency programs, highly competitive programs were more likely to rank applicants with publications, research experience, AOA membership, higher Step 1 scores, and excellent personal statements.[18]

How important is the USMLE?

Dr. Scherer, former program director at the University of California-Davis, states that their program puts "significant value on Step 1 scores."[19] The mean USMLE Step 1 score for 2014 U.S. allopathic applicants who matched was 232, considerably higher than the mean score of unmatched applicants (213).[1] "Although each program varies in their approach to screening applicants, generally speaking a minimum score of 210 needs to be achieved for the least competitive programs," writes the Department of Surgery at SUNY Downstate.[20] Dr. Potts, former program director at the University of Texas-Houston, states that "many university programs screen out those who made less than the 50th percentile on the USMLE Step 1."[21]

When should I take the USMLE Step 2 CK?

A 2012 NRMP survey of nearly 96 general surgery residency programs revealed that 39.8% of programs required passage of Step 2 CK for granting interviews.[22]

Did you know?

One study sought to determine the relationship between different application variables and the global rating score (GRS) of applicants to a single general surgery residency program. Researchers found that higher USMLE Step 2 CK scores, higher overall PS score and PS Written Expression score, and LORs from surgeons in leadership positions had a significant effect on the GRS.[23]

How important is research experience?

In a survey of 134 general surgery PDs, approximately 90% considered research experience almost always or all the time in their evaluation of applications. Nearly 30%, though, reported giving research experience little or no credit unless the work had been published. Respondents were also asked to rate the importance of research experience on a scale of 1 (low importance) to 5 (high importance). While 11 PDs gave research a 5 score, 93 directors rated it a 3, showing that most directors attach moderate importance to this selection variable. Of note, in this survey an applicant's demonstrated interest in surgery was an important selection factor, with 78 directors giving this factor a 5 score. The authors wrote that a "student's participation in research demonstrates considerable interest in the surgical field, which is a selection factor at the top of most program directors' lists."[24] Among the 871 U.S. senior applicants who matched in 2014, 47 had no prior research experience during medical school, and 158 reported no abstracts, publications, or presentations.[1]

How important is the personal statement?

Most general surgery programs place significant value on the personal statement. Recommendations from programs are described in the table on the following page.

Recommendations for General Surgery Personal Statement	
Surgery Program	**Comments**
Department of Surgery University of Colorado	"...write about your career goals, your strengths, and what attracts you to their 'type' of program...Furthermore, including several experiences or personal traits that make you unique and an interesting candidate is important. Ask yourself, 'Would I want to seek this person out in a crowd to talk to based upon this statement?' Remember that the field of surgery is generally pretty conservative. Save the melodramatic stories and infamous quotes for another time. Surgeons are interested in what **you** have to say, not what Shakespeare said in the late 18th century."[25]
Department of Surgery University of Utah	The personal statement "demonstrates your ability to use the language and organize your thoughts in a succinct fashion."[26]
Department of Surgery University of Virginia	"Write it as a means of persuading someone that you are a good candidate for their residency. Do not tell about all the little subtle things that made you want to be a surgeon, and don't tell them why you think surgery is swell...The thesis of this statement is that you will be a good resident. The thesis is not that you like surgery or that surgery is great. Most program directors do not care all that much about your research, your future plans, what made you go into surgery, or why surgery is great. They do care about what there is about you that will make you a good resident."[27]
Department of Surgery University of Washington	"The purpose of the personal statement is two-fold...to indicate that you have what the hospital needs in terms of abilities, experiences, skills, and maturity...that you are indeed the person the program is looking for with similar values and philosophies; in other words, that you are a good 'match.'"[28]

How important is the interview?

According to the NRMP, interactions with the faculty and house staff during the interview day were considered the most important factor in making the rank-order list.[7] In Melendez's survey, among selection criteria, the interview received the highest ranking from 93 of the 134 program directors.[24]

In a recent study, faculty at the Medical University of South Carolina found that faculty evaluations of personal characteristics through the interview were predictive of subsequent resident performance. This study also provided some insight into the selection process at one program. Each applicant has 3 one-on-one interviews with faculty members, as well as shorter interviews with the chairman, program director, and chief of general surgery. Interviewers are then asked to complete a "personal characteristics" form describing and rating the applicant's "attitude, motivation, integrity, interpersonal relationships, and response to specific life challenges...During a designated meeting, all surgical faculty members are given equal input, with individual members providing insight into the applicants whom they interviewed."[29]

Advice for the General Surgery Residency Interview	
Department of Surgery University of North Dakota	It is important to follow the program's interview schedule. "All sessions of the interview process are considered to be important in assessing and evaluating applicants as well as giving each applicant the appropriate exposure to the UND Surgical Residency Program. Therefore applicants that cannot attend all portions of the interview process will not be considered for NRMP ranking."[30]
Department of Surgery UT San Antonio	Do not underestimate the importance of the residents in the selection process. "Applicants have the opportunity to get to know the residents and vice versa. The current residents' input is valued highly in the selection process."[31]
Dr. L.D. Britt Chairman of Surgery Eastern Virginia Medical School	"Turnoffs include sloppy appearance, tardiness, argumentative nature, rudeness to staff, strong prejudices, overaggressiveness, condemnation of other specialties, mention of 'connections', noting influential individuals, and looking at watch during the interview."[32]
Dr. Karen Horvath Program Director Department of Surgery University of Washington	"You WILL be asked "What questions do you have for me?" numerous times, be prepared and thoughtful! You may have to guide your own interview. Do not ask questions about work hour violations. You may be asked about work hour restrictions, and should have a thoughtful opinion. You should be ready to explain what YOU would bring to the program, which would improve things for the program somehow."[33]

Did you know?

In one study, researchers sought to determine variables in the application process that might predict future success. In an 18-year review of all matched applicants to a single university-based general surgery program, the interview and USMLE Step 1 score predicted successful completion of residency. Overall attrition rate was 23.7%.[34]

References

[1]Charting Outcomes in the Match (2014). Available at: http://www.nrmp.org/wp-content/uploads/2014/09/Charting-Outcomes-2014-Final.pdf. Accessed March 3, 2014.
[2]General Surgery Residency Program at Carolina HealthCare System. Available at: http://www.carolinashealthcare.org/general-surgery-application-process-medical-education. Accessed May 2, 2015.
[3]Osteopathic GME Match Report (2014). Available at: file:///C:/Users/labme/Downloads/DO_GME_match_2014.pdf. Accessed March 3, 2014.
[4]Advance Data Tables: 2016 Main Residency Match. Available at: http://www.nrmp.org/match-data/main-residency-match-data/. Accessed April 23, 2016.
[5]Brotherton S, Etzel S. Graduate Medical Education, 2014-2015. *JAMA* 2015; 314 (22): 2436-2454.
[6]Brotherton S, Etzel S. Graduate Medical Education, 2008-2009. *JAMA* 2009; 302 (12): 1357-1372.
[7]Results of the 2014 NRMP Program Director Survey. Available at: http://www.nrmp.org/wp-content/uploads/2014/09/PD-Survey-Report-2014.pdf. Accessed March 3, 2015.
[8]American College of Surgeons. Available at: http://www.facs.org. Accessed December 8, 2008.
[9]Jacobsen R, Daly S, Schmidt J, Fleming B, Krupin A, Luu M, Anderson M, Myers J. The impact of visiting student electives on surgical Match outcomes. *J Surg Res* 2015; 196(2): 209-215.
[10]Texas Tech University Department of Surgery. Available at: https://www.ttuhsc.edu/som/studentaffairs/documents/CA_Surgery.pdf. Accessed March 4, 2015.
[11]Falcone J. Home-field advantage: the role of selection bias in the general surgery national residency matching program. *J Surg Educ* 2013; 70 (4): 461-5.
[12]Go P, Klaasen Z, Chamberlin R. Attitudes and practices of surgery residency program directors toward the use of social networking profiles to select residency candidates: a nationwide survey analysis. *J Surg Educ* 2012; 69 (3): 292-300.
[13]General Surgery News. Available at: http://www.generalsurgerynews.com/ViewArticle.aspx?d=Editorial+Page&d_id=66&i=December+2011&i_id=797&a_id=19775. Accessed May 16, 2012.
[14]AMSA Essentials of Getting into a Surgical Residency. Available at: http://www.amsa.org/AMSA/Libraries/Committee_Docs/Essentials_of_a_Getting_into_a_Surgical_Residency.sflb.ashx. Accessed April 30, 2012.
[15]Washington University Department of Surgery. Available at: http://surgery.wustl.edu/Surgery_M.aspx?id=682&menu_id=124. Accessed April 30, 2012.
[16]University of Washington Department of Surgery. Available at: students.washington.edu/.../Surgery_Med_Student_Advice_%20Final. Accessed May 18, 2012.
[17]Laster L. *Life After Medical School: Thirty-Two Doctors Describe How They Shaped Their Medical Careers*. W. W. Norton & Company; New York, NY: 1996.
[18]Stain S, Hiatt J, Ata A, Ashley S, Roggin K, Potts J, Moore RA, Galante J, Britt L, Deveney K, Ellison E. Characteristics of highly ranked applicants to general surgery residency programs. *JAMA Surg* 2013; 148 (5): 413-7.
[19]Scherer L. A guide to the perplexed: residency guide. Available at: http://www.ucdmc.ucdavis.edu. Accessed December 8, 2008.
[20]SUNY Downstate Department of Surgery. Available at: http://www.downstate.edu/college_of_medicine/pdf/care/Career-Booklet-Surgery.pdf. Accessed March 4, 2015.

[21]Potts J. Career counseling: general surgery. Available at: http://www.uth.tmc.edu/med/administration/student/ms4/2003CCC.htm. Accessed December 8, 2008.
[22]Program Requirements around Passage of USMLE Step 2 CK and USMLE Step 2 CS. Available at: http://www.student.med.umn.edu/osr/wp-content/uploads/2012/09/Program-Requirements-around-Passage-of-USMLE-Step-2CK-and-USMLE-Step-2CS-11.pdf. Accessed March, 3, 2014.
[23]Sharp C, Plank A, Dove J, Woll N. Hunsinger M, Morgan A, Blansfield J, Shabahang M. The predictive value of application variables on the global rating of applicants to a general surgery residency program. *J Surg Educ* 2015; 72 (1): 148-55.
[24]Melendez M, Xu X, Sexton T, Shapiro M, Mohan E. The importance of basic science and clinical research as a selection criterion for general surgery residency programs. *J Surg Educ* 2008; 65 (2): 151-4.
[25]University of Colorado Department of surgery. Available at: http://www.ucdenver.edu/academics/colleges/medicalschool/education/studentaffairs/studentgroups/SurgicalSociety/Pages/FAQ.aspx. Accessed April 30, 2012.
[26]University of Utah Department of Surgery. Available at: http://utahhealthsciences.net/pageview.aspx?menu=4971&id=16902. Accessed April 30, 2012.
[27]University of Virginia. *Obtaining a Surgical Residency: A Guide for University of Virginia Medical Students*. Available at: http://surgery.umc.edu/facultystaff/medstudents/documents/ApplicationGuide-UMMC.doc. Accessed April 30, 2012.
[28]University of Washington Department of Surgery. Available at: *students.washington.edu/.../Surgery_Med_Student_Advice_%20Final. Accessed May 18, 2012.*
[29]Brothers T, Wetherholt S. Importance of the faculty interview during the resident application process. *J Surg Educ* 2007; 64 (6): 378-85.
[30]University of North Dakota Department of Surgery. Available at: http://www.med.und.edu/residency/surgery/residency_app.html#interviews. Accessed September 13, 2012.
[31]University of Texas San Antonio Department of Surgery. Available at: http://surgery.uthscsa.edu/gsresidency/applications.asp. Accessed September 2, 2012.
[32]Britt L. How to interview for a residency position. Available at: https://www.facs.org/~/media/files/education/medicalstudents/britt.ashx. Accessed March 4, 2015.
[33]University of Washington Department of Surgery. Available at: http://students.washington.edu/uwsig/resources/Surgery_Med_Student_Advice_%20Final.pdf. Accessed September 3, 2012.
[34]Alterman D, Jones T, Heidel R, Daley B, Goldman M. The predictive value of general surgery application data for future resident performance. *J Surg Educ* 2011; 68 (6): 513-518.

Chapter 28

Internal Medicine

How competitive is the specialty?

The number of U.S. allopathic medical students entering categorical internal medicine (IM) residencies has risen every year for the past 5 years. According to the NRMP, 3,167 U.S. allopathic medical students matched into the specialty in 2014. However, this number remains significantly below the peak reached in 1985 (3,884). Securing a residency position in IM is not difficult for U.S. allopathic medical students. There are many more positions than interested applicants. In the 2016 NRMP Match, there were 7,024 total positions. Only 2.3% of allopathic students failed to match. Securing positions is considerably more difficult for osteopathic and international medical graduates. The NRMP designates these two groups as independent applicants. In 2014, 45.9% of independent applicants were unable to land positions in the field.[1]

Did you know?

There are programs in which you can combine IM residency training with another specialty (IM/anesthesiology, IM/dermatology, IM/emergency medicine, IM/family medicine, IM/medical genetics, IM/neurology, IM/pediatrics, IM/preventive medicine, IM/primary care, and IM/psychiatry).

Did you know?

Despite efforts to encourage IM residents to pursue careers in primary care, most residents choose to pursue subspecialty training. In 1998, over 50% of IM residents entered the primary care workforce. In recent years, however, only 20-25% of IM residency graduates become primary care physicians.

Did you know?

Although U.S. allopathic students have had great success matching into IM, it can be very difficult to match with a highly coveted program. "We are a competitive university program and receive over 2,000 applications per year," writes the Department of Medicine at Indiana University School of Medicine. "We extend interviews to just over 200 students."[2]

Did you know?

Osteopathic applicants may also apply to 129 AOA-approved internal medicine residency programs.

Highlights of the 2016 NRMP Internal Medicine Match[3]

- There were a total of 7,024 positions.
- 46.9% of positions were filled with allopathic medical student applicants.
- 498 osteopathic applicants matched.
- 1016 U.S. IMG applicants matched.
- 2013 non-U.S. IMG applicants matched.
- 117 U.S. graduates matched.
- 86 positions went unfilled.

How many years of training are required to become an internist?

To become an internist, a minimum of 3 years of residency training is required.

What percentage of available positions is filled by U.S. seniors? What about other applicants?

In 2013 – 2014, there were 23,258 total residents training in a total of 396 internal medicine residency programs.[4] 52% were U.S. MDs, 40.3% were international medical graduates, and 7.5% were osteopathic graduates.

Residents Training in U.S. Internal Medicine Residency Programs[4-5]

Year	Residency Programs	Total # residents	% US MDs	% IMGs	% DO
2013-2014	396	23,258	52.2%	40.3%	7.5%
2007-2008	382	22,132	49.4%	44.6%	5.9%

How do programs select residents?

Every few years, the NRMP conducts a survey of PDs. In 2014, the NRMP surveyed 194 internal medicine PDs to determine the factors that are important in selecting applicants to interview.[6] The top three factors are USMLE Step 1/COMLEX Level 1 score, MSPE, and USMLE Step 2 CK/COMLEX Level 2 CE score. These factors are categorized into tiers of importance in the table on the next page.

Factors Identified As Important in Selecting Applicants to Interview by Internal Medicine Residency Program Directors	
Top Tier Factors (Cited by 70-99% of programs)	USMLE Step 1/COMLEX Level 1 score MSPE USMLE Step 2 CK/COMLEX Level 2 score LORs in the specialty U.S. allopathic graduate Grades in required clerkships Class rank Gaps in medical education Pass USMLE Step 2 CS / COMLEX Level PE
Middle Tier Factors (Cited by 40-69% of programs)	Honors in clinical clerkships Perceived commitment to specialty Audition elective within your department Leadership qualities Honors in clerkship in desired specialty Grades in clerkship in desired specialty AOA membership Professionalism and ethics Personal statement Personal prior knowledge of the applicant Perceived interest in program Consistency of grades Graduate of well-regarded U.S. med school Visa status
Lowest Tier Factors (Cited by < 40% of programs)	Away rotation in your specialty at another institution Demonstrated involvement and interest in research Volunteer/extracurricular experiences Honors in basic sciences Interest in academic career Gold Society membership Fluency in language spoken by your patient population USMLE Step 3 score / COMLEX Step 3 score
Adapted from Results of the 2014 NRMP Program Director Survey. Available at: http://www.nrmp.org/wp-content/uploads/2014/09/PD-Survey-Report-2014.pdf.	

How important are audition electives?

Audition electives are not essential to match into internal medicine. We recommend considering audition electives if you want to better assess your fit with a particular program. If you're considering residency training in a part of the country you're unfamiliar with, an audition elective will allow you to make a more informed decision. Some advisors consider away rotations to be risky.

"There are only a handful of discrete circumstances where away rotations are advantageous," writes Dr. Susan Lane, Program Director at Stony Brook University Hospital. "If you have received advice that the target program would be a 'stretch' (meaning you are unlikely to get an interview at a program unless you go there and show the program your commitment). You absolutely need to be at a particular institution because of a personal relationship or proximity to family."[7]

How important are the letters of recommendation?

Letters of recommendation are an important component of the internal medicine residency application. At least one of your letters, and preferably two, should be written by a faculty member from the Department of Medicine or one of its subspecialties. One of your letters should be the chairman's letter (see box below).

Did you know?

Medical students seeking residency positions in internal medicine will often require a Department of Medicine (DOM) letter, also known as the "chair's letter." These letters are not always written by the chair. Departments may designate a particular faculty member to write this letter, such as the vice chair, clerkship director, or associate clerkship director. Most students haven't worked with these individuals, and therefore wonder why residency programs would ask for such letters. Programs seek to understand how your performance compares to other applicants, and the DOM letter is essentially a summary letter that incorporates the perspectives of multiple faculty members with whom you have worked. Often included in these letters:

- Description of clerkship structure
- Grading policy
- Grade distributions for core clerkship and subinternship
- Clarification of student's performance
- Synthesis of key narrative comments from clinical evaluations
- Specific circumstances impacting clerkship grades[8]

How important is AOA?

In a 2006 survey of PDs, AOA membership was seventh in importance among a group of 16 criteria.[9] However, most applicants who secure positions in internal medicine residency programs are not AOA members. The NRMP reports that 16.4% of U.S. seniors who matched to internal medicine in 2014 were members of AOA.[1]

How important is the personal statement?

The NRMP reported that 66% of PDs find the personal statement useful in making interview decisions.[6]

> **Did you know?**
>
> In a piece written in the *Annals of Internal Medicine*, Dr. Turi McNamee, Vice Chair of Education and Program Director at the University of Missouri, writes about common themes she encounters among the hundreds of statements she reads every year. "The statement usually follows 1 of 3 scripts:
>
> - The candidates relay a medical catastrophe that afflicted them or their family. Curiosity is piqued. They indulge their curiosity by poring over endless tomes of biologic sciences and end up in medical school.
> - Or, they know that they've wanted to be a doctor since conception. They were always exceptionally skilled in the sciences but really wanted to help people. Medical school was the natural conclusion.
> - Or, lastly, the curious case of Mr. X, who tells me a great deal about the unfortunate patient but surprisingly little about the candidate."
>
> No matter which approach is taken, she finds that all applicants have some sort of epiphany during their internal medicine clerkship, leading them to pursue a career in the field. "I hate them all," says Dr. McNamee. "Not the candidates, but their personal statements. Because there's really very little that's personal about them. The major thing they've told me about themselves is that they are very much like 90% of the other candidates for my program..."[10]

How important is the USMLE?

The mean USMLE Step 1 score for 2014 U.S. senior applicants who matched was 231.[1] 92% of PDs cited the Step 1 score as a factor used to make interview decisions.[6] Dr. Henderson, Program Director at University of California-Davis, states that his program doesn't "pay much attention to Step 1 unless it's very low (below 200 or so)…The most competitive programs may use Step 1 scores because they can, having many excellent applicants."[11]

> **When should I take the USMLE Step 2 CK?**
>
> A 2012 NRMP survey of 160 internal medicine residency programs revealed that 31.3% of programs required passage of Step 2 CK for granting interviews. A much higher percentage (72%) required passage for placement on the rank-order list.[12]

How important is research experience?

Among 16 academic criteria, Green found that published medical school research was last in importance.[9] Participation in research is not necessary, although research experience, especially if it leads to publication, may enhance competitiveness at the more competitive programs.

How important is the interview?

According to a survey of PDs conducted by the NRMP, the interview is the most important factor used to make ranking decisions.[6] It received a rating of 4.7 on a scale of 1 (not at all important) to 5 (very important).

Advice for the Internal Medicine Residency Interview	
Dr. Roy Ziegelstein Professor of Medicine Johns Hopkins University	"Applicants who stand out in the interview are able to communicate confidence without arrogance; sincere interest in the program that does not appear disingenuous; good speaking and also good listening skills; and an enthusiasm for medicine. Applicants stand out when they make me feel that the interview flew by rather than dragged. Applicants stand out if I can envision them taking care of my patients when they need to be hospitalized and/or if the interview leaves me feeling eager to teach and work with them."[13]
Dr. Philip Masters Vice Chair of Education Department of Medicine Penn State University	"Remember the purpose of the interview. If you have been asked to visit the program, then you are an acceptable candidate on paper. The interviewers will be paying attention to your interpersonal skills, professionalism, and how well they think you would fit into the program."[14]
Dr. John McConville Program Director Department of Medicine University of Chicago	"Prepare for your interviews by learning about the program through the web or other information materials. Ask questions that reflect you've studied the program (i.e. do not ask questions that are easily answered by the website or program materials). Do not talk poorly of your own institution as this is a 'red flag' to the interviewer. Such students come across as either 'not loyal' or extremely needy."[15]
Dr. Gopi Astik Former Chief Resident Department of Medicine UMKC	"Look your interviewers in the eye and offer your hand…Please look the interviewer in the eye even it's not in your nature to do so normally. When interviewees don't look at me, it makes me feel awkward myself– I feel like they are being evasive for some reason… We don't just want to hear what you have to say; we are also watching how you interact with your peers. In our program, being social is very important because we tend to spend a lot of time together outside of work. Being antisocial or extremely introverted is a negative in our eyes."[16]

References

[1]Charting Outcomes in the Match (2014). Available at: http://www.nrmp.org/wp-content/uploads/2014/09/Charting-Outcomes-2014-Final.pdf. Accessed March 3, 2014.

[2]Department of Medicine at Indiana University School of Medicine. Available at: http://medicine.iupui.edu/RESIDENCY/application/selection. Accessed July 22, 2015.

[3]Advance Data Tables: 2016 Main Residency Match. Available at: http://www.nrmp.org/match-data/main-residency-match-data/. Accessed April 23, 2016.

[4]Brotherton S, Etzel S. Graduate Medical Education, 2014-2015. *JAMA* 2015; 314 (22): 2436-2454.

[5]Brotherton S, Etzel S. Graduate Medical Education, 2008-2009. *JAMA* 2009; 302 (12): 1357-1372.

[6]Results of the 2014 NRMP Program Director Survey. Available at: http://www.nrmp.org/wp-content/uploads/2014/09/PD-Survey-Report-2014.pdf. Accessed March 3, 2015.

[7]Stony Brook Medicine Career Advisement Manual. Available at: http://medicine.stonybrookmedicine.edu/system/files/neofiles/Career%20Counseling%20Manual%20for%20Advisors%202014.pdf. Accessed March 3, 2015.

[8]Lang V, Aboff B, Bordley D, Call S, Dezee K, Fazio S, Fitz M, Hemmer P, Logio L, Wayne D. Guidelines for writing department of medicine summary letters. *Am J Med* 2013; 126 (5): 458-63.

[9]Green M, Jones P, Thomas J. Selection criteria for residency: results of a national program director survey. *Acad Med* 2009; 84 (3): 362-7.

[10]McNamee T. In defense of the personal statement. *Ann Intern Med* 2012; 157(9): 675.

[11]Henderson M. A guide to the perplexed: residency guide. Available at: http://www.ucdmc.ucdavis.edu. Accessed December 8, 2008.

[12]Program Requirements around Passage of USMLE Step 2 CK and USMLE Step 2 CS. Available at: http://www.student.med.umn.edu/osr/wp-content/uploads/2012/09/Program-Requirements-around-Passage-of-USMLE-Step-2CK-and-USMLE-Step-2CS-11.pdf. Accessed March, 3, 2014.

[13]The Successful Match: Interview with Dr. Roy Ziegelstein. Available at: http://studentdoctor.net/2009/06/the-successful-match-interview-with-dr-roy-ziegelstein/. Accessed September 5, 2012.

[14]Penn State University Department of Medicine. Available at: http://www.pennstatehershey.org/c/document_library/get_file?uuid=4561a5f4-7ec5-4f0f-9dba-66638e6e054a&groupId=133445. Accessed September 12, 2012.

[15]University of Chicago Residency Process Guide. Available at: http://pritzker.uchicago.edu/current/students/ResidencyProcessGuide.pdf. Accessed September 3, 2012.

[16]KevinMD Blog. Available at: http://www.kevinmd.com/blog/2012/03/residency-interview-tips-chief-resident.html. Accessed September 5, 2012.

Chapter 29

Internal Medicine/Pediatrics

How competitive is the specialty?

Combined Internal Medicine and Pediatrics or Med-Peds is a relatively new specialty. In 1980, there were fewer than 10 positions in the field. Since then, the number of positions has increased significantly, to about 350. Most, but not all, positions are filled with U.S. senior allopathic medical students. "It is important to note, however, that the most 'coveted' programs nationally can be quite competitive, particularly in light of the small number of residents accepted to each program," write Drs. Heather Nash and Bradley Monash, Career Advisors at UCSF.[1] Securing positions in Med-Peds residency programs is considerably more difficult for osteopathic and international medical graduates. The NRMP designates these two groups as independent applicants. In 2014, 44% of independent applicants were unable to land positions in the field.[2]

Highlights of the 2016 NRMP Internal Medicine/Pediatrics Match[3]

- There were a total of 386 positions.
- 85% of positions were filled with allopathic medical student applicants.
- 25 osteopathic applicants matched.
- 17 U.S. IMG applicants matched.
- 8 non-U.S. IMG applicants matched.
- 4 U.S. graduates matched.
- 2position went unfilled.

How many years of training are required to become board-eligible in Med-Peds?

To become board-eligible, a minimum of 4 years of residency training is required.

What percentage of available positions is filled by U.S. seniors? What about other applicants?

In 2013 – 2014, there were 1,439 total residents training in a total of 79 Med-Peds residency programs.[4] 83% were U.S. MDs, 9.5% were international medical graduates, and 7.8% were osteopathic graduates.

Residents Training in U.S. Med-Peds Residency Programs[4-5]					
Year	Residency Programs	Total # residents	% US MDs	% IMGs	% DO
2013-2014	79	1,439	82.6%	9.5%	7.8%
2007-2008	81	1,411	78.7%	14.2%	7.1%

How do programs select residents?

Every few years, the NRMP conducts a survey of PDs. In 2014, the NRMP surveyed 34 Med-Peds PDs to determine the factors that are important in selecting applicants to interview.[6] The top three factors are USMLE Step 1/COMLEX Level 1 score, USMLE Step 2 CK/COMLEX Level 2 CE score, and grades in required clerkships. These factors are categorized into tiers of importance in the following table.

Factors Identified as Important in Selecting Applicants to Interview by Med-Peds Residency Program Directors	
Top Tier Factors (Cited by 70-99% of programs)	USMLE Step 1/COMLEX Level 1 score USMLE Step 2 CK/COMLEX Level 2 score Grades in required clerkships MSPE Personal statement U.S. allopathic graduate Class rank Leadership qualities AOA membership
Middle Tier Factors (Cited by 40-69% of programs)	LORs in the specialty Gaps in medical education Honors in clinical clerkships Perceived commitment to specialty Professionalism and ethics Personal prior knowledge of the applicant Honors in clerkship in desired specialty Grades in clerkship in desired specialty Pass USMLE Step 2 CS / COMLEX Level PE Perceived interest in program Consistency of grades Graduate of well-regarded U.S. med school Volunteer/extracurricular experiences Gold Society membership
Lowest Tier Factors (Cited by < 40% of programs)	Audition elective within your department Visa status Away rotation in your specialty at another institution Demonstrated interest and involvement in research Honors in basic sciences Interest in academic career Fluency in language spoken by your patient population USMLE Step 3 score / COMLEX Step 3 score
Adapted from Results of the 2014 NRMP Program Director Survey. Available at: http://www.nrmp.org/wp-content/uploads/2014/09/PD-Survey-Report-2014.pdf.	

How important are audition electives?

Audition electives are not essential to match into Med-Peds. In the NRMP survey of PDs, only 38% cited an audition elective within the department as a factor in selecting applicants to interview. On a scale of 1 (not at all important) to 5 (very important), PDs gave the audition elective a mean rating of 3.2. Twenty-eight of the 32 factors used by programs in deciding whom to interview had higher mean ratings than the audition elective.[6] That said, there may be situations in which students should complete away electives. "Whether or not a student should do an away rotation depends upon the student," writes Dr. Rita Rossi-Foulkes, Program Director of the Med-Peds Residency Program at the University of Chicago. "If you wish to match at a specific program, AND you make a great first impression AND you adapt well to new situations, then consider rotating at the institution where you wish to match. If, however, you are quiet, and take a while to adapt to new situations, then doing an away rotation may not be a good idea. Away rotations can hurt as well as help your chances."[7]

How important are the letters of recommendation?

Letters of recommendation are an important component of the Med-Peds residency application. Programs require 3 or 4 letters of recommendation. Note that some programs do require or recommend letters from the Chairs of both Internal Medicine and Pediatrics Departments. The remaining letters should be written by physicians in Internal Medicine and/or Pediatrics with whom you have directly worked in a clinical capacity.

How important is AOA?

AOA membership is highly valued by Med-Peds programs. However, most applicants who secure positions are <u>not</u> AOA members. The NRMP reports that 22.1% of U.S. seniors who matched to Med-Peds in 2014 were members of AOA.[2]

How important is the personal statement?

The NRMP reported that 71% of PDs find the personal statement useful in making interview decisions.[6]

How important is the USMLE?

The mean USMLE Step 1 score for 2014 U.S. senior applicants who matched was 233.[2] 94% of PDs cited the Step 1 score as a factor used to make interview decisions.[7]

How important is the interview?

According to a survey of PDs conducted by the NRMP, the interview is the most important factor used to make ranking decisions.[6] It received a rating of 4.7 on a scale of 1 (not at all important) to 5 (very important).

References

[1]University of California San Francisco. Available at: http://meded.ucsf.edu/ume/career-information-medicine-pediatrics. Accessed September 30, 2015.

[2]Charting Outcomes in the Match (2014). Available at: http://www.nrmp.org/wp-content/uploads/2014/09/Charting-Outcomes-2014-Final.pdf. Accessed March 3, 2014.

[3]Advance Data Tables: 2016 Main Residency Match. Available at: http://www.nrmp.org/match-data/main-residency-match-data/. Accessed April 23, 2016.

[4]Brotherton S, Etzel S. Graduate Medical Education, 2014-2015. *JAMA* 2015; 314 (22): 2436-2454.

[5]Brotherton S, Etzel S. Graduate Medical Education, 2008-2009. *JAMA* 2009; 302 (12): 1357-1372.

[6]Results of the 2014 NRMP Program Director Survey. Available at: http://www.nrmp.org/wp-content/uploads/2014/09/PD-Survey-Report-2014.pdf. Accessed March 3, 2015.

[7]University of Chicago Residency Process Guide. Available at: http://pritzker.uchicago.edu/current/students/ResidencyProcessGuide.pdf. Accessed September 30, 2015.

Chapter 30

Neurology

How competitive is the specialty?

Securing a residency position in neurology is not difficult for U.S. allopathic medical students. There are many more positions than interested applicants. In the 2015 NRMP Match, there were 747 total positions at both the PGY1 and PGY2 levels. Only 2.5% of allopathic students failed to match. Independent applicants (osteopathic and international medical graduates) find it more difficult to land positions. In 2014, 40.4% of independent applicants failed to match.[1] With that said, neurology is among the top 5 specialties filled with the highest numbers of independent applicants.

Did you know?

Osteopathic applicants may also apply to 11 AOA-approved neurology residency programs.

Highlights of the 2016 NRMP Neurology Match[2]

- There were a total of 747 positions at the PGY1 and PGY2 levels.
- 58.5% of positions were filled with allopathic medical student applicants.
- 70 osteopathic applicants matched.
- 44 U.S. IMG applicants matched.
- 176 non-U.S. IMG applicants matched.
- 10 U.S. graduates matched.
- 9 positions went unfilled.

Did you know?

Although U.S. allopathic medical students have had success matching into neurology, it can be very difficult to match with a highly coveted program. "We typically receive about 400 applications and interview about 65 candidates for 6 positions," writes the Department of Neurology at the University of Michigan.[3]

How many years of training are required to become a neurologist?

To become a neurologist, a minimum of 4 years of residency training is required. The first year of training is usually completed in internal medicine. Neurology residency programs can be divided into two groups:

- Categorical

  In categorical programs, all 4 years of training take place within a single program.

- Advanced

  In advanced programs, only the last 3 years of training are included. The applicant must apply separately to programs for internship positions.

What percentage of available positions is filled by U.S. seniors? What about other applicants?

In 2013 – 2014, there were 2,246 total residents training in a total of 133 neurology residency programs.[4] 55% were U.S. MDs, 36.5% were international medical graduates, and 8.2% were osteopathic graduates.

Residents Training in U.S. Neurology Residency Programs[4-5]					
Year	**Residency Programs**	**Total # residents**	**% US MDs**	**% IMGs**	**% DO**
2012-2013	133	2246	55.2%	36.5%	8.2%
2007-2008	125	1743	56.3%	36.7%	6.5%

How do programs select residents?

Every few years, the NRMP conducts a survey of PDs. In 2014, the NRMP surveyed 59 neurology residency PDs to determine the factors that are important in selecting applicants to interview.[6] The top three factors are LORs in the specialty, USMLE Step 1/COMLEX Level 1 score, and MSPE. These factors are categorized into tiers of importance in the table on the next page.

How important is AOA?

The NRMP reports that 12.8% of U.S. seniors who matched to neurology in 2014 were members of AOA.[1]

How important is the USMLE?

The mean USMLE Step 1 score for 2014 U.S. senior applicants who matched was 230.[1] Should you take the USMLE Step 2 CK exam before applying to neurology? The decision should be based on your Step 1 performance and the requirements of the programs to which you're applying. Traditionally, applicants have been told that if the Step 1 score is competitive for matching, then you can take the Step 2 CK later. However, an increasing number of programs are requiring the Step 2 CK score prior to the Match. Applicants are urged to research programs of interest well in advance of application submission. If you have a low USMLE Step 1 score, you should consider taking the USMLE Step 2 CK exam in the July – September time period.

Factors Identified as Important in Selecting Applicants to Interview by Neurology Residency Program Directors	
Top Tier Factors (Cited by 70-99% of programs)	LORs in the specialty USMLE Step 1/COMLEX Level 1 score MSPE USMLE Step 2 CK/COMLEX Level 2 score U.S. allopathic graduate Personal statement Class rank Gaps in medical education Perceived commitment to specialty
Middle Tier Factors (Cited by 40-69% of programs)	Grades in required clerkships Honors in clinical clerkships Audition elective within your department Leadership qualities Honors in clerkship in desired specialty Grades in clerkship in desired specialty AOA membership Professionalism and ethics Personal prior knowledge of the applicant Pass USMLE Step 2 CS / COMLEX Level PE Perceived interest in program Consistency of grades Volunteer/extracurricular experiences Graduate of well-regarded U.S. med school Involvement and interest in research
Lowest Tier Factors (Cited by < 40% of programs)	Away rotation in your specialty at another institution Visa status Honors in basic sciences Interest in academic career Gold Society membership Fluency in language spoken by your patient population USMLE Step 3 score COMLEX Step 3 score
Adapted from Results of the 2014 NRMP Program Director Survey. Available at: http://www.nrmp.org/wp-content/uploads/2014/09/PD-Survey-Report-2014.pdf.	

How important are audition electives?

For most applicants, away electives are not necessary for a successful match. When Dr. Helene Rubiez, Program Director of the Neurology Residency Program at the University of Chicago, was asked, "Should applicants do away rotations," she responded emphatically with "NOT REQUIRED."[7] Although this advice holds true for most allopathic students, applicants with red flags in their background may find it worthwhile to boost their chances of receiving interview invitations. "If you are interested in a very specific program, then it may be a good idea, but you cannot do a rotation in every program that you are interested in," writes Dr. Ramadevi Goureneni, Neurology Career Advising Coordinator at the Feinberg School of Medicine at Northwestern University."[8]

Did you know?

Dr. Maggie Waung, a resident in the Department of Neurology at UCSF, offers some excellent advice on how to impress during the away elective. In addition to working hard, showing enthusiasm, and being dependable, she recommends taking ownership of patients. "Research your patient's conditions during your free time. Be tenacious about obtaining prior medical records. Offer to take call if it is not already expected. Participate in discussions. If you give a wrong answer, don't sweat it. It is more important to show that you are thinking. Keep in touch with the attendings you worked with. Offer to write up case reports if you are interested."[9]

Did you know?

In one study of medical student performance during the neurology clerkship, in nearly 75% of patient encounters, researchers found that students "were able to identically or closely localize the likely site of the lesion."[10] What were the common errors made by students?

- Poor understanding of the functions of the cerebellum and incorrect localization of lesions to the cerebellum were among the most common errors. Other frequently reported errors included mislocalization to the muscle, parietal cortex, and peripheral nerve.
- Many students had difficulty recommending proper diagnostic testing. In only 1/3 of the time were students in agreement with faculty.
- Formulating a management plan was also a difficult area with students often failing to discuss issues beyond pharmacology such as education, lifestyle modifications, support group referral, and recommendations for equipment for the prevention of complications.

Before your neurology elective, we recommend that you strengthen these areas to stand out from the average student.

How important are letters of recommendation?

Letters of recommendation are a very important component of the neurology residency application, consistently ranked as one of the top factors used to make interview decisions. According to the NRMP, LORs were rated more important than test scores.[6] Although test scores are important, Dr. Scheiss of the University of Texas-Houston states that "test scores assume secondary importance. Far more important are letters from physicians…that speak to the character, intellectual curiosity, diligence and the passion for neurology of the applicant. These letters should be based on direct observation of the applicant."[11] "Not having a letter from a neurologist" is one of the most common mistakes according to Dr. Eric Krauss, Clerkship Director at the University of Washington.[12] Most programs request 1-2 letters from neurologists.

Tip # 164

Some programs are very specific in their instructions. "One should be from the Department of Neurology chair or designee; the second should be from a Neurology faculty member who has worked closely with you and the third should be from a faculty member of your choosing," writes the Department of Neurology at the University of California Irvine.[13] If programs you covet have specific requirements, strategize on how you will meet these requirements. Note that most programs don't require a Chairman's letter.

Tip # 165

Should you submit a letter written by a research advisor or mentor? "Neurology programs look for letters from faculty who have worked closely with students clinically," writes Dr. Helene Rubiez, Program Director of the Neurology Residency Program at the University of Chicago.[14] That said, there are times when a research letter may be recommended. Some neurology residency programs place considerable emphasis on research. "If you are a PhD student, it is recommended one of the letters be from your PhD mentor," writes the Department of Neurology at UCSF.[15]

How important is the personal statement?

According to the NRMP, the personal statement is used by 71% of neurology residency programs in making interview decisions.[6] "Please submit a brief personal statement telling us something about yourself, your interest in neurology, your plans for residency training, and your career goals in neurology," writes the Department of Neurology at the University of Washington.[16] Dr. Scheiss feels that it is of "utmost importance" for applicants to communicate their desire to be a neurologist.[11]

How important is research experience?

"Research is not required, but often adds strength to your application," writes Dr. Cara Harth, Program Director at Stony Brook University Hospital.[17] Applicants seeking positions at the most competitive programs may find that research experience provides a boost to their application, particularly if it has led to publication.

How important is the interview?

As with other specialties, the interview is the most important factor used by neurology programs to rank applicants.

References

[1]Charting Outcomes in the Match (2014). Available at: http://www.nrmp.org/wp-content/uploads/2014/09/Charting-Outcomes-2014-Final.pdf. Accessed March 3, 2014.
[2]Advance Data Tables: 2016 Main Residency Match. Available at: http://www.nrmp.org/match-data/main-residency-match-data/. Accessed April 23, 2016.
[3]Department of Neurology at the University of Michigan. Available at: http://www.med.umich.edu/Neurology/edu/application.htm. Accessed March 9, 2015.
[4]Brotherton S, Etzel S. Graduate Medical Education, 2014-2015. *JAMA* 2015; 314 (22): 2436-2454.
[5]Brotherton S, Etzel S. Graduate Medical Education, 2008-2009. *JAMA* 2009; 302 (12): 1357-1372.
[6]Results of the 2014 NRMP Program Director Survey. Available at: http://www.nrmp.org/wp-content/uploads/2014/09/PD-Survey-Report-2014.pdf. Accessed March 3, 2015.
[7]University of Chicago Pritzker School of Medicine. Available at: pritzker.uchicago.edu/current/students/ResidencyProcessGuide.pdf. Accessed March 3, 2013.
[8]Northwestern University Department of Neurology. Available at: http://www.feinberg.northwestern.edu/education/current-students/career-development-residency/career-development-program/career-advising-specialties/neurology.html. Accessed March 2, 2013.
[9]Alpha Omega Alpha at UT Southwestern Medical School. Available at: http://utswaoa.wordpress.com/guides/away-rotations/. Accessed March 4, 2013.
[10]Davis L, King M. Assessment of medical student clinical competencies in the neurology clinic. *Neurology* 2007; 68 (8): 597-9.
[11]Scheiss M. Career counseling: neurology. Available at: http://www.uth.tmc.edu/med/administration/student/ms4/2003CCC.htm. Accessed December 8, 2008.
[12]University of Washington School of Medicine Career Advisors FAQ List. Available at: http://www.uwmedicine.org/education/documents/md-program/Departmental-Career-Advisors-FAQs.pdf. Accessed March 9, 2015.
[13]University of California Irvine Department of Neurology. Available at: http://www.neurology.uci.edu/residency.asp. Accessed March 3, 2013.
[14]University of Chicago Pritzker School of Medicine. Available at: pritzker.uchicago.edu/current/students/ResidencyProcessGuide.pdf. Accessed March 3, 2013.
[15]UCSF Department of Neurology. Available at: http://www.ucsfneuroresidency.com/public_html/Applicant/Applicant_Adult.html. Accessed March 3, 2013.
[16]Department of Neurology at the University of Washington School of Medicine. Available at: http://depts.washington.edu/neurolog/education/residency/application-information.html. Accessed March 6, 2015.
[17]Stony Brook Medicine Career Advisement Manual. Available at: http://medicine.stonybrookmedicine.edu/system/files/neofiles/Career%20Counseling%20Manual%20for%20Advisors%202014.pdf. Accessed March 3, 2015.

Chapter 31

Neurosurgery

How competitive is the specialty?

Neurosurgery is a highly competitive specialty. In the 2014 NRMP Match, over 20% of U.S. allopathic medical students failed to match. The numbers are significantly worse for independent applicants (osteopathic and international medical graduates). 79% of independent applicants failed to match.[1]

> **Did you know?**
>
> Osteopathic applicants may also apply to 11 AOA-approved neurosurgery residency programs.

> **Highlights of the 2016 NRMP Neurosurgery Match[2]**
>
> - There were a total of 216 positions.
> - 93% of positions were filled with allopathic medical student applicants.
> - 0 osteopathic applicants matched.
> - 3 U.S. IMG applicants matched.
> - 8 non-U.S. IMG applicants matched.
> - 3 U.S. graduates matched.
> - 2 positions went unfilled.

> **Did you know?**
>
> Most neurosurgery programs interview 30 – 40 applicants for just a few positions.

How many years of training are required to become a neurosurgeon?

To become a neurosurgeon, a minimum of 6 years of residency training is required. The first year of training is usually completed in general surgery.

What percentage of available positions is filled by U.S. seniors? What about other applicants?

In 2013 – 2014, there were 1,315 total residents training in a total of 105 neurosurgery residency programs.[3] 91% were U.S. MDs, 8.3% were international medical graduates, and 0.5% were osteopathic graduates.

Residents Training in U.S. Neurosurgery Residency Programs[3-4]					
Year	**Residency Programs**	**Total # residents**	**% US MDs**	**% IMGs**	**% DO**
2013-2014	104	1272	91.2%	8.3%	0.5%
2007-2008	99	961	87.8%	11.4%	0.4%

How do programs select residents?

In a 2011 survey of neurosurgery PDs, researchers determined the criteria used by programs to select residents. The study had a response rate of 46%.[5]

Neurosurgery Residency Program Directors' Rankings of Selection Criteria	
Criteria	**Mean**
Interview	3.80
USMLE Step 1 score	3.58
Letters of recommendation	3.56
Class rank	3.36
Interactions with residents at dinner	3.32
Publications/research	3.18
Clinical honors	3.18
USMLE Step 2 CK score	3.13
Performance on away elective	2.82
Extramural activities	2.37
Medical school attended	2.69
Presentation at neurosurgical conferences	2.56
Personal statement	2.51
Advanced degree	2.20
On-site presentation	2.00
Khalili A, Chalouhi N, Tjoumakaris S, Gonzalez L, Starke R. Rosenwasser R, Jabbour P. Programs selection criteria for neurological surgery applicants in the United States: a national survey of neurological surgery program directors. *World Neurosurg* 2014; 81 (3-4): 473-477.	

Every few years, the NRMP conducts its own survey of PDs. In 2014, the NRMP surveyed 54 neurosurgery PDs to determine the factors important in selecting applicants to interview (see table on following page).[6] The top 4 factors are letters of recommendation in the specialty, USMLE Step 1/COMLEX Level 1 score, MSPE, and AOA membership. The findings are shown in the table on the next page.

Factors Identified as Important in Selecting Applicants to Interview by Neurosurgery Residency Program Directors	
Top Tier Factors (Cited by 70-99% of programs)	LORs in the specialty USMLE Step 1/COMLEX Level 1 score MSPE AOA membership Personal statement U.S. allopathic graduate Perceived commitment to specialty Leadership qualities Professionalism and ethics Involvement and interest in research
Middle Tier Factors (Cited by 40-69% of programs)	USMLE Step 2 CK/COMLEX Level 2 score Audition elective within your department Grades in required clerkships Gaps in medical education Class rank Clinical clerkship honors Honors in clerkship in desired specialty Grades in clerkship in desired specialty Honors in basic sciences Interest in academic career Away rotation in your specialty at another institution Personal prior knowledge of the applicant Perceived interest in program Consistency of grades Volunteer/extracurricular experiences Graduate of well-regarded U.S. med school
Lowest Tier Factors (Cited by < 40% of programs)	Pass USMLE Step 2 CS Pass COMLEX Level PE Visa status Gold Society membership Fluency in language spoken by your patient population USMLE Step 3 score / COMLEX Step 3 score
Adapted from Results of the 2014 NRMP Program Director Survey. Available at: http://www.nrmp.org/wp-content/uploads/2014/09/PD-Survey-Report-2014.pdf.	

How important are letters of recommendation?

Letters of recommendation, particularly from neurosurgeons who know you well, are very important. In the 2014 NRMP Program Directors Survey, letters were rated most important in making interview decisions.[6] The American Association of Neurological Surgeons considers "letters from 'famous' individuals that do not speak of you in a personalized fashion" as less useful.[7] Applicants should have at least two letters written by neurosurgeons. Dr. Shaver of the Medical College of Georgia states that "it is also important to get a letter of recommendation from the chairman of the Neurosurgery department at your medical school."[8]

How important is the personal statement?

Program directors recommend that applicants clearly describe the reasons that led them to choose a career in neurosurgery. Applicants often underestimate the importance of the statement. The American Association of Neurological Surgeons encourages applicants to "take the time to do it well. It is important to your future."[7] In screening applications, the Department of Neurosurgery at University of Buffalo evaluates the "quality of the personal statement, which should indicate effective written communication skills as well as a commitment to a career in neurosurgery."[9]

How important is the USMLE?

Nearly 50% of programs have a minimum cut-off USMLE Step 1 score. Applicants with scores below this threshold are removed from consideration. The average USMLE Step 1 score for 2014 matched applicants was 244. The average score for unmatched applicants was 232.[1] Dr. Muizelaar, former program director at University of California-Davis, writes that "grades and numbers must be high."[10]

When should I take the USMLE Step 2 CK?

A 2012 NRMP survey of 40 neurosurgery residency programs revealed that 24% of programs required passage of Step 2 CK for granting interviews. A higher percentage (30%) required passage for placement on the rank-order list.[11]

How important are away electives?

Many neurosurgery PDs recommend audition electives. "We consider each applicant on an individual basis," writes the Department of Neurological Surgery at Washington University. "Completing a clerkship allows faculty members, as well as residents to get to know you better, and may highlight your skills and abilities, strengthening your application. Currently, approximately 75% of active residents completed a clerkship as a medical student."[12]

When should you do the away rotations? If you are hoping to secure LORs from the rotation that will benefit your residency application to all programs, then it's best to complete the rotations in July through September. This will allow for the letters to be written and available for programs at a time when interview decisions are made. If your plan is to enhance your candidacy at a single institution, then you could consider doing the rotation as late as December.

Be strategic in how you choose away electives. Your advisor will often have valuable information to help you in your decision-making. "It is important to get advice on picking programs for these rotations," writes the Department of Neurological Surgery at Drexel University. "Many students choose the 'top' programs in an effort to get a good letter of recommendation from the Chairman. Unfortunately many times there is little contact with the Chairman and this is obvious in the cursory letters of 'support' which end up being written."[13]

Did you know...

Excellent tips to excel during an away elective in neurosurgery were offered in a recent article published in *World Neurosurgery*. Among the tips:

- Spend time reviewing the images before surgery so that you can identify as many anatomical structures as possible.
- "It is advisable to not participate in discussion unless you are invited," writes Dr. Shamim, lead author of the article. "Your idea may seem brilliant to you, but there is a good chance it isn't. I don't mean to scare you into being a mute nonparticipating member of the team; your time to speak up will come. The faculty encourages you to ask questions; however, please do so when the air is relaxed. How do you know when the air is NOT relaxed? Trust me, you will know!"
- Bluffing is to be avoided at all costs. "Either when guessing a patient's examination or answering a question about the anatomy, a bluff will destroy your reliability," writes Dr. Shamim.[14]

How important is research experience?

Dr. Muizelaar writes "Research in medical school is highly desirable, especially in basic or clinical sciences related to neurosurgery."[10]

How important is the interview?

As with other competitive specialties, the interview is of great importance. The Department of Neurological Surgery at the University of Chicago states that "all faculty interview each applicant and questions vary from assessment of medical knowledge to more general aspects of preparedness for residency, knowledge of requirements and commitment, maturity, and prior skills."[15] Research indicates that qualities viewed favorably by neurosurgery program directors include honesty, verbal skills, cooperative personality, empathy, and social skills. Having an anxious or aggressive personality was rated negatively.[5]

What happens after the interview?

According to one study, there was considerable variability in how neurosurgery residency programs developed the rank-order list:

- Program director alone (15%)
- Program director and chairman (30.5%)
- Committee of core faculty (32.6%)
- All faculty members (38%)[5]

References

[1]Charting Outcomes in the Match (2014). Available at: http://www.nrmp.org/wp-content/uploads/2014/09/Charting-Outcomes-2014-Final.pdf. Accessed March 3, 2014.
[2]Advance Data Tables: 2016 Main Residency Match. Available at: http://www.nrmp.org/match-data/main-residency-match-data/. Accessed April 23, 2016.
[3]Brotherton S, Etzel S. Graduate Medical Education, 2014-2015. *JAMA* 2015; 314 (22): 2436-2454.
[4]Brotherton S, Etzel S. Graduate Medical Education, 2008-2009. *JAMA* 2009; 302 (12): 1357-1372.
[5]Khalili A, Chalouhi N, Tjoumakaris S, Gonzalez L, Starke R. Rosenwasser R, Jabbour P. Programs selection criteria for neurological surgery applicants in the United States: a national survey of neurological surgery program directors. *World Neurosurg* 2014; 81 (3-4): 473-477.
[6]Results of the 2014 NRMP Program Director Survey. Available at: http://www.nrmp.org/wp-content/uploads/2014/09/PD-Survey-Report-2014.pdf. Accessed March 3, 2015.
[7]American Association of Neurological Surgeons. Available at: http://www.neurosurgery.org. Accessed December 8, 2008.
[8]Shaver E. Neurosurgery. Available at: http://www.womensurgeons.org. Accessed December 8, 2008.
[9]Department of Neurosurgery at University of Buffalo. Available at: http://www.ubns.com/residency-and-fellowship/residency-program/selection-process/. Accessed March 4, 2015.
[10]Muizelaar J. A guide to the perplexed: residency guide. Available at: http://ucdmc.ucdavis.edu. Accessed March 5, 2015.
[11]Program Requirements around Passage of USMLE Step 2 CK and USMLE Step 2 CS. Available at: http://www.student.med.umn.edu/osr/wp-content/uploads/2012/09/Program-Requirements-around-Passage-of-USMLE-Step-2CK-and-USMLE-Step-2CS-11.pdf. Accessed March, 3, 2014.
[12]University of Washington Department of Neurological Surgery. Available at: http://neurosurgery.washington.edu/education/residency/faq.asp#clerkship. Accessed February 22, 2016.
[13]Drexel University Department of Neurological Surgery. Available at: http://webcampus.drexelmed.edu/cdc/medSpecialtyNeurologicalSurgery.asp. Accessed February 22, 2016.
[14]Shamim M, Sobani Z. Neurosurgical electives: operating room survival guide. *World Neurosurg* 2012; 78 (1-2): 18-9.
[15]University of Chicago Pritzker School of Medicine. Available at: pritzker.uchicago.edu/current/students/ResidencyProcessGuide.pdf. Accessed March 3, 2013.

Chapter 32

Obstetrics & Gynecology

How competitive is the specialty?

Obstetrics and gynecology is a moderately competitive specialty. In the 2014 NRMP Match, over 7% of U.S. allopathic medical students failed to match. The numbers are significantly worse for independent applicants (osteopathic and international medical graduates). 52% of independent applicants failed to match.[1] In an NRMP survey of obstetrics and gynecology residency programs performed in 2010, programs reported receiving an average of 356 applications for an average of 5 available resident positions. From this large group of applicants, programs interviewed about 60 applicants to fill their spots.[2]

Did you know?

Osteopathic applicants may also apply to 33 AOA-approved obstetrics and gynecology residency programs.

Highlights of the 2016 NRMP Obstetrics & Gynecology Match[3]

- There were a total of 1,265 positions.
- 78% of positions were filled with allopathic medical student applicants.
- 128 osteopathic applicants matched.
- 68 U.S. IMG applicants matched.
- 47 non-U.S. IMG applicants matched.
- 32 U.S. graduates matched.
- 8 positions went unfilled.

Did you know?

Obstetrics and gynecology residency programs examine all components of the residency application to ensure that applicants are committed to the specialty and to their program. Research indicates that there is significant attrition in obstetrics and gynecology residency programs. In one study, almost 22% of residents failed to complete training over a six-year period.[4] When a resident leaves a program, it affects the educational experience of the other residents and challenges the PD to adjust schedules, maintain duty hour compliance, and find another resident to replace the departing one.

How many years of training are required to become an obstetrician/gynecologist?

To become an obstetrician/gynecologist, a minimum of 4years of residency training is required.

What percentage of available positions is filled by U.S. seniors? What about other applicants?

In 2013 – 2014, there were 5,018 total residents training in a total of 242 obstetrics and gynecology residency programs. 76% were U.S. MDs, 12.8% were international medical graduates, and 10.9% were osteopathic graduates.[5]

Residents Training in U.S. Obstetrics & Gynecology Residency Programs[5-6]					
Year	**Residency Programs**	**Total # residents**	**% US MDs**	**% IMGs**	**% DO**
2013-2014	242	5018	76.2%	12.8%	10.9%
2007-2008	247	4815	71.8%	19.9%	8.1%

How do programs select residents?

Every few years, the NRMP conducts a survey of PDs. In 2014, the NRMP surveyed 117 obstetrics & gynecology PDs to determine the factors important in selecting applicants to interview.[7] The top 3 factors are USMLE Step 1/COMLEX Level 1 score, letters of recommendation in the specialty, and USMLE Step 2 CK/COMLEX Level 2 score. The findings are shown in the table on the following page.

How important is AOA?

The NRMP reports that of 12.6% of U.S. seniors who matched to obstetrics and gynecology in 2014 were members of AOA.[1]

How important is the USMLE?

The mean USMLE Step 1 score for 2014 U.S. senior applicants who matched was 226. Note that many applicants with lower scores are still able to match. In the 2014 Match, 178 of 224 applicants with scores below 210 matched.[1] Dr. Clara Paik, program director at the University of California Davis, states that "a low USMLE score does not preclude someone from going into obstetrics and gynecology."[8]

Did you know?

Researchers have found a strong statistically significant correlation between USMLE and Council of Resident Education in Obstetrics and Gynecology (CREOG) In-Training examinations.[9]

When should I take the USMLE Step 2 CK?

A 2012 NRMP survey of 94 obstetrics and gynecology residency programs revealed that 23.2% of programs required passage of Step 2 CK for granting interviews. A higher percentage (65%) required passage for placement on the rank-order list.[10]

Factors Identified as Important in Selecting Applicants to Interview by Obstetrics & Gynecology Residency Program Directors	
Top Tier Factors (Cited by 70-99% of programs)	USMLE Step 1/COMLEX Level 1 score LORs in the specialty USMLE Step 2 CK/COMLEX Level 2 score MSPE Personal statement Grades in required clerkships Class rank Gaps in medical education Honors in clinical clerkships
Middle Tier Factors (Cited by 40-69% of programs)	Audition elective within your department Leadership qualities Honors in clerkship in desired specialty Grades in clerkship in desired specialty AOA membership Professionalism and ethics Perceived commitment to specialty U.S. allopathic graduate Personal prior knowledge of the applicant Pass USMLE Step 2 CS / Pass COMLEX Level PE Perceived interest in program Consistency of grades Volunteer/extracurricular experiences Involvement and interest in research
Lowest Tier Factors (Cited by < 40% of programs)	Graduate of well-regarded U.S. med school Visa status Away rotation in your specialty at another institution Honors in basic sciences Interest in academic career Gold Society membership Fluency in language spoken by your patient population USMLE Step 3 score COMLEX Step 3 score
Adapted from Results of the 2014 NRMP Program Director Survey. Available at: http://www.nrmp.org/wp-content/uploads/2014/09/PD-Survey-Report-2014.pdf.	

How important are audition electives?

To determine a particular program's philosophy on the audition elective, visit the Association of Professors of Gynecology and Obstetrics (APGO) website. You'll find a directory of residency programs. The APGO has asked each program to answer the following questions:

- Elective as student in department required for resident selection?
- Elective as student recommended for resident selection?
- Elective as student discouraged for resident selection?
- If not required, elective is beneficial in obtaining residency position?

This information will help you make an informed decision. Dr. Tony Ogburn, former program director at the University of New Mexico, recommends an audition elective if an applicant is particularly interested in a certain program.[11] The Department of Obstetrics and Gynecology at the University of Chicago states that "completing an elective at a desired program can be very helpful. This is especially applicable for very competitive positions."[12] Applicants with poor academic records or USMLE scores may also benefit from away electives. A discussion with your advisor is recommended.

How important are letters of recommendation?

Letters of recommendation are one of the most important factors used by PDs to make interview decisions. Most programs request that one or two letters be written by obstetrics and gynecology faculty. Many programs require a letter from the Chair of the Department. What if you have never worked with the Chairman? We asked Dr. Eugene Toy, Program Director of the Obstetrics and Gynecology Residency Program at the Houston Methodist Hospital, for his thoughts. "As much as possible, a student should try to get a letter of recommendation from one of these individuals, since these faculty members have great insight into what type of student is appropriate for the field of ob/gyn. Even if the student doesn't have a chance to work clinically with these people, a student can set up one or two meetings. For instance I have written plenty of letters of recommendation on the basis of meeting with students, learning about their interests and passions, and reading their evaluations."[13]

Did you know?

How important is academic rank of the letter writer? "The fact of the matter is that senior people often write better letters and have a broader range/duration of exposure to students," writes Dr. Patricia Garza, Career Counseling Coordinator in the Department of Obstetrics and Gynecology at Northwestern University. "So, when a senior person writes, 'this is the best student I have seen in 5 years' it is usually from a denominator of hundreds of students. When a junior person writes the same sentence, it may not carry the same weight. HOWEVER, a person who knows you well and can speak to your specific, personal attributes may be more important than an impersonal form letter from a departmental 'heavyweight.'"[14]

Recommendations for Away Electives in Obstetrics & Gynecology	
OB/GYN Program	**Comments**
Dr. Patricia Garcia Professor Department of OB/GYN Northwestern University	According to Dr. Garza, audition rotations are not necessary. "Sometimes, when rotating quickly through various divisions and departments, you may not hit it off with everyone or make a good first impression. Proceed cautiously. If you want to see what a particular program is really like from an internal perspective, consider doing an elective in Ob anesthesia or Neonatology at the institution at which you are interested. This allows you some up close observation of them without their scrutiny of you."[14]
Department of OB/GYN Emory University	Students performing audition electives hope to increase their chances of receiving an interview at the program. However, rotating at an institution does not guarantee an interview offer. "Medical student participation in an elective does not guarantee an interview for a residency position in our department," writes the Department of Obstetrics and Gynecology at Emory University.[15] We recommend consulting the APGO directory before applying for audition electives if your main goal is to secure an interview.
Department of OB/GYN UAB	When deciding whether to do away electives, the competitiveness of your application should be considered in the decision-making process. "Audition Elective in Obstetrics and Gynecology at another institution is strongly recommended if you are certain of your top selection and you rank in the bottom third of the class."[16]
Dr. Carol Major Program Director UC Irvine	"Doing well during an externship will only help regardless of a student's class standing. For very competitive programs, it is helpful for even the top students to do an externship…Students in the middle of their class definitely should do an externship at competitive programs that they are interested in…Students at the lower end of their class should consider doing more than one externship at the less competitive programs to be strongly considered."[17]
Dr. Eugene Toy Program Director The Methodist Hospital	"The audition elective can be both an excellent way for the student to learn about the program, and also for the faculty and residents of a program to learn about the student. This can be a double-edged sword. For instance, a student who goes into a new hospital system has to learn an entire medical record system, the hospital logistics, and the medical school specifics; this puts a visiting student at a disadvantage as compared to local students. Nevertheless, with sufficient preparation and dedication, a student can overcome these obstacles. I always advise a student doing an audition elective to be prepared to work harder than any other student in the history of the hospital, to put off any leisure during that month until after the rotation is over, and to do more research, read more, arrive earlier, and stay later than any other student."[13]

How important is the personal statement?

Although the importance of the personal statement varies from one program to another, most programs consider it an important part of the application. The Department of Obstetrics and Gynecology at the University of Virginia offers valuable advice for personal statement preparation. "Make your personal statement personal. Make it say something about yourself: a unique life experience, a formative event, what gets you excited about entering a field in women's health. Write something memorable. Application reviewers may read over 200 – 300 personal statements, so keep it concise (less than one typed single page), professional, and creative."[18]

"More than anything else," says Dr. Eugene Toy. "I look at the personal statement to answer the questions: 'Why is this student interested in ob/gyn, and does this interest seem to ring true?' Certainly if the personal statement tastefully and artfully presents some unique aspects of the student without being awkward or bizarre, then all the better. As a program director, I am looking for a solid responsible resident who will be committed in a demanding specialty to the end. I am not looking for a literary or creative genius. Grammar, spelling, and diction, however, are important."[13]

What should you address in the personal statement? According to the Association of Professors of Gynecology and Obstetrics, some suggestions include:

- Provide a brief description of your background.
- Explain why you developed a specific interest in obstetrics and gynecology.
- Discuss what makes you unique as an individual.
- Explain unusual constraints in the selection of a residency program (e.g., couples match, special geographical considerations).
- Discuss your future plans (preferred geographic location, private practice versus academic medicine, fellowship interest).
- Describe extracurricular activities.[19]

Did you know?

Should you address a weakness or deficiency in the personal statement? "If relevant, include an explanation for a suboptimal academic performance or deceleration (illness, pregnancy, family member's death)," writes Dr. Cathy Callahan, Chair of the Department of Obstetrics and Gynecology at the Edward via Virginia College of Osteopathic Medicine.[20] However, we recommend that you discuss your approach with your advisor, as there are many potential variables.

How important is research experience?

In a 2006 survey of obstetrics and gynecology residency program directors, PDs were asked to rate the importance of 16 criteria on a scale of 1 (unimportant) to 5 (critical).[7] Among 16 academic criteria, Green found that published medical school research was last in importance.[21] Among 2014 applicants, 210 of 236 applicants with no publications or presentations matched.[1]

Did you know?

In a review of applications to one obstetrics and gynecology residency program, researchers determined the rate of erroneous and unverifiable publications. The notable findings included:

- 25.5% of applicants listing peer reviewed articles or abstracts made major errors.
- 12.5% committed minor errors.
- 24.1% had articles or abstracts that could not be verified.[22]

Take care in how you cite your research, and bring copies of your work with you to the interview.

How important is the interview?

The interview is rated as the most important factor used to make rank-order list decisions. "Other than the grades and USMLE scores, the interview is the single most important factor in the ranking of a candidate," says Dr. Toy. "The student should do adequate homework ahead of time to learn about the program and the hospital, being prompt to the interview, going to the social event, and making the most of the entire interview day…Students sometimes forget that in a field such as ob/gyn, it is a small world, and one act of poor judgment in one program can be broadcast to many different programs. In other words, there is not the same anonymity as there was as an undergraduate student."[13]

Some programs utilize behavioral interviews. Examples of behavioral interview questions include "Tell me about a time when you had to deal with a difficult attending physician" or "Describe a situation in which you had to deal with an angry or upset patient." Behavioral questions such as these are specific, and require you to respond with an example. In asking you these types of questions, the interviewer hopes to learn how you handled or reacted to the situation in the past, as it may be an indicator of how you might handle the situation in the future. Behavioral interviewing is based on the premise that future behavior is best predicted by past behavior. We discuss behavioral interviews in more detail in Chapter ???

Programs will ask why you are interested in their program, and it is crucial that you deliver a specific response based on research. Dr. Patrick Duff is the Associate Dean of Student Affairs and Program Director of the obstetrics and gynecology residency program at the University of Florida, and he offers this advice to medical students. "Do your homework beforehand. Be able to explain in detail exactly why you chose the program — i.e., suggestion of your adviser, national reputation, recommendations from recent graduates of that program who are now house officers at UF, unique training opportunities, job opportunities for your significant other. Do not just say you chose a given program because you like warm weather, have a relative in the area, or like the proximity of the program to the ocean or to an attraction like Disney World."[23]

Every applicant needs to be prepared with questions to ask interviewers. Dr. Elizabeth Ann Micks, a faculty member in the Department of Obstetrics and Gynecology at the University of Washington, echoes this advice. "At every interview I went on, people asked about a billion times: 'Do you have any more questions?' The most important part of your interview process is coming up with a countless number of intelligent, original, personalized questions. Get started."[24]

Did you know?

Dr. Eric Strand is the PD of the obstetrics and gynecology residency program at St. Vincent Hospital in Indianapolis. He offers valuable advice for applicants with red flags in their application. "Don't try to hide deficiencies—be prepared to discuss them instead. If you took a leave of absence, failed a course, repeated the USMLE's, etc, understand that we will ask about that. Oftentimes, individual failures can be turned into a positive if the event became an opportunity for significant personal insight or growth."[25]

Did you know?

Illegal questions are common during residency interviews. In a survey of all applicants from U.S. medical schools applying to five specialties (internal medicine, general surgery, orthopedic surgery, obstetrics-gynecology, emergency medicine), researchers found that applicants were often asked about age, marital status, current children, intent to have children, ethnicity, religion, and sexual orientation. Over 7,000 applicants completed the survey, and 64.8% reported being asked at least one potentially illegal question. Obstetrics and gynecology applicants reported a high prevalence of such questions (21.4%), second only to general surgery.[26]

Did you know?

In a survey of 137 obstetrics and gynecology PDs, 29% reported that they would view an applicant more positively if the applicant expressed interest beyond a routine thank you. 30% of programs indicated that applicants who did not communicate with programs following the interview would be at a disadvantage.[27]

References

[1]Charting Outcomes in the Match (2014). Available at: http://www.nrmp.org/wp-content/uploads/2014/09/Charting-Outcomes-2014-Final.pdf. Accessed March 3, 2014.
[2]Results of the 2010 NRMP Program Directors Survey. Available at: http://www.nrmp.org/wp-content/uploads/2013/08/programresultsbyspecialty2010v3.pdf. Accessed July 22, 2015.
[3]Advance Data Tables: 2016 Main Residency Match. Available at: http://www.nrmp.org/match-data/main-residency-match-data/. Accessed April 23, 2016.
[4]McAlister R, Andriole D, Brotherton S, Jeffe D. Attrition in residents entering US obstetrics and gynecology residencies: analysis of National GME Census data. *Am J Obstet Gynecol* 2008; 199 (5): 574.
[5]Brotherton S, Etzel S. Graduate Medical Education, 2014-2015. *JAMA* 2015; 314 (22): 2436-2454.
[6]Brotherton S, Etzel S. Graduate Medical Education, 2008-2009. *JAMA* 2009; 302 (12): 1357-1372.
[7]Results of the 2014 NRMP Program Director Survey. Available at: http://www.nrmp.org/wp-content/uploads/2014/09/PD-Survey-Report-2014.pdf. Accessed March 3, 2015.
[8]Residency Advice – UC Davis Health System. Available at: www.ucdmc.ucdavis.edu. Accessed July 22, 2015.
[9]Spellacy W, Downes K. United states medical licensing examination scores as a predictor of performance on the annual council of resident education in obstetrics and gynecology examinations. *Am J Obstet Gynecol* 2014; 211 (4): 344-50.
[10]Program Requirements around Passage of USMLE Step 2 CK and USMLE Step 2 CS. Available at: http://www.student.med.umn.edu/osr/wp-content/uploads/2012/09/Program-Requirements-around-Passage-of-USMLE-Step-2CK-and-USMLE-Step-2CS-11.pdf. Accessed March, 3, 2014.
[11]Espey E, Ogburn T. Guidelines for pursuing a residency in obstetrics and gynecology: 2005-2006. Available at: http://obgyn.unm.edu/clerkship. Accessed July 2, 2008.
[12]Blanchard A, Gilmore-Bradford E. Pritzker residency process guide: obstetrics and gynecology. Available at: http://pritzker.uchicago.edu/current/students/Residency ProcessGuide.pdf. Accessed November 22, 2008.
[13]The Successful Match: Getting into Obstetrics and Gynecology. Available at: http://studentdoctor.net/2010/05/the-successful-match-getting-into-obstetrics-and-gynecology/. Accessed February 10, 2013.
[14]Northwestern University Department of Obstetrics and Gynecology. Available at: http://www.feinberg.northwestern.edu/education/current-students/career-development-residency/career-development-program/career-advising-specialties/ob-gyn.html. Accessed February 10, 2013.
[15]Emory University Department of Obstetrics and Gynecology. Available at: http://www.gynob.emory.edu/education/residency_program/application_info.html. Accessed February 10, 2013.
[16]University of Alabama Birmingham Department of Obstetrics and Gynecology. Available at: http://www.obgyn.uab.edu/medicalstudents/obgyn/uasom/documents/Final2012Guidelines.pdf. Accessed February 10, 2013.
[17]University of California Irvine Department of Obstetrics and Gynecology. Available at: http://www.meded.uci.edu/education/residencyselection/obgyn.html. Accessed February 10, 2013.
[18]University of Virginia Department of Obstetrics and Gynecology. Available at: http://www.medicine.virginia.edu/clinical/departments/obgyn/Clerkship/medstudentquestions.pdf. Accessed February 10, 2013.

[19]Association of Professors of Gynecology and Obstetrics. Available at: http://www.apgo.org/binary/ResidencyProgram.htm. Accessed February 10, 2013.
[20]Department of Obstetrics and Gynecology at the Edward via Virginia College of Osteopathic Medicine. Available at: www.vcom.vt.edu/obgyn/files/Presentation.ppt. Accessed February 10, 2013.
[21]Green M, Jones P, Thomas J. Selection criteria for residency: results of a national program director survey. *Acad Med* 2009; 84 (3): 362-7.
[22]Simmons H, Kim S, Zins A, Chiang S, Amies Oelschlager A. Unverifiable and erroneous publications reported by obstetrics and gynecology residency applicants. *Obstet Gynecol 2012; 119 (3): 498-503.*
[23]University of Florida College of Medicine. Available at: http://osa.med.ufl.edu/faq/student-advice/. Accessed September 4, 2012.
[24]Jefferson Medical College. Available at: http://jeffline.jefferson.edu/Students/residency/pdf/Ob-Gyn.pdf. Accessed September 12, 2012.
[25]Tips for Residency Interviews. Available at: http://hcp.obgyn.net/residency/content/article/1760982/1921219. Accessed September 24, 2012.
[26]Hern H, Alter H, Wills C, Snoey E, Simon B. How prevalent are potentially illegal questions during residency interviews? *Acad Med* 2013; 88 (8): 1116-21.
[27]Frishman G, Matteson K, Bienstock J, George K, Ogburn T, Rauk P, Schnatz P, Learman L. Postinterview communication with residents: a call for clarity! *J Reprod Med* 2014; 59 (1-2): 17-19.

Chapter 33

Ophthalmology

How competitive is the specialty?

Ophthalmology is a highly competitive specialty. Ophthalmology does not participate in the NRMP but rather utilizes the Ophthalmology Residency Matching Program (OMP) established by the Association of University Professors of Ophthalmology (AUPO). In the 2016 OMP, there were 726 participants for 469 positions. 36% of all applicants failed to match. Past U.S. graduates and IMGs have considerably more difficulty landing positions.[1]

Highlights of the 2016 Ophthalmology Residency Match[1]

- There were a total of 469 positions.
- 92% of positions were filled with allopathic medical student applicants.
- 13 IMG applicants matched.
- 25 U.S. graduates matched.
- 2 residency positions were unfilled.

Did you know?

Results of the Ophthalmology Residency Matching Program are announced in January, several months before the NRMP Match.

Results of Ophthalmology Residency Match: 2015 vs 2016[1]

	2015 Match	2016 Match
Number of CAS participants	753	726
US seniors matched	413	429
US medical school graduates matched	34	25
IMGs matched	17	13
Matched applicants (total #)	464	467
Unmatched applicants	289	259

Did you know?

Osteopathic applicants may also apply to 15 AOA-approved ophthalmology residency programs.

How many years of training are required to become an ophthalmologist?

To become an ophthalmologist, 3 years of training in ophthalmology are required following one year of postgraduate clinical training. This initial year can be completed in a transitional or preliminary year program.

What percentage of available positions is filled by U.S. seniors? What about other applicants?

In 2013 – 2014, there were 1,348 total residents training in a total of 116 ophthalmology residency programs. 93% were U.S. MDs, 5.2% were international medical graduates, and 1.6% were osteopathic graduates.[2]

Residents Training in U.S. Ophthalmology Residency Programs[2-3]					
Year	**Residency Programs**	**Total # residents**	**% US MDs**	**% IMGs**	**% DO**
2013-2014	116	1348	93.0%	5.2%	1.6%
2007-2008	118	1220	91.7%	7.0%	1.0%

How do programs select residents?

In 2006, Green surveyed ophthalmology residency program directors about the residency selection process. Of the 106 surveys sent, responses were received from 46 directors (43%). Program directors were asked to rate the importance of 16 criteria on a scale of 1 (unimportant) to 5 (critical).[4] The findings are shown in the table on the following page.

How important are audition electives?

Although the Association of University Professors of Ophthalmology does not recommend audition electives, not all ophthalmology faculty advisors agree with this position. The Texas Tech University Department of Ophthalmology writes that audition electives are "very strongly recommended. If we see how you are to work with, this will factor strongly into the decision making process."[5] Dr. Susan Ksiazek, Program Director at the University of Chicago, states that "if you are really interested in a particular program, an on-site rotation is a must."[6] Dr. Nicholas Volpe, Chair of the Department of Ophthalmology at Northwestern University, feels that audition electives should be considered in certain situations. "In some cases, an away rotation may be considered (for example: need to match in a geographic location).[7] Applicants should understand that doing an away rotation does not guarantee an interview. Only 50% of programs routinely interview most applicants who complete audition rotations at their institution.[8]

Ophthalmology Residency Program Directors' Rankings of Academic Criteria Used in the Residency Selection Process	
Criteria	**Mean**
Recommendation Letters	4.02
USMLE Step 1 Score	4.00
Required Clerkship Grades	3.91
No. of Clerkship Honors	3.91
Membership in Alpha Omega Alpha	3.82
Grades in Senior Elective in Specialty	3.67
Class Rank	3.64
Medical School Academic Awards	3.52
Published Research	3.48
USMLE Step 2 CK Score	3.30
Medical School Reputation	3.22
Grades in Senior Electives not in Specialty	3.20
Audition Electives	3.20
Grades in Preclinical Courses	3.12
Step 2 CS Pass	3.06
Value of Medical Student Performance Evaluation	2.66
Green M, Jones P, Thomas J. Selection criteria for residency: results of a national program director survey. *Acad Med* 2009; 84 (3): 362-7.	

How important is the personal statement?

Dr. Ksiazek encourages applicants to "place great attention on the personal statement. This is your chance to paint a picture of yourself for the reader and to differentiate yourself from everyone else...Often the personal statement is the deciding factor in granting an interview."[6] Dr. Natalie Kerr, Professor of Ophthalmology at the University of Tennessee, offers additional advice. "Tell us something unique/interesting, special about you...Please don't tell us why ophthalmology is the best specialty ever."[9]

How important are the letters of recommendation?

Two letters from academic ophthalmologists are recommended. The specialty does not require applicants to submit a Chairman's Letter. Dr. Jennifer Simpson, former program director at the University of California-Irvine feels it is "critical" for applicants to obtain letters from ophthalmology professors who truly "know you. If he/she is famous, or has connections to a particular program, it does help – but a letter from a renowned ophthalmologic academic that states: 'I understand from my residents that this student was good...' would be a real negative."[10]

How important is the USMLE?

The USMLE Step 1 score is very important. The average score among 2015 matched applicants was 243. Among unmatched applicants, the mean score was 228.[1] Approximately 30% of programs use a USMLE cut-off score in the screening process.[8]

Did you know?

International medical graduates have considerable difficulty matching into ophthalmology. In one study, researchers analyzed all successful IMG applications to U.S. ophthalmology residency programs over a five-year period. Factors associated with increased odds of matching were having 3 letters of recommendation written by U.S. ophthalmologists, higher USMLE Step 1 scores, academic awards, high-impact journal publications, and U.S. research experience.[11]

Did you know?

Ophthalmology applicants should be aware of geographical considerations in the application process. Research indicates that applicants in all regions tend to land positions within their own geographic region. In a recent study, 61% of applicants from the South matched in the South. Some of this has to do with the desire of applicants to stay within a particular region. Other factors may also be in play, including the relationships that faculty within a region have with one another, and how these relationships may affect the student's chances of matching when faculty advocate for them. It is also possible that programs may interview and rank applicants from the same region higher because they perceive that the applicant has a stronger interest in their program.[12]

How important is research experience?

Most applicants have participated in some type of research. For prestigious programs, lack of research experience or even a publication can remove an applicant from further consideration.

Did you know?

In a study of 201 applicants to a single ophthalmology residency program, 15 applicants were found to have misrepresented published articles. The most common type of misrepresentation was self-promotion on the author list followed by omission of other authors, nonexistent articles, and nonauthorship. The author concluded that "residency program directors should request copies of published articles from interviewing applicants."[13]

How important is the interview?

The interview is the most important factor in determining a program's rank list. Dr. Ksiazek urges applicants to "research the program before you get there and ask program-specific questions. You do not want to blend into a sea of other applicants by asking the same old questions."[6]

Receiving an interview doesn't guarantee placement on the program's rank-order list, although one survey showed that 57% of programs will rank at least 90% of interviewed applicants.[8]

What are programs looking for in applicants? "Major factors we consider in selecting residents include the applicant's record in medical school, communication and interpersonal skills and our assessment of his/her maturity and suitability for our program and likelihood of high levels of future professional achievement," writes the Department of Ophthalmology at the University of Wisconsin.[14]

James Dunn, Professor of Ophthalmology and Director of the Wilmer Eye Institute Ophthalmology Program at Johns Hopkins, feels that applicants can definitely ruin their chances of matching with a poor interview. "For the most part, an applicant can sink themselves with a bad attitude (condescension toward the staff who organize our interview days is the kiss of death) or by appearing clueless about what is in their application (I've written off applicants who couldn't tell me about articles on which they were a co-author, and even had one applicant last year who, when asked about an intriguing-sounding article she had published in AJO just in the previous year, actually said, 'Oh, that was a while ago; I don't really remember anything about that.').[15]

Dr. Andrew Lee is the Chairman of the Department of Ophthalmology at Houston Methodist Hospital. He has written extensively about the ophthalmology residency selection process. In an interview with Dr. Lee, we asked him to tell us what impresses him most about an applicant during an interview. "I am looking for three things in a resident interview. First, eliminate the people who may have looked 'great on paper' but are terrible in person (e.g., psychopathic or sociopathic types, hermits or hotdogs, socially inappropriate duds, or selfish, arrogant jerks). Second, elevate the people who look mediocre on paper but are superstars in person (e.g., charismatic, engaging, enthusiastic, well spoken, and passionate). Third, and perhaps less tangible, I am looking for philosophical and personality 'fit'. Applicants should understand their own, as well as the prospective program's learning environment, institutional culture, and teaching philosophy. Hard work, intelligence, teamwork, leadership, communication and interpersonal skills and professionalism are welcome attributes in most programs, and demonstrating these qualities can be a challenge in a short conversation. I am most impressed by applicants who are comfortable with themselves and with emphasizing their achievements in a credible manner, who can communicate clearly and concisely their career goals, and who can make the interview time 'fly by' and who make me want to keep talking with the person beyond the assigned time."[16]

Did you know?

In a recent survey of ophthalmology residency programs, researchers learned that PDs interview every applicant in 87% of programs. The chairman is also heavily involved, interviewing every applicant in 71% of programs.[17] Although most interviews will be one-on-one, be prepared for panel interviews. "Some interviewers will be paired up and the residency program director will interview candidates one-on-one," writes the Cleveland Clinic Department of Ophthalmology.[18] To prepare for varying interview structures and formats, it helps to make inquiries with the program coordinator on what to expect on interview day.

Did you know?

Asking the program coordinator about the interview day schedule/itinerary will prepare you for any "unusual events" taking place on interview day. Note that 9.2% of programs require an eye examination, and 3.1% of programs test manual dexterity.[17]

Did you know?

In a study of nearly 3,500 ophthalmology applicants over a five-year period, researchers found that an applicant's likelihood of matching plateaued after ranking 11 programs. Among those who ranked 11 programs, 96% landed positions in ophthalmology. There was no difference in the match rate between those who ranked 11 programs and those who ranked more. This information may be helpful to applicants who are concerned about the cost of interviewing but fearful of not matching.[12]

References

[1]SF Match. Available at: https://www.sfmatch.org/SpecialtyInsideAll.aspx?id=6&typ=2&name=Ophthalmology. Accessed April 3, 2016.
[2]Brotherton S, Etzel S. Graduate Medical Education, 2014-2015. *JAMA* 2015; 314 (22): 2436-2454.
[3]Brotherton S, Etzel S. Graduate Medical Education, 2008-2009. *JAMA* 2009; 302 (12): 1357-1372.
[4]Green M, Jones P, Thomas J. Selection criteria for residency: results of a national program director survey. *Acad Med* 2009; 84 (3): 362-367.
[5]Texas Tech University Department of Ophthalmology. Available at: http://www.ttuhsc.edu/som/studentaffairs/documents/CA_Ophthalmology.pdf. Accessed May 21, 2012.
[6]Ksiazek S, Taylor T. Pritzker residency process guide: ophthalmology. Available at: http://pritzker.uchicago.edu/current/students/ResidencyProcessGuide.pdf. Accessed November 22, 2008.
[7]Northwestern University Feinberg School of Medicine Department of Ophthalmology. Available at: http://www.feinberg.northwestern.edu/education/current-students/career-development-residency/career-advising-specialties/ophthalmology.html. Accessed January 2, 2014.
[8]Ophthalmology Residency Medical Student Information Session. Available at: http://www.feinberg.northwestern.edu/education/docs/Ophthalmology-M3-Info-Session-Feb-8-2012.pdf. Accessed January 4, 2016.
[9]So You Think You Want To Be An Ophthalmologist. Available at: http://www.uthsc.edu/eye/sigio/documents/SIGIO2009.pdf. Accessed January 4, 2016.
[10]Simpson J. Residency selection handbook: ophthalmology. Available at: http://www.ucihs.uci.edu. Accessed July 22, 2008.
[11]Driver T, Loh A, Joseph D, Keenan J, Naseri A. Predictors of matching in ophthalmology residency for international medical graduates. *Ophthalmology* 2014; 121 (4): 974-5.
[12]Loh A, Joseph D, Keenan J, Lietman T, Naseri A. Predictors of matching in an ophthalmology residency program. *Ophthalmology* 2013; 120 (4): 865-70.
[13]Wiggins M. Misrepresentation by ophthalmology residency applicants. *Arch Ophthalmol* 2010; 128 (7): 906-10.
[14]University of Wisconsin Department of Ophthalmology. Available at: http://www.ophth.wisc.edu/education/residency/apply. Accessed September 13, 2012.
[15]Pearls in Ophthalmology. Available at: http://www.medrounds.org/ophthalmology-pearls/2009/09/matching-in-ophthalmology-and-then.html. Accessed September 20, 2012.
[16]The Successful Match: Getting into Ophthalmology. Available at: http://studentdoctor.net/2009/08/the-successful-match-interview-with-dr-andrew-lee-ophthalmology/. Accessed September 20, 2012.
[17]Nallaswamy S, Uhler T, Nallasamy N, Tapino P, Volpe N. Ophthalmology resident selection: current trends in selection criteria and improving the process. *Ophthalmology* 2010; 117 (5): 1041-7.
[18]Cleveland Clinic Department of Ophthalmology. Available at: http://my.clevelandclinic.org/eye/physicians/education/residents/default.aspx. September 12, 2012.

Chapter 34

Orthopedic Surgery

How competitive is the specialty?

Orthopedic surgery is a highly competitive specialty. Many residency programs receive over 100 applications per available position. In the 2014 NRMP Match, 23% of U.S. allopathic medical students failed to match. The numbers are significantly worse for independent applicants (osteopathic and international medical graduates). 72% of independent applicants failed to match.[1]

Did you know?

Osteopathic applicants may also apply to 42 AOA-approved orthopedic surgery residency programs.

Highlights of the 2016 NRMP Orthopedic Surgery Match[2]

- There were a total of 717 positions.
- 91% of positions were filled with allopathic medical student applicants.
- 4 osteopathic applicants matched.
- 14 IMG applicants matched (6 US IMG and 8 non-US IMG)
- 49 U.S. graduates matched.
- 0 positions went unfilled.

How many years of training are required to become an orthopedic surgeon?

To become an orthopedic surgeon, a minimum of 5 years of residency training is required.

What percentage of available positions is filled by U.S. seniors? What about other applicants?

In 2013 – 2014, there were 3,581 total residents training in a total of 156 orthopedic surgery residency programs. 97% were U.S. MDs, 1.8% were international medical graduates, and 0.9% were osteopathic graduates.[3]

Residents Training in U.S. Orthopedic Surgery Residency Programs[3-4]					
Year	**Residency Programs**	**Total # residents**	**% US MDs**	**% IMGs**	**% DO**
2013-2014	156	3581	97.3%	1.8%	0.9%
2007-2008	153	3303	96.5%	2.6%	0.9%

How do programs select residents?

Every few years, the NRMP conducts a survey of PDs. In 2014, the NRMP surveyed 85 orthopedic surgery PDs to determine the factors that are important in selecting applicants to interview.[5] The top 3 factors are USMLE Step 1/COMLEX Level 1 score, letters of recommendation in the specialty, and honors in clinical clerkships.

Factors Identified as Important in Selecting Applicants to Interview by Orthopedic Surgery Residency Program Directors	
Top Tier Factors (Cited by 70-99% of programs)	USMLE Step 1/COMLEX Level 1 score LORs in the specialty Honors in clinical clerkships MSPE Personal statement U.S. allopathic graduate Grades in required clerkships Class rank Professionalism and ethics Leadership qualities AOA membership
Middle Tier Factors (Cited by 40-69% of programs)	USMLE Step 2 CK/COMLEX Level 2 score Audition elective within your department Honors in clerkship in desired specialty Grades in clerkship in desired specialty Perceived commitment to specialty Personal prior knowledge of the applicant Perceived interest in program Consistency of grades Volunteer/extracurricular experiences Involvement and interest in research Gaps in medical education Honors in basic sciences
Lowest Tier Factors (Cited by < 40% of programs)	Graduate of well-regarded U.S. med school Visa status Away rotation in your specialty at another institution Interest in academic career Gold Society membership Fluency in language spoken by your patient population USMLE Step 3 score COMLEX Step 3 score Pass USMLE Step 2 CS / Pass COMLEX Level PE
Adapted from Results of the 2014 NRMP Program Director Survey. Available at: http://www.nrmp.org/wp-content/uploads/2014/09/PD-Survey-Report-2014.pdf.	

How important are audition electives?

For applicants to orthopedic surgery, audition electives are very important. In a survey of orthopedic surgery PDs, among criteria used to make interview decisions, performing an elective at the program director's institution was rated 4.6 on a scale of 1 (not at all important) to 5 (very important).[5] No other factor was rated higher.

Dr. Bernstein, the lead author, stated that "60% of programs reported that 50% or more of their matching residents over the previous three years had performed medical student orthopedic surgery rotations at the program prior to matching for residency."[6] Drs. Peabody and Manning of the University of Chicago strongly recommend audition electives. "It's almost mandatory to do an away elective and shine."[7]

Faculty in the Department of Orthopedic Surgery at the University of Pennsylvania describe the benefits of away rotations. "First, it allows applicants the opportunity to impress residents and attendings with their work ethic and ability to fit into the team. Second, it allows the student to get letters of recommendation from the orthopedic staff at that institution, which, if written in strong support of the student, could help the student's chance of matching not only at that school but at other programs as well. Third, it may allow the applicant to get involved in research projects or mentorship that they otherwise would not have had access to."[8]

How important are letters of recommendation?

Letters of recommendation are very important in the selection process. According to the NRMP, 92% of orthopedic surgery programs cited letters as a factor used to make interview decisions.[5] Many programs require applicants to submit a Chairman's Letter. Letters from orthopedic surgeons are rated considerably higher than those from non-orthopedic surgeons. In Bernstein's survey, the most important aspect of a letter, according to 54% of the directors, was that it was written by someone they know.[6] The University of Washington states, "input from senior orthopedists are particularly helpful" but only if the applicant is well known to the individual.[9]

How many of your letters should be written by orthopedic surgeons? This varies from program to program. The Department of Orthopedic Surgery at the University of Florida asks for three letters of reference. "At least one letter should be from an orthopedic surgeon associated with your medical school and familiar with your work."[10] The University of California Irvine also asks for three letters but indicates that at least two must be from orthopedic surgeons and/or Chair or Program Director.[11] Drexel University requires "three letters of recommendation from orthopedic surgeons who are familiar with your rotations and under whom you have spent time in medical school."[12]

How important is AOA?

The NRMP reports that 32.2% of U.S. seniors who matched to orthopedic surgery in 2014 were members of AOA.[1] Although AOA membership is valued, it is certainly not a requirement. According to Bernstein, only 1% of PDs agreed with the statement that "only applicants that are AOA are offered an interview."[6]

How important is the USMLE?

USMLE Step 1 scores are clearly important. The average score among U.S. allopathic seniors who matched in 2014 was 245. Note that high scores are no guarantee of match success in this field. In 2014, unmatched U.S. seniors had a mean score of 231. One hundred applicants with scores > 230 failed to match. While applicants with lower scores can match successfully, the odds of matching significantly decrease. Among applicants with scores less than 230, only 72 of 155 were able to land positions in the field.[1]

When should I take the USMLE Step 2 CK?

A 2012 NRMP survey of orthopedic surgery residency programs revealed that 18% of programs required passage of Step 2 CK for granting interviews. A higher percentage (26%) required passage for placement on the rank-order list.[13]

How important is research experience?

In this field, research experience is important. Among 2014 U.S. senior allopathic applicants, over 98% had participated in a research project. 87% claimed at least one abstract, publication, or presentation.[1] This represents a significant change from 2007 when only 60% claimed at least one abstract, publication, or presentation. Dr. Gary Phipps, former program director at the University of California Irvine, states that doing research in the field will "definitely" improve the chances of obtaining a residency.[14]

How important is the personal statement?

According to the NRMP, 82% of programs cited the personal statement as a factor used to make interview decisions.[5] In Bernstein's survey, 43% of directors felt that the most important aspect of the statement was "to learn about the candidate's personal interests and background," while 32% felt that it was "to gain insight into an applicant's ability to write and communicate effectively."[6] Dr. Kevin Coupe, former program director at the University of Texas Houston, states that the "personal statement is read by each of our orthopedic faculty members, and is considered by our faculty to be a very important part of the application process. It is often used as a point of departure for interviewing the student."[15]

Recommendations for Orthopedic Surgery Personal Statement	
Orthopedic Program	**Comments**
Dr. Laith Jazrawi Chief Division of Sports Medicine NYU	What should you address in the personal statement? In his book *Orthopedic Residency and Fellowship: A Guide to Success*, Dr. Jazrawi has compiled questions applicants may wish to address. A few of these include:[16] • Why are you pursuing a career in orthopedic surgery? Why are you particularly suited for this field? • What special leadership abilities do you have, and what have you done to exemplify them? • What are your major research accomplishments and interests? Do you plan to pursue research in the future? • What is your passion? What makes you interesting? How much more of you is there than the numbers and grades that are found in your application?"
Dr. Howard Luks Chief of Sports Medicine Associate Professor New York Medical College	"Avoid the habit of describing how great the field of X is or perseverating about a lengthy patient story without mentioning much about yourself…We generally recommend a 'hook' to open, followed by 2-3 paragraphs describing one or two experiences or activities that helped cultivate your interest or prepared you for the field you are entering…For memorable 'hooks,' think about what makes you unique and what might be a good conversation starter. This could be the 'a-ha' moment you experienced while volunteering abroad or something interesting about yourself such as your first career, an unusual hobby, an athletic or professional achievement. Your job is to relate this to your passion for the field"[17]
Dr. Aki Puryear Associate Professor Dept. of Orthopedic Surgery Saint Louis University	"Most of the statements say similar things like: • The applicant or a family member had some interaction with an orthopedic surgeon and that is what made them interested in it. • The applicant was an athlete. • The applicant likes to work with his/her hands. • On a rotation, the applicant had an experience which shaped his/her decision. So, for me, I read the statement and if I start to see this theme, no bonus points." However, he cautions applicants from being too creative. "It is tricky if you decide to go outside of the norm. If it is too artsy and you sound crazy, minus; if you are creative and interesting, plus. But this is tricky and I would only recommend this for the literary inclined."[18]

How important is the interview?

The interview is the most important factor used by programs to make rank-order list decisions. Once invited for an interview, 22% of orthopedic surgery programs place candidates on equal footing with ranking decisions based solely on interview performance.[6]

Advice for Re-applicants to Orthopedic Surgery

Since so many U.S. allopathic medical students fail to match into orthopedic surgery, a group of researchers studied factors associated with match success in previously unsuccessful applicants. This survey of 91 programs revealed important findings:

- Although 11% reported that they often interview previously unmatched applicants, 35% indicated that they never or rarely offer interviews.
- 75% agreed or strongly agreed that an unsuccessful applicant should complete a preliminary year in surgery.
- 65% agreed or strongly agreed that they would be more likely to extend an interview to a previously unmatched applicant who elected to do an internship.
- All programs indicated that they were more likely to extend an interview to an intern at their own institution.
- How do programs view applicants who choose to perform a research year rather than a preliminary year in surgery? Research years are viewed less favorably overall, but academic programs place more weight on the research year. If you're considering a research year, it would be preferable to complete the year at an academic program. Academic institutions tend to favor applicants who had performed the research at their own institutions.
- New letters of recommendation can significantly enhance your application. 78% ranked new letters as important or extremely important.
- Step scores remain important to programs when evaluating re-applicants. 37% of programs reported requiring a minimum score of 220 on the Step 1 exam. Only 17% of programs indicated that they would interview applicants with lower scores.

Amin N, Jakoi A, Cerynik D, Kumar N, Johanson N. How should unmatched orthopedic surgery applicants proceed? *Clin Orthop Relat Res* 2013; 471 (2): 672-679.

References

[1]Charting Outcomes in the Match (2014). Available at: http://www.nrmp.org/wp-content/uploads/2014/09/Charting-Outcomes-2014-Final.pdf. Accessed March 3, 2014.
[2]Advance Data Tables: 2016 Main Residency Match. Available at: http://www.nrmp.org/match-data/main-residency-match-data/. Accessed April 23, 2016.
[3]Brotherton S, Etzel S. Graduate Medical Education, 2014-2015. *JAMA* 2015; 314 (22): 2436-2454.
[4]Brotherton S, Etzel S. Graduate Medical Education, 2008-2009. *JAMA* 2009; 302 (12): 1357-1372.
[5]Results of the 2014 NRMP Program Director Survey. Available at: http://www.nrmp.org/wp-content/uploads/2014/09/PD-Survey-Report-2014.pdf. Accessed March 3, 2015.
[6]Bernstein A, Jazrawi L, Elbeshbeshy B, Della Valle C, Zuckerman J. Orthopedic resident-selection criteria. *J Bone Joint Surg Am* 2002; 84-A (11): 2090-2096.
[7]Peabody T, Manning D. Pritzker residency process guide: orthopedic surgery. Available at: http://pritzker.uchicago.edu/current/students/ResidencyProcessGuide.pdf. Accessed November 2, 2008.
[8]Baldwin K, Weidner Z, Ahn J, Mehta S. Are away rotations critical for a successful match in orthopedic surgery? *Clin Orthop Relat Res* 2009; 467 (12): 3340-5.
[9]University of Washington Department of Orthopedic Surgery. Available at: http://www.orthop.washington.edu/?q=education/residency/applicants.html. Accessed
[10]University of Florida Department of Orthopedic Surgery. Available at: http://www.ortho.ufl.edu/residency-program/application. Accessed April 30, 2012.
[11]University of California Department of Orthopedic Surgery. Available at: http://www.orthopaedicsurgery.uci.edu/do.html. Accessed April 30, 2012.
[12]Drexel University Department of Orthopedic Surgery. Available at: http://www.drexelmed.edu/Home/ResidenciesandFellowships/ResidencyPrograms/OrthopaedicSurgery/HowtoApply.aspx.Accessed April 30, 2012.
[13]AAMC Report - Program Requirements around Passage of USMLE Step 2CK and USMLE Step 2CS Results. Available at: http://www.student.med.umn.edu/osr/wp-content/uploads/2012/09/Program-Requirements-around-Passage-of-USMLE-Step-2CK-and-USMLE-Step-2CS-11.pdf. Accessed February 13, 2013.
[14]Phipps G. Residency selection handbook: orthopedic surgery. Available at: http://www.ucihs.uci.edu. Accessed November 2, 2008.
[15]Coupe K. Career counseling: orthopedic surgery. Available at: http://www.uth.tmc.edu/med/administration/student/ms4/2003CCC.htm. Accessed November 2, 2008.
[16]Jazrawi L, Egol K, Zuckerman J. *Orthopedic residency and fellowship*. Slack Incorporated; Thorofare, NJ: 2010.
[17]Dr. Howard Luks. Available at: http://www.howardluksmd.com/sports-medicine/personal-statement-do%E2%80%99s-and-don%E2%80%99ts-%C2%AB-futuredocs/. Accessed April 30, 2012.
[18]Dr. Aki Puryear. Available at: http://orthopaedic-residency.blogspot.com/2007_01_01_archive.html. Accessed April 30, 2012.

Chapter 35

Otolaryngology

How competitive is the specialty?

Otolaryngology is a highly competitive specialty. In the 2014 NRMP Match, approximately 25% of U.S. allopathic medical students failed to match. The numbers are significantly worse for independent applicants (osteopathic and international medical graduates). 72% of independent applicants failed to match.[1]

> **Did you know?**
>
> Osteopathic applicants may also apply to 20 AOA-approved otolaryngology surgery residency programs.

> **Highlights of the 2016 NRMP Otolaryngology Match[2]**
>
> - There were a total of 304 positions.
> - 89% of positions were filled with allopathic medical student applicants.
> - 1 osteopathic applicant matched.
> - 11 IMG applicants matched (3 US IMG and 8 non-US IMG).
> - 18 U.S. graduates matched.
> - 2 positions went unfilled.

> **Did you know?**
>
> In one study, researchers looked for factors predictive of future success as an otolaryngologist. This was a retrospective review of residency applications over a 10-year period at a single program. Objective factors in the residency application showed no correlation with higher faculty ranking. What was shown to be associated with a higher rating? Having excelled in a team sport.[3]

How many years of training are required to become an otolaryngologist?

To become an otolaryngologist, a minimum of 5 years of residency training is required.

What percentage of available positions is filled by U.S. seniors? What about other applicants?

In 2013 – 2014, there were 1,464 total residents training in a total of 106 otolaryngology residency programs. 98% were U.S. MDs, 1.6% were international medical graduates, and 0.2% were osteopathic graduates.[4]

Residents Training in U.S. Otolaryngology Residency Programs[4-5]					
Year	**Residency Programs**	**Total # residents**	**% US MDs**	**% IMGs**	**% DO**
2013-2014	106	1464	98.1%	1.6%	0.2%
2007-2008	103	1372	96.1%	3.4%	0.3%

How do programs select residents?

In a survey of otolaryngology residency programs during the 2009 and 2010 match cycles, researchers asked PDs and applicants to rank the importance of 10 criteria used in residency selection. Factors were ranked on a 20-point scale from 1 (of utmost importance) to 20 (not important at all). For PDs, interview and personal knowledge of the applicant were the most important criteria. For applicants, interview and letters of recommendation were the most important. The results of this study are presented in the following table. The overall rank given by PDs and applicants is shown, followed by the mean rank score in parentheses.[6]

Rankings of Criteria Used in the Otolaryngology Residency Selection Process: Comparison Between Program Directors and Applicants		
Criteria	**Program Director Rank**	**Applicant Rank**
Interview	1 (2.63)	1 (2.55)
Personal knowledge of the applicant	2 (3.63)	5 (5.65)
USMLE scores	3 (4.63)	4 (5.42)
Letters of recommendation	4 (5.07)	2 (3.65)
Medical school grades	5 (5.54)	3 (5.06)
Research experience	6 (7.02)	6 (7.55)
Reputation of medical school	7 (8.54)	8 (10.96)
Extracurricular activities	8 (10.0)	7 (8.45)
Likelihood to rank program highly	9 (14.28)	9 (13.48)
Ethnicity/gender	10 (17.15)	10 (16.31)
Puscas L, Sharp S, Scwab B, Lee W. Qualities of residency applicants: comparison of otolaryngology program critiera with applicant expectations. *Arch Otolaryngol Head Neck Surg* 2012; 138 (1):.10-4.		

Every few years, the NRMP conducts its own survey of PDs. In 2014, the NRMP surveyed 46 otolaryngology PDs to determine the factors that are important in selecting applicants to interview.[7] The top 3 factors are letters of recommendation in the specialty, USMLE Step 1/COMLEX Level 1 score, and honors in clinical clerkships. Factors are presented in the table below.

Factors Identified As Important in Selecting Applicants to Interview by Otolaryngology Surgery Residency Program Directors	
Top Tier Factors (Cited by 70-99% of programs)	LORs in the specialty USMLE Step 1/COMLEX Level 1 score Honors in clinical clerkships MSPE Personal statement Grades in required clerkships Personal prior knowledge of the applicant Honors in clerkship in desired specialty Leadership qualities AOA membership Volunteer/extracurricular experiences Involvement and interest in research
Middle Tier Factors (Cited by 40-69% of programs)	U.S. allopathic graduate Class rank USMLE Step 2 CK/COMLEX Level 2 score Audition elective within your department Grades in clerkship in desired specialty Perceived interest in program Consistency of grades Professionalism and ethics Perceived commitment to specialty Gaps in medical education Graduate of well-regarded U.S. med school
Lowest Tier Factors (Cited by < 40% of programs)	Visa status Away rotation in your specialty at another institution Interest in academic career Gold Society membership Fluency in language spoken by your patient population Honors in basic sciences USMLE Step 3 score COMLEX Step 3 score Pass USMLE Step 2 CS / Pass COMLEX Level PE
Adapted from Results of the 2014 NRMP Program Director Survey. Available at: http://www.nrmp.org/wp-content/uploads/2014/09/PD-Survey-Report-2014.pdf.	

How important are audition electives?

Most applicants pursuing a career in otolaryngology complete audition electives. Personal knowledge of an applicant is highly valued by PDs, and the audition elective is one way to become known to a program. Faculty advisors generally recommend no more than two away electives. The website for the Boston University program states that "although it is not an absolute requirement that the clerkship be taken in our institution, it is advantageous to the candidate and to the program if it is taken in one of our hospitals."[8] Dr. Dana Suskind of the University of Chicago echoes these comments. "As an evaluator of the application process, it is hard to distinguish among the many strong medical student candidates. For this reason…we strongly encourage sub-internship…An away sub-internship at the program of your choice is recommended."[9] "Given the utmost importance placed on personal interaction (either through the interview or personal knowledge of the applicant) by PDs, applicants interested in a particular residency program may want to consider doing a rotation at that site," writes Dr. Liana Puscas of Duke University.[6]

Recommendations for Away Electives in Otolaryngology	
ENT Program	**Comments**
Department of Otolaryngology Oregon Health Sciences University	"If there is a specific program you are interested in, an early 'away rotation' at that program prior to October/ November of your fourth year will allow you to learn more about the program and improve your chances of matching at that particular institution."[10]
Dr. William Armstrong Program Director UC Irvine	"Externships at an outside institution can help an applicant with board scores or grades that are suboptimal, as strong work ethic, teamwork, and conscientiousness are critical characteristics of successful practitioners that are not well assessed in standardized applications. It can also backfire for a bright applicant with poor work habits."[11]
Dr. John Del Gaudio Program Director Emory University	"Students that perform well on a rotation at a particular program have a better chance of matching at that program than an equally qualified or even better qualified candidate who didn't rotate there."[12]

Did you know?

In one study, applicants to a single otolaryngology residency program were searched on the Facebook website. Following review of these profiles, a professionalism score was generated. In 11% of profiles, reviewers found pictures or text that at least one reviewer felt was unprofessional.[13]

How important are letters of recommendation?

Letters of recommendation are very important in the selection process. According to the NRMP, 100% of otolaryngology residency programs cited letters as a factor used to make interview decisions.[7] Applicants should generally aim to submit at least two letters from otolaryngology faculty members.

> **Did you know?**
>
> Should you request a letter from the Chairman of your Department of Otolaryngology? A letter from the "chair of the parent institution's department of otolaryngology is important," writes Dr. William Armstrong, Program Director of the Otolaryngology Residency Program at the University of California Irvine.[11] "Every student should have a letter from the chair," writes Dr. Alan Micco, Otolaryngology Career Advising Coordinator at Northwestern University.[14] "Chair's letter is STRONGLY recommended," writes the Department of Otolaryngology at Wayne State University.[15] In the 2008 NRMP Program Director Survey, 94% of respondents indicated that the letter from the otolaryngology department chair was a factor in deciding whom to interview.[16]

> **Did you know?**
>
> Many applicants do not have the opportunity to work closely with the chairman. Since the chairman's letter is required by most programs, applicants are understandably concerned about the quality of this letter. However, this letter often ends up being a summary of your clinical performance in their department. To develop this letter, the chairman or his/her designee will seek the input of those with whom you have worked, review your clinical evaluations, and even interview you. Every department has a system set in place for the development of this letter. At the University of Chicago, students are urged to "set up an appointment to speak with Dr. Naclerio. The letter is a summary of the student's clinical performance during the ENT Sub-Internship."[17]

Make it as easy as possible for the letter writer to develop a strong letter of recommendation. Ask early, while your performance is fresh in his or her mind, provide enough time for the development of the letter, and supply the professor with key information (curriculum vitae, personal statement). Include any involvement in team sports, particularly if you have a track record of excellence. Why? In one recent study assessing factors predictive or indicative of success as an otolaryngology resident, researchers found that "serious participation in athletic activities was the best determiner of a good clinician." Dr. Richard A. Chole, Chairman of the Department of Otolaryngology at Washington University, was involved in the study and offered his thoughts on these findings. "The way medicine goes now, a lot of kids go through high school, college, medical school and residency without having any experiences in which they learn to interact with their peers and supervisors in a productive manner," he said. "They're usually spending all of their time studying and working on good grades, often in relative isolation." Dr. Anna Messner is the program director of the otolaryngology residency program at Stanford University, and she weighed in on the results of this study. "In a team sport, you learn how to support your colleagues, you learn how to interact with your colleagues, you work hard and you achieve a positive outcome together—and those are the same things we do in medicine."[18]

How important is the personal statement?

According to the NRMP, 74% of programs cited the personal statement as a factor used to make interview decisions.[7]

Recommendations for Otolaryngology Personal Statement	
ENT Program	**Comments**
Dr. Henry Ou Assistant Professor of Otolaryngology University of Washington	"In countless personal statements for residency, medical students have described their first experience seeing the facial nerve or a neck dissection as the pivotal moment they became interested in otolaryngology."[19] Avoid overused statements in the personal statement. Having your statement read by an advisor will allow you to make this determination.
Dr. Robert Naclerio Section Chief of Otolaryngology University of Chicago	"Otolaryngology programs are just looking to see if you are able to write. A bad personal statement can hurt an applicant."[17]

How important is AOA?

The NRMP reports that 38.9% of U.S. seniors who matched to otolaryngology in 2014 were members of AOA. AOA membership doesn't guarantee a successful match, as a significant percentage of applicants who were AOA members in 2014 failed to match (18.6%).[1]

How important is the USMLE?

USMLE Step 1 scores are clearly important. The average score among U.S. allopathic seniors who matched in 2014 was 252. Note that high scores are no guarantee of match success in this field. In 2014, unmatched U.S. seniors had a mean step 1 score of 245. 20% of applicants with scores higher than 230 failed to match. That said, applicants with lower scores can match successfully but the odds of matching significantly decrease. Among applicants with scores less than 230, only 20 of 45 were able to land positions in the field.[1]

When should I take the USMLE Step 2 CK?

The USMLE Step 2 CK score is also a factor used by some otolaryngology residency programs in deciding whom to invite for interviews. A recent survey of otolaryngology PDs shed some light on how programs use the Step 2 CK score. Programs were asked, "Do you require USMG applicants to pass USMLE Step 2 CK before granting an interview?" 18% require passage of the exam in order to receive an interview invitation. Note also that some programs will not place you on their rank-order list unless they have proof of a passing USMLE Step 2 CK score. In the aforementioned survey, 17% required a passing score for placement of applicants on their rank-order list. Research your programs of interest early so that you can make well informed decisions regarding when to take the Step 2 CK exam.[20]

How important is research experience?

Almost every applicant has participated in a research project and/or published. According to the NRMP, over 99% of U.S. seniors who applied in 2014 had some research experience, and 95% claimed at least one abstract, publication, or presentation.[1] Highly academic or research-oriented programs may not extend interview invitations to applicants with no research experience.

Did you know?

In research done at a single institution, researchers examined peer-reviewed journal publications reported as "provisionally accepted," "accepted," or "in print" by residency applicants. Reviewers verified these publications using PubMed, Google Scholar, and electronic journals. When publications were unverifiable, reviewers contacted applicants by e-mail before interview invitations were extended. In the study, erroneously reported or unverifiable publications were designated "misrepresented." Among the 400 plus publications reported by 53.2% of applicants, 5.1% were found to be misrepresented by 17 applicants.[21]

Did you know?

An article published in *JAMA Otolaryngology* highlights the challenges that programs face in screening residency applications. As the median number of applications per U.S. graduate has increased from 40 in 2006 to 60 in 2014, the average number of submitted applications per otolaryngology program has nearly doubled, from 159 in 2008 to 278 in 2014. Programs find it difficult to determine which applicants have a strong and genuine interest in their program. "What is missing is the ability to determine who is genuinely interested in a specific program," wrote the authors. "Without that information, the selection of which candidates to invite for an interview is based on the objective information in the application and not on personal information or the applicant's degree of interest in the program. This results in invitations to some less interested candidates and no invitations to some with strong interest in a specific program…In recent years, we have observed that the percentage of applicants who accept interviews has risen. Traveling to multiple interviews for fear of not receiving a match is costly to the applicants, and unfair to other applicants who might be more interested in the slot…"[22]

How important is the interview?

As with other highly competitive specialties, the interview takes on immense importance. Dr. Suskind states that "interviews are a major determinant in the decision process."[10] Interviewees should note that some programs do not use the traditional interview approach. For example, the Department of Otolaryngology at Duke University utilizes behavioral-based interviewing to assess applicants for five core qualities – initiative, integrity, self-discipline, responsibility, and accountability. One question the program uses to assess integrity is "Describe a situation in which your integrity was challenged. How did you resolve it?"[23]

Did you know?

In a survey done to identify qualities of the <u>unsuccessful</u> resident, researchers surveyed 40 PDs. Researchers defined the unsuccessful resident as one who quit the program, was terminated by the program, or whose actions led to criminal action or citation against their medical license. Factors more commonly associated with the unsuccessful resident included poor interpersonal and communication skills with healthcare professionals and poor clinical judgment.[24]

References

[1]Charting Outcomes in the Match (2014). Available at: http://www.nrmp.org/wp-content/uploads/2014/09/Charting-Outcomes-2014-Final.pdf. Accessed March 3, 2014.
[2]Advance Data Tables: 2016 Main Residency Match. Available at: http://www.nrmp.org/match-data/main-residency-match-data/. Accessed April 23, 2016.
[3]Chole R, Ogden M. Predictors of future success in otolaryngology residency applicants. *Arch Otolaryngol Head Neck Surg* 2012; 138 (8): 707-12.
[4]Brotherton S, Etzel S. Graduate Medical Education, 2014-2015. *JAMA* 2015; 314 (22): 2436-2454.
[5]Brotherton S, Etzel S. Graduate Medical Education, 2008-2009. *JAMA* 2009; 302 (12): 1357-1372.
[6]Puscas L, Sharp S, Scwab B, Lee W. Qualities of residency applicants: comparison of otolaryngology program critiera with applicant expectations. *Arch Otolaryngol Head Neck Surg* 2012; 138 (1): 10-4.
[7]Results of the 2014 NRMP Program Director Survey. Available at: http://www.nrmp.org/wp-content/uploads/2014/09/PD-Survey-Report-2014.pdf. Accessed March 3, 2015.
[8]Boston University School of Medicine Department of Otolaryngology. Available at: http://www.bumc.bu.edu/orl/application-for-resident-training/. Accessed February 2, 2015.
[9]Suskind D. Pritzker residency process guide: otolaryngology. Available at http://pritzker.uchicago.edu/current/students/ResidencyProcessGuide.pdf.
[10]Oregon Health Sciences University Department of Otolaryngology. Available at: http://www.ohsu.edu/xd/health/services/ent/training/medical-student-education/career_guide.cfm. Accessed March 29, 2013.
[11]University of California Irvine Department of Otolaryngology. Available at: http://www.meded.uci.edu/education/residencyselection/ent.html. Accessed March 25, 2013.
[12]Emory University Department of Otolaryngology. Available at: www.panamorl.com.ar/DelGaudio%20US%20Oto%20Requirements. Accessed March 29, 2013.
[13]Golden J, Sweeny L, Bush B, Carroll W. Social networking and professionalism in otolaryngology residency applicants. *Laryngoscope* 2012; 122 (7): 1493-6.
[14]Northwestern University Department of Otolaryngology. Available at: http://www.feinberg.northwestern.edu/education/current-students/career-development-residency/career-development-program/career-advising-specialties/otolaryngology.html. Accessed March 27, 2013.
[15]Wayne State University Department of Otolaryngology. Available at: http://studentaffairs.med.wayne.edu/oto-advising.php. Accessed March 23, 2013.
[16]NRMP 2008 Program Director Survey. Available at: http://www.nrmp.org/data/programresultsbyspecialty.pdf. Accessed March 24, 2013.
[17]University of Chicago Department of Otolaryngology. Available at: pritzker.uchicago.edu/current/students/ResidencyProcessGuide.pdf. Accessed March 24, 2013.
[18]ENT Today. Available at: http://www.enttoday.org/details/article/4170771/Participation_in_Athletics_May_Make_for_a_Better_Otolaryngologist.html. Accessed March 26, 2013.
[19]Otomatch (Henry Ou, MD). Available at: http://www.otomatch.com/why/index.html. Accessed March 29, 2013.
[20]Program Requirements around Passage of USMLE Step 2CK and USMLE Step 2CS. Available at: http://www.student.med.umn.edu/osr/wp-

content/uploads/2012/09/Program-Requirements-around-Passage-of-USMLE-Step-2CK-and-USMLE-Step-2CS-11.pdf. Accessed April 1, 2013.

[21]Beswick D, Man L, Johnston B, Johnson J, Schaitkin B. Publication misrepresentation among otolaryngology residency applicants. *Otolaryngol Head Neck Surg* 2010; 143 (6): 815-9.

[22]Naclerio R, Pinto J, Baroody F. Drowning in applications for residency training: a program's perspective and simple solutions. *JAMA Otolaryngology Head Neck Surg* 2014; 140 (8): 695-6.

[23]Lee W, Esclamado R, Puscas L. Selecting among otolaryngology residency applicants to train as tomorrow's leaders. *JAMA Otolaryngol Head Neck Surg* 2013; 139 (8): 770-1.

[26]Badran K, Kelley K, Conderman C, Mahboubi H, Armstrong W, Bhandarkar N. Improving applicant selection: Identifying qualities of the unsuccessful otolaryngology resident. *Laryngoscope* 2014; Aug 5.

Chapter 36

Pathology

How competitive is the specialty?

Pathology is among the less competitive specialties for U.S. medical students. In the 2014 NRMP Match, only 5 students failed to secure a position. The numbers are significantly worse for independent applicants (osteopathic and international medical graduates). 41% of independent applicants failed to match.[1] As with other specialties, securing a position in one of the top programs in the field is difficult. "Please keep in mind that this is a highly competitive program that receives a large number of applications, and we typically accept less than 3% of those applying," writes the Department of Pathology at Brigham and Women's Hospital.[2]

Highlights of the 2016 NRMP Pathology Match[3]

- There were a total of 579 positions.
- 43% of positions were filled with allopathic medical student applicants.
- 52 U.S. IMG applicants matched.
- 167 non-U.S. IMG applicants matched.
- 51 osteopathic applicants matched.
- 29 U.S. graduates matched.
- 30 positions went unfilled.

How many years of training are required to become a pathologist?

To become a pathologist trained in anatomic and clinical pathology, a minimum of 4 years of residency training is required. There are also 3-year programs for training in only anatomic or clinical pathology.

What percentage of available positions is filled by U.S. seniors? What about other applicants?

In 2013 – 2014, there were 2,270 total residents training in a total of 142 pathology residency programs. 54% were U.S. MDs, 37.6% were international medical graduates, and 8.5% were osteopathic graduates.[4]

Residents Training in U.S. Pathology Residency Programs[4-5]					
Year	Residency Programs	Total # residents	% US MDs	% IMGs	% DO
2013-2014	142	2270	53.8%	37.6%	8.5%
2007-2008	149	2312	63.7%	30.7%	5.5%

How do programs select residents?

Every few years, the NRMP conducts a survey of PDs. In 2014, the NRMP surveyed 84 pathology PDs to determine the factors that are important in selecting applicants to interview.[6] The top 3 factors are letters of recommendation in the specialty, USMLE Step 1/COMLEX Level 1 score, and perceived commitment to the specialty.

Factors Identified as Important in Selecting Applicants to Interview by Pathology Residency Program Directors	
Top Tier Factors (Cited by 70-99% of programs)	LORs in the specialty USMLE Step 1/COMLEX Level 1 score Perceived commitment to specialty MSPE USMLE Step 2 CK/COMLEX Level 2 score Personal statement Gaps in medical education Pass USMLE Step 2 CS/COMLEX Level PE
Middle Tier Factors (Cited by 40-69% of programs)	U.S. allopathic graduate Grades in required clerkships Honors in clinical clerkships Class rank Professionalism and ethics Personal prior knowledge of the applicant Audition elective within your department Honors in clerkship in desired specialty Leadership qualities Grades in clerkship in desired specialty AOA membership Perceived interest in program Consistency of grades Volunteer/extracurricular experiences Graduate of well-regarded U.S. med school Involvement and interest in research Visa status Honors in basic sciences Away rotation in your specialty at another institution
Lowest Tier Factors (Cited by < 40% of programs)	Interest in academic career Gold Society membership Fluency in language spoken by your patient population USMLE Step 3 score/COMLEX Step 3 score
Adapted from Results of the 2014 NRMP Program Director Survey. Available at: http://www.nrmp.org/wp-content/uploads/2014/09/PD-Survey-Report-2014.pdf.	

How important are letters of recommendation?

Letters of recommendation are important, and applicants are urged to follow program directions carefully. One letter from a pathologist may suffice for some programs. Other programs, especially the more competitive ones, may prefer additional letters. "Our program likes to see a few letters (2-3) from pathologists," writes the Department of Pathology at SUNY Downstate. "Once you have made the decision to apply to pathology programs, it is advisable to get to know the department chair who will usually be willing to write a letter on your behalf. In addition, seek letters from more senior faculty and division directors, e.g. director of surgical pathology, director of cytopathology, etc. Those you ask should be individuals you have gotten to know through elective rotations or through career discussions with them."[7]

How important are audition electives?

Audition electives are not required, but should be considered if you're seeking a position in one of the competitive programs. Dr. Mara Rendi, Career Advisor in the Department of Pathology at the University of Washington, recommends an away elective "only if there is one main institution they want to go to in which case it can be helpful to do an elective there. Also, if their record is weak, it can help. But really, people do not expect you to do a rotation at another institution and it's definitely not necessary."[8]

How important is the personal statement?

According to the NRMP, 83% of programs consider the statement to be useful for selecting an applicant to interview.[6] "Your Personal Statement should summarize your particular background and interests and depict you as a unique person," writes the Wayne State University Department of Pathology. "You should indicate in your personal statement why you are interested in pathology as a career, what kind of experiences you have had in pathology, and what career path you plan to follow after training."[9] Submit "a personal statement, not more than one page, indicating why pathology is your preference and what have you got to offer to the world of pathology and our training program that others may not be able to," writes the University of Tennessee Department of Pathology and Laboratory Medicine.[10]

How important is AOA?

AOA members accounted for 11% of U.S. seniors who matched in 2014.[1]

How important is the USMLE?

In the NRMP Program Directors Survey, 94% of programs reported using the USMLE Step 1 score to make interview decisions.[6] The mean USMLE Step 1 score for U.S. seniors who matched in 2014 was 231.[1] Some programs will utilize cutoff scores in the screening process, but others will take a more holistic approach. “Because we take a holistic approach to candidate selection, we do not have a cutoff for Step scores,” writes the Indiana University Department of Pathology and Laboratory Medicine. “However, the average Step 1 and Step 2 scores for the candidates interviewed during the 2014-2015 recruitment season were 238 and 243 respectively.”[11]

When should I take the USMLE Step 2 CK?

Pathology residency programs have differing requirements with respect to the USMLE Step 2 CK exam for U.S. medical students. “Step 2 & 3 scores are not required for application; however, successful completion of Step 2 (CK & CS) is required before the start of residency,” writes the University of Wisconsin Department of Pathology and Laboratory Medicine.[12] USMLE Step 2 CK scores must be available before ranking for applicants seeking consideration by the Department of Pathology at UCSF. Applicants are encouraged to review program websites early in the process so they can make informed decisions.

How important is the interview?

According to a survey conducted by the NRMP, “interactions with the faculty during the interview and visit” was rated the top factor for ranking applicants.[6] “The invitation to schedule an interview is a clear indication that you are competitive for the residency program,” writes the Department of Pathology at New York Medical College. “However, most programs will interview 10 to 20 candidates for every available position. Therefore, prepare carefully for each interview. Use the interview as an opportunity to demonstrate you are a mature, articulate, and friendly individual.”[13]

References

[1]Charting Outcomes in the Match (2014). Available at: http://www.nrmp.org/wp-content/uploads/2014/09/Charting-Outcomes-2014-Final.pdf. Accessed March 3, 2014.
[2]Brigham and Women's Hospital Department of Pathology. Available at http://www.brighamandwomens.org/Departments_and_Services/pathology/ResidencyProgram/HowToApply.aspx?sub=6. Accessed September 30, 2015.
[3]Advance Data Tables: 2016 Main Residency Match. Available at: http://www.nrmp.org/match-data/main-residency-match-data/. Accessed April 23, 2016.
[4]Brotherton S, Etzel S. Graduate Medical Education, 2014-2015. *JAMA* 2015; 314 (22): 2436-2454.
[5]Brotherton S, Etzel S. Graduate Medical Education, 2008-2009. *JAMA* 2009; 302 (12): 1357-1372.
[6]Results of the 2014 NRMP Program Director Survey. Available at: http://www.nrmp.org/wp-content/uploads/2014/09/PD-Survey-Report-2014.pdf. Accessed March 3, 2015.
[7]SUNY Downstate Department of Pathology. Available at http://www.downstate.edu/college_of_medicine/pdf/care/Career-Booklet-Pathology.pdf. Accessed September 29, 2015.
[8]University of Washington Department of Pathology. Available at: http://www.uwmedicine.org/education/Documents/2015%20Career%20Advisors%20FAQ.pdf. Accessed September 30, 2015.
[9]Wayne State University Department of Pathology. Available at: http://pathology.med.wayne.edu/education/faq.php. Accessed September 30, 2015.
[10]University of Tennessee Department of Pathology and Laboratory Medicine. Available at: https://www.uthsc.edu/pathology/residents-fellows/application.php. Accessed September 30, 2015.
[11]Indiana University Department of Pathology and Laboratory Medicine. Available at: http://pathology.medicine.iu.edu/residency-and-fellowship-programs/resident-programs/application/. Accessed September 30, 2015.
[12]University of Wisconsin Department of Pathology and Laboratory Medicine. Available at: http://www.pathology.wisc.edu/education/residency/application-process. Accessed September 30, 2015.
[13]Guidelines for Pursuing a Residency in Pathology. Available at: https://www.nymc.edu/clubs/ghhs/PathGuide_forNYMC-UPDATED2014.pdf. Accessed September 30, 2015.

Chapter 37

Pediatrics

How competitive is the specialty?

Pediatrics is one of the less competitive specialties for U.S. allopathic medical students. Only 3.8% of U.S. seniors failed to match in 2014. Osteopathic and international medical graduates have less success. These groups of applicants are designated independent applicants by the NRMP. In 2014, 42% of independent applicants failed to match.[1] "Acceptance into our residency program is highly competitive with an average of 1,500 applications for the 12 spots per year," writes the Department of Pediatrics at the St. Joseph's Healthcare System.[2]

Did you know?

Osteopathic applicants may also apply to 20 AOA-approved pediatrics residency programs.

Highlights of the 2016 NRMP Pediatrics Match[3]

- There were a total of 2,689 positions.
- 68% of positions were filled with allopathic medical student applicants.
- 353 osteopathic applicants matched.
- 201 U.S. IMG applicants matched.
- 250 non-U.S. IMG applicants matched.
- 41 U.S. graduates matched.
- 14 positions went unfilled.

How many years of training are required to become a pediatrician?

To become a pediatrician, a minimum of 3 years of residency training is required.

What percentage of available positions is filled by U.S. seniors? What about other applicants?

In 2013 – 2014, there were 8,529 total residents training in a total of 199 pediatrics residency programs. 68% were U.S. MDs, 21.4% were international medical graduates, and 10.9% were osteopathic graduates.[4]

Residents Training in U.S. Pediatrics Residency Programs[4-5]					
Year	**Residency Programs**	**Total # residents**	**% US MDs**	**% IMGs**	**% DO**
2013-2014	199	8529	67.7%	21.4%	10.9%
2007-2008	194	8089	67.5%	24.0%	8.1%

How do programs select residents?

Every few years, the NRMP conducts a survey of PDs. In 2014, the NRMP surveyed 121 pediatrics PDs to determine the factors important in selecting applicants to interview.[6] The top 3 factors are USMLE Step 1/COMLEX Level 1 score, MSPE, and USMLE Step 2 CK/COMLEX Level 2 score.

Factors Identified As Important in Selecting Applicants to Interview by Pediatrics Residency Program Directors	
Top Tier Factors (Cited by 70-99% of programs)	USMLE Step 1/COMLEX Level 1 score MSPE USMLE Step 2 CK/COMLEX Level 2 score Personal statement LORs in the specialty U.S. allopathic graduate Class rank Gaps in medical education
Middle Tier Factors (Cited by 40-69% of programs)	Honors in clinical clerkships Grades in required clerkships Perceived commitment to specialty Audition elective within your department Professionalism and ethics Personal prior knowledge of the applicant Honors in clerkship in desired specialty Grades in clerkship in desired specialty Leadership qualities AOA membership Consistency of grades Pass USMLE Step 2 CS/COMLEX Level PE Volunteer/extracurricular experiences Graduate of well-regarded U.S. med school
Lowest Tier Factors (Cited by < 40% of programs)	Honors in basic sciences Involvement and interest in research Perceived interest in program Visa status Interest in academic career Away rotation in your specialty at another institution Gold Society membership Fluency in language spoken by your patient population USMLE Step 3 score/COMLEX Step 3 score
Adapted from Results of the 2014 NRMP Program Director Survey. Available at: http://www.nrmp.org/wp-content/uploads/2014/09/PD-Survey-Report-2014.pdf.	

How important are letters of recommendation?

Most pediatric residency programs ask applicants to submit three letters of recommendation. LORs are important to programs, and we recommend that you submit at least one from pediatrics faculty. A small but growing number of programs require a Chair's letter. It's best to review program websites in advance so that you can arrange for this letter if your programs of interest require it. A study of pediatric PDs shed some light on the importance of the source of the letter. Researchers asked directors to rate the source on a scale of 1 (not at all relevant) to 5 (very highly relevant).[7]

Importance of the Source of the Pediatric Letter of Recommendation in the Selection Process

Type of Letter Writer	Mean score
Pediatric chair who has worked directly with student	4.40
Pediatric attending on inpatient 4th year subinternship	4.38
Pediatric attending on clerkship	4.15
Pediatric clerkship director	3.93
Pediatric attending on outpatient 4th year subinternship	3.90
Pediatric community preceptor	3.20
Research mentor	2.91
Pediatric chair who has not worked directly with student	2.57

Stoffer M, Slavin S, Chung P, Fall L, Lawless M. Letters of recommendation for residency: can we do better? Platform presentation. Pediatric Academic Societies Meeting, May 2003, Seattle, WA.

Did you know?

"Advisors can guide the process of obtaining letters of recommendation; they are sometimes familiar with other students' experiences and may have a sense of the quality of letters offered by their faculty colleagues. This can be a huge benefit."[8]

Dr. David Levine
Professor of Pediatrics
Morehouse School of Medicine

How important are audition electives?

For most U.S. allopathic students, audition electives are not required to match to pediatrics. The Department of Pediatrics at the University of North Carolina states that the audition elective is "helpful if your heart is set on one program or one geographic area."[9] Obviously, the student must do well in this rotation, and that can be challenging for a variety of reasons.

How important is the personal statement?

According to the NRMP, 70% of programs considered the statement to be useful for selecting an applicant to interview.[6] "Theoretically, the personal statement is important, communicating a candidate's personal commentary on his or her strengths, passions, and other personal beliefs and sentiments to the resident selection committee in a way that the more structured and less personal elements of the application do not permit," writes Dr. Deepak Kamat, Vice Chair of Education in the Department of Pediatrics at Wayne State University. "The personal statement could be a valuable tool for program directors in formulating the tone and laying the groundwork for a personal interview with a candidate."[10]

Did you know...

"The personal statement enables the applicant to add a new dimension to the application, to persuade those who read it that the applicant will be an asset to the program and will fit in, while reflecting special qualities and interests that separate the applicant from his/her peers."[8]

Dr. James Stallworth
Professor of Pediatrics
University of South Carolina School of Medicine

Dr. Cynthia Christy
Professor of Pediatrics
University of Rochester School of Medicine & Dentistry

How important is AOA?

AOA members accounted for 12.9% of U.S. seniors who matched in 2014.[1]

How important is the USMLE?

In the NRMP Program Directors Survey, 98% of programs reported using the USMLE Step 1 score to make interview decisions.[6] The mean USMLE Step 1 score for U.S. seniors who matched in 2014 was 226. 89% of U.S. allopathic seniors with lower USMLE scores (< 210) successfully matched.[1] Dr. Daniel West, Program Director at University of California San Francisco, advises students "not to worry too much about boards, but to work very hard during their clerkships." He does note, however, that students "who barely pass" the USMLE may have difficulty with the pediatric board exam, and that failing the pediatric boards reflects poorly on a residency program.[11]

When should I take the USMLE Step 2 CK?

A 2012 NRMP survey of 94 pediatrics residency programs revealed that 24.7% of programs required passage of Step 2 CK for granting interviews. A higher percentage (68%) required passage for placement on the rank-order list.[12]

How important is research experience?

In 2006, Green surveyed pediatrics PDs about the residency selection process. Of the 131 surveys sent, responses were received from 82 directors (63%). Program directors were asked to rate the importance of 16 criteria on a scale of 1 (unimportant) to 5 (critical).[13] Among 16 academic criteria, Green found that published medical school research was last in importance. Research involvement is certainly not required, but can be helpful.

How important is the interview?

The interview is ranked as the most important factor used to make rank-order list decisions. A study performed at the Children's Hospital of Philadelphia residency program offered some insight into the importance of the interview. The authors wrote that "interview scores were the most important variable for candidate ranking on the NRMP list."[14] We interviewed Dr. Su-Ting Li, Program Director of the Pediatrics residency program at the University of California Davis. We asked her the following question: "As you think back to applicants who really impressed you during the interview, what do you believe distinguishes these applicants from others?"

If personal statements are a first date, interviews are a second date. The program is interested enough in the applicant to want to get to know the applicant better...For the program, interviews are a time to assess the applicant outside of their paper application. In particular, interviews allow programs to assess the applicant's interpersonal and communication skills, and sometimes their critical thinking skills. I particularly enjoy interviews where the time seems to fly and I'm asking my residency coordinator for a few more minutes with the applicant. Great interviews feel much more like a conversation with a new interesting friend than an interview – topics flow naturally from one to another and there are no lulls in the conversation. These applicants are genuinely enthusiastic about pediatrics and about your residency training program. They have stellar interpersonal and communication skills. They can thoughtfully describe their previous experiences, and articulate what they learned from the experiences, how they shaped who they are, and how they influenced their career trajectory. They can clearly communicate how they utilized the medical literature to help them approach the diagnosis or management of a challenging patient they took care of. They ask intelligent questions and listen attentively to your responses. At the end of the conversation, I can't wait to talk to the applicant again – hopefully as one of my new interns.[15]

Advice for the Pediatrics Residency Interview	
Dr. Laura Stewart Associate Program Director St. John Hospital	What does Dr. Sterwart look for in the interview? "Most importantly, I like to get an idea of how passionate they are about Pediatrics. They need to have relevant, thoughtful questions about the program."[16]
University of Connecticut Department of Pediatrics	At the University of Connecticut, 30% of the applicant's total score is based on interpersonal relations, maturity, professionalism, and program fit. During the interview, the applicant is assessed for the following characteristics / qualities: • Patient • Tolerant and able to handle stress • Able with problem solving and decision making • Able to confront failure and errors successfully • Teamwork and communication • Initiative and eagerness to learn • Leadership and teaching ability[11] Consider how you would highlight these qualities in a residency interview.[17]
Dr. Terry Kind Director of Pediatric Medical Student Education George Washington University	"Make sure you can discuss anything and everything on there. And that you can say something you learned or something meaningful about any of those things you've listed." She also feels that candidates are often not prepared for the "Please tell me something about yourself" question. Finally, she recommends that by having "a few key points that you want to convey about yourself during the interview, you can work those in at some point during the interview."[18]
Dr. R. Franklin Trimm Program Director University of South Alabama	"My goal for the interview is to get beyond the scores and formal descriptions of the applicant, and get to know her or him as a person to be able to form an opinion about how likely the individual is to succeed as a pediatrician and how good a fit our program may be for that person."[19]

Did you know?

What are some common interview pitfalls? The American Academy of Pediatrics Medical Student Subcommittee interviewed 5 faculty members heavily involved in the residency selection process. They found that interview day pitfalls included "showing disinterest during the interview, falling asleep at morning report, dressing inappropriately, asking logistical questions that can easily be answered on the program's website or handouts, and talking poorly of the program in comparison to your home program. Despite the common sense nature of some of these suggestions, our panel had a wide array of stories of students doing all of these."[19]

References

[1]Charting Outcomes in the Match (2014). Available at: http://www.nrmp.org/wp-content/uploads/2014/09/Charting-Outcomes-2014-Final.pdf. Accessed March 3, 2014.
[2]St. Joseph's Healthcare System Department of Pediatrics. Available at: https://www.stjosephshealth.org/education/item/1444-pediatrics. Accessed September 28, 2015.
[3]Advance Data Tables: 2016 Main Residency Match. Available at: http://www.nrmp.org/match-data/main-residency-match-data/. Accessed April 23, 2016.
[4]Brotherton S, Etzel S. Graduate Medical Education, 2014-2015. *JAMA* 2015; 314 (22): 2436-2454.
[5]Brotherton S, Etzel S. Graduate Medical Education, 2008-2009. *JAMA* 2009; 302 (12): 1357-1372.
[6]Results of the 2014 NRMP Program Director Survey. Available at: http://www.nrmp.org/wp-content/uploads/2014/09/PD-Survey-Report-2014.pdf. Accessed March 3, 2015.
[7]Stoffer M, Slavin S, Chung P, Fall L, Lawless M. Letters of recommendation for residency: can we do better? Platform presentation. Pediatric Academic Societies Meeting, May 2003, Seattle, WA.
[8]American Academy of Pediatrics. Available at http://www.aap.org/en-us/about-the-aap/Committees-Councils-Sections/Medical-Students/Documents/AP140_BecomingAPediatrician_vF.pdf. Accessed September 28, 2015.
[9]University of North Carolina Preparing for Pediatrics Residency Training. Available at https://www.med.unc.edu/pedclerk/resources/pedsres/PreparingforPedsResidency2008-9_001.ppt. Accessed September 28, 2015.
[10]Mathur A, Kamat D. The personal statement. *J Pediatr* 2014; 164 (4): 682.
[11]West D. A guide to the perplexed: residency guide. Available at: http://www.ucdmc.ucdavis.edu. Accessed June 2, 2009.
[12]Program Requirements around Passage of USMLE Step 2CK and USMLE Step 2CS. Available at: http://www.student.med.umn.edu/osr/wp-content/uploads/2012/09/Program-Requirements-around-Passage-of-USMLE-Step-2CK-and-USMLE-Step-2CS-11.pdf. Accessed April 1, 2013.
[13]Green M, Jones P, Thomas J. Selection criteria for residency: results of a national program director survey. *Acad Med* 2009; 84 (3): 362-7.
[14]Swanson W, Harris M, Master C, Gallagher P, Maruo A, Ludwing S. The impact of the interview in pediatric residency selection. *Amb Pediatr* 2005; 5 (4): 216-220.
[15]The Successful Match: Getting into Pediatrics. Available at: http://studentdoctor.net/2011/05/the-successful-match-getting-into-pediatrics/. Accessed September 2, 2012.
[16]American University of the Caribbean. Available at: http://www.aucmed.edu/news/?p=873. Accessed September 27, 2012.
[17]University of Connecticut Department of Pediatrics. Available at: http://www.uchc.edu/md/pediatrics/Selection%20Policy%20for%20Residents.pdf. Accessed September 4, 2012.
[18]Pediatric Career Blog. Available at: http://www.pediatriccareer.org/2011_09_01_archive.html. Accessed September 28, 2012.
[19]AAP Medical Student Newsletter. Available at: http://www2.aap.org/sections/ypn/ms/educ_resources/newsletter.html. Accessed September 5, 2012.

Chapter 38

Physical Medicine & Rehabilitation

How competitive is the specialty?

Physical medicine and rehabilitation (PM&R) is a moderately competitive specialty. In the 2014 NRMP Match, 13% of U.S. allopathic medical students failed to match. The numbers are worse for osteopathic and international medical graduates. These groups of applicants are designated independent applicants by the NRMP. In 2014, 47% of independent applicants failed to match.[1] "From the more than 200 completed applications we receive, the review committee typically selects 60-75 applicants for interview," writes the combined Baylor College of Medicine/University of Texas at Houston Medical School PM&R Alliance Residency Program. "We recruit to fill 10-12 residency slots."[2]

Did you know?

Osteopathic applicants may also apply to 6 AOA-approved physical medicine and rehabilitation residency programs.

Highlights of the 2016 NRMP Physical Medicine and Rehabilitation Match[3]

- There were a total of 402 positions at the PGY1 and PGY2 levels.
- 56% of positions were filled with allopathic medical student applicants.
- 114 osteopathic applicants matched.
- 37 U.S. IMG applicants matched.
- 12 non-U.S. IMG applicants matched.
- 8 U.S. graduates matched.
- 9 positions went unfilled.

How many years of training are required to become a physiatrist?

To become a physiatrist, a minimum of 4 years of residency training is required. Training begins with either a transitional or preliminary year followed by 3 years of training in PM&R. There are two types of PM&R programs:

- Categorical 4-year program

  Some PM&R residency programs offer 4 years of training with an internship (akin to a preliminary medicine year) embedded within the training period. One benefit of these programs is that the trainee is not required to move after the first year.

- Advanced 3-year program

  These programs require a separate internship. Applicants applying to these programs must also apply to preliminary or transitional year programs.

What percentage of available positions is filled by U.S. seniors? What about other applicants?

In 2013 – 2014, there were 1212 total residents training in a total of 78 PM&R residency programs. 54% were U.S. MDs, 17.6% were international medical graduates, and 28.9% were osteopathic graduates.[4]

Residents Training in U.S. PM&R Residency Programs[4-5]					
Year	**Residency Programs**	**Total # residents**	**% US MDs**	**% IMGs**	**% DO**
2013-2014	78	1212	53.5%	17.6%	28.9%
2007-2008	79	1203	56.2%	18.6%	25.0%

How do programs select residents?

Every few years, the NRMP conducts a survey of PDs. In 2014, the NRMP surveyed 34 PM&R PDs to determine the factors that are important in selecting applicants to interview.[6] The top 3 factors are USMLE Step 1/COMLEX Level 1 score, LORs in the specialty, and MSPE. Factors are shown in the table on the following page.

How important are letters of recommendation?

According to the NRMP, LORs were cited by 91% of PDs as a factor used to make interview decisions.[6] Most PM&R residency programs ask applicants to submit 3 letters of recommendation. We recommend that you submit at least one from PM&R faculty. In a survey of PM&R PDs, most highly valued was a letter from a faculty member in the PD's department, followed by a letter written by a chairman of a PM&R department.[7] However, a Chair's letter is not required, and applicants are urged to obtain letters from faculty who have worked with them closely.

How important are audition electives?

For most U.S. allopathic students, audition electives are not required to match to physiatry. You may consider an away rotation if you have a strong need to match at a particular program but there is concern that the paper record is not competitive for that particular program. "Away electives at sites where you are most interested allow the programs there to 'interview' you prior to the Match interview process," writes Dr. Margaret Turk of SUNY Upstate. "Audition electives are not common in PM&R, so not typically expected."[8]

Factors Identified As Important in Selecting Applicants to Interview by PM&R Residency Program Directors	
Top Tier Factors (Cited by 70-99% of programs)	USMLE Step 1/COMLEX Level 1 score LORs in the specialty MSPE USMLE Step 2 CK/COMLEX Level 2 score Personal statement Gaps in medical education Grades in required clerkships Perceived commitment to specialty Professionalism and ethics Pass USMLE Step 2 CS/COMLEX Level PE
Middle Tier Factors (Cited by 40-69% of programs)	U.S. allopathic graduate Honors in clinical clerkships Class rank Audition elective within your department Personal prior knowledge of the applicant Honors in clerkship in desired specialty Grades in clerkship in desired specialty Leadership qualities AOA membership Perceived interest in program Consistency of grades Volunteer/extracurricular experiences Involvement and interest in research Fluency in language spoken by your patient population
Lowest Tier Factors (Cited by < 40% of programs)	Graduate of well-regarded U.S. med school Honors in basic sciences Visa status Interest in academic career Away rotation in your specialty at another institution Gold Society membership USMLE Step 3 score/COMLEX Step 3 score
Adapted from Results of the 2014 NRMP Program Director Survey. Available at: http://www.nrmp.org/wp-content/uploads/2014/09/PD-Survey-Report-2014.pdf.	

How important is the personal statement?

According to the NRMP, 79% of programs considered the statement to be useful for selecting an applicant to interview.[6] "PMR programs are looking for students to discuss their specific interest in PMR and what experiences led to their decision to pursue this particular specialty," writes Dr. Susan Stickevers, Program Director at Stony Brook University.[9]

How important is AOA?

AOA members accounted for 5.5% of U.S. seniors who matched in 2014.[1]

How important is the USMLE?

In the NRMP Program Directors Survey, 91% of programs reported using the USMLE Step 1 score to make interview decisions.[6] The mean USMLE Step 1 score for U.S. seniors who matched in 2014 was 220.[1]

When should I take the USMLE Step 2 CK?

A 2012 NRMP survey of 20 PM&R residency programs revealed that 10.5% of programs required passage of Step 2 CK for granting interviews. A higher percentage (47%) required passage for placement on the rank-order list.[10]

How important is research experience?

In 2006, Green surveyed PM&R residency program directors about the selection process. PDs were asked to rate the importance of 16 criteria on a scale of 1 (unimportant) to 5 (critical).[11] Among 16 academic criteria, Green found that published medical school research was last in importance. "Research is not required for an interview invitation or matching," writes Dr. Margaret Turk of SUNY Upstate. "However, having engaged in research relevant to the field allows good conversation during the interview process, and allows you to demonstrate your understanding of PM&R."[8]

How important is the interview?

The interview is ranked as the most important factor used to make rank-order list decisions. DeLisa asked PDs about the importance of various applicant characteristics assessed during interviews.[7] The findings are shown in the table on the next page.

Importance of Applicant Characteristics Assessed During PM&R Residency Interview	
Characteristic	**Mean**
Compatibility with the program	4.4
Ability to articulate thoughts	4.2
Ability to work with the team	4.2
Ability to listen	4.1
Commitment to hard work	4.1
Ability to grow in knowledge	4.1
Maturity	3.9
Ability to solve problems	3.9
Fund of medical knowledge	3.8
Sensitivity to others' psychosocial needs	3.7
Relevant questions asked	3.7
Personal appearance and professionalism	3.6
Level of confidence	3.6
Realistic self-appraisal	3.6
Knowledge of the specialty	3.5
DeLisa J, Jain S, Campagnolo D. Factors used by physical medicine and rehabilitation program directors to select their residents. *Am J Phys Med Rehabil* 1994; 73 (3): 152-156.	

References

[1]Charting Outcomes in the Match (2014). Available at: http://www.nrmp.org/wp-content/uploads/2014/09/Charting-Outcomes-2014-Final.pdf. Accessed March 3, 2014.
[2]Baylor College of Medicine Physical Medicine and Rehabilitation Residency. Available at: https://www.bcm.edu/departments/physical-medicine-and-rehabilitation/education/physical-medicine-rehabilitation-residency/admissions. Accessed September 28, 2015.
[3]Advance Data Tables: 2016 Main Residency Match. Available at: http://www.nrmp.org/match-data/main-residency-match-data/. Accessed April 23, 2016.
[4]Brotherton S, Etzel S. Graduate Medical Education, 2014-2015. *JAMA* 2015; 314 (22): 2436-2454.
[5]Brotherton S, Etzel S. Graduate Medical Education, 2008-2009. *JAMA* 2009; 302 (12): 1357-1372.
[6]Results of the 2014 NRMP Program Director Survey. Available at: http://www.nrmp.org/wp-content/uploads/2014/09/PD-Survey-Report-2014.pdf. Accessed March 3, 2015.
[7]DeLisa J, Jain S, Campagnolo D. Factors used by physical medicine and rehabilitation program directors to select their residents. *Am J Phys Med Rehabil* 1994; 73 (3): 152-156.
[8]SUNY Upstate Medical Center Department of Physical Medicine & Rehabilitation. Available at: http://www.upstate.edu/currentstudents/document/pm_r_advising.pdf.
[9]StonyBrook Medicine Career Advisement Manual 2014. Available at: http://medicine.stonybrookmedicine.edu/system/files/neofiles/Career%20Counseling%20Manual%20for%20Advisors%202014.pdf. Accessed September 28, 2015.
[10]Program Requirements around Passage of USMLE Step 2CK and USMLE Step 2CS. Available at: http://www.student.med.umn.edu/osr/wp-content/uploads/2012/09/Program-Requirements-around-Passage-of-USMLE-Step-2CK-and-USMLE-Step-2CS-11.pdf. Accessed April 1, 2013.
[11]Green M, Jones P, Thomas J. Selection criteria for residency: results of a national program director survey. *Acad Med* 2009; 84 (3): 362-7.
Accessed September 28, 2015.

Chapter 39

Plastic Surgery

How competitive is the specialty?

Plastic surgery is a highly competitive specialty. In 2014, out of 178 U.S. allopathic seniors applying to plastic surgery, 52 failed to match. In other words, approximately 30% of U.S. allopathic seniors applying to plastic surgery failed to match. The numbers are worse for osteopathic and international medical graduates. These groups of applicants are designated independent applicants by the NRMP. In 2014, 65% of independent applicants failed to match.[1]

Highlights of the 2016 NRMP Plastic Surgery Match[2]

- There were a total of 152 positions (Integrated Pathway).
- 88% of positions were filled with allopathic medical student applicants.
- 1 osteopathic applicant matched.
- 3 U.S. IMG applicant matched.
- 3 non-U.S. IMG applicants matched.
- 11 U.S. graduates matched.
- 1 positions was unfilled.

How many years of training are required to become a plastic surgeon?

There are two types of plastic surgery residency programs:

- Integrated pathway

  These are 6-year training programs that accept students immediately following medical school graduation.

- Independent pathway

  These are 3-year training programs open to graduates of general surgery, neurological surgery, orthopedic surgery, oral and maxillofacial surgery, otolaryngology, and urology residency programs.

What percentage of available positions is filled by U.S. seniors? What about other applicants?

In 2013 – 2014, there were 573 total residents training in a total of 65 integrated plastic surgery residency programs.[3] 95% were U.S. MDs and 4.0% were international medical graduates.

Residents Training in U.S. Plastic Surgery Residency Programs (Integrated)[3-4]					
Year	**Residency Programs**	**Total # residents**	**% US MDs**	**% IMGs**	**% DO**
2013-2014	65	573	95.3%	4.0%	0.7%
2007-2008	15	189	96.3%	3.2%	0%

How do programs select residents?

In a recent survey of nearly 300 members of the American Association of Plastic Surgeons, researchers determined the metrics most important to respondents in the plastic surgery residency selection process. Respondents were asked to rate criteria on a scale of 1 (irrelevant) to 5 (very important). The criteria are presented below in descending order of importance:

- Letter from known recommender
- Intelligence
- Dexterity
- Spatial sense
- Clerkship grades
- USMLE scores
- Extracurriculars
- Potential for research
- School rank
- Research productivity
- Artistic
- Letter from unknown recommender

Of note, the top 3 (letter from known recommender, intelligence, and dexterity) each received a rating above 4.00. The three least important criteria still received a mean score above 3.00.[5]

Every few years, the NRMP conducts a survey of program directors. In 2014, the NRMP surveyed 39 plastic surgery PDs to determine the factors important in selecting applicants to interview.[6] The top 3 factors are USMLE Step 1/COMLEX Level 1 score, LORs in the specialty, and personal statement. Factors are shown in the table on the following page.

Factors Identified As Important in Selecting Applicants to Interview by Plastic Surgery Residency Program Directors	
Top Tier Factors (Cited by 70-99% of programs)	USMLE Step 1/COMLEX Level 1 score LORs in the specialty Personal statement Involvement and interest in research U.S. allopathic graduate Honors in clinical clerkships Perceived commitment to specialty Personal prior knowledge of the applicant Leadership qualities Honors in clerkship in desired specialty AOA membership
Middle Tier Factors (Cited by 40-69% of programs)	MSPE USMLE Step 2 CK/COMLEX Level 2 score Grades in required clerkships Class rank Audition elective within your department Professionalism and ethics Grades in clerkship in desired specialty Perceived interest in program Volunteer/extracurricular experiences Graduate of well-regarded U.S. med school Visa status Interest in academic career
Lowest Tier Factors (Cited by < 40% of programs)	Honors in basic sciences Away rotation in your specialty at another institution Gold Society membership USMLE Step 3 score/COMLEX Step 3 score Gaps in medical education Pass USMLE Step 2 CS/COMLEX Level PE Consistency of grades Fluency in language spoken by your patient population
Adapted from Results of the 2014 NRMP Program Director Survey. Available at: http://www.nrmp.org/wp-content/uploads/2014/09/PD-Survey-Report-2014.pdf.	

Did you know?

"As a medical student, the first thing you need to do is to be honest with yourself: Do you have the basic prerequisites to be in the running for an integrated program position? If you are already a fourth-year medical student and you cannot clear this bar, there is likely not enough time to improve your grade point average and United States Medical Licensing Examination scores – or to compensate for them with more publications. You may be best served by pursuing the independent pathway."[7]

Dr. Rod Rohrich
Professor of Plastic Surgery
University of Texas Southwestern Medical School

How important are letters of recommendation?

Most plastic surgery residency programs ask applicants to submit 3 LORs. According to the NRMP, LORs were cited by 94% of PDs as a factor used to make interview decisions.[6] Although the same percentage of programs utilized LORs and USMLE Step 1 scores to make interview decisions, the letters were more important. Particularly important are letters written by colleagues known to the residency program. "If possible a letter from a nationally recognized plastic surgeon will help as their letters are well known and easier to interpret," writes the Department of Plastic Surgery at SUNY Downstate. "Letters should come from people that are best able to write meaningful letters that demonstrate a real understanding of the applicant, rather than just a reiteration of a file."[8] Most programs <u>do</u> require a Chief's or Chair's letter.

Did you know?

"When a respected plastic surgeon vouches that you possess the qualities of an excellent resident, program directors take notice...Some applicants fall into the trap of thinking that they need a letter – any letter – from a well-known plastic surgeon. The truth is that a letter from someone who does not know you well is the opposite of a high-quality letter – program directors can smell a generic letter of recommendation from a mile away."[7]

Dr. Rod Rohrich
Professor of Plastic Surgery
University of Texas Southwestern Medical School

How important are audition electives?

Most advisors recommend that applicants complete one or two audition electives to maximize the chances of a successful match.

How important is the personal statement?

According to the NRMP, 85% of programs considered the statement to be useful for selecting an applicant to interview.[6]

How important is AOA?

AOA members accounted for 39% of U.S. seniors who matched in 2014. Of note, AOA membership does not guarantee success. Among the unmatched group of applicants, 15% were AOA members.[1]

How important is the USMLE?

High scores do not guarantee success as the mean score among unmatched applicants was 236. In the NRMP Program Directors Survey, 94% of programs reported using the USMLE Step 1 score to make interview decisions.[6] The mean USMLE Step 1 score for U.S. seniors who matched in 2014 was 245.[1] "Having a high USMLE score is essential in qualifying for an interview," writes the Department of Plastic Surgery at SUNY Downstate. "Average USMLE step 1 scores are typically the highest for plastic surgery applicants. A competitive score would be higher than 240."[8]

How important is research experience?

Research experience is important for plastic surgery applicants. In 2014, the mean number of abstracts, presentations, and publications for matched applicants was 12.5, significantly higher than the number for unmatched applicants (6.4).[1] In 2006, Green surveyed plastic surgery PDs about the selection process. PDs were asked to rate the importance of 16 criteria on a scale of 1 (unimportant) to 5 (critical). Among 16 academic criteria, Green found that published medical school research was fifth in importance.[9]

How important is the interview?

In 2003, Dr. LaGrasso of the University of South Carolina surveyed PDs to learn about the criteria that programs use to select residents. PDs were asked to rank 20 items that were used in the evaluation of applicants during the interview process. The results are shown in the table on the next page.[10]

Did you know?

A more recent survey of 295 members of the American Association of Plastic Surgeons revealed important information about personality attributes valued in residents. Highly rated were honesty and hard work, followed by commitment to patients, being a team player, having maturity, and having compassion (in descending order of importance). Negative attributes included dishonesty, laziness, arrogance, being a non-team player, money-oriented attitude, sycophantic qualities, and being overly aggressive.[7]

Subjective Resident Selection Criteria Used By Plastic Surgery Residency Directors		
Rank	**Criteria**	**Mean***
1	Leadership qualities	4.60
2	Apparent maturity	4.47
3	Answers to questions	4.07
4	Candidate's interest in teaching/academics	4.07
5	Attitude toward questions	3.93
6	Questions that candidate poses	3.80
7	Overall appearance	3.73
8	Statement of candidate's goals	3.73
9	General knowledge	3.47
10	Attire	3.00
11	Family obligations	2.87
12	Interest in specialty area	2.87
13	Age	2.47
14	Participation in ASPS activities	2.13
15	Family in plastic surgery field	1.73
16	Apparent ethnicity	1.53
17	Accent	1.47
18	Gender	1.40
19	Sexual preference	1.27
20	Religious preference	1.07

*Survey participants were asked to rank each item on a scale of 1 (least important) to 5 (most important).

LaGrasso J, Kennedy D, Hoehn J, Ashruf S, Pryzbyla A. Selection criteria for the integrated model of plastic surgery residency. *Plast Reconstr Surg* 2008; 121 (3): 121e-125e.

References

[1]Charting Outcomes in the Match (2014). Available at: http://www.nrmp.org/wp-content/uploads/2014/09/Charting-Outcomes-2014-Final.pdf. Accessed March 3, 2014.
[2]Advance Data Tables: 2016 Main Residency Match. Available at: http://www.nrmp.org/match-data/main-residency-match-data/. Accessed April 23, 2016.
[3]Brotherton S, Etzel S. Graduate Medical Education, 2014-2015. *JAMA* 2015; 314 (22): 2436-54.
[4]Brotherton S, Etzel S. Graduate Medical Education, 2008-2009. *JAMA* 2009; 302 (12): 1357-72.
[5]Liang F, Rudnicki P, Prince N, Lipsitz S, May J, Guo L. An evaluation of plastic surgery resident selection factors. *J Surg Educ* 2015; 72 (1): 8-15.
[6]Results of the 2014 NRMP Program Director Survey. Available at: http://www.nrmp.org/wp-content/uploads/2014/09/PD-Survey-Report-2014.pdf. Accessed March 3, 2015.
[7]Nagarkar P, Pulikkottil B, Patel A, Rohrich R. So you want to become a plastic surgeon? What do you need to do and know to get into a plastic surgery residency. *Plast Reconstr Surg* 2013; 131 (2): 419-22.
[8]SUNY Downstate Department of Plastic Surgery. Available at http://www.downstate.edu/college_of_medicine/pdf/care/Career-Booklet-Plastic-Surgery.pdf. Accessed September 28, 2015.
[9]Green M, Jones P, Thomas J. Selection criteria for residency: results of a national program director survey. *Acad Med* 2009; 84 (3): 362-7.
[10]LaGrasso J, Kennedy D, Hoehn J, Ashruf S, Pryzbyla A. Selection criteria for the integrated model of plastic surgery residency. *Plast Reconstr Surg* 2008; 121 (3): 121e-125e.

Chapter 40

Psychiatry

How competitive is the specialty?

Psychiatry is among the less competitive specialties. However, the top programs in the field are quite competitive. "We received nearly 800 completed applications in 2013," writes the Department of Psychiatry at Thomas Jefferson University. "We expect to conduct about 110 interviews this year."[1] Many positions in psychiatry are filled with osteopathic and international medical graduate applicants. That said, 51% of these applicants failed to match in 2014.[2]

Highlights of the 2016 NRMP Psychiatry Match[3]

- There were a total of 1,384 positions.
- 61% of positions were filled with allopathic medical student applicants.
- 188 osteopathic applicants matched.
- 162 U.S. IMG applicants matched.
- 132 non-U.S. IMG applicants matched.
- 41 U.S. graduates matched.
- 11 positions went unfilled.

How many years of training are required to become a psychiatrist?

To become a psychiatrist, a minimum of 4 years of residency training is required. This includes a preliminary year of training in clinical medicine.

What percentage of available positions is filled by U.S. seniors? What about other applicants?

In 2013 – 2014, there were 4,966 total residents training in a total of 193 psychiatry residency programs.[4] 56% were U.S. MDs, 32.6% were international medical graduates, and 11.5% were osteopathic graduates.

Residents Training in U.S. Psychiatry Residency Programs[4-5]					
Year	**Residency Programs**	**Total # residents**	**% US MDs**	**% IMGs**	**% DO**
2013-2014	193	4966	55.9%	32.6%	11.5%
2007-2008	182	4751	58.8%	32.9%	7.9%

How do programs select residents?

Every few years, the NRMP conducts a survey of PDs. In 2014, the NRMP surveyed 84 psychiatry PDs to determine the factors important in selecting applicants to interview.[6] The top 3 factors are MSPE, personal statement, and gaps in medical education. Factors are shown in the table on the following page.

Factors Identified As Important in Selecting Applicants to Interview by Psychiatry Residency Program Directors	
Top Tier Factors (Cited by 70-99% of programs)	MSPE Personal statement Gaps in medical education LORs in the specialty USMLE Step 1/COMLEX Level 1 score USMLE Step 2 CK/COMLEX Level 2 score U.S. allopathic graduate Grades in required clerkships Perceived commitment to specialty Professionalism and ethics Personal prior knowledge of the applicant Grades in clerkship in desired specialty Pass USMLE Step 2 CS/COMLEX Level PE
Middle Tier Factors (Cited by 40-69% of programs)	Honors in clinical clerkships Class rank Audition elective within your department Honors in clerkship in desired specialty Leadership qualities AOA membership Perceived interest in program Consistency of grades Volunteer/extracurricular experiences Involvement and interest in research Graduate of well-regarded U.S. med school Visa status Gold Society membership Fluency in language spoken by your patient population
Lowest Tier Factors (Cited by < 40% of programs)	Interest in academic career Away rotation in your specialty at another institution USMLE Step 3 score/COMLEX Step 3 score Honors in basic sciences
Adapted from Results of the 2014 NRMP Program Director Survey. Available at: http://www.nrmp.org/wp-content/uploads/2014/09/PD-Survey-Report-2014.pdf.	

How important are letters of recommendation?

Letters of recommendation are cited by 84% of psychiatry residency programs as an important factor used to make interview decisions.[6] For most applicants, one letter from a psychiatrist with whom you've worked closely is sufficient.

How important is the personal statement?

According to the NRMP, 92% of programs considered the statement to be useful for selecting an applicant to interview.[6] Many applicants begin their statements by answering the question, "Why psychiatry?" Often, these statements start with the story of a patient that served as an impetus to pursue a career in psychiatry. Dr. Mina Bak recommends that applicants not spend more than "a brief paragraph about such a vignette. Readers want the statement to give a sense of the applicant as a total person. Thus, applicants should feel empowered to expand on 'how," in addition to 'why,' they ended up applying to psychiatry."[7] In addition to answering "Why psychiatry?" Dr. Deborah Spitz, Program Director at the University of Chicago, encourages applicants to personalize the statement. "Why do you want to interview at a specific residency program?"[8]

How important is AOA?

AOA members accounted for 4.9% of U.S. seniors who matched in 2014.[2]

How important is the USMLE?

Although 87% of psychiatry residency programs use the USMLE Step 1 score as a factor to make interview decisions, the score takes on less importance for ranking purposes.[6] The mean USMLE Step 1 score for U.S. seniors who matched in 2014 was 220.[2] Dr. Mark Servis, Program Director at University of California-Davis, states that "we don't usually talk about scores in selection committee unless the students either have an unusually high score or failed their first time. If they failed first try, they may not be invited to interview."[9] Dr. Jon Lehrmann, Chairman of the Department of Psychiatry at the Medical College of Wisconsin, writes that "if a candidate failed two or more times, the application goes on a 'no interview' pile; however, if something else stands out positively on the application, it may end up on a 'maybe' pile. Applications showing scores of 200 or higher go on a 'yes' pile. Applications with passing scores less than 200 go on the 'maybe' pile."[10]

When should I take the USMLE Step 2 CK?

A 2012 NRMP survey of 63 psychiatry residency programs revealed that 30.6% of programs required passage of Step 2 CK for granting interviews. A higher percentage (66.7%) required passage for placement on the rank-order list.[11]

How important is research experience?

Bak writes that "most residents, even at top academic programs, primarily tend to become clinicians; thus, research experience is not essential for applicants to successfully match."[7]

How important is the interview?

The interview is ranked as the most important factor used to make rank-order list decisions. Dr. Edward Reilly, former residency program director at the University of Texas – Houston, states that interviews are "critical. The good interview can save someone with the less than perfect application. A bad interview cannot always be salvaged by a paper record."[12] Applicants should ready themselves for somewhat personal questions. Feedback we've received from our mock interview clients has shown that some programs, particularly those with a psychodynamic bent, tend to ask about family background and relationships.

Did you know?

How important is the psychiatry residency interview? According to Dr. David Bienenfeld, Vice Chair and Director of Residency Training at Wright State University, "the interview is the centerpiece of the application for psychiatric residency. Be prepared to demonstrate that you have thought clearly about your career decision, and about selecting the programs to which you are applying. Come with questions about the characteristics that define the program, such as its philosophies about teaching and learning and about psychiatric practice."[13]

Did you know?

You must have questions for the interviewer. Dr. Julie Niedermier is the Psychiatry Program Director at Ohio State University. What does Dr. Niedermier hate to be told? "I don't have any questions...they've all been answered already" is at the top of her list. "Candidates should have multiple questions prepared for any given interview." Good questions to ask, according to her, include:

- "Those suggesting the applicant has good insight into both residency and their career choice and beyond.
- Those referring to a sense of direction in a career or at least possible ideas about their future, as well as the future of the profession.
- Applicants showing self-awareness and able to reflect on this as it relates to patient interactions, communication and relationships with mentors (i.e., What changes have you anticipated or did not anticipate happening in the field of psychiatry? How has the profession changed since you were a resident?)"[14]

Advice for the Psychiatry Residency Interview	
Department of Psychiatry Texas Tech University	"Your interview affords the best opportunity for us to show off our program and for you to meet our residents and faculty and see our facilities. The interview will allow you to become acquainted with both our philosophy and practice for resident education and for you to determine if this philosophy meets your needs."[15]
Dr. Elana Miller Department of Psychiatry UCLA	"If you come across as arbitrarily having checked off a box on your ERAS program, however, — especially at a formidable program like UCLA — it won't reflect well. There was an applicant a few weeks ago, who despite having great scores and grades, came across as so disinterested in UCLA that she was ranked low enough as to have no chance of matching. You should be able to state why you're interested in the program, such as the reputation, the people, the research opportunities, the therapy training, etc. You're allowed to say the weather plays a part (let's be honest – it does!), but don't make this your sole reason for applying."[16]
Department of Psychiatry University of Michigan	"Following interviews, the Selection and Evaluation Committee will review candidates' application materials and comments of faculty, house officers, and staff who have interacted with the candidates to assess their potential for the program."[17]
Dr. Marcia Verduin Associate Dean/Professor Department of Psychiatry University of Central Florida	"Make sure you come up with 2 or 3 psychiatry patients you found interesting or challenging. I was asked about that a number of times. What did you learn from the patient? How did they influence your decision to go into psychiatry?"[18]
Dr. Deborah Spitz Program Director University of Chicago	"Be prepared to engage with the interviewers. They will want to know who you are and what you are passionate about in the field. Students should be prepared to be asked somewhat personal questions by some interviewers. Some more psychodynamic programs ask about family background and relationships; if you do not want to reveal much, you should not apply to those places."[19]
Dr. Mina Bak	"Interviewers have sometimes read the applicant's materials (not blinded interviews), but others have intentionally not (blinded interviews)."[12] In your interview preparation, consider how you would sell yourself to an interviewer who has not read your application. What are the key points you must get across?[7]

Did you know?

In one study, researchers asked residency training coordinators to complete a rating form about interviewed applicants. Coordinators were asked to rate candidates' attentiveness, communication, attitude, and professionalism. The question "Would you feel comfortable seeing this person as your doctor?" was also posed to the respondents. Residency candidates rated highly by coordinators were more likely to be ranked at the institution represented by the authors of the study. The authors wrote that "a 'No' answer to the question 'Would you feel comfortable seeing this person as your doctor?' was especially predictive of failure to match."[20]

References

[1]Thomas Jefferson University Department of Psychiatry. Available at http://www.jefferson.edu/university/jmc/departments/psychiatry/education/residency.html. Accessed May 2, 2013.

[2]Charting Outcomes in the Match (2014). Available at: http://www.nrmp.org/wp-content/uploads/2014/09/Charting-Outcomes-2014-Final.pdf. Accessed March 3, 2014.

[3]Advance Data Tables: 2016 Main Residency Match. Available at: http://www.nrmp.org/match-data/main-residency-match-data/. Accessed April 23, 2016.

[4]Brotherton S, Etzel S. Graduate Medical Education, 2014-2015. *JAMA* 2015; 314 (22): 2436-2454.

[5]Brotherton S, Etzel S. Graduate Medical Education, 2008-2009. *JAMA* 2009; 302 (12): 1357-1372.

[6]Results of the 2014 NRMP Program Director Survey. Available at: http://www.nrmp.org/wp-content/uploads/2014/09/PD-Survey-Report-2014.pdf. Accessed March 3, 2015.

[7]Bak M, Louie A, Tong L, Coverdale J, Roberts L. Applying to psychiatry residency. *Acad Psychiatry* 2006; 30 (3): 239-247.

[8]Spitz D, Penna N. Pritzker residency process guide: psychiatry. Available at http://pritzker.uchicago.edu/current/students/ResidencyProcessGuide.pdf. Accessed June 2, 2009.

[9]Servis M. A guide to the perplexed: residency guide. Available at http://www.ucdmc.ucdavis.edu. Accessed June 2, 2008.

[10]Lehrmann J, Walaszek A. Assessing the quality of residency applicants in psychiatry. *Acad Psychiatry* 2008; 32 (3): 180-182.

[11]Program Requirements around Passage of USMLE Step 2CK and USMLE Step 2CS. Available at: http://www.student.med.umn.edu/osr/wp-content/uploads/2012/09/Program-Requirements-around-Passage-of-USMLE-Step-2CK-and-USMLE-Step-2CS-11.pdf. Accessed April 1, 2013.

[12]Reilly E. Career counseling: psychiatry. Available at: http://www.uth.tmc.edu/med/administration/student/ms4/2003CCC.htm. Accessed June 2, 2009.

[13]Wright State University Department of Psychiatry. Available at: https://www.medu.wright.edu/2012/M3/Psy/CareersPsychiatry. Accessed September 22, 2012.

[14]Ohio State University Department of Psychiatry. Available at: http://medicine.osu.edu/students/life/career_advising/toolkit/Documents/Interviewing2012-2013.pdf. Accessed September 13, 2012.
[15]Texas Tech University Department of Psychiatry. Available at: http://www.ttuhsc.edu/som/psychiatry/residency/program.aspx. Accessed September 24, 2012.
[16]Zen Psychiatry. Available at: http://www.psych.med.umich.edu/education/general_psychiatry/howto.asp. Accessed September 24, 2012.
[17]University of Michigan Department of Psychiatry. Available at: http://zenpsychiatry.com/how-to-rock-your-psychiatry-residency-interview/. Accessed September 22, 2012.
[18]UCLA Psychiatry Student Interest Group. Available at: http://www.medstudent.ucla.edu/psychsig/?page_id=29. Accessed September 28, 2012.
[19]University of Chicago Department of Psychiatry. Available at: http://pritzker.uchicago.edu/current/students/ResidencyProcessGuide.pdf. Accessed September 22, 2012.
[20]Robinson S, Roberts N, Dzara K. Residency-coordinator perceptions of psychiatry residency candidates: a pilot study. *Acad Psychiatry* 2013; 37 (4): 265-267.

Chapter 41

Radiation Oncology

How competitive is the specialty?

Radiation oncology is a highly competitive specialty. In 2014, out of 188 U.S. seniors applying to radiation oncology, 20 failed to match (11%). Very few osteopathic and IMG applicants match successfully into the field. In 2014, 67% of these independent applicants failed to match.[1]

Highlights of the 2016 NRMP Radiation Oncology Match[2]

- There were a total of 183 positions at the PGY1 and PGY2 levels.
- 92% of positions were filled with allopathic medical student applicants.
- 4 osteopathic applicants matched.
- 1 U.S. IMG applicant matched.
- 3 non-U.S. IMG applicants matched.
- 5 U.S. graduates matched.
- 1 position was unfilled.

How many years of training are required to become a radiation oncologist?

To become a radiation oncologist, a minimum of 5 years of residency training is required. The first year of training can be completed in an accredited family medicine, internal medicine, pediatrics, surgery, or transitional year program.

What percentage of available positions is filled by U.S. seniors? What about other applicants?

In 2013 – 2014, there were 706 total residents training in a total of 88 radiation oncology residency programs.[3] 96% were U.S. MDs, 2.3% were international medical graduates, and 1.8% were osteopathic graduates.

Residents Training in U.S. Radiation Oncology Residency Programs[3-4]

Year	Residency Programs	Total # residents	% US MDs	% IMGs	% DO
2013-2014	90	706	95.9%	2.3%	1.8%
2007-2008	81	588	94.6%	3.7%	1.5%

How do programs select residents?

Every few years, the NRMP conducts a survey of PDs. In 2014, the NRMP surveyed 44 radiation oncology residency PDs to determine the factors important in selecting applicants to interview.[5] The top 4 factors are LORs in the specialty, USMLE Step 1/COMLEX Level 1 score, involvement and interest in research, and MSPE. Factors are shown in the table on the following page.

Factors Identified As Important in Selecting Applicants to Interview by Radiation Oncology Residency Program Directors	
Top Tier Factors (Cited by 70-99% of programs)	LORs in the specialty USMLE Step 1/COMLEX Level 1 score Involvement and interest in research MSPE Personal statement Audition elective within your department Perceived interest in program Honors in clinical clerkships Grades in required clerkships
Middle Tier Factors (Cited by 40-69% of programs)	Class rank AOA membership U.S. allopathic graduate USMLE Step 2 CK/COMLEX Level 2 score Honors in clerkship in desired specialty Grades in clerkship in desired specialty Perceived commitment to specialty Leadership qualities Professionalism and ethics Personal prior knowledge of the applicant Consistency of grades Volunteer/extracurricular experiences Graduate of well-regarded U.S. med school Interest in academic career Away rotation in your specialty at another institution
Lowest Tier Factors (Cited by < 40% of programs)	Visa status Gaps in medical education Honors in basic sciences Pass USMLE Step 2 CS/COMLEX Level PE Gold Society membership Fluency in language spoken by your patient population USMLE Step 3 score/COMLEX Step 3 score
Adapted from Results of the 2014 NRMP Program Director Survey. Available at: http://www.nrmp.org/wp-content/uploads/2014/09/PD-Survey-Report-2014.pdf.	

Did you know?

In 2014, approximately 45% of U.S. allopathic seniors who matched into radiation oncology had an additional graduate degree (Ph.D., MBA, MPH, M.S.).[1]

How important are audition electives?

Dr. Jeffrey Kuo, Program Director at the University of California-Irvine, states that "audition electives...are considered very helpful by most students and residency program directors so that one can become acquainted with the other."[6] Dr. Janice Ryu, former program director at the University of California-Davis, strongly recommends an audition elective, stating that "an elective rotation at the program of choice and a superb performance during that rotation is of foremost importance."[7]

How important are letters of recommendation?

Letters of recommendation are an essential component of the radiation oncology residency application. Residency programs heavily use these letters to make interview decisions. In a recent survey of radiation oncology PDs, 97% cited a LOR from a colleague in the specialty as an important factor in selecting applicants to interview.[5] Dr. Kuo states that "program directors have come to expect at least one audition elective in clinical radiation oncology with two to three letters from radiation oncology faculty."[6] "It is a good idea to get a mix of letters from nationally prominent faculty members, faculty who know you well, and those who have worked with you clinically," writes the Department of Radiation Oncology at the University of Chicago.[8]

Did you know?

"The best letters of recommendation are from faculty with whom you have had a long professional relationship. It is best to try to forge those relationships early. In our program, some of our faculty view the quality of the letters of recommendation as very important. At our program, we want at least 2 letters from radiation oncologists. More would be great, but a truly outstanding letter from a primary care physician is better than a mediocre letter from a radiation oncologist. We want to train outstanding physicians who happen to specialize in radiation oncology."[9]

Department of Radiation Oncology at the University of Washington

How important is the personal statement?

Dr. Phillip Connell of the University of Chicago states that the personal statement is "of moderate importance at some programs, while of major importance at others."[10]

Recommendations for Radiation Oncology Personal Statement	
Radiation Oncology Program	**Comments**
Dept. of Radiation Oncology Harvard University	"Explain any interruptions in your education. Tell us why you have chosen radiation oncology as your specialty."[11]
Dept. of Radiation Oncology University of Chicago	"The personal statement should be carefully thought out and well written. Be careful not to send up red flags suggesting that you may be unbalanced or difficult for one reason or another. It's best to be fairly conservative."[12]
Dept. of Radiation Oncology Loyola University Chicago Stritch School of Medicine	"The selection committee is most interested in what special qualities and experiences you have and what you hope to do with your radiation oncology training. The personal statement helps us to know you, and we read it with great care."[13]
Dept. of Radiation Oncology Virginia Commonwealth University School of Medicine	"Personal statements should include reasons why the applicant wishes to enter the field of radiation oncology and is best used to explain any discrepancies on their ERAS application."[14]

How important is AOA?

The NRMP reports that 23.6% of U.S. seniors who matched to radiation oncology in 2014 were members of AOA.[1]

How important is the USMLE?

Very important. The mean USMLE Step 1 score for 2014 applicants who matched was 241.[1]

When should I take the USMLE Step 2 CK?

A 2012 NRMP survey of 25 radiation oncology programs revealed that 4.8% of programs required passage of Step 2 CK for granting interviews. A higher percentage (13.6%) required passage for placement on the rank-order list.[15]

How important is research experience?

In 2006, Green surveyed radiation oncology PDs about the residency selection process. Program directors were asked to rate the importance of 16 criteria on a scale of 1 (unimportant) to 5 (critical).[5] Among 16 academic criteria, Green found that published research was tied for first in importance.[16] This is understandable given the emphasis radiation oncology residency programs place on research during residency. Many programs have up to one year of protected research time for their trainees.

Among 2014 U.S. senior applicants who matched, only 3 of the 169 applicants reported not having a single abstract, publication, or presentation. For U.S. seniors who matched, the mean number of abstracts, publications, and presentations was 12.2.[1] Dr. Ryu feels that research experience is highly desirable, increasing the strength of a candidate's application.[7]

Did you know?

There are other ways to gain exposure to radiation oncology during medical school. Students interested in policy and advocacy should consider the government relations internship program sponsored by the AMA and ASTRO. Known as GRIP, this is a 6-week program in Washington, D.C., which typically takes place during the summer between the first and second year of medical school.[17]

How important is the interview?

As is the case with other competitive specialties, the interview is of immense importance.

References

[1]Charting Outcomes in the Match (2014). Available at: http://www.nrmp.org/wp-content/uploads/2014/09/Charting-Outcomes-2014-Final.pdf. Accessed March 3, 2014.
[2]Advance Data Tables: 2016 Main Residency Match. Available at: http://www.nrmp.org/match-data/main-residency-match-data/. Accessed April 23, 2016.
[3]Brotherton S, Etzel S. Graduate Medical Education, 2014-2015. *JAMA* 2015; 314 (22): 2436-2454.
[4]Brotherton S, Etzel S. Graduate Medical Education, 2008-2009. *JAMA* 2009; 302 (12): 1357-1372.
[5]Results of the 2014 NRMP Program Director Survey. Available at: http://www.nrmp.org/wp-content/uploads/2014/09/PD-Survey-Report-2014.pdf. Accessed March 3, 2015.
[6]Kuo J. Residency selection handbook: radiation oncology. Available at http://www.ucihs.uci.edu. Accessed June 2, 2009.
[7]Ryu J. A guide to the perplexed: residency guide. Available at http://www.ucdmc.ucdavis.edu. Accessed June 2, 2009.
[8]University of Chicago Department of Radiation Oncology. Available at: http://pritzker.uchicago.edu/current/students/ResidencyProcessGuide.pdf. Accessed March 21, 2013.
[9]University of Washington Department of Radiation Oncology. Available at: www.uwmedicine.org/.../Dept-Career-Advisors-Survey04072011.pdf. Accessed March 4, 2013.
[10]Connell P. Pritzker residency process guide: radiation oncology. Available at http://pritzker.uchicago.edu/current/students/ResidencyProcessGuide.pdf. Accessed June 2, 2009.
[11]Harvard University Department of Radiation Oncology. Available at: http://www.harvardradonc.org/apply.asp. Accessed March 3, 2013.
[12]University of Chicago Department of Radiation Oncology. Available at: http://pritzker.uchicago.edu/current/students/ResidencyProcessGuide.pdf. Accessed March 21, 2013.
[13]Loyola University Chicago Department of Radiation Oncology. Available at: http://www.stritch.luc.edu/depts/radonc/resident/applying.htm. Accessed March 24, 2013.
[14]VCU Department of Radiation Oncology. Available at: http://www.massey.vcu.edu/radiation-oncology-clinical-residency-program.htm. Accessed March 24, 2013.
[15]Program Requirements around Passage of USMLE Step 2CK and USMLE Step 2CS. Available at: http://www.student.med.umn.edu/osr/wp-content/uploads/2012/09/Program-Requirements-around-Passage-of-USMLE-Step-2CK-and-USMLE-Step-2CS-11.pdf. Accessed April 1, 2013.
[16]Green M, Jones P, Thomas J. Selection criteria for residency: results of a national program director survey. *Acad Med* 2009; 84 (3): 362-7.
[17]Agarwal A, DeNunzio N, Ahuja D, Hirsch A. Beyond the standard curriculum: a review of available opportunities for medical students to prepare for a career in radiation oncology. *Int J Radiat Oncol Bio Phys* 2014; 88 (1): 39-44.

Chapter 42

Radiology

How competitive is the specialty?

Interest in radiology as a career among U.S. allopathic medical students has declined considerably over the past 5 years, mainly due to concerns about the job market. The 7th most competitive specialty in 2009, radiology fell to 15th among a group of 21 specialties in 2014.[1]

In the 2014 match, there were 81 unfilled positions, a number exceeded only by pathology.[2] Despite this, positions in coveted programs remain difficult to secure. "We typically receive over 700 applications for 12 residency positions," wrote Dr. Evan Siegelman, Chair of the Radiology Residency Selection Committee at the University of Pennsylvania.[3] Although osteopathic and IMG applicants have more difficulty matching successfully, only 30% of these independent applicants failed to match in 2014.[1] As a point of comparison, in 2009, 66% of independent applicants failed to match.

> **Did you know?**
>
> Osteopathic applicants may also apply to 16 AOA-approved radiology residency programs.

> **Highlights of the 2016 NRMP Radiology Match[2]**
>
> - There were a total of 1,133 positions at the PGY1 and PGY2 levels.
> - 67% of positions were filled with allopathic medical student applicants.
> - 108 osteopathic applicants matched.
> - 76 U.S. IMG applicants matched.
> - 107 non-U.S. IMG applicants matched.
> - 43 U.S. graduates matched.
> - 45 positions went unfilled.

How many years of training are required to become a radiologist?

To become a radiologist, a minimum of 5 years of residency training is required. This includes a preliminary year of training in clinical medicine.

What percentage of available positions is filled by U.S. seniors? What about other applicants?

In 2013 – 2014, there were 4,386 total residents training in a total of 185 radiology residency programs.[4] 84% were U.S. MDs, 9.0% were international medical graduates, and 6.2% were osteopathic graduates.

Residents Training in U.S. Radiology Residency Programs[4-5]					
Year	**Residency Programs**	**Total # residents**	**% US MDs**	**% IMGs**	**% DO**
2013-2014	185	4386	84.4%	9.4%	6.2%
2007-2008	188	4455	88.3%	7.6%	3.9%

How do programs select residents?

Every few years, the NRMP conducts a survey of PDs. In 2014, the NRMP surveyed 75 radiology PDs to determine the factors that are important in selecting applicants to interview.[6] The top 3 factors are USMLE Step 1/COMLEX Level 1 score, MSPE, and class rank. The findings are shown in the table on the next page.

How important is the USMLE?

99% of programs cited the USMLE Step 1 score as a factor used in selecting applicants to interview.[6] The mean USMLE Step 1 score for U.S. seniors who matched in 2014 was 241. Of note, although there were few applicants with USMLE Step 1 scores below 210 who applied to radiology, most matched.[1]

When should I take the USMLE Step 2 CK?

A 2012 NRMP survey of 90 radiology programs revealed that 22.9% of programs required passage of Step 2 CK for placement on the rank-order list.[7]

Did you know?

In a survey of 140 radiology PDs, researchers learned that "programs use an applicant's location as a proxy for true interest in the program, and interest in the program is important for granting interviews and final ranking." The survey also revealed that most programs will invite local applicants even if applicants do not clearly signal their interest.[8]

Factors Identified As Important in Selecting Applicants to Interview by Radiology Residency Program Directors	
Top Tier Factors (Cited by 70-99% of programs)	USMLE Step 1/COMLEX Level 1 score MSPE Class rank LORs in the specialty AOA membership Personal statement U.S. allopathic graduate Honors in clinical clerkships Grades in required clerkships Gaps in medical education
Middle Tier Factors (Cited by 40-69% of programs)	USMLE Step 2 CK/COMLEX Level 2 score Audition elective within your department Honors in clerkship in desired specialty Grades in clerkship in desired specialty Honors in basic sciences Perceived commitment to specialty Leadership qualities Professionalism and ethics Involvement and interest in research Personal prior knowledge of the applicant Perceived interest in program Consistency of grades Volunteer/extracurricular experiences Graduate of well-regarded U.S. med school Visa status
Lowest Tier Factors (Cited by < 40% of programs)	Interest in academic career Away rotation in your specialty at another institution Pass USMLE Step 2 CS/COMLEX Level PE Gold Society membership Fluency in language spoken by your patient population USMLE Step 3 score/COMLEX Step 3 score
Adapted from Results of the 2014 NRMP Program Director Survey. Available at: http://www.nrmp.org/wp-content/uploads/2014/09/PD-Survey-Report-2014.pdf.	

How important are letters of recommendation?

Letters of recommendation are cited by most radiology residency programs as an important factor used to make interview decisions. For most applicants, one letter from a radiologist with whom you have worked closely is sufficient. The other letters can come from other departments such as internal medicine, pediatrics, obstetrics & gynecology, and surgery. Dr. Judith Amorosa, former program director at the UMDNJ/Robert Wood Johnson Medical School, cautions applicants about obtaining letters from well-known faculty. "Someone who is well known but who doesn't know the student very well may be less enthusiastic about her."[9] Additional advice for LORs is presented in the table below.

Advice for Radiology Letters of Recommendation	
Dr. Donna Magid Director of Undergraduate Medical Education in Imaging Johns Hopkins University	"..plan to get 4-5 letters of reference. You can submit up to 4 letters per program. Plan on 4 in case one writer doesn't get it done, you have a back-up letter."[10]
Dr. Sandeep Deshmukh Chairman Residency Selection Committee Department of Radiology Thomas Jefferson University	"I expect every letter of recommendation to be good; if there is anything negative or weak in the letter, it reflects poorly on the applicant (i.e., you had bad judgment in asking someone who wasn't going to write an awesome letter). As far as radiology goes, letters from radiologists tend to be weak, unless you have spent a significant amount of time working with the radiologist…I would much rather read a letter from a medicine, surgery, pediatrics, OB/GYN, or psychiatry attending who spent a significant amount of time with you during a clerkship and can comment on your fund of knowledge, work ethic, and logical reasoning skills, as well as your personality."[11]
Dr. Sandra Oldham Program Director Department of Radiology University of Texas Houston	"I want to read about something special about you….how you came in early, stayed late, were enthusiastic, a description of an event during the rotation that demonstrated to the writer your sense of curiosity, that you knew not only your patients but your colleagues' patients, when you did not know an answer you looked it up and learned about it, how you treated a patient on your service devotedly and stayed up all night regulating their insulin doses. That is personal stuff not on your CV which makes for a very good read."[12]
Department of Radiology University of Michigan	"It is almost always better to have a letter from a department chairman or full professor than one from assistant professors and young faculty, unless of course that person is able to write a significantly stronger recommendation. In addition, it is better to get letters of recommendation from strong academic medical centers than from smaller, less well-known medical schools and medical centers. In other words, the higher up and more senior the letter writer and the better the medical school or institution that that letter writer is from, the more effective the letter will be."[13]

How important is the personal statement?

According to the NRMP, 74% of programs considered the statement to be useful for selecting an applicant to interview.[6]

In an analysis of personal statements submitted to one radiology residency program, Dr. Smith of the Wayne State University School of Medicine sought to determine the components of a statement considered most important to members of the selection committee. Most important was that an applicant clearly expressed his reasons for pursuing a career in radiology. Also considered important were the applicant's perception of radiology, defined as the applicant explicitly stating "what he/she feels are the important characteristics of either radiologists or the practice of radiology...and mention of applicant's personality traits or skills that would affect their training in a positive manner."[14]

Dr. Rosenbaum, former program director at the University of Chicago, states that "if you are applying out of state, make sure it is clear why you would be interested in coming to that city or state. With the number of applicants, if a program does not think you are likely to want to come there, they probably will not grant you an interview."[15] Consider using the personal statement to express your specific interest.

Advice for the Radiology Personal Statement	
Dr. Nolan Kagetsu Program Director Department of Radiology St. Luke's – Roosevelt Hospital	Dr. Kagetsu encourages applicants to include specific examples in the statement. "If you state that you handle stress well, you should describe a situation where you handled stress well…For example, 'I like the high tech aspects of neuroradiology.' vs. describing a case with a diffusion/perfusion mismatch, the neurointerventional team lysed the clot, and the patient had no permanent deficit."[16]
Dr. Sravanthi Reddy Chief of Emergency Radiology University of Southern California	"It will increase your odds of getting an interview at certain locations, if you include a few lines on why you want to go to the area or to a specific program."[17]
Dr. Donna Magid Assistant Program Director Johns Hopkins University	"Trust me, committees will not overlook the misspelled word or poorly phrased thought. Radiologists worship precision, accuracy, and the written and spoken word."[10]
Department of Radiology University of California Davis	"The personal statement is important in the decision to extend an interview invitation. It should be personal, addressing the candidates' attributes and personal characteristics that would make them enjoyable to work with. The candidate should try to avoid generic explanations of what Radiology encompasses, as this does not add to their application."[18]
Dr. Sandra Oldham Program Director Department of Radiology University of Texas Houston	"Tell me a story about yourself or your family that gives me a glimpse about your true self. Tell me about things that have happened in your life that demonstrate your enthusiasm, curiosity, resilience, ability to be a team player, and ability to be a team leader. Tall order? You bet, but it's a tough residency to get into and putting a lot of thought into the personal statement can make the difference."[12]
Dr. Vicki Marx Program Director Department of Radiology University of Southern California	"The personal statement is hard to write because no one gets taught how to write well about themselves…ERAS application components (transcript, MSPE, etc) do a pretty good job of explaining each applicant's who, what, where, and when. The personal statement gives you the opportunity to talk about your "why", to explain your past, your stumbles, your dreams for the future, your motivations for living the life you live, and your reasons for working towards the goals you have set for yourself. A successful personal statement answers "why" in a way that is sincere and succinct. You don't need quotes from obscure literature. You don't need references to "Where's Waldo?" You do need honest reflection, clear communication, and ruthless editing."[19]

How important is AOA?

AOA members accounted for 21.8% of U.S. seniors who matched in 2014 (25.8% in 2007).[1]

How important are away electives in the specialty?

Away electives in radiology are not as highly valued as other selection criteria. In a survey of radiology PDs, an audition elective was ranked fifteenth among a group of 16 criteria.[6] "An 'away' rotation is neither required nor expected of our applicants," writes the University of California San Francisco Department of Radiology.[10]

Advice for Radiology Away Electives	
Dr. Sravanthi Reddy Chief of Emergency Radiology University of Southern California	"Aim at your high target programs, i.e., not your 'reach' programs, where you are likely to get an interview anyway."[17]
Department of Radiology University of Michigan	"If you happen to be at a medical school with a very strong radiology department, then a rotation in that department with recommendations from the radiologists in that department would probably serve you better than doing an away rotation at a less strong radiology department. If you happen to be at a small medical school or a medical school that does not have a well-recognized radiology department, then an away rotation at a better medical school (or one with a stronger radiology department or a more well recognized radiology staff) would prove quite useful, chiefly because of the recommendations you could potentially garner during that rotation."[13]
Dr. Vicki Marx Program Director University of Southern California	"The away rotation is a mixed bag because the student is in the position of being interviewed by the program over a period of weeks instead of minutes. For most people this is great but for a few it isn't. The investment and anxiety are most likely to be worthwhile when the student has a well-informed opinion that the program is where s/he wants to do residency. The drive could be geographic or academic…The student should explain the reasons for doing the away rotation openly and honestly with the clerkship director and the residency program director early in the rotation. The rest of the clerkship should be spent in sustained effort to do a good job and to learn more about the program. The student should meet with the program director a second time near completion of the rotation as a courtesy and to remind the PD about his/her interest. We are old. If you don't remind us (politely and without being pushy) we will forget."[19]

How important is research experience?

Although research is among the least important criteria in the selection process, note that some radiology programs seek to recruit candidates who will pursue careers in academic radiology. These programs may place more emphasis on published research. One study showed that pre-residency academic productivity in the form of multiple publications was associated with an increased likelihood of future academic success.[20] Dr. Judith Amorosa states that "starting a research elective near the end of the third year in medical school can be challenging. If there is adequate infrastructure and close mentoring, it is possible to accomplish a project that may even be submitted to a national meeting and eventually be published."[9]

Did you know?

In a study at a single institution, researchers examined publications listed on the residency application as "accepted," "in press," "provisionally accepted," or "submitted." One-third of manuscripts listed were unpublished at the time of the residency application. Two years later, slightly more than half of those listed as "submitted" and even less of those listed as "accepted", "in press," or "submitted" were published. "Residency selection committees should consider these publication rates when assessing applicants," wrote the authors.[21]

Did you know?

In one study, researchers determined the rate of misrepresentation of publications among applicants for radiology residency during one application cycle. Among 138 applicants citing one or more publications, there were 5 misrepresentations. These included:

- An article not found in the journal listed.
- A listed journal that could not be found.
- An article in which the author's name did not appear
- Several articles in which the author's name was not listed in the correct position.

"It is reasonable to request that applicants bring to their interviews a copy of each cited article and to assess their knowledge of all other listed research activities," wrote the authors.[22]

How important is the interview?

The interview is ranked as the most important factor used to make rank-order list decisions. A study performed at one radiology program demonstrated a strong correlation between interview scores and final applicant ranking, but a poor correlation between pre-interview scores and final applicant ranking. This highlights the importance of the interview in the ranking of applicants.[23]

Did you know?

In an interview with Dr. Vicki Marx, Program Director at the University of Southern California, we asked Dr. Marx about the personal qualities associated with success in radiology:[19]

A successful radiology resident first and foremost recognizes the critical role that radiology plays in patient care and enjoys the responsibility of that role. Successful residents behave professionally in all work activities and put the needs of patients above their own, within the constraints imposed by ACGME work hour rules. Successful residents interpret as many studies as possible and work hard to learn the clinical judgment, decision-making skills, and communication skills (spoken and written) necessary to ensure that their interpretations are meaningful in real time. A successful resident is a positive contributor to a team that includes the residency class, the residency as a whole, the faculty, the non-physician members of the department, the referring physicians, and the institution. A successful radiology resident is smart, hardworking, honest, and focused. That focus must be maintained in three spheres: clinical work, home study, and relaxation time with friends and family away from work. All of these personal attributes require an underlying positive energy for being a physician and specific enthusiasm for the specialty of Diagnostic Radiology that is easy to communicate to an interviewer.

Advice for Radiology Residency Interview	
Department of Radiology Stanford University	"Radiology faculty and residents work one-on-one every day, all day, throughout the residency program. Therefore, the interview is our most important factor in resident selection. When the dust has settled and USMLE and clerkship grades have been tabulated, MSPE and recommendation letters have been decrypted, and personal statements have been deconstructed, the selection process comes down to whether we feel applicants' character and personality are a good fit for our program."[24]
Dr. James Silberzweig Program Director Beth Israel Medical Center	"We plan to discuss your strengths, goals, values, professional and personal interests, research, and other aspects of your background and training. We are interested in what you consider important in a training program."[25]
Dr. Sandeep Deshmukh Chairman of the Residency Selection Committee for Radiology Thomas Jefferson University	"In my eyes, it is bad judgment for you not to ask questions; in half a day, or a full day, there is no way you could possibly know everything about our residency. Ask intelligent questions; it definitely gets noticed. This means you may need to do some homework on the program in advance. Check out their website and see what you can find out online."[11]

Did you know?

Many residency programs tend to prefer students located in the same geographical region because of the belief that students with a connection to the area are likely to perform better as residents. In an interview with Dr. Vicki Marx, Program Director at the University of Southern California, we asked Dr. Marx what she thought would be the best way for applicants to communicate an interest in a specific program:[19]

The applicant's primary goal is to make sure the program director (or designee) knows that the student has a sincere and focused interest in this particular program. The secondary goal is to avoid being annoying during this effort! Two points in the application process create natural opportunities for such interest to be brought to the application screener's attention. The first is a focused personal statement where the interest in a particular program is clearly articulated for the reader. This strategy requires careful attention to detail – don't send a tailored personal statement intended for one program to all the programs! The second is an email to the program director and program coordinator after being rejected or waitlisted for an interview. The email serves the same purpose as the focused personal statement: to articulate clearly the reasons the applicant has for being interested in the program and the willingness to interview on short notice should an opportunity become available. If no response comes to the email, a phone call to the program coordinator is a reasonable step – to make sure the email was received. Then you wait. You may get an interview and you may not. There are no guarantees in this difficult process.

Speaking from my own experience as a program director, I do have a bit of advice about actions to avoid if you want to increase your interview opportunities. First, do not make multiple phone calls to the department. Listen carefully to what is said in the first phone call and live with it. Second, do not trash the program in question on a public internet forum. Your username may be less anonymous than you think! Finally, do not let one of your parents, or one of their friends who has connections with the institution, call the department on your behalf. Those phone calls are uncomfortable for all involved and do nothing to change the content of your application.

References

[1]Charting Outcomes in the Match (2014). Available at: http://www.nrmp.org/wp-content/uploads/2014/09/Charting-Outcomes-2014-Final.pdf. Accessed March 3, 2014.
[2]Advance Data Tables: 2016 Main Residency Match. Available at: http://www.nrmp.org/match-data/main-residency-match-data/. Accessed April 23, 2016.
[3]University of Pennsylvania Department of Radiology. Available at http://www.uphs.upenn.edu/radiology/education/residency/hup/apply.html. Accessed September 28, 2015.
[4]Brotherton S, Etzel S. Graduate Medical Education, 2014-2015. *JAMA* 2015; 314 (22): 2436-2454.
[5]Brotherton S, Etzel S. Graduate Medical Education, 2008-2009. *JAMA* 2009; 302 (12): 1357-1372.
[6]Results of the 2014 NRMP Program Director Survey. Available at: http://www.nrmp.org/wp-content/uploads/2014/09/PD-Survey-Report-2014.pdf. Accessed March 3, 2015.
[7]Program Requirements around Passage of USMLE Step 2CK and USMLE Step 2CS. Available at: http://www.student.med.umn.edu/osr/wp-content/uploads/2012/09/Program-Requirements-around-Passage-of-USMLE-Step-2CK-and-USMLE-Step-2CS-11.pdf. Accessed April 1, 2013.
[8]Deloney L, Rozenshtein A, Deitte L, Mullins M, Robbin M. What program directors think: results of the 2011 annual survey of the Association of Program Directors in Radiology. *Acad Radiol* 2012; 19 (12): 1583-8.
[9]Amorosa J. How do I mentor medical students interested in radiology. *Acad Radiol* 2003; 10: 527-535.
[10]Apps of Steel. Available at: www.rad.jhmi.edu/residents/documents/apps-of-steel.pdf. Accessed April 26, 2012.
[11]StudentDoc. Available at: http://www.studentdoc.com/medical-training.html. Accessed April 26, 2012.
[12]University of Texas Houston Medical School Guide to the Radiology Match. Available at: http://www.uth.tmc.edu/radiology/radiology-match-guide/index.html. Accessed April 26, 2012.
[13]University of Michigan Department of Radiology. Available at: http://sitemaker.umich.edu/radiologyintgroup/frequently_asked_questions#9. Accessed April 23, 2012.
[14]Smith E, Weyhing B, Mody Y, Smith W. A critical analysis of personal statements submitted by radiology residency applicants. *Acad Rad* 2005; 12: 1024-8.
[15]Rosenblum J. Pritzker residency process guide: radiology. Available at http://pritzker.uchicago.edu/current/students/ResidencyProcessGuide.pdf.
[16]St. Luke's – Roosevelt Department of Radiology. Available at: http://www.stlukesrooseveltradiology.org/application-procedures. Accessed April 12, 2012.
[17]AMSER Guide to Applying for Radiology Residency. Available at: *xray.stanford.edu/.../AMSER_Guide_Applying_for_Radiology_Residency_2010_.pdf.* Accessed April 26, 2012.
[18]University of California Davis Department of Radiology. Available at: http://www.ucdmc.ucdavis.edu/mdprogram/class-information/pdfs/ElectiveSuggestions.pdf. Accessed April 20, 2012.
[19]The Successful Match: Getting into Radiology. Available at: http://studentdoctor.net/2010/10/the-successful-match-getting-into-radiology/. Accessed April 26, 2012.
[20]Rezek I, McDonald R, Kallmes D. Pre-residency publication rate strongly predicts future academic radiology potential. *Acad Radiol* 2012; 19 (5): 632-4.

[21]Grimm L, Maxfield C. Ultimate publication rate of unpublished manuscripts listed on radiology residency applications at one institution. *Acad Med* 2013; 88 (11): 1719-22.
[22]Eisenberg R, Cunningham M, Kung J, Slanetz P. Misrepresentation of publications by radiology residency applicants: is it really a problem? *J Am Coll Radiol* 2013; 10 (3): 195-7.
[23]Mt. Sinai School of Medicine Secrets of the Match. Available at: students.mssm.edu/groups/radiology/files/Match2010.doc. Accessed April 26, 2012.
[24]Stanford University Department of Radiology. Available at: http://xray.stanford.edu/AP/timeline.html.
Accessed April 19, 2012.
[25]Beth Israel Medical Center Department of Radiology. Available at: http://www.bethisraelradiology.com/contact-us/frequently-asked-questions. Accessed August 18, 2012.

Chapter 43

Urology

How competitive is the specialty?

Urology is a highly competitive specialty. In 2016, 23% of U.S. seniors failed to match. Matching successfully is considerably more difficult for osteopathic and international medical graduates. In 2016, 83% of international medical graduate applicants failed to match.[1] Programs typically receive hundreds of applications for just a few positions. In 2014, the Brady Urological Institute at Johns Hopkins University received 260 applications. From this group, 39 were interviewed to fill a class of three.[2] Of note, Urology has its own matching program – Urology Residency Match Program – administered by the American Urological Association. The Urology Match takes place in January.

Highlights of the 2016 Urology Residency Match[1]

- There were a total of 295 positions.
- 77% of U.S. seniors matched.
- 47% of previous U.S. graduates matched.
- 17% of IMG applicants matched.

Did you know?

Osteopathic applicants may also apply to 11 AOA-approved urology residency programs.

How many years of training are required to become a urologist?

To become a urologist, a minimum of 5 years of residency training is required. The first year or two of training must be completed in an accredited general surgery training program. Note that some programs have added an additional year devoted to research.

What percentage of available positions is filled by U.S. seniors? What about other applicants?

In 2013 – 2014, there were 1,201 total residents training in a total of 126 urology residency programs.[3] 94% were U.S. MDs, 4.1% were international medical graduates, and 1.2% were osteopathic graduates.

Residents Training in U.S. Urology Residency Programs (Allopathic)[3-4]					
Year	**Residency Programs**	**Total # residents**	**% US MDs**	**% IMGs**	**% DO**
2013-2014	126	1201	93.9%	4.7%	1.2%
2007-2008	118	1031	94.2%	4.6%	1.2%

How do programs select residents?

In 2014, researchers from the University of Pennsylvania surveyed 76 urology PDs to determine factors important in selecting applicants for interviewing and matching.[5]

Importance of Factors in Selecting Urology Applicants for Interviewing and Matching	
Factor	**Mean Importance Rating***
Urology references	8.6
USMLE scores	8.6
Grade in urology	7.4
AOA status	7.4
Class rank	7.1
Research publications	7.1
Grade in surgery	7.0
Grades in nonsurgical clinical rotations	6.1
Dean's letter of recommendation	5.4
Community service	5.2
College/university prestige	5.2
Nonsurgical references	4.9
Athletic prowess	4.6

*Survey participants were asked to rank each item on a scale of 1 (no importance) to 10 (most important).

Weissbart S, Stock J, Wein A. Program directors' criteria for selection into urology residency. *Urology* 2015; 85 (4): 731-6.

The authors also inquired about factors that would lead programs to downgrade applicants. The following factors were considered to be a significant downgrade by at least 50% of respondents:

- USMLE Step 1 score < 220
- USMLE Step 2 CK score < 220
- Previous match failure

- Not being in the top 40% of the class
- Current postgraduate year 1 (PGY1) for any reason
- Zero research publications or presentations
- No honors in surgery

Applicants with one or more of these factors should discuss their credentials with a specialty-specific advisor, and develop a strategy to overcome any obstacles.

How important are audition electives?

In Weissbart's study, 86.8% of PDs reported giving special consideration to applicants who had completed an audition elective at their institution.[5] Most advisors recommend performing 1 – 2 away electives, preferably in the summer before applying for residency.

How important are letters of recommendation?

Letters of recommendation are an essential component of the urology residency application. In fact, letters written by urologists are as highly valued as USMLE Step 1 scores in the selection process. Dr. Joseph Schmidt, former chairman of the urology department at University of California San Diego, considers LORs to be one of the most important components of the application. "They are especially significant when coming from practicing urologists and particularly important if those urologists are in academic health centers and well known to my faculty or me."[6] This sentiment is substantiated by the results of Weissbart's study in which references from urologists were much more valued than nonsurgical references.[5]

Did you know?

"A letter of recommendation from the Chair of Urology is desirable; some residency programs may ask for this specifically. After you have met with your advisor and selected those programs to which you will apply, you should make an appointment with the Chair so that he or she can meet with you in anticipation of writing a letter on your behalf."[7]

Northwestern University Department of Urology

How important is the personal statement?

Dr. Charles Brendler, former chairman of the Section of Urology at the University of Chicago, encourages applicants to "emphasize some unique aspect of your life which will catch the interest of the reader. Remember that the reviewer will probably be reading at least 200 of these statements."[8] Dr. Michael Ritchey, a faculty member in the Department of Pediatric Urology at Phoenix Children's Hospital, writes that "the personal statement should be short and concise. Some programs like applicants to indicate a preference for an academic career."[9]

How important is the USMLE?

The two most highly rated factors in the selection process are USMLE scores and urology references. Dr. Chad Ritenour, Program Director at Emory, states "honestly, at most programs, I believe board scores, as they are the only objective standard, carry the most initial weight."[10] Low-scoring applicants must strengthen every component of the application to maximize chances of a successful match. Working closely with a urology-specific advisor is highly recommended.

How important is research experience?

Dr. Martha Terris, Program Director at the Medical College of Georgia, states that "participation in a research project will improve the chances of matching with a program high on their list. The more in depth the research, the more the application is enhanced. Research does not necessarily have to be in the field of urology to boost one's application."[11] Dr. Bernard Fallon, former program director at the University of Iowa, encourages applicants to participate in research. Starting early in medical school is preferable, with the goal being to "get at least one publication from this involvement."[12] Dr. Roger Low, former program director at the University of California Davis, writes that "research is highly desirable; most invited for interview are involved in past research."[13]

Did you know?

Several studies have examined the rate of publication misrepresentation among urology residency applicants. In one review of applications submitted to a single program during one cycle, researchers found misrepresentation in 3.5% of published articles. Among the findings was self-promotion to first-authorship and non-existent articles.[14] In another analysis of applications received by a single program, 19% of applicants had at least one unverifiable publication.[15]

How important is the interview?

Very important. Dr. Arieh Shalhav, Chief of the Section of Urology at the University of Chicago, urges applicants to "listen carefully to the information provided and presented by the program prior to your actual interview and formulate your questions based on the information provided."[16] Of note, programs may ask you to return for second look interviews. In one survey of applicants, 79% of respondents returned for such interviews at least once.[17]

Did you know?

How much money do urology residency applicants spend in their efforts to match? In a survey of 173 applicants, researchers learned that the average per interview cost was approximately $ 500. Applicants had a mean of 14 interviews.[18]

References

[1]American Urological Association. Available at https://www.auanet.org/education/urology-and-specialty-matches.cfm. Accessed April 8, 2016.
[2]Brady Urological Institute at Johns Hopkins University. Available at http://bradyurology.blogspot.com/2014/12/application-season-for-urology.html. Accessed September 28, 2015.
[3]Brotherton S, Etzel S. Graduate Medical Education, 2014-2015. *JAMA* 2015; 314 (22): 2436-2454.
[4]Brotherton S, Etzel S. Graduate Medical Education, 2008-2009. *JAMA* 2009; 302 (12): 1357-1372.
[5]Weissbart S, Stock J, Wein A. Program directors' criteria for selection into urology residency. *Urology* 2015; 85 (4): 731-736.
[6]Urology Match. Available at: http://www.urologymatch.com/node/354. Accessed December 14, 2015.
[7]Application for Urology Residency: Information for medical students. Available at: http://www.feinberg.northwestern.edu/education/docs/current-students/Urology-2013-MS4-match-guide.pdf. Accessed December 14, 2015.
[8]Urology Match. Available at: http://www.urologymatch.com/node/188. Accessed December 14, 2015.
[9]Ritchey M. Career counseling: urology. Available at: http://www.uth.tmc.edu//med/administration/student/ms4/2003CCC.htm. Accessed January 2, 2008.
[10]Urology Match. Available at: http://www.urologymatch.com/node/356. Accessed December 14, 2015.
[11]Urology Match. Available at: http://www.urologymatch.com/faculty-survey-results?page=4. Accessed December 14, 2015.
[12]Urology Match. Available at: http://urologymatch.yuku.com/topic/1361/Iowa-University-of-Iowa-Program. Accessed December 14, 2015.
[13]Low R. A guide to the perplexed: residency guide. Available at: http://ucdmc.ucdavis.edu. Accessed September 2, 2008.
[14]Hsi R, Hotaling J, Moore T, Joyner B. Publication misrepresentation among urology residency applicants. *World J Urol* 2013; 31 (3): 697-702.
[15]Nosnik I, Friedmann P, Nagler H, Dinlenc C. Resume fraud: unverifiable publications of urology training program applicants. *J Urol* 2010; 183 (4): 1520-1523.
[16]Pritzker residency process guide: urology. Available at: http://pritzker.uchicago.edu/current/students/Residency ProcessGuide.pdf. Accessed September 2, 2008.
[17]Nikonow T, Lyon T, Jackman S, Averch T. Survey of applicant experience and cost in the urology match: opportunities for reform. *J Urol* 2015; 194 (4): 1063-1067.

Chapter 44

Vascular Surgery

How competitive is the specialty?

Traditionally, applicants interested in vascular surgery were required to complete general surgery residency training first. However, there are now several training pathways for aspiring vascular surgeons. In 2006, the ACGME approved the integrated track, allowing medical students to match during medical school. Within this 0 + 5 model are two years devoted to core surgical training and three years devoted to vascular surgery. Vascular surgery is a competitive specialty. "Applicants to 0 + 5 programs are comparable to the top tier of General Surgery applicants at our institution," writes Dr. John Rectenwald, Program Director of the Vascular Surgery Residency Program at the University of Michigan.[1] In the 2014 NRMP Match, there were 90 applicants seeking positions for only 44 spots.[2] Applicants who fail to match still have the option to enter the specialty following five years of general surgery residency training (5 + 2 model).

How many years of training are required to become a vascular surgeon?

To become a vascular surgeon through the integrated pathway, a minimum of five years of residency training is required.

What percentage of available positions is filled by U.S. seniors? What about other applicants?

In 2013 – 2014, there were 211 total residents training in a total of 51 integrated vascular surgery residency programs.[3] 88% were U.S. MDs, 8.5% were international medical graduates, and 3.8% were osteopathic graduates.

How do programs select residents?

Every few years, the NRMP conducts its own survey of PDs. In 2014, the NRMP surveyed 22 vascular surgery PDs to determine factors important in selecting applicants to interview.[4] The top 4 factors are LORs in the specialty, USMLE Step 1/COMLEX Level 1 score, USMLE Step 2 CK/COMLEX Level 2 score, and personal statement. The findings are shown in the following table.

Factors Identified As Important in Selecting Applicants to Interview by Vascular Surgery Residency Program Directors	
Top Tier Factors (Cited by 70-99% of programs)	LORs in the specialty USMLE Step 1/COMLEX Level 1 score USMLE Step 2 CK/COMLEX Level 2 score Personal statement Perceived commitment to specialty MSPE Honors in clinical clerkships Honors in clerkship in desired specialty Involvement and interest in research
Middle Tier Factors (Cited by 40-69% of programs)	U.S. allopathic graduate Grades in required clerkships Class rank Professionalism and ethics Personal prior knowledge of the applicant Audition elective within your department Grades in clerkship in desired specialty Leadership qualities AOA membership Pass USMLE Step 2 CS/COMLEX Level PE Perceived interest in program Consistency of grades Volunteer/extracurricular experiences Graduate of well-regarded U.S. med school Visa status Interest in academic career
Lowest Tier Factors (Cited by < 40% of programs)	Away rotation in your specialty at another institution Gold Society membership Fluency in language spoken by your patient population USMLE Step 3 score/COMLEX Step 3 score Honors in basic sciences Gaps in medical education
Adapted from Results of the 2014 NRMP Program Director Survey. Available at: http://www.nrmp.org/wp-content/uploads/2014/09/PD-Survey-Report-2014.pdf.	

Did you know?

In an analysis of 190 applicants to the integrated vascular surgery residency program at Stanford University from 2008 to 2011, researchers examined the credentials and accomplishments of applicants. Among the notable findings:

- 48% had honored their surgery clerkship.
- 27% were members of AOA.
- 40% were in the top quartile of their graduating class.
- 72% reported at least one publication.
- On average applicants listed 4.4 publications.[5]

How important is the USMLE?

95% of programs cite the USMLE Step 1 score as an important factor in making interview decisions. The Step 1 score is second only to letters of recommendation, which were cited as a factor by 100% of programs.[4] In the 2014 NRMP Match, the mean USMLE Step 1 score was 237 among matched U.S. senior applicants.[6]

How important is the interview?

According to the NRMP, "interactions with faculty during interview visit" and "interpersonal skills" were the two most important factors used by programs to make rank-order list decisions. On a scale of 1 (not at all important) to 5 (very important), interactions with faculty received an average rating of 4.9.[4]

References

[1]Vascular 0 + 5 residency: Lessons learned from the first five years. Available at: https://www.vascularweb.org/APDVS/Documents/2012%20Spring%20Meeting%20Presentations/19%20APDVS%20Lessons%20Learned%202012.pdf. Accessed January 22, 2016.

[2]Sheahan M, Bray J, Sheahan C, Gerdes J, Brooke E, Palit T, Torrance B, Batson R, Hollier L. Integrated vascular surgery residency: A look at ERAS applicant numbers and NRMP Match outcomes. Available at: http://symposium.scvs.org/abstracts/2015/17.cgi. Accessed January 22, 2016.

[3]Brotherton S, Etzel S. Graduate Medical Education, 2014-2015. *JAMA* 2015; 314 (22): 2436-54.

[4]Results of the 2014 NRMP Program Director Survey. Available at: http://www.nrmp.org/wp-content/uploads/2014/09/PD-Survey-Report-2014.pdf. Accessed March 3, 2015.

[5]Zayed M, Dalman R, Lee J. A comparison of 0 + 5 versus 5 + 2 applicants to vascular surgery training programs. *J Vasc Surg* 2012; 56 (5): 1448-1452.

[6]Charting Outcomes in the Match (2014). Available at: http://www.nrmp.org/wp-content/uploads/2014/09/Charting-Outcomes-2014-Final.pdf. Accessed March 3, 2014.

Chapter 45

Fellowship Match

Note: The following chapter is excerpted from the book Resident's Guide to the Fellowship Match: Rules for Success

What does it take to secure a position in the subspecialty and fellowship program of your choice?

As the years have passed, subspecialty training has increased in popularity. In 1987, 46% of graduating ophthalmology residents chose fellowship training. By 2003, the percentage had risen to 64%.[1] In some specialties, over 90% of residency graduates pursue fellowship training. "The fellowship year is now chosen by more than 90% of radiology residents," writes Dr. Stephen Baker, Chair of Radiology at the UMDNJ School of Medicine.[2] In 2012, the American Society for Clinical Pathology surveyed over 1,200 pathology residents about attitudes towards fellowship training and experiences with the application process. The authors wrote that "fellowship training in pathology is sought after by 95% of residents."[3]

Competition is intense, and some applicants are unsuccessful. In the 2013 NRMP Fellowship Match, nearly 25% of applicants failed to match into one of 48 participating subspecialties. As you might expect, some subspecialties are more competitive than others. In competitive fields such as gastroenterology and gynecologic oncology, over 40% of applicants failed to match.[4]

Percentage of Fellowship Applicants who Failed to Match in 2013[4]	
Specialty	**% of applicants unmatched**
Abdominal Transplant Surgery	47.4%
Gastroenterology	40.9%
Gynecologic Oncology	40.3%
Pediatric Surgery	38.4%
Cardiovascular Disease	34.4%
Hematology and Oncology	33.9%
Reproductive Endocrinology	33.8%
Colon and Rectal Surgery	31.0%
Maternal – Fetal Medicine	28.8%
Female Pelvic Medicine and Reconstructive Surgery	26.2%
Allergy and Immunology	26.2%
Hand Surgery	24.6%
Pediatric Cardiology	21.1%
Interventional Radiology	17.1%

Graduates of U.S. allopathic medical schools fare better than osteopathic and international medical graduates.

Failure to Match % by Applicant Type (2013 NRMP Fellowship Match)[4]	
Applicant Type	**Failure to Match %**
Graduates of U.S. Allopathic Medical School	13.4%
Graduates of Osteopathic Medical Schools	23.2%
International Medical Graduates (Non-U.S. Citizen)	36.1%
International Medical Graduates (U.S. Citizen)	41.6%

As an applicant, you seek to secure a position in your preferred subspecialty. You also hope to gain acceptance into your most coveted program. That makes the process even more challenging. We review "approximately 400 fellowship applications every year," writes the Division of Hematology & Oncology at the University of Pennsylvania. From those applicants, approximately 50 candidates are interviewed...There are 8 fellows accepted per year."[5] The percentage of applicants matching with their first-choice program is shown below for some subspecialties.

% of Applicants Matching with their First-Choice Program (2013 NRMP Match)[4]	
Subspecialty	**Percentage**
Pediatric Surgery	16.4%
Gynecologic Oncology	19.5%
Colon and Rectal Surgery	25.6%
Abdominal Transplant Surgery	29.3%
Hand Surgery	31.5%
Female Pelvic Medicine and Reconstructive Surgery	32.3%
Gastroenterology	32.7%
Cardiovascular Disease	35.2%
Hematology and Oncology	35.7%
Maternal – Fetal Medicine	38.4%
Pediatric Cardiology	42.9%

What does it actually take to secure a position in the subspecialty and program of your choice? In the following 300 plus pages, we answer this important question. As with our book, *The Successful Match: 200 Rules to Succeed in the Residency Match*, we provide specific evidence-based advice to maximize your chances of success.

Having successfully matched into a residency program, you may believe that the same strategy will serve you well in the fellowship application process. It is true that there are similarities between the two processes but there are significant differences. Being well informed about the fellowship application and selection process will help you develop the "right" strategy and implement a plan for success.

Our recommendations are based on evidence whenever possible. We have scoured the literature to present you evidence obtained from scientific study and published in academic medical literature. Who actually chooses the fellows? What do these decision makers care about? We review the data on the criteria that matter to them. How can you convince them that you would be the right fellow for their program? We provide concrete, practical recommendations based on this data.

Starting on page 148 we present specialty-specific data. Given the high failure to match rates for certain subspecialties, is there any literature available to applicants to guide them through the fellowship application process? Data is not available for every subspecialty but research in this area has accelerated over the past 5 to 10 years, and we provide the results of these studies. For example, in pediatric emergency medicine, a survey of fellowship program directors obtained data from 40 of 43 directors. Which criteria did these directors rank as most important in granting interviews? Which characteristics were most important in determining an applicant's place on the program's rank order list?[6] This evidence-based information is critical to developing a strategy that maximizes your chances of success.

Residency Program Director

The residency program director will have significant impact on your chances of securing a position in a fellowship program. Surveys of fellowship programs have consistently demonstrated the importance of the program director letter of recommendation in the selection process. Therefore, it is essential to make the program director a strong advocate for you.

How should you proceed? Chief in importance is delivering high quality care to your patients. Fellowship programs are searching for applicants who are dedicated to excellence in patient care, and seek evidence of this in program director letters. What are the qualities that make an outstanding resident? We discuss these qualities in chapter 2.

The problem resident is defined as a "trainee who demonstrates a significant enough problem that requires intervention by someone of authority, usually the program director or chief resident."[7] In a survey of 298 internal medicine residency program directors, Yao and Wright found that the mean point prevalence of problem residents was 6.9% for the academic year 1998 – 1999.[8] In a more recent study of problem residents, 73.5% of programs reported having residents in difficulty.[9] Problem residents can negatively impact a program by compromising patient care and increasing the workload of their resident colleagues. In addition, to remediate the problem, considerable time, support, and guidance is required from the faculty, including the program director. What are the behaviors, attitudes, and actions that would label you a "problem resident?" Why is it surprisingly easy to become a problem resident? Which problem resident behaviors are worse than others? How will this affect your fellowship chances? Most importantly, how can you avoid being a problem resident? You will find the answers to these questions in Chapter 2.

In writing your letter of recommendation, the program director will rely heavily on the contents of your resident file. What is the resident file? What are the typical contents of the file? How can you protect it from harm? You'll also find the answers to these questions in Chapter 2.

Letters of Recommendation

You will recall that letters of recommendation were an important component of the residency application. How important are letters of recommendation in the selection process for fellowship programs? Multiple surveys of fellowship programs have demonstrated that letters are critical. "Plastic surgery is a small community, with only approximately 500 academic plastic surgeons in the United States," writes Dr. Rod Rohrich, Chair of the University of Texas Southwestern Medical Center Plastic Surgery. "When a respected plastic surgeon vouches that you possess the qualities of an excellent resident, program directors take notice."[10]

Who you choose to write the letter can make a major difference in the strength of your application. A letter written by a faculty colleague who is well known to the fellowship program can carry considerable weight. In a survey of fellowship directors of internal medicine subspecialties, letters written from known specialists were ranked # 2 in importance, considerably higher than letters written by attendings not in the fellowship field (# 16).[11]

Of course, this requires you to develop a strong relationship with the letter writer. How do you develop such relationships with faculty in your chosen subspecialty field? Whom should you target? How will you know if the writer is capable of writing the type of letter you require? These important questions are answered in chapter 3.

How can you help the faculty member write a glowing letter of recommendation? We discuss the type of information to provide, and the manner in which to provide it.

Our chapter on letters of recommendation reviews strategies to locate letter writers who will be most helpful to your candidacy. We review how to identify these writers, approach them, and develop relationships with them. More importantly, we describe the type of evidence you can provide to the writer and the professional manner in which you provide it. Your letter writers want to write the best letter possible, and you can do much more than you realize to make this a reality.

Research

Research has always been an important part of the selection process for the most competitive specialties. As competition for fellowship positions has increased overall, even less competitive specialties and programs are placing more value on resident research. Applicants are urged to speak with advisors about the importance of research in the selection process for their specialty of interest.

Involvement in research, particularly work that leads to publication, is a means to gain recognition among of a sea of qualified applicants. "Many fellowship programs look for students who have published because it shows academic initiative, which is pretty important to fellowship directors," explained Dr. Eric Milbrandt, former Chair of the ACP Council of Associates. "The articles don't have to be groundbreaking cases; a simple case review published in a small journal will do. The important thing is to gain the research experience and to have your name on the study as a lead author."[12]

Research that is published or presented is more highly regarded than participation alone. Bringing research to publication or presentation is not easy, particularly for residents. To maximize the chances of publication or presentation, you must recognize the major barriers residents face in completing projects. What are the major barriers? How you can overcome these obstacles? In chapter 4, we present you this important information.

Given the importance of research in the fellowship selection process, your choice of research mentor will have significant impact on your chances of success. "The right research mentor and appropriate projects are crucial for successful completion of projects," writes Dr. Mitchell Cappell, Chief of Gastroenterology at William Beaumont Hospital.[13] Careful thought and consideration are necessary in choosing among the available mentors. What are the key qualities of a research mentor? What should you discuss in your initial meeting with potential mentors? What are red flags that should make you reconsider your choice?

Also of importance is selection of the right project. A study of medical student research serves to emphasize this point even further. When researchers examined the productivity of students who had spent one year fully immersed in research following their third year of medical school, they found that only 23% had publications in print by 6 months post-research fellowship. This date was chosen to indicate publications that could be included in residency applications. These were students mentored by well-regarded faculty as part of the Clinical Research Training Program at the National Institutes of Health or the Doris Duke Clinical Research Fellowship Program.[14] The key point here is that considerable time is often required to perform the research and complete the peer-review and publication process. It is possible to accelerate this process, and we discuss this further in chapter 4.

Personal Statement

The personal statement plays an important role in the fellowship selection process. "This is your opportunity to let us get to know you and take your application out of the very large stack of competing applications," writes the Department of Pediatric Cardiology at Stanford University. "What makes you special? Why are you a particularly good candidate for us? Why is Stanford a good fit for you? What in your background has prepared you to excel in fellowship? Our screening process puts a great deal of weight on the personal statement so make sure yours gets noticed."[15]

In your application for residency, you may have submitted one statement to all programs. There is evidence to suggest that this approach may not be ideal for the fellowship application. Many fellowship programs seek to understand why you have specifically applied to their program. The clinical neurophysiology fellowship program at Wayne State University informs applicants that the personal statement should describe "your career goals, the reasoning behind your choice of the field and the fellowship program."[16] The Cardiovascular Disease Fellowship at the University of Washington has similar language at their department website. "The personal statement is limited to 300 words, and for the UW program, must contain the following information…type of research you are interested…potential mentors at the UW…Why are you interested in training in our program in Seattle?"[17]

Dr. Catherine Nelson, Assistant Professor of Surgery at the University of Rochester, emphasizes the importance of "fit." "If they have an ultrasound course and this interests you, tell them why. If they have specific rotations or patient populations that you want training with, spend time talking about it. Programs not only have to figure out if you are a good match for them but also if they are a good match for you. You want to show them why their program is ideal for your needs."[18]

In chapter 5, we provide detailed information to help you develop a powerful and compelling statement. What content should you include? How can you develop a statement that sets you apart from other candidates? What do program directors and other key decision-makers prefer to see in statements? You'll find the answers to these questions and more in our personal statement chapter.

Standardized Exams

USMLE scores are a factor of importance in the fellowship selection process. The emphasis placed on the USMLE varies from specialty to specialty, and even among programs within a specialty. In a survey of radiology fellowship program directors, most respondents viewed medical test scores (e.g., USMLE) as moderately to very important factors in the selection process.[19]

As with residency programs, some fellowship programs will have minimum score requirements. The Division of Gastroenterology at the University of Colorado requires applicants to have "taken and passed USMLE parts I and II, or equivalent test, with minimum of average score on both tests (typically about 200)."[20] Some programs will not have a minimum score, preferring to review applications in a more holistic manner.

Low-scoring applicants should understand that scores remain an important factor, and make every effort to strengthen credentials in other areas. Doing so will help you make a more convincing case to program directors. We have seen that low-scoring applicants can receive interviews at institutions where they do not meet the threshold score if other components of the application are particularly compelling.

In-Training Examinations are exams administered to residents during the training period. Like the USMLE, these exams are standardized and objective, and are thought to be excellent measures of medical knowledge. Results allow the examinee to compare his performance with that of other residents at the same level of training. Although intended to be used as an educational tool, programs in certain subspecialties do request these scores.

Which specialties utilize In-Training exam scores in the selection process? How important are these scores? What percentile should you aim for? You'll find the answers to these questions in chapter 6.

Audition Elective

If you are a resident in a program that permits away electives at other institutions, one very effective way to communicate your interest and demonstrate your excellence to fellowship programs is through an audition rotation. “Internal candidates always have an advantage. People who've come to visit and spent a month training are known so they're more likely to get a break,” writes Dr. Dennis Ahnen, Director of the Gastroenterology Program at the University of Colorado. “It's hard for program directors and residents to evaluate somebody when they just see them for a day."[12]

An audition elective essentially serves as an extended interview, and should be regarded as such. Audition electives are valued by programs as a means to more reliably assess an applicant’s cognitive and noncognitive skills and traits. Residents can showcase their clinical acumen, their skills in patient interaction, their abilities to work with colleagues and faculty, and their enthusiasm for the particular program.

These audition electives should not be taken lightly. Your performance will certainly be a major factor in the program’s consideration of you as an applicant. Less well appreciated among applicants is the importance of these electives to other institutions. The Galloway and Rutledge Fellowship Programs are short-term rotations in gynecologic oncology open to obstetrics and gynecology residents at the Memorial Sloan – Kettering Cancer Center and M.D. Anderson Cancer Center, respectively. Residents at other institutions may apply for these fellowships. Fellowship programs in gynecologic oncology often request grades or letters from such experiences. “If you do a rotation such as Galloway or Rutledge Fellowship, we would like a letter from this rotation,” writes the Gynecologic Oncology Fellowship Program at the University of North Carolina.[21] In chapter 7, you’ll learn more about the pros and cons of audition electives.

Teaching

Teaching is an important responsibility of fellows. “Fellows are expected to vigorously pursue teaching medical students and residents,” writes the University of Missouri Kansas City Critical Care Medicine Fellowship Program. “Regularly scheduled conference presentations by the Fellows are included in this teaching responsibility.”[22]

Programs will assess your interest and commitment to teaching through review of your application, analysis of your letters of recommendation, and interview.

How can you be recognized as a teacher at your institution? What are the awards available to residents for teaching excellence? We’ll discuss this in chapter 8.

Specialty Organizations

Attending a national conference in your subspecialty of interest will allow you to learn more about the field. Often, there are sessions and workshops geared to young physicians. Networking opportunities abound, and many residents have opportunities to meet key fellowship program personnel, including fellowship program directors, at different institutions.

National scientific meetings are an excellent venue to present your research findings. Many residents have presented their work in the form of posters.

Opportunities for resident involvement beyond research also exist at national meetings. Many organizations not only offer membership to residents but also invite residents to participate on committees, run for leadership positions, and locate mentors outside of their home institutions. In chapter 9, we describe how you can become more actively involved in specialty organizations, and how this involvement can enhance your chances of securing a fellowship position.

Curriculum Vitae

The CV is an important component of the fellowship application. Few program administrators have seen more CVs than Annabeth Borg, former secretary to the Chairman and Program Director at the Nassau County Medical Center Department of Medicine. She was heavily involved in the hiring process for trainees, and became quite familiar with how CVs were used in the selection process. Because of her expertise, the American College of Physicians asked her to provide tips for writing a CV for residents. Below, she describes the importance of the CV:

Generally, your CV is the first contact you may have with a prospective program director. Therefore, you would surely want a C.V. that does more than simply impart information about your personal history, and educational and professional qualifications and achievements. Strive for a CV that establishes a favorable image of your professionalism in the mind of the reader. It should emphasize your areas of strength and create an interest about you sufficient to result in a personal interview. Make your C.V. work for you![23]

As a fellowship applicant, you are undoubtedly familiar with the CV, having written one for your residency application. Whether you applied to residency programs utilizing ERAS or the Central Application Service, you probably recall not being able to attach your unique CV to the application. Instead, you were asked to enter information from your CV directly by computer into the ERAS CV format.

Over 50 subspecialties utilize ERAS, and you will follow the same process for the CV if you applying to one of these ERAS participating specialties. Even though you won't be able to attach your CV to your ERAS application, you will still need to create a professional-looking paper version of your CV for the following reasons:

- Many subspecialties don't participate in ERAS. These programs will request a paper CV.
- Even within ERAS participating specialties, there are some programs that do not utilize ERAS.
- The CV will help you complete different sections of the fellowship application.
- The CV can be of considerable help to you as you being to draft your personal statement.
- Mentors and faculty in your specialty of interest will review your CV to provide you with informed advice about how to strengthen your credentials.
- Your letter writers will rely on your CV to help them write strong letters of recommendation.
- Reviewing your CV prior to the interview will remind you of your strengths and accomplishments, helping to boost confidence.
- Interviewers may request a copy of your CV at the start of an interview in order to help structure the interview. This provides an ideal opportunity to emphasize your strengths and highlight the skills you would bring as a fellow.

The overall appearance of your CV is important as well. Fellowship programs must whittle down a large group of applications, and therefore every piece of the application becomes magnified in importance. Before reviewing your CV, the reader will form an impression of you based on its overall appearance.

How can you create a powerful and professional CV? What should you include? What should you not include? What are the common and damaging mistakes CV mistakes? In chapter 10, you'll receive CV tips directly from program directors and other key decision-makers.

Interview

Over the years, many surveys of fellowship program directors have inquired about the importance of the interview in the selection process. These surveys have consistently found the interview to be a major factor. In fact, the results of multiple studies indicate that the interview is *the most* important factor.

In a survey of internal medicine subspecialty fellowship directors, the candidate interview was found to be the most important selection factor among a group of 18 criteria.[11] "Most fellowship program directors consider the fellowship interview the most crucial aspect of the selection process," writes

Dr. Eleanor Summerhill, Program Director of the Internal Medicine Residency Program at the Memorial Hospital of Rhode Island.[24] The interview is never just a formality. It can absolutely make or break your chances of matching.

Researching the program thoroughly before your visit is crucial. In our experience conducting mock interviews with fellowship applicants, this is perhaps one of the most common and serious mistakes applicants make. Inadequate research prevents applicants from responding to questions with specific answers. These are the types of answers that help applicants stand out. "Nothing strikes a better chord than a candidate who knows about the center at which he or she is interviewing, and can articulate what it is that attracted him or her to that particular center," writes Dr. Steven J. Cohen, Program Director of the Fox Chase/Temple University Hematology - Oncology Fellowship.[25]

What type of research should you perform? How do you incorporate your research into your interview answers? How do you communicate that you are the right "fit" for the program? What are common interview pitfalls? Turn to chapter 11 for detailed preparation for your fellowship interview.

Chapter excerpted from the book Resident's Guide to the Fellowship Match: Rules for Success

References

[1]Gedde S, Budenz D, Haft P, et al. Factors influencing career choices among graduating ophthalmology residents. *Ophthalmology* 2005; 112: 1247–1254.
[2]Baker S, Luk L, Clarkin K. The trouble with fellowships. J Am Coll Radiol 2010; 7 (6): 446-51.
[3]ASCP Fellowship and Job Market Survey. Available at: http://www.ascp.org/PDF/Fellowship-Reports/Fellowship-Job-Market-2012.pdf. Accessed May 24, 2013.
[4]NRMP Match. Available at http://www.nrmp.org/. Accessed May 22, 2013.
[5]Penn Medicine Division of Hematology/Oncology. Available at: http://www.pennmedicine.org/hematology-oncology/academics/fellowship/how-to-apply.html. Accessed May 23, 2013.
[6]Poirier M, Pruitt C. Factors used by pediatric emergency medicine program directors to select their fellows. *Pediatr Emerg Care* 2003; 19 (3): 157-61.
[7]American Board of Internal Medicine. Association of Program Directors in Internal Medicine (APDIM) Chief Residents' Workshop on Problem Residents; 1999.
[8]Yao D, Wright S. National survey of intenral medicine residency program directors regarding problem residents. *JAMA* 2000; 284 (9): 1099-1104.
[9]Dupras D, Edson R, Halvorsen A, Hopkins R, McDonald F. "Problem residents": prevalence, problems and remediation in the era of core competencies. *Am J Med* 2012; 125 (4): 421-5.
[10]Nagarkar P, Pulikkottil B, Patel A, Rohrich R. So You Want to Become a Plastic Surgeon? What You Need to Do and Know to Get into a Plastic Surgery Residency. *Plast Reconstr Surg* 2013; 131 (2): 419-22.
[11]Mikhail S, Bernstein P. Selection criteria for fellowship: are we all on the same page? *Academic Internal Medicine Insight* 2007; 5 (1): 1, 10-11.
[12]Palmer I. Tips to find a fellowship in a competitive market. *ACP Internist*. Available at: http://www.acpinternist.org/archives/2000/07/fellowship.htm. Accessed May 2, 2013.
[13]Cappell M. Advice to program directors and applicants for gastroenterology fellowship application and selection. *Gastrointest Endosc* 2011; 74 (1): 155-8.
[14]Cohen B, Friedman E, Zier K. Publications by students doing a year of full-time research: what are realistic expectations? *Am J Med* 2008; 121 (6): 545-8.
[15]Stanford University Department of Pediatric Cardiology. Available at: http://pedcard.stanford.edu/education/application.html. Accessed May 12, 2013.
[16]Neurophysiology Fellowship Program at Wayne State University. Available at: http://neurology.med.wayne.edu/epilepsy/app-info.php. Accessed June 23, 2013.
[17]University of Washington Cardiovascular Disease Fellowship. Available at: http://depts.washington.edu/cardweb/fellowship/application.shtml. Accessed May 12, 2013.
[18]Chiu W, Reilly P, Asensio J, Tisherman S, Minshall C. A Guide to Fellowship Training Programs in Trauma, Surgical Critical Care, and Acute Care Surgery. Developed by the Eastern Association for the Surgery of Trauma Careers in Trauma Committee. Available at: www.east.org/content/documents/eastfell7.pdf. Accessed May 13, 2013.
[19]Mulcahy H, Chew F, Mulcahy M. The radiology fellowship application and selection process in the United States: experiences and perceptions from both sides. *Radiology Res Pract* 2012 (epub).

[20]University of Colorado Department of Gastroenterology. Available at: http://www.ucdenver.edu/academics/colleges/medicalschool/departments/medicine/Gastroenterology/Fellowship/Pages/FellowshipApplicationProcess.aspx. Accessed May 12, 2013.

[21]University of North Carolina Department of Gynecologic Oncology. Available at: https://www.med.unc.edu/obgyn/Patient_Care/specialty-services/gynecologic-oncology/education-research/fellowship#application. Accessed May 2, 2013.

[22]UMKC Critical Care Fellowship Program. Available at: http://www.med.umkc.edu/fellowships/critical_care/overview.shtml. Accessed May 2, 2013.

[23]Borg, A. How to write a CV. Available at: http://www.acponline.org/medical_students/residency/borg.htm. Accessed May 30, 2013.

[24]Williams F. *A Textbook for Today's Chief Medical Resident* (20th edition). Association of Program Directors in Internal Medicine; 2012.

[25]Bruck L. Interviewing 101: Tips for landing your first post-fellowship position. Available at: http://www.targetedhc.com/publications/oncology-fellows/2011/december-2011/Interviewing-101-Tips-for-Landing-Your-First-Post-Fellowship-Position. Accessed May 15, 2013.

The Medical School Interview: Winning Strategies from Admissions Faculty

By Samir Desai MD and Rajani Katta MD

ISBN # 9781937978013

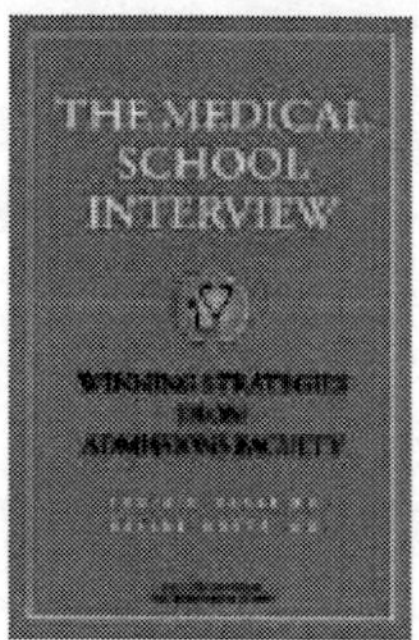

The medical school interview is the most important factor in the admissions process. Our detailed advice, based on evidence from research in the field and the perspectives of admissions faculty, will provide you with an insiders' perspective.

How can you best prepare for the traditional interview, group interview, panel interview, and behavioral interview? What qualities would make applicants less likely to be admitted? What personal qualities are most valued by admissions faculty? What can students do to achieve maximum success during the interview?

This book shows medical school applicants how to develop the optimal strategy for interview success.

"…this is an extremely thorough handbook, covering the questions applicants are likely to be asked and the appropriate and inappropriate answers…likely to be found indispensable by readers embarking on the arduous process of applying to medical school."

- Kirkus Reviews

Multiple Mini Interview (MMI): Winning Strategies from Admissions Faculty

By Samir Desai MD
ISBN # 9781937978051

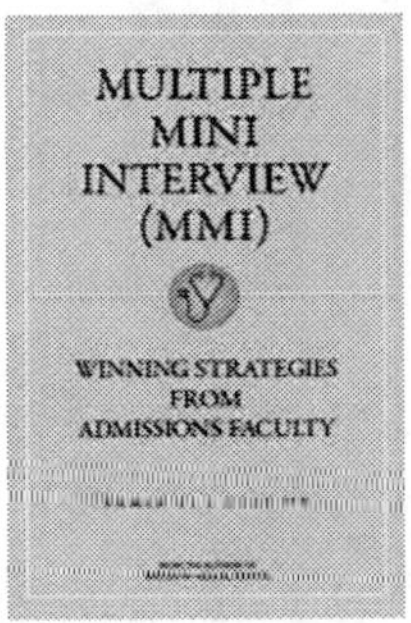

The Multiple Mini Interview (MMI) has become the preferred interview format at many health professions programs and medical schools. Applicants seeking admission to these schools face considerable anxiety preparing for these interviews because of a lack of resources available for guidance.

Our detailed advice, based on evidence from research in the field and perspectives of admissions faculty, will provide you with an insiders' perspective. How can you best prepare for the MMI? What is required to deliver a winning interview performance? Which behaviors, attitudes, and answers are prized by interviewers? Includes sample answers to MMI questions and advice to help you avoid common mistakes.

This book shows applicants how to develop the optimal strategy for MMI success - an invaluable resource to help applicants gain that extra edge.

“I am a health communication professor and I work closely with the university's premed program. I sometimes do trainings prepping the students for their med school interviews and many of my students have been successfully admitted to med school. I have found this book, along with The Medical School Interview: Winning Strategies from Admissions Faculty to be the 2 essential books of prepping for med school. The best thing you can do for yourself is buying these 2 books, reading them thoroughly, and practicing more than once.”

- Christine (Amazon Review)

Hopes and Fears, Dreams and Tears: A County Memoir

By Niraj Mehta MD

ISBN # 9781937978037

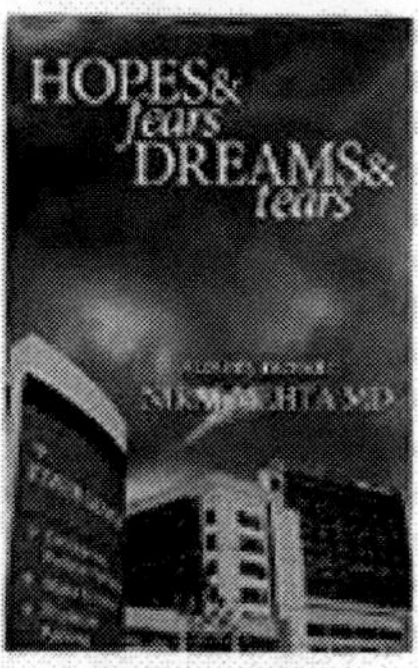

Every destination has a journey and every journey has a story.

Hopes and Fears, Dreams and Tears: A County Memoir traces the story of a young medical student full of idealism as he starts his training. Lacking in knowledge, he embarks on a confusing journey full of Hopes and Fears, Dreams and Tears at a County Hospital similar to one that most doctors in the United States train at today.

Using humor to deal with triumphs and tragedies, both personal as well as those involving his patients, the young doctor in training finally achieves wisdom decades later as a full-time medical educator teaching at the same County Hospital. Having come full circle, he finally realizes that perhaps all he ever needed to know to be a successful healer he already knew as a naive young medical student.

"Dr. Niraj Mehta's medical memoir is at once honest and thought provoking. He has a great sense of humor: the book will keep you laughing even as it helps you understand the difficult and stressful challenges faced by medical students and interns, and also the exhilaration of being able to save lives. The book teaches us several important lessons about compassion as well. A great read!"

- Chitra Banerjee Divakaruni, Author of *Palace of Illusions* and *Oleander Girl*

Success in Medical School: Insider Advice for the Preclinical Years

By Samir P. Desai MD and Rajani Katta MD

ISBN # 9781937978006

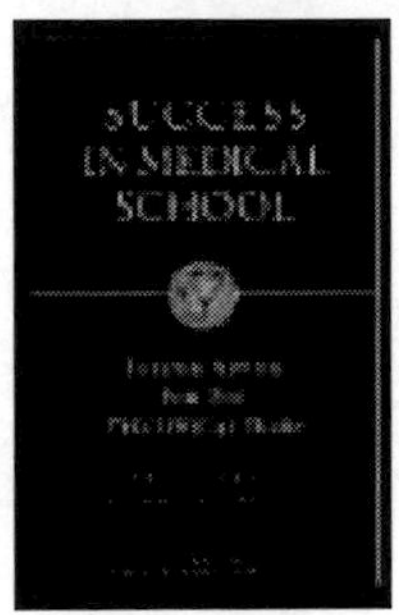

According to the AAMC, the United States will have a shortage of 90,000 physicians by 2020. In the mid-1990s, the AAMC urged medical schools to expand enrollment. Class sizes have increased, and new schools have opened their doors. Unfortunately, rising enrollment in medical schools has not led to a corresponding increase in the number of residency positions.

As a result, medical students are finding it increasingly difficult to match with the specialty and program of their choice. "Competition is tightening," said Mona Signer, Executive Director of the National Resident Matching Program. "The growth in applicants is more than the increase in positions."

Now more than ever, preclinical students need to be well informed so that they can maximize their chances of success. The decisions you make early in medical school can have a significant impact on your future specialty options.

To build a strong foundation for your future physician career, and to match into your chosen field, you must maximize your preclinical education. In *Success in Medical School*, you'll learn specific strategies for success during these important years of medical school.

"…I recommend this book...The book has so much information about everything that there has to be a part of the book that will satisfy your interests."

- Medical School Success website

Medical School Scholarships, Grants & Awards: Insider Advice On How To Win Scholarships

By Samir P. Desai MD and Anand Trivedi MD

ISBN # 9781937978044

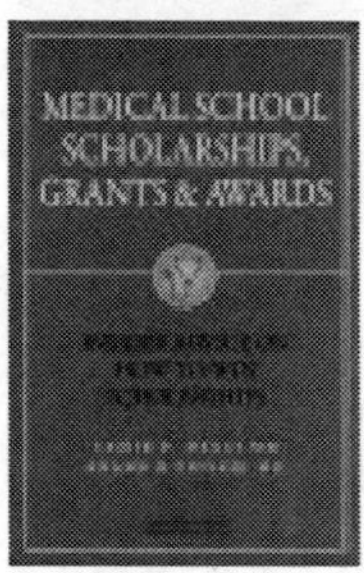

****Named a high-value resource by the AAMC Group on Student Affairs****

Residency match expert Dr. Samir Desai has helped students win medical school scholarships, grants, and awards, and now shares his perspectives in this new resource.

Over 1,000 awards are featured along with profiles of winners, proven strategies for success, and crucial tips. Learn how to craft a powerful scholarship application, write compelling essays, secure strong letters of recommendation, and stand out from the competition. Discover the best scholarships for you with awards for research, leadership, writing, global health, service, extracurricular activities, ethnicity, and gender.

Winning can:

- Significantly reduce your debt.
- Provide a major boost to your residency application, and set you apart from your peers. Awards can be placed in the application, MSPE, letters of recommendation, and CV.
- Elevate your profile with competitive specialties and residency programs.
- Raise your stature in medical school.
- Make you more attractive for other awards and scholarships.
- Further your professional reputation and enhance your credibility in the areas that form the basis for the award.
- Solidify the support of faculty who become reference letter writers. Strengthening these relationships over time allows faculty members to write strong letters of recommendation for residency.

Clinician's Guide to Laboratory Medicine: Pocket

By Samir P. Desai MD
ISBN # 9780972556187

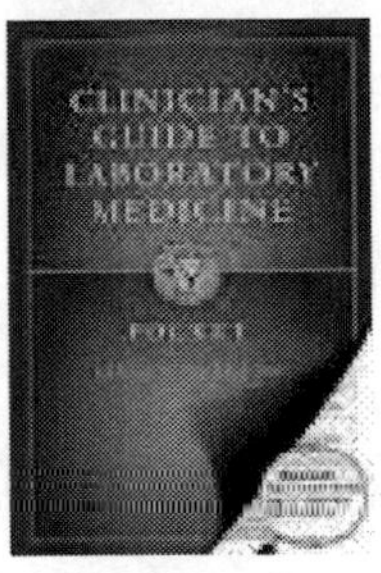

This book offers practical approaches to lab test interpretation. It includes differential diagnoses, step-by-step approaches, and algorithms, all designed to answer your lab test questions in a flash. Listed as one of the "Best Medical Books of All Time" by The Medical Media Review, see why so many consider it a "must-have" book.

"In our Medicine Clerkship, the Clinician's Guide to Laboratory Medicine has quickly become one of the two most popular paperback books. Our students have praised the algorithms, tables, and ease of pursuit of clinical problems through better understanding of the utilization of tests appropriate to the problem at hand."

- Greg Magarian, MD, Director, 3rd Year Internal Medicine Clerkship, Oregon Health & Science University

"It provides an excellent practical approach to abnormal labs."

- Northwestern University Feinberg School of Medicine Internal Medicine Clerkship website.

Success on the Wards: 250 Rules for Clerkship Success

By Samir P. Desai MD and Rajani Katta MD
ISBN # 9780972556194

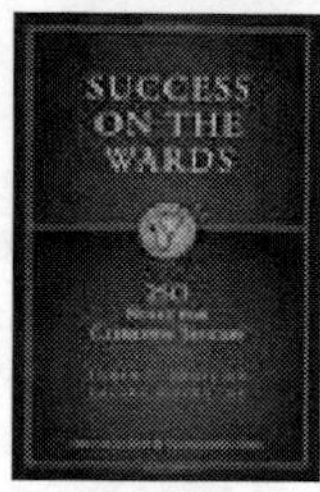

The authors of *The Successful Match: 200 Rules to Succeed in the Residency Match* bring their same combination of practical recommendations and evidence-based advice to clerkships.

The book begins as a how-to guide with clerkship-specific templates, along with sample notes and guides, for every aspect of clerkships. The book reviews proven strategies for success in patient care, write-ups, rounds, and other vital areas.

Grades in required rotations are one of the most important academic criteria used to select residents, and this critical year can determine career choices. This book shows students what they can do now to position themselves for match success. An invaluable resource for medical students - no student should be without it.

"I strongly recommend this book. It should be a must-read for any motivated student doctor."

- AMSA *New Physician*

"*Success on the Wards: 250 Rules for Clerkship Success* is an excellent reference for any 3rd year medical student and some is probably great reading for advanced students and even residents and interns."

- Review by Medfools.com

"*Success on the Wards* is easily the best book I have read on how to succeed in clerkship. It is comprehensive, thorough and jam-packed with valuable information. Dr. Desai and Dr. Katta provide an all-encompassing look into what clerkship is really like."

- Review by Medaholic.com

The Resident's Guide to the Fellowship Match

By Samir P. Desai MD
ISBN # 9781937978020

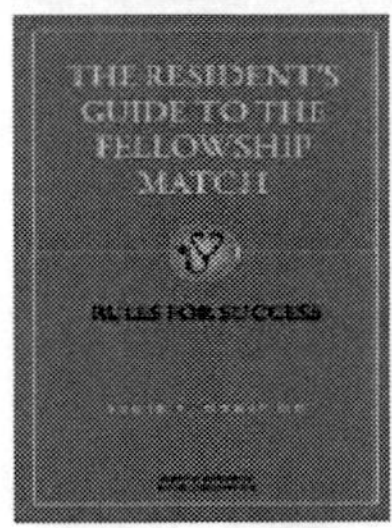

What does it take to match into the subspecialty and fellowship program of your choice?

Our detailed advice, based on evidence from research in the field and the perspectives of fellowship program directors, will provide you with an insiders' perspective.

What are the criteria most important to decision-makers? What can you do to have the best possible letters of recommendation written on your behalf? How can you develop a powerful and compelling personal statement? How can you overcome the obstacles of residency to publish research? What can you do to achieve maximum success during the interview?

This book shows fellowship applicants how to develop the optimal strategy for success - an invaluable resource to help applicants gain that extra edge.

"The Resident's Guide to The Fellowship Match is a great book…It helps you prepare for the fellowship application starting on the first day of residency. I personally learned a lot from it…The book is very systematic and covers everything you need to ace your fellowship interviews. I would strongly recommend this book…"

- Huda Khaleel (Amazon Review)

The Successful Match website

Our website, TheSuccessfulMatch.com, provides residency applicants with a better understanding of the selection process. You'll find:

- Inside look at the residency selection process
- Advice from the decision-makers
- Information to position yourself for residency match success

Consulting services

We also offer expert one-on-one consulting services to medical students and IMGs. Whether you seek an overall strategy for match success, accurate assessment of your candidacy for a particular specialty or program, review of your curriculum vitae or personal statement, or thorough preparation for interviews, you can rest assured we have the knowledge, expertise, and insight to help you achieve your goals. All applicants work directly with Dr. Samir Desai. If you are interested in our consultation services, please visit us at www.TheSuccessfulMatch.com. The website provides further details, including pricing and specific services.

MD2B Titles

The Medical School Interview: Winning Strategies from Admissions Faculty

Multiple Mini Interview: Winning Strategies from Admissions Faculty

Hopes and Fears, Dreams and Tears: A County Memoir

Medical School Scholarships, Grants, & Awards: Insider Advice on How to Win Scholarships

Success in Medical School: Insider Advice for the Preclinical Years

Success on the Wards: 250 Rules for Clerkship Success

The Successful Match 2017: Rules to Succeed in the Residency Match

The Resident's Guide to the Fellowship Match: Rules for Success

Clinician's Guide to Laboratory Medicine: Pocket

Available at TheSuccessfulMatch.com

Bulk Sales

MD2B is able to provide discounts on any of our titles when purchased in bulk. The discount rate depends on the quantity ordered. For more information, please contact us at info@md2b.net or (713) 927-6830.